Practitioner's Guide to Evaluating Change
with Neuropsychological Assessment Instruments

CRITICAL ISSUES IN NEUROPSYCHOLOGY

Series Editors

Antonio E. Puente
University of North Carolina at Wilmington

Cecil R. Reynolds
Texas A&M University and Bastrop Mental Health Associates

A Continuation Order Plan is available for this series. A continuation order will bring delivery of each new volume immediately upon publication. Volumes are billed only upon actual shipment. For further information please contact the publisher.

Practitioner's Guide to Evaluating Change with Neuropsychological Assessment Instruments

Edited by

Robert J. McCaffrey

University at Albany
State University of New York
Albany, New York

Kevin Duff

University at Albany
State University of New York
Albany, New York

and

Holly James Westervelt

Brown University School of Medicine
Providence, Rhode Island

Kluwer Academic / Plenum Publishers
New York, Boston, Dordrecht, London, Moscow

Library of Congress Cataloging-in-Publication Data

Practitioner's guide to evaluating change with neuropsychological assessment
instruments / edited by Robert J. McCaffrey, Kevin Duff, and Holly James Westervelt.
   p. ; cm. -- (Critical issues in neuropsychology series)
  Includes bibliographical references and index.
  ISBN 0-306-46361-X
  1. Neuropsychological tests. I. McCaffrey, Robert J. II. Duff, Kevin, 1968- III.
Westervelt, Holly James, 1969- IV. Critical issues in neuropsychology
  [DNLM: 1. Neuropsychological Tests. 2. Nervous System Diseases--diagnosis. 3.
Neuropsychology--methods. 4. Practice (Psychology). WL 141 P8955 2000]
  RC386.6.N48 P73 2000
  616.8'0475--dc21

                                                                99-057688

ISBN 0-306-46361-X

©2000 Kluwer Academic / Plenum Publishers
233 Spring Street, New York, N.Y. 10013

http://www.wkap.nl

10 9 8 7 6 5 4 3 2 1

A C.I.P. record for this book is available from the Library of Congress.

All rights reserved

No part of this book may be reproduced, stored in a retrieval system, or transmitted in any form or by any means, electronic, mechanical, photocopying, microfilming, recording, or otherwise, without written permission from the Publisher

Printed in the United States of America

For my parents, Robert and Dorothy, and to the memory of
Antonia Suarez de Ortiz.—RJM

To my loving wife, Ali, who keeps it all in perspective.—KD

To Brian, for all of your love and support.—HJW

Preface

The impetus for this volume began with our research in the 1980's involving serial neuropsychological evaluation with various patient populations. At that time, reports on the practice effects associated with routinely utilized clinical neuropsychological instruments were sparse. While test-retest data were available for almost all assessment instruments, this was usually in the form of correlation coefficients and not changes in mean performance between or across assessment periods (see McCaffrey & Westervelt, 1995 for a detailed discussion of these and related issues). Clinical neuropsychological practitioners had few guidelines to assist them in determining if a change in a patient's performance across assessments was due to an intervention, maturation, practice effects, or a combination of factors.

This volume represents our efforts at reviewing the literature between 1970 and 1998 and extracting the reported information on practice effects. The tables include the assessment instrument used, information on the subject/patient groups, the sample size (n), gender, age, intervention, interval between the assessments, scores at both assessment points, and the citation. Those studies that reported data on more than two assessment points are indicated by a notation; however, any data beyond the second assessment are not reported and the interested reader should refer to the original article. The tables are arranged alphabetically for the most widely used assessment instruments. Those instruments for which there was limited data on practice effects are grouped by "domain" (e.g., attention tests, paired associate tests). The test index is arranged by the name of the test as reported in the specific article.

Notably absent from this volume is the data on intellectual assessment instruments. A companion volume focusing on intellectual tests is under preparation. Two factors contributed to this decision. First, the sheer volume of information was beyond a single practitioner's guide. Second, the information relating to intelligence tests (e.g., Wechsler tests, Stanford-Binet tests) is likely to be applicable to a broader range of professionals (e.g., clinical psychologists, school psychologists, educational psychologists, etc.).

A project of this scope cannot be undertaken without considerable help. We would like to thank the following individuals for their assistance in the successful completion of this project (names are presented alphabetically and not necessarily in order of contribution): Leatt Beder, Eleni Dimoulas, Lucia DiSimone, Nory Gonzalez, Tammy Inco, Edie Kaunack, Rachael Landau, Numayra Mubdi, Tanisha Rosa, Danielle White, and Thomas Youllar. Finally, the support, assistance, and encouragement of our editor, Mariclaire Cloutier, was instrumental in the completion of this project.

Contents

List of Tables

Introduction

Clinical neuropsychological practitioners are often involved in conducting serial neuropsychological assessments in order to monitor the progression of a disease process (e.g., dementia), to document recovery of function following insult (e.g., stroke), or to evaluate the therapeutic efficacy of a specific treatment (e.g., medications). In these instances, practitioners are often faced with a variety of questions when attempting to interpret the changes in an individual's neuropsychological performance across assessments. For example, how much fluctuation in test performance may be due to the psychometric characteristics of this test (e.g., reliability)? Is the observed improvement/decline an artifact of statistical regression? To what extent is this patient's performance improved merely by prior exposure to the testing material? To what extent is the patient's performance across time affected by demographic variables, such as age, gender, or education? Do different disease processes (e.g., traumatic brain injury, Alzheimer's disease, and stroke) impact serial neuropsychological performance in different ways? When administering neuropsychological measures across time, how important are variables inherent in the testing situation, such as test-retest interval or test sophistication? These are commonplace questions; however, resources to assist the clinical neuropsychological practitioner when interpreting the results of serial neuropsychological assessments have been lacking.

Reliability

Reliability may be defined as the extent to which an instrument is free from measurement error. In its broadest sense, it indicates the extent to which an obtained score represents the "true" score of the characteristic being measured, rather than the extent to which an obtained score is attributable to chance errors (Anastasi, 1988).

Knowledge of the reliability of an instrument is informative in serial assessments in that it provides an indication of the extent to which an instrument may be influenced by non-systematic error. In addition, reliability provides some estimate of what proportion of the change in a score may reflect random fluctuations or alterations in moment-specific factors. Chance fluctuations or situation-specific factors, which potentially influence scores, may arise from a variety of sources. These include, but are not restricted to, changes in the examinee's motivation, interceding aspects of personal history, changes in rapport with the assessor, different assessors, momentary fluctuations in the examinee's attention or mood, temporary fatigue, and alterations in the assessment environment (e.g., room temperature, lighting, ventilation, noise, etc.). There are reports in the literature that even factors which seem relatively benign, such as the presence of third party observers (McCaffrey, Fisher, Gold, & Lynch, 1996) may have a measurable effect on an individual's performance. Other factors which may influence the outcome of an examination include familiarity with the assessor (Sacks, 1952; Tsudzuki, Hata, & Kuze, 1957), the general manner of the assessor (Wickes, 1956) the type of seating (Kelley, 1943, Traxler & Hilkert, 1942), or response sheet (Bell, Hoff, & Hoyt, 1964). In short, chance errors may arise from any condition that is irrelevant to the purpose of testing or involves nonstandard administration of a test. Despite an assessor's best efforts to adhere to standardized administration and to maintain uniform testing conditions, random error is likely to occur to some extent in all measures, because no instrument is perfectly reliable.

Some measures are not expected to remain stable across assessments given the nature of the characteristic being measures. For example, a measure of "state" (rather than "trait") anxiety may be expected to fluctuate between and across assessments given changes in the examinee's psychological status. Such changes in mood represent the characteristic being measured and would not be considered sources of error. In contrast, a measure of attention in a healthy adult, for example, may be expected to remain relatively stable across assessments. In this case, a change in the examinee's performance from one testing session to the next due to alterations in his/her psychological state introduces a source of unwanted error.

The reliability of an instrument is defined by a correlation coefficient between two sets of scores. A variety of methods exist to evaluate the reliability of an instrument, though for the purposes of evaluating the stability of a measure over time (rather than the consistency of items within a measure), test-retest and alternate forms reliability provide the most valuable data. The most obvious method of obtaining these data involves readministering a test on a second occasion to the same group of examinees (test-retest reliability). The higher the test-retest reliability, the less susceptible the measure is to random changes in the examinee's state or the testing environment. With respect to serial assessment, the higher the test-retest reliability, the less likely it is that any observed change across assessments is due to chance. Nonetheless, test-retest correlation coefficients reflect nothing more than the relative ranking of examinees' performances between two assessments.

Alternate forms reliability involves retesting the same group of examinees with an equivalent form of the instrument. In order for the reliability index to provide meaningful data, the tests must be truly parallel, with the same number of items, same format, same content type, and, ideally, identical psychometric properties (e.g., mean, standard deviation, etc.). Unfortunately, parallel forms are not available for most tests, and few available alternate forms meet these criteria.

The length of the retest interval poses a challenge when interpreting the impact of reliability in assessing change. It is generally accepted that test-retest correlations will decrease as the length of the test-retest interval increases, resulting in a potentially infinite number of test-retest reliability coefficients for any one measure (Anastasi, 1988). The reliability coefficients reported in test manuals are often based on relatively brief test-retest intervals (e.g., 7 or 14 days). For this reason, they may not be particularly informative to clinical neuropsychological practitioners, as the length of the test-retest intervals in clinical practice often far exceed those reported in test manuals.

Regression to the Mean

Regression to the mean is a statistical phenomenon which refers to the tendency for extreme scores to revert (or regress) toward the mean of a distribution when the measure is readministered (Kazdin, 1992). If examinees are selected for investigation because they are extreme on a given measure, one can predict on statistical grounds alone that on a subsequent administration of an instrument, those scores will revert toward the mean of the distribution of scores. In other words, subjects who initially scored above the mean would be expected to regress downward toward the mean, whereas subjects who initially scored below the mean would be expected to regress upward toward the mean, absent any intervening factors. As Hayes (1988) notes, regression to the mean is not "some immutable law of nature. Rather, it is, at least in part, a statistical consequence of our choosing to predict in this linear way…" (p.560). This statistical phenomenon is related in large part to the correlation between initial test and retest scores (i.e., test-retest reliability coefficient). The lower the correlation, the greater the amount of measurement error, and the greater the regression to the mean (Kazdin, 1992). Kazdin adds that, in general, regression is of greatest concern in the case of extreme scores, suggesting that, particularly in cases of poor reliability of the measurement instrument, chance plays some role in the examinee's obtaining an extreme score. When evaluating change in *group* means, unless scores are specifically selected on the criterion that they are extreme, regression influences would push each group member's score toward the group mean (up or down depending upon the initial score), theoretically resulting in no mean change in the group. Observed changes in overall group mean performance, therefore, would likely reflect some other systematic force.

Practice Effects

In addition to the impact of random, chance fluctuations or regression to the mean, changes in scores across assessments may reflect *systematic* variance, such as practice effects. "Practice effects" refer to the impact of repeated exposure to an instrument on an examinee's performance. In general, neuropsychological assessment instruments with a speeded component, those requiring an infrequently practiced response, or those having a single, easily conceptualized solution, are most susceptible to the effects of practice (Lezak, 1995). Measures of learning and memory, such as the California Verbal Learning Test (CVLT), are also likely to show large practice effects. Anastasi (1988) differentiates between "learning" and "practice" in that *learning* is a broader experience that may affect future performance, but does not invalidate it insofar as the retest score adequately reflects the examinee's standing in the abilities under consideration. In contrast, *practice* is a more narrow influence, which affects performance on certain items or certain types of items without appreciably affecting the behavioral domain being measured.

Although practice effects tend to be most pronounced with repetition of the same test, sheer test taking exposure can improve subsequent performances, a phenomenon referred to as "test sophistication" (Anastasi, 1988). Although alternate forms of an instrument are often developed to avoid or minimize the effects of practice, improvement in scores may be obtained across alternate forms. As Anastasi points out, the impact of test-taking practice, however, is not limited to retest with alternate forms or the same measure. For example, Coutts et al. (1987) found that mere exposure to testing situations can improve performance on the Category Test as much as repeated exposure to the test itself. In addition, Dirks (1982) found that exposure to a commercially available game (Trac 4) significantly increased the performance of 10-year-old children on the Block Design subtest of the Wechsler Intelligence Scale for Children-Revised (WISC-R).

Unfortunately, the current neuropsychological literature offers little guidance on the interpretation of practice effects. Within the existing literature, there is little consensus regarding how practice effects may vary as a function of the first score (e.g., ceiling effects, regression to the mean), type of task, length of the retest interval, or population. Moreover, although the necessary information to determine the extent of practice effects is collected by test developers in order to compute reliability coefficients, the data on practice effects are rarely presented in test manuals. As noted above, reliability coefficients provide useful psychometric data, and they may be informative in evaluating changes in scores across assessments insofar as they indicate the likelihood of fluctuations due to measurement error. They are meaningless, however, in evaluating the impact of practice, in that practice effects are a reflection of changes in the *total scores*, whereas a reliability coefficient reflects the stability of the *relative ranking* of each examinee's score. For example, a test-retest correlation of 0.93 indicates excellent stability of the relative rankings of each member of the group studied but does not necessarily imply that the group mean is highly stable from one test administration to the second. The same test-retest reliability coefficient could be obtained under several scenarios while the mean performance between assessments could be markedly different. For example, if examinees systematically made mild, moderate, or substantial increases or decreases in their performances at the second administration of an instrument compared with the first administration, but maintained their relative rank ordering on the two administrations, the test-retest reliability coefficient would remain unchanged despite marked changes in group means between assessments.

Controlling Practice Effects

Statistical Procedures

Several researchers have devised statistical procedures for the evaluation of change in clinical trials (see Brouwers & Mohr, 1989; Knight & Shelton, 1983; Meredith & Tisak, 1990; Mohr & Brouwers, 1991; Tisak & Meredith, 1989; Welford, 1985, 1987, for details). In addressing interpretation of change in individual scores, a number of researchers have suggested that the standard error of measurement (SEM) of an instrument be used to set up confidence intervals around an individual's score. This would then be used to partial out practice effects from other factors which may be related to improvement in performance across assessments (e.g., recovery of function; Sattler, 1990; Shatz, 1981). Because the calculation of the standard error of measurement is based on the reliability coefficient ($SEM = SD_t \sqrt{1 - r_{tt}}$

), it provides a range in which the true score is expected to fall, given the observed score, standard deviation, and measurement error. A score obtained outside of that range, therefore, is less likely to reflect the effects of measurement error. Instead, the score would more likely reflect the impact of some *systematic* force (such as treatment, recovery, a disease process, or practice), making use of the SEM an imperfect method for assessing practice effects.

In addition to SEM, several statistical methods have been developed and implemented in an attempt to control and/or correct for measurement error and/or practice effects. Bruggemans, Van de Vijver, and Huysmans (1997) reviewed five traditional statistical approaches and proposed a new method for assessing change across time. The five traditional approaches were: the standard Deviation Index, the Reliable Change Index (Jacobson & Truax, 1991), a second Reliable Change Index (Zegers & Hafkenscheid, 1994), the Reliability-Stability Index (Chelune, Naugle, Luders, Sedlak, & Awad, 1993), and a second Reliability-Stability Index (McSweeny, Naugle, Chelune, & Luders, 1993). The new method, the proposed Reliability-Stability Index, attempts to correct for individual difference variables that may impact on or interact with practice effects. Another approach that attempts to control for practice effects is the standardized regression-based change scores (Sawrie, Marson, Boothe, & Harrell, 1999). This method, which is an extension of the second Reliability-Stability Index noted above, allows for control of demographic variables and regression-to-the-mean. Although no one statistical approach has become "the standard," each attempts to control for important differences that affect change over time.

Methodological Procedures

In addition to statistical manipulations for controlling the effects of practice, several methodological manipulations have been employed. These include, but are not limited to, the use of adequate control groups, dual baseline approach, alternate forms, and test-retest intervals.

Control groups. The selection of an appropriate control group is an essential component of good research methodology (Kazdin, 1998) and is paramount to the accurate interpretation of change across assessment points. Identifying the most appropriate control group(s) should not be an afterthought; it requires the careful weighting of numerous variables and the hypotheses to be investigated. For example, what is the appropriate control group for a study of patients undergoing a temporal lobectomy? Are healthy individuals an appropriate control group? Are temporal lobe epilepsy patients who are not receiving lobectomies? Are other non-temporal lobectomy brain surgery patients? Are other non-brain surgery surgical patients? Often the selection of a control group is made for pragmatic reasons (e.g., what additional groups do we have access to?) rather than to more fully test the hypotheses. The more closely matched the groups are in terms of demographic variables, test-retest intervals, as so on, the more confident one can be in attributing the differences between the groups to the independent variable (e.g., treatment, disease processes, etc.).

Although it is tempting for researchers to forego the use of control groups in serial assessment studies under the assumption that the initial assessment point can serve as a baseline and adequate control for future evaluation, results from such studies should be viewed cautiously. In such instances, researchers often fail to address the potential influence of practice, or summarily negate the impact of practice without empirical support for their claims.

Dual baseline approach. In addition to the use of appropriate control groups at every assessment point, some investigators further attempt to control for practice effects by employing a dual baseline approach in which the entire neuropsychological battery is administered twice prior to the introduction of any independent variable. The initial administration serves as a methodological procedure to reduce the influence of practice effects on subsequent assessments. The second administration is then used as the baseline comparison for following evaluations. This approach has been utilized in our laboratory since 1986 and has been found to be a viable means of reducing practice effects in studies involving multiple assessment points, even in instruments with robust practice effects such as the CVLT (Duff, Westervelt, Haase, & McCaffrey, 1999). The viability of the dual baseline approach, however, needs to be empirically investigated with other measures and other populations.

Alternate forms. An additional method for controlling/minimizing practice effects is to administer alternate forms of the test during subsequent evaluations. As noted earlier, alternate forms of a test should also be "parallel" (e.g., possess the same format and content type, yield identical psychometric properties, etc.) to the original form of the test. If an alternate form is sufficiently parallel/comparable to its original form, it may minimize practice effects. For example, Crawford, Stewart, and Moore (1989) developed an alternate form of the Rey Auditory Verbal Learning

Test (RAVLT) and compared the results of a group of subjects given the original form twice to a group given the original form first and the alternate form on retest. In this study, significant gains were made when the original test was given twice, but those gains were minimized when an alternate form was used at retest.

In other instances, the differences between two forms of a test are not sufficient to eliminate the practice effects. In a comparison of the Rey-Osterrieth Complex Figure Test (ROCFT) and the Taylor Complex Figure Test (TCFT), DeLaney, Prevey, Cramer, Mattson, and colleagues (1992) administered the ROCFT followed by the TCFT to a group of normal subjects. Immediate and delayed recall scores of the TCFT were significantly greater than the scores on the ROCFT. The authors note that the subjects' experience with the format of the ROCFT (i.e., "surprise" immediate and delayed recall trials) may prepare them for the TCFT. The authors also note that alternative explanations for the effect (e.g., that the TCFT is easier than the ROCFT) cannot be ruled out given that they did not counterbalance the administration of the two tests. Anastasi and Urbina (1997) refer to the practice effects on alternate forms as "test sophistication effects." Unfortunately, little empirical work has been completed on alternate forms or test sophistication effects.

Increasing test-retest interval. As noted earlier, the length of the test-retest interval is an important variable to consider when interpreting reliability data. As the retest interval increases, the correlation between test and retest scores decrease. Although the test-retest interval's effect on reliability is fairly well documented, its impact on actual test scores and practice effects has been seldom studied.

In two studies investigating the effects of various test-retest intervals, Catron (1978) and Catron and Thompson (1979) administered the Wechsler Adult Intelligence Scale (WAIS) to college students with the following intervals: immediate, 1 week, 1 month, 2 months, or 4 months. For both Performance Intelligence Quotient (PIQ) and Full Scale Intelligence Quotient (FSIQ), a clear trend was observed, in that, the longer the test-retest interval, the smaller the gains at retesting.

Despite answering the initial question "can test-retest intervals impact practice effects?," many additional questions remain. Do these same trends appear with other neuropsychological measures? Are these same trends observed across longer periods of time? Is there an interval that optimally minimizes practice effects? How do various person-specific variables (e.g., age, gender, and intelligence) interact with the test-retest interval effect?

Clinical folklore and practice effects. Unfortunately, some researchers have made assumptions about how practice effects interact with a particular population or research design methodology and these assumptions guide current research. For example, it may be assumed that certain patient populations (e.g., Alzheimer's disease) are immune to practice effects. Empirical evidence, however, disputes this assumption (Eagger, Morant, Levy, & Sahakian, 1992). Similarly, clinical folklore indicates that 6 months is an adequate length of time to negate practice effects. Again, empirical evidence does not completely support this notion [e.g., Burgess et al., (1994) reported practice effects among patients with HIV after a 12-month retest]. These assumptions, which are rarely based on data, may lead to research design decisions (e.g., exclusion of control groups because a 6-month test-retest interval is used) which might minimize the significance of the findings.

Several other person-specific variables are thought to impact serial assessments and practice effects. The following section will outline a number of those variables and present relevant literature addressing their impact on serial assessment and practice effects. It should be noted that this review is intended to be neither all-inclusive (i.e., containing all possible person-specific variables) nor exhaustive (i.e., containing all relevant literature on those variables). Rather, it is intended as an impetus for further debate and future research.

Person-Specific Variables

Person-specific variables are those variables that are inherent in the individual and include age, gender, education, intelligence, and disease processes. Many of these variables have been shown to affect performance on neuropsychological measures during a single assessment. For example, age and/or disease process has been shown to impinge on neuropsychological functioning (Grant & Adams, 1996; Lezak, 1995). Their effects on repeated assessments of neuropsychological functioning are, however, unclear.

Age

Age may be one of the most widely researched person-specific variables. Its impact on neuropsychological functioning has also received considerable attention (Grant & Adams, 1996; Lezak, 1995). Many standardized neuropsychological measures rely on age-corrected scores for the accurate interpretation of performance. Unfortunately, the impact of age on serial neuropsychological functioning has received less attention.

Despite limited research directly assessing the effect of age on serial neuropsychological performance, several studies have supported the expectation that it does have a mediating effect. In a review of several empirical works, Shatz (1981) notes that "age is probably an important variable" (p. 176) in determining the extent of practice effects on neuropsychological measures such as the WAIS. Additionally Shatz notes that age impacts on the test-retest interval effect (i.e., older adults benefit less from practice effects with longer test-retest intervals).

Hamby, Bardi, and Wilkins (1993) reported on a group of younger HIV+ subjects who displayed a greater practice effect compared to older HIV+ subjects on a processing speed composite score. Age effects on practice were not found, however, on the composite scores of verbal memory or visuospatial abilities. This study highlights two areas for future research: 1) the selective effects of age on serial neuropsychological performance (i.e., age may affect some measures/domains but not others), and 2) the interaction of age and disease process on practice effects and serial assessments (i.e., age may affect some diseases/disorders but not others).

Lehmann, Ban, & Kral (1968) studied the effects of practice in a group of geriatric patients from two psychiatric hospitals and compared their results to those of a younger control and two older control groups.

Unexpectedly, *older* subjects (70 + years) showed improvement due to practice across more measures than younger subjects (< 70 years). Although not noted by the authors, a possible explanation for these findings may be due to ceiling effects (i.e., younger subjects had already reached the maximum score and could not improve any further whereas older subjects may have had more room to improve), though the data were lacking to test this hypothesis.

Although less representative, some studies indicate that serial assessment performance is only minimally affected by the age the examinees. MacInnes, Paull Uhl, and Schima (1987) report on a "normal" elderly sample of subjects examined twice with the Luria-Nebraska Neuropsychological Battery (LNNB) across a three- to four-year period. The results showed improvement on only one clinical scale (Expressive Language) and declines on three indices (Arithmetic Scale, Profile Elevation Index, and Impairment Index) of the LNNB. A further comparison of older versus younger elderly subjects revealed no significant differences across time. Similarly, Denney and Heldrich (1990) observed no differential improvement on the Raven's Progressive Matrices (RPM) for three age groups across time.

In sum, age has been observed to have a significant effect on some neuropsychological measures. When those measures are given repeatedly, this effect may be compounded. Many of the studies that have directly investigated this person-specific variable have supported the hypothesis that age has an effect on neuropsychological performance across time. The studies reviewed do not, however, provide consensus as to which measures are likely to be affected (e.g., verbal, visuospatial, processing speed) or to what extent. A limited number of studies do not support an age by serial assessment interaction. These "dissenting" studies, however, were not designed to test the effect of age on serial assessment. These studies may provide better evidence for other, interactive effects (e.g., MacInnes, et al.,1987 may provide more information on the interaction of age and test-retest interval effect).

Gender

Whereas age effects on single assessments are more widely accepted, gender differences on single neuropsychological assessments are less clear. Males have traditionally been reported to show superiority for visuospatial tasks and arithmetic skills. Females, on the other hand, have been reported to show superiority for verbally oriented tasks and tasks that employ perceptual speed. These differences, however, tend to be small and less consistent compared to the age-related differences. These differences have also not been fully explored longitudinally.

When Lehmann, Ban, and Kral (1968) divided their geriatric sample by gender, they reported minor differences in practice effects. Males tended to display a greater practice effect on reaction time and females displayed a greater improvement across time on a forward digit span task. With a considerably younger sample and a more experimental task, Payne (1989) observed that female subjects displayed less of a practice effect across trials compared to male subjects on a mirror-tracking task.

A study by Trenerry et al. (1996) highlights the interaction between gender and disease process on serial assessments of neuropsychological functioning. Unilateral, temporal lobectomy patients were assessed pre- and post-operatively with an extensive neuropsychological battery. Results indicate that, regardless of the site of surgery, females' Wechsler Memory Scale-Revised (WMS-R) Visual Reproduction savings score improved post-operatively whereas scores for male patients declined. The effects of gender versus disease process versus intervention are difficult to partial out, as are their potential interactions.

To some degree, the studies noted above support a gender effect on serial neuropsychological assessments. Not all studies, however, lend support to the gender effect hypothesis. MacInnes, Paull, Uhl, and Schima (1987), for example, noted only one scale differed between "normal" elderly males and females on the LNNB across time. Many more studies appear to ignore this variable and either do not make comparisons between genders or do not even report the gender breakdown of the samples. Clearly, further exploration of this person-specific variable is needed to assess its effect on serial assessment. As with the effect of age, different studies report different findings concerning which tests are affected and to what degree those tests are affected by this person-specific variable.

Intelligence

The effect of intelligence on neuropsychological performance is equivocal and will only be reviewed briefly. Whereas some clinicians expect to find a positive correlation between intelligence and neuropsychological functioning, others have noted that there is little empirical evidence to support the strong relationship between IQ and neuropsychological functioning. Likewise, studies investigating the impact of intelligence on serial neuropsychological performance are also sparse. Recently, however, several studies have addressed this topic.

Rapport, Brines, Axelrod, and Theisen (1997b) conducted a brief longitudinal investigation with normal, healthy adults to explore the role of IQ on practice effects of the Wechsler Adult Intelligence Scale-Revised (WAIS-R). Subjects were categorized into one of three groups based on an initial WAIS-R FSIQ (High Average, Average, Low Average). Subjects were then tested four times at two-week intervals. Results indicated those subjects in the Average and High Average groups made greater retest gains across time compared to the subjects in the Low Average group. The authors conclude that, although all subjects improved with prior exposure to the test, subjects with higher initial IQ scores improved more.

In a similar study investigating the effect of intelligence on memory functioning, Rapport, Axelrod, Theisen, Brines, Kalechstein, and Ricker (1997a) divided a group of adults by WAIS-R FSIQ scores (High Average, Average, Low Average). The subjects were administered the WMS-R and the CVLT twice within a two-week interval. Results indicate that all three groups showed significant practice effects across time on the memory measures. Although not statistically significant, greater practice effects were evident for the Average and High Average groups compared to the Low Average group on the WMS-R General Memory Index and the CVLT Total Words Trials 1-5. The lack of statistical significance for these and other memory measures may have been due to a ceiling effect in Average and High Average subjects.

Additionally, Hamby, Bardi, and Wilkins (1993) noted that HIV+ subjects with higher WAIS-R Vocabulary scores exhibited greater practice effects compared to subjects with lower Vocabulary scores. Practice effects were noted on two of three neuropsychological composite scores assessed. Although it was not investigated in this study, the inclusion of an HIV- group could have examined another possible interaction of person-specific variables: intelligence and disease process.

Whereas few studies have directly investigated the effect of intelligence on serial assessment, comparisons of several different studies with similar methodologies reveal the expected trend. In two studies using the WISC-R, normal schoolchildren (Tuma & Appelbaum, 1990) improved on the VIQ (+1.09), PIQ (+7.82), and FSIQ (+4.73) whereas children diagnosed with either a Learning Disability (LD) or history of Mental Retardation (MR) (Vance, Blixt, Ellis, & Debell, 1981) showed a different pattern at retest (VIQ = -1.87, PIQ = +2.04, FSIQ = 0.0).

The studies noted above, along with clinical intuition, suggest that intelligence has an effect on serial neuropsychological functioning. As with age and gender, systematic research is currently lacking. At present, it is unknown which neuropsychological domains are affected by intelligence and to what extent.

Education

The hypothesis that level of education affects neuropsychological performance is somewhat supported in the clinical literature. Heaton, et al. (1996) report that several subtests of the Wechsler intelligence tests (e.g., Vocabulary, Information, Similarities, Comprehension) are affected by the subject's educational level. On the other hand, measures from the Halstead-Reitan Neuropsychological Battery (HRNB) appear to be less sensitive to the effects of education (Heaton et al., 1996). Given these findings, it is expected that when some tests are given repeatedly to subjects, there may be a variety of education-related performance effects. However, support for this expectation is mixed. Selnes et al. (1990), for example, observed that education (and age) predicted change in neuropsychological performance across time in a longitudinal study of HIV. Conversely, Hamby, Bardi, and Wilkins (1993) did not find an education effect in their study of patients with HIV. Since many of the effects (or lack of effects) are post-hoc findings, more direct research into this area is needed.

Disease Process

Patients who suffer from different neurological conditions perform differently on measures of neuropsychological functioning. The memory deficits associated with Alzheimer's disease are different from the memory deficits associated with Parkinson's disease. Differential diagnoses are commonly based, in part, on the differential results of neuropsychological evaluations. Given the specific deficits of each patient group, it is possible that these groups will also respond differently to the effects of practice.

In a review of practice effects in clinical neuropsychology, Shatz (1981) concludes that different patient populations are unlikely to show the same patterns of improvement on neuropsychological measures. An absence of practice effects may set apart different patient populations. In one study, Dodrill and Troupin (1975) administered the HRNB four times to a sample of chronic epileptics across 18 to 29 months and noted that significant practice effects were absent until the fourth testing session, whereas Matarazzo, Matarazzo, Gallo, & Weins (1979) observed practice effects on HRNB measures in healthy controls and chronic schizophrenic patients after a single retest. Similarly, Coutts et al. (1987) concluded that children diagnosed as learning-disabled did not benefit as much from practice on the Category Test as non-learning disabled children.

Practice effects may also appear where they are not expected. In studies with certain patient populations, such as Alzheimer's disease, researchers often do not feel the need to control for practice effects because the patients are identified in part by their severe memory dysfunction and are not expected to benefit from practice. In some instances, however, this expectation is unfounded. For example Eagger, Morant, Levy, and Sahakian (1992) demonstrated practice effects on the Abbreviated Mental Test Score with brief test-retest intervals in a group of placebo-treated Alzheimer's patients. The extent to which this group may show practice effects with longer test-retest intervals or improvement on other measures, however, remains unclear.

The effects of practice may also be seen as "no change" when deterioration is expected over time. For example, a patient with a progressive neurological disorder may be expected to show a gradual decline in memory functioning based on the natural history of the disorder. If this patient is enrolled in a non-controlled clinical research trial designed to evaluate the efficacy of a new drug thought to slow the progression of disorder, repeated testing with the WMS-R Logical Memory may occur monthly. Initially, the expected decline in memory scores is evident but over the course of several months the decline in memory scores diminishes and eventually ceases. The patient demonstrates no decline in memory. The clinician happily reports to the family that the expected further decline in memory has been halted due to the drug. Unfortunately, the clinician may not have considered the role of practice effects. In this case, the practice effects may have offset the decline associated with the natural course of the disorder. The additive as well as interactive effects due to both practice and the disease need to be considered by the clinician.

The few studies mentioned above lend some preliminary support to the hypothesis that different disease processes may have differential rates and patterns of practice effects. For example, minimal or absent practice effects may be a noteworthy finding. When improvement is expected, this pattern of performance may indicate that the patient cannot benefit from practice. Alternatively, practice effects may appear as "no change" when practice effects offset a deteriorating disease process. Lastly, practice effects may appear among patients in which they are not expected (e.g., Alzheimer's disease). Unfortunately, there has been little systematic study of any of these patterns in the different disease processes commonly seen by clinical neuropsychological practitioners.

An Illustrative Example

The following study illustrates the potential for misinterpretation of serial neuropsychological assessment in the absence of a control group. Additionally, this example will highlight one use of the current manual, with specific reference to the subsequent tables. Halperin et al. (1988) tested 17 patients with Lyme disease complaining of memory or other cognitive difficulties. All patients were tested before antibiotic treatment and retested 5 to 28 weeks following treatment. Significant improvement was found on tests of verbal and visual recall, a test of problem solving (Booklet Category Test), and measures defined as psychomotor speed (WAIS-R Block Design and Purdue Pegboard). Halperin et al. attempted to control for practice effects by utilizing alternate forms with the CVLT and the WMS. Nonetheless, without the inclusion of a control group, the relative contributions of practice/test sophistication and improvements in cognitive functioning due to treatment are almost impossible to tease apart. This may be particularly true for these findings, in that all of the measures which showed improvement are among those most likely to be affected by practice (i.e., memory tasks, those with a single, easily conceptualize response [if solved on initial assessment], and those with a speeded component, Lezak, 1995).

To illustrate this point (and the use of this manual), the results of Halperin et al. (1988) are presented below. Change scores (post-treatment mean minus pre-treatment mean) were calculated for several of the measures used in the study. These change scores were compared to change scores for "control" subjects based on the accumulated data in the subsequent tables. Although control subjects could not be matched identically to those from the Halperin et al. study, comparable controls (i.e., similar age, test-retest interval) were often found in the subsequent tables. Between-group comparisons of Halperin et al.'s patients with Lyme disease and the comparable controls from the clinical literature revealed three types of results: results that continue to support the original within-subjects comparisons, results that dispute the original within-subjects comparisons, and non-significant results that might be significant. Examples of the first type (i.e., results that continue to support the original results) include results from measures of the CVLT. On one such measure, Trial 5 of the CVLT, Halperin et al. found a mean increase of 2.81 on post-treatment assessment for the study's patients ($p<.001$). Based on information from Table 12 (p. 106), Hanly, et al.

(1994) found a mean increase of 0.71 for 17 controls over a 12- month interval. Despite the discrepancy between test-retest intervals (Halperin et al.'s = 5-28 weeks), the post-treatment scores of the patients with Lyme disease surpassed that found in healthy controls by almost fourfold. Such between-group comparisons provide additional strength to the conclusions drawn by Halperin et al.

As noted above, some comparisons with control subjects were not as favorable to the conclusions drawn in the original article. For example, Halperin et al. (1988) observed a mean improvement on the Booklet Category Test of 19.65 during the post-treatment assessment ($p<.01$). Several studies from the subsequent tables call this "significant improvement" into question. Saykin et al. (1991) observed a mean improvement of 8.15 on the Booklet Category Test across an 18-month interval in control subjects (see Table 15, p. 115). Despite the longer interval in Saykin et al.'s study, approximately half of Halperin et al.'s pre-post difference may be attributable to practice effects based on this between-group comparison. Additionally, Bornstein et al. (1987) and Matarazzo et al. (1979) reported improvements for control subjects on the Category Test of 22.9 and 11.6 points, respectively, for intervals of 3 and 20 weeks, respectively (see Table 15, pp. 116 and 117, respectively). Despite the questionable equivalence of the Booklet Category Test and the Category Test, practice effects either completely or substantially subsume the differences reported by Halperin et al. For the above mentioned neuropsychological measures, the addition of a control/comparison group (albeit an imperfectly matched control/comparison group) served to alter the conclusions drawn in the original article.

One additional result that may be entertained from the between-group comparisons of Halperin et al.'s (1988) patients and "our" control subjects is that non-significant findings from the original article may actually be significant when compared to the control group. For example, post-treatment Controlled Oral Word Association Test (COWAT) scores improved only 0.17 for the patients with Lyme disease (non-significant). Comparable control data indicates that at a 3-month interval, Macciocchi (1990) observed a mean improvement of 4.5 for control subjects on the COWAT (Table 68, p. 398). Taking these two findings together, Halperin et al. should have expected an approximately 4.5 point increase for their patients, yet a much smaller increase was actually observed. This lack-of-adifference-when-one-is-expected (based on practice effects) could have lead Halperin et al. to posit a deficit in verbal fluency for these patients that is not ameliorated with treatment.

The above illustrative example applied the information from subsequent tables to research findings. Additionally, a practitioner could apply the information from the tables to an individual patient. The procedure would follow the research example closely (i.e., find the appropriate comparison group [e.g., comparable age, gender, test-retest interval, etc.] and compare "change scores").

For both clinical and research comparisons, the information presented in the following tables may best be used prospectively rather than retrospectively. That is, the researcher or clinician may choose the appropriate comparison group a priori and then conduct the experiment or clinical assessment following similar parameters (e.g., similar measures, similar test-retest intervals, etc.). By equating the comparison group and the "experimental" group or individual ahead of time, error due to mismatched methodologies can be minimized and comparisons can be more informative.

By aggregating this information, we are not, however, advocating for methodological shortcuts. When searching for a reliable effect, there is no substitute for an appropriately designed research project that maximizes internal validity. In some cases, however, an appropriate comparison group is neither available nor feasible. This should not absolve the researcher/clinician from considering variables that impact serial neuropsychological performance.

Tables

Abbreviations used in Group column

AAMI = Age Associated Memory Impairment
abstin = abstinence
ADHD = Attention Deficit Hyperactivity Disorder
AIDS = Acquired Immunodeficiency Syndrome
ALL = Acute Lymphocytic Leukemia
ALS = Amyotrophic Lateral Sclerosis
APOE-E4 = apolipoprotein ε4
ARC = AIDS Related Complex
asx = asymptomatic
avg = average
AVM = Arteriovenous Malformation
BMT = Bone Marrow Transplant
BZ = Benzodiazepine
CAD = Carotid Artery Disease

CDR = Clinical Dementia Rating
CVD = Cerebrovascular Disease
CVA = Cerebral Vascular Accident
D/O = Disorder
DAT = Dementia of the Alzheimer's Type
EMR = Educable Mental Retardation
Enceph = Encephalopathy
HD = Huntington's Disease
Hemorr = Hemorrhage
HIV = Human Immunodeficiency Virus
Hydroceph = Hydrocephalus
Inpts = Inpatients
IQ = Intelligence Quotient
IVDU = Intravenous Drug User
LD = Learning Disability
MID = Multi-Infarct Dementia
min = minimal
mod = moderate
MR = Mental Retardation
MS = Multiple Sclerosis
PCP = Phencyclidine
PD = Parkinson's Disease
PLG = persistent generalized lymphadenopathy
PTA = Post-Traumatic Amnesia
Pts = Patients

PVD = Peripheral Vascular Disease
SES = Socio-Economic Status
sev = severe
SLE = Systemic Lupus Erythematosus
sx = symptom, symptomatic
sz = seizures
TBI = Traumatic Brain Injury
TIA = Transient Ischemic Attack
VA = Veteran's Administration
w/ = with
yr = year
yrs = years

Abbreviations used in Instrument column

[#] = maximum score
% forg = percent forgotten
% ret = percent retained
%ile = percentile
2-D = 2-Dimensional
3-D = 3-Dimensional
3D CP = Benton 3-Dimensional Constructional Praxis Test
AAT = Aachen Aphasia Test
ACI = Attention Concentration Index
Acquis = Acquisition

AMNART = American National Adult Reading Test
AMTC = Attention/Mental Tracking Composite
ASS = Age Scaled Score
AST = Aphasia Screening Examination
avg = average
BDAE = Boston Diagnostic Aphasia Examination
Beery VMI = Beery Test of Visual Motor Integration
BH = Both Hands
BIMCT = Blessed Information Memory Concentration Test
BNT = Boston Naming Test
BSID = Bayley Scales of Infant Development
BSRT = Buschke Selective Reminding Test
BSSS = Bilateral Simultaneous Sensory Stimulation
B-W DCT = Bourdon-Wiersma Dot Cancellation Test
C = Color
Cancell = Cancellation
CANTAB = Cambridge Automated Neuropsychological Test Assessment Battery
CCC = Auditory Consonant Trigrams
CDRT = Cognitive Drug Research Test
CERAD = Consortium to Establish a Registry for the Assessment of Dementia
CFF = Critical Flicker Fusion
CFT = Complex Figure Test
CHIPASAT = Children's Paced Auditory Serial Addition Test
CLTR = Consistent Long-Term Retrieval
comiss = comissions

Comp = Comprehension
Cons = Consistency
COWAT = Controlled Oral Word Association Test
COWAT = Controlled Oral Word Association Test
CPT = Continuous Performance Test
CPT-A = Auditory Continuous Performance Test
CPT-V = Visual Continuous Performance Test
CQ = Conceptual Quotient
CR = Cued Recall
CRMT = Continuous Recognition Memory Test
CVLT = California Verbal Learning Test
CVMT = Continuous Visual Memory Test
CVS = Crichton Vocabulary Scale
CW = Color-Word
D Span = Digit Span
D Sym = Digit Symbol
DDEL = Design Delay Retention
DH = dominant hand
Discrim = Discriminability
DMtS = Delay Match to Sample
DPLI = Delayed Position Learning Index
DR = Delayed Recall
DRI = Delayed Recall Index
DRS = Mattis Dementia Rating Scale
DSUM = Design Learning over trials

EFT = Embedded Figures Test
FM = Figural Memory
FP = False Positives
FR = Free Recall
freq = frequency
FRT = Benton Facial Recognition Test
FTT = Finger Tapping Test
GCI = General Cognitive Index
GMI = General Memory Index
GMT = Guild Memory Test
GORT = Gray Oral Reading Test
gr = grade level
hr = hour
HVLT = Hopkins Verbal Learning Test
HVOT = Hooper Visual Organization Test
Imm = Immediate
Imp = Impairment
Info = Information
Intrus = Intrusions
IQ = Intelligence Quotient
JLOT = Benton Judgment of Line Orientation Test
KTEA = Kaufman Test of Educational Achievement
L = Left
LDCR = Long Delay Cued Recall
LDE = Lateral Dominance Examination

LDFR = Long Delay Free Recall
LE (as in Auditory LE) = Left Ear
LE (as in Visual LE) = Left Eye
LFH = Left Face and Hand
LH = Left Hand
LM = Logical Memory
LM x = Logical Memory (not specified)
LNNB = Luria Nebraska Neuropsychological Battery
LTR = Long-Term Retrieval
LTS = Long-Term Storage
LVF = Left Visual Field
MAE = Multilingual Aphasia Examination
mBNT = modified Boston Naming Test
MC = Mental Control
MC = Multiple Choice
mD Sym = modified Digit Symbol
med = medium
MFFT = Matching Familiar Figures Test
MHV = Mill Hill Vocabulary Test
min = minute
MKMSB = Matthews-Klove Motor Steadiness Battery
mMMSE = modified Mini Mental State Examination
MMSE = Mini Mental State Examination
MQ = Memory Quotient
MQ = Memory Quotient

MSCA = McCarthy Scales of Children's Abilities
msec = milliseconds
mSpeech Sounds Perception Test = modified Speech Sounds Perception Test
mStroop = modified Stroop
mToken Test = modified Token Test
mTower of London = modified Tower of London
NART = North American Reading Test
NDH = non-dominant hand
NES = Neurobehavioral Evaluation System
NPE = Nonperseverative Errors
omiss = omissions
Orient = Orientation
PA = Paired Associates
PA x = Paired Associates (not specified)
PAL = Paired Associate Learning
PALT = Paired Associate Learning Test
PASAT = Paced Auditory Serial Addition Test
PAT = Paired Associate Test
PE = Perseverative Errors
Pegb = Pegboard
Percep = Perceptual
Percept-Perform = Perceptual-Performance
Persev = Perseverations
PIAT = Peabody Individual Achievement Test
PLI = Position Learning Index over trials

PPVT = Peabody Picture Vocabulary Test
PPVT-IIIA = Peabody Picture Vocabulary Test-III Form A
PPVT-IIIB = Peabody Picture Vocabulary Test-III Form B
PPVT-R = Peabody Picture Vocabulary Test-Revised
PR = Perseverative Responses
R = Right
RAVLT= Rey Auditory Verbal Learning Test
RB = Response Bias
RBMT = Rivermead Behavioural Memory Test
RCPM = Raven's Colored Progressive Matrices
RCPMB = Repeatable Cognitive Perceptual Motor Battery
RE (as in Auditory RE) = Right Ear
RE (as in Visual RE) = Right Eye
Recog = Recognition
RFH = Right Face and Hand
RH = Right Hand
RLB = Right Left Both
RLTR = Random Long-Term Retrieval
RMT = Randt Memory Test
ROCFT = Rey-Osterrieth Complex Figure Test
RPAB = Rivermead Perception Assessment Battery
RPM = Raven's Progressive Matrices
rpm = revolutions per minute
RT = Reaction Time
RVF = Right Visual Field

SDCR = Short Delay Cued Recall
SDFR = Short Delay Free Recall
SDMT = Symbol Digit Modalities Test
SeaRT = Seashore Rhythm Test
sec = seconds
Sem = Semantic
Seq = Sequence
Ser = Serial
SHILS = Shipley Hartford Institute of Living Scale
SRT = Selective Reminding Test
SSPT = Speech Sounds Perception Test
ST = Benton Stereognosis Test
std = standard score
STR = Short-Term Recall
Sym Dig = Symbol Digit
t = t-score
TFPT = Benton Tactile Form Perception Test
TMT-A = Trail Making Test Part A
TMT-B = Trail Making Test Part B
TMT-C = Trail Making Test Part C
TMT-D = Trail Making Test Part D
TOT = Benton Temporal Orientation Test
TOVA = Test of Visual Attention
TPT = Tactual Performance Test
TPT-6 = Tactual Performance Test (Six Block Version)

TQ = Test Quotient
V Span = Visual Span
VeMI = Verbal Memory Index
Vigil = Vigilance
ViMI = Visual Memory Index
VR = Visual Reproduction
VR x = Visual Reproduction (not specified)
VRT = Benton Visual Retention Test
VRT-F = Benton Visual Retention Test Form F
VRT-G = Benton Visual Retention Test Form G
VST = Visual Search Task/Test
W = Word
WAB = Western Aphasia Battery
WCST = Wisconsin Card Sorting Test
WJ-R = Woodcock Johnson-Revised
WMI = Working Memory Index
WMS = Wechsler Memory Scale
WMS x = Wechsler Memory Scale (version not specified)
WMS-III = Wechsler Memory Scale-III
WMS-R = Wechsler Memory Scale-Revised
WRAT = Wide Range Achievement Test
WRAT-3 = Wide Range Achievement Test-3
WRAT-R = Wide Range Achievement Test-Revised

Abbreviations used in Intervention column

ABMT = autologous bone marrow transplant
admin = administered
antidepress = antidepressant
bendrofluaz = bendrofluazide
BMT = bone marrow transplant
BZ = benzodiazepine
CABG = coronary artery bypass graph
carbamaz = carbamazepine
cb = counterbalanced
CDP = cytdine diphosphoryl
CE = carotid endarterectomy
chlorpromaz = chlorpromazepine
CPB = coronary bypass
d/c = discharged
DGAVP = des-gly-arg vassopressin
diphenhydram = diphenhydramine
ECT = electroconvulsive therapy
F/T = full-time
g = grams
inpt = inpatient
LCE = left carotid endarterectomy
LTL = left temporal lobectomy

meds = medications
methylphen = methylphenidate
mg = milligrams
min = minimal
MSR = sustained-release methylphenidate
n/a = not applicable
NSAID = non-steriod anti-inflammatory drug
outpt = out patient
P/T = part-time
PVD = peripheral vascular disease
RCE = right carotid endarterectomy
rehab = rehabilitation
rHuEpo = recombinant human erythropoietin
RTL = right temporal lobectomy
std = standard
TDB = tripostassium dicitrato bismuthate
TIPSS = check in Jalan (1995)
trihexphen = check in Koller (1984)
tx = treatment
wk = week
zdv = zidovudine

Abbreviations for Interval column

~ = approximately
d = day(s)
h = hour(s)
m = month(s)
min = minute(s)
w = week(s)
y = year(s)

Abbreviations for t1 and t2 columns
%c = percent change from baseline
ac = absolute change from baseline
c = change score from baseline
NR = not reported

Abbreviations for Note column
* = more than two assessments reported in original article
4-lett C = 4 letter words beginning with c
A = Form/Part A
AF = Alternate Forms used (not further specified)
alt = alternate form
anim = category fluency (animals)
auto = automated administration
B = Form/Part B

Bab/Term = Babcock/Terman
bird = category fluency (birds)
C = Form/Part C
categ = category fluency (not further specified)
CB = forms Counterbalanced
CFL = letters c, f, and l used
city = category fluency (cities)
cloth = category fluency (clothing)
color = category fluency (colors)
comp = computer administration
D = Form/Part D
F = letter f used
FAS = letters f, a, and s used
food = category fluency (food)
fruit = category fluency (fruit)
H = letter h used
I = Form I
II = Form II
lett = letters (not further specified)
MPD = letters m, p, and d used
presid = category fluency (presidents)
prof = category fluency (professions)
PRW = letters p, r, and w used
PS = letters p and s used
round = category fluency (round objects)

SP = letters s and p used
std = standard administration
street = category fluency (things seen on a street)
town = category fluency (towns)
veg = category fluency (vegetables)
ver = version
wood = category fluency (objects made of wood)

Table 1. Achievement Tests

instrument	group	n	m/f	age	intervention	inter	t #1	t #2	note	citation
GORT (gr)	LD	29	24/5	10.83 (1.40)	methylphen	8 w	2.17 (0.11)	2.42 (0.15)		Gittleman-Klein, et al (1976)
GORT (gr)	LD	32	23/9	10.67 (1.30)	placebo	8 w	2.13 (0.11)	2.28 (0.14)		Gittleman-Klein, et al (1976)
KTEA Math Applications	Control	20	10/10	~11.00	n/a	12-16 d	115.6 (16.4)	121.3 (16.2)		Shull-Senn, et al (1995)
KTEA Math Applications	Control	20	10/10	~7.00	n/a	12-16 d	97.8 (16.1)	101.7 (17.4)		Shull-Senn, et al (1995)
KTEA Math Applications	Control	20	10/10	~9.00	n/a	12-16 d	107.3 (19.0)	112.3 (20.8)		Shull-Senn, et al (1995)
KTEA Math Composite	Control	20	10/10	~7.00	n/a	12-16 d	95.6 (17.3)	98.8 (19.0)		Shull-Senn, et al (1995)
KTEA Math Composite	Control	20	10/10	~11.00	n/a	12-16 d	111.5 (15.9)	118.8 (16.7)		Shull-Senn, et al (1995)
KTEA Math Composite	Control	20	10/10	~9.00	n/a	12-16 d	104.1 (18.9)	109.4 (20.3)		Shull-Senn, et al (1995)
KTEA Math Computations	Control	20	10/10	~11.00	n/a	12-16 d	106.6 (16.0)	112.9 (17.3)		Shull-Senn, et al (1995)
KTEA Math Computations	Control	20	10/10	~7.00	n/a	12-16 d	98.4 (16.9)	99.9 (17.8)		Shull-Senn, et al (1995)
KTEA Math Computations	Control	20	10/10	~9.00	n/a	12-16 d	101.1 (16.5)	105.0 (18.2)		Shull-Senn, et al (1995)
KTEA Reading Composite	Control	20	10/10	~11.00	n/a	12-16 d	107.5 (20.5)	112.0 (22.7)		Shull-Senn, et al (1995)

instrument	group	n	m/f	age	intervention	inter	t #1	t #2	note	citation
KTEA Reading Composite	Control	20	10/10	~7.00	n/a	12-16 d	96.0 (20.5)	98.9 (22.3)		Shull-Senn, et al (1995)
KTEA Reading Composite	Control	20	10/10	~9.00	n/a	12-16 d	102.9 (17.3)	108.1 (18.2)		Shull-Senn, et al (1995)
KTEA Reading Comp	Control	20	10/10	~7.00	n/a	12-16 d	97.3 (20.3)	99.9 (20.6)		Shull-Senn, et al (1995)
KTEA Reading Comp	Control	20	10/10	~11.00	n/a	12-16 d	111.1 (17.6)	114.6 (19.2)		Shull-Senn, et al (1995)
KTEA Reading Comp	Control	20	10/10	~9.00	n/a	12-16 d	102.1 (19.0)	106.3 (19.4)		Shull-Senn, et al (1995)
KTEA Reading Decoding	Control	20	10/10	~9.00	n/a	12-16 d	103.9 (15.3)	109.3 (16.5)		Shull-Senn, et al (1995)
KTEA Reading Decoding	Control	20	10/10	~7.00	n/a	12-16 d	95.1 (20.4)	98.0 (22.7)		Shull-Senn, et al (1995)
KTEA Reading Decoding	Control	20	10/10	~11.00	n/a	12-16 d	103.2 (21.6)	107.4 (23.3)		Shull-Senn, et al (1995)
KTEA Spelling	Control	20	10/10	~9.00	n/a	12-16 d	94.1 (16.1)	96.4 (17.4)		Shull-Senn, et al (1995)
KTEA Spelling	Control	20	10/10	~11.00	n/a	12-16 d	98.7 (20.7)	101.9 (24.3)		Shull-Senn, et al (1995)
KTEA Spelling	Control	20	10/10	~7.00	n/a	12-16 d	91.5 (14.5)	92.6 (15.8)		Shull-Senn, et al (1995)
PIAT Reading Comp	Brain Tumor	7	3/4	10.33	surgery	1 m	108.5 (5.7)	113.0 (5.7)		Bordeaux, et al (1988)
PIAT Reading Comp	Brain Tumor	7	4/3	9.83	radiotherapy	11 m	104.3 (20.2)	99.0 (14.2)		Bordeaux, et al (1988)

instrument	group	n	m/f	age	intervention	inter	t #1	t #2	note	citation
PIAT Reading Comp (raw)	PD	4	3/1	53.50	fetal tissue implanted	12 m	67.1	63.5		Sass, et al (1995)
PIAT Reading Recog	Brain Tumor	7	4/3	9.83	radiotherapy	11 m	106.8 (19.8)	100.2 (16.0)		Bordeaux, et al (1988)
PIAT Reading Recog	Brain Tumor	7	3/4	10.33	surgery	1 m	108.3 (5.5)	110.5 (3.5)		Bordeaux, et al (1988)
PIAT Spelling (raw)	PD	4	3/1	53.50	fetal tissue implanted	12 m	65.5	68.3		Sass, et al (1995)
Reading Age	Williams Syndrome	23	12/11	12.90 (1.90)	n/a	8.8 (0.2) y	7.83	8.74	Neale/ Word	Udwin, et al(1996)
Reading Comp Age	Williams Syndrome	23	12/11	12.90 (1.90)	n/a	8.8 (0.2) y	7.77	7.23	Neale/ Word	Udwin, et al (1996)
Spelling Age	Williams Syndrome	23	12/11	12.90 (1.90)	n/a	8.8 (0.2) y	6.62	7.57	Vernon / Word	Udwin, et al (1996)

Table 2. Aphasia Screening Test (AST)

instrument	group	n	m/f	age	intervention	inter	t #1	t #2	note	citation
AST (drawing errors)	Cardiac	90	77/13	59.00 (10.59)	CABG/CPB	8 d	3.8 (1.9)	4.8 (2.6)	*	Townes, et al (1989)
AST (drawing errors)	Control	47	35/12	59.00 (9.81)	n/a	8 d	3.7 (2.0)	3.4 (2.0)	*	Townes, et al (1989)
AST (errors)	Alcoholic (1 yr abstin)	23	23/0	36.80 (6.30)	n/a	1 y	1.74	2.13		Adams, et al (1980)
AST (errors)	Alcoholic (2.5 yrs abstin)	25	25/0	36.50 (6.30)	n/a	1 y	1.52	1.12		Adams, et al (1980)

instrument	group	n	m/f	age	intervention	inter	t #1	t #2	note	citation
AST (errors)	CAD	20	n/a	57.20 (7.20)	CE	6 m	8.8	7.4		Parker, et al (1983)
AST (errors)	CAD	17	n/a	57.20 (7.20)	n/a	6 m	8.6	7.6		Parker, et al (1983)
AST (errors)	CAD	36	n./a	61.10 (8.30)	CE	6 m	9.0	7.9	*	Parker, et al (1986)
AST (errors)	CAD	17	n/a	57.90 (8.40)	n/a	6 m	7.4	6.6	*	Parker, et al (1986)
AST (errors)	Control	21	21/0	36.90 (5.90)	n/a	1 y	1.33	0.76		Adams, et al (1980)
AST (errors)	Depression	33	14/19	37.40	antidepress	7 w	2.0 (2.3)	1.1 (1.1)		Fromm, et al (1984)
AST (errors)	Surgical	17	n/a	57.20 (7.20)	surgery	6 m	4.6	4.1		Parker, et al (1983)
AST (errors)	Surgical	26	n/a	55.30 (6.80)	surgery (non-CE)	6 m	4.9	3.8	*	Parker, et al (1986)
AST (verbal errors)	Cardiac	90	77/13	59.00 (10.59)	CABG/CPB	8 d	7.9 (5.2)	10.1 (11.7)	*	Townes, et al (1989)
AST (verbal errors)	Control	47	35/12	59.00 (9.81)	n/a	8 d	7.3 (4.9)	5.0 (3.7)	*	Townes, et al (1989)
AST (verbal errors)	Mountain climbers	35	34/1	24.00 - 45.00	climb of 5,000-8,000 meters	~1 m	0.52 (0.80)	1.03 (1.10)		Hornbein, et al (1989)
AST (verbal errors)	Mountain climbers	6	6/0	21.00 - 31.00	progressive decompression	~43 d	6.17 (3.60)	7.50 (3.39)		Hornbein, et al (1989)
AST (visual motor errors)	Mountain climbers	6	6/0	21.00 - 31.00	progressive decompression	~43 d	1.71 (1.25)	2.83 (1.33)		Hornbein, et al (1989)

instrument	group	n	m/f	age	intervention	inter	t #1	t #2	note	citation
AST (visual motor errors)	Mountain climbers	35	34/1	24.00 - 45.00	climb of 5,000-8,000 meters	~1 m	0.58 (0.71)	0.58 (0.87)		Hornbein, et al (1989)

Table 3. Attention Tests

instrument	group	n	m/f	age	intervention	inter	t #1	t #2	note	citation
BIMCT	Control	70	26/44	29.30 (1.15)	n/a	4 y	33.81 (0.6)	33.87 (0.4)		Amato, et al (1995)
BIMCT	DAT	40	n/a	50.00 - 90.00	n/a	1 w	16.05 (5.32)	14.87 (5.3)	*	Thal, et al (1986)
BIMCT	DAT (declining)	12	3/9	56.20 (6.40)	n/a	1 y	NR	-6.8 (3.8)c		Piccini, et al (1995)
BIMCT	DAT (stable)	19	3/16	61.00 (6.40)	n/a	1 y	NR	-2.9 (1.5)c		Piccini, et al (1995)
BIMCT	Dementia (mod-sev)	57	25/32	80.40 (7.50)	n/a	8 w	26.9 (7.4)	28.8 (6.8)		Lloyd, et al (1995)
BIMCT	MS	50	18/32	29.90 (8.48)	n/a	4 y	32.32 (3.3)	32.82 (9.8)		Amato, et al (1995)
Counting	Control	10	5/5	60.00 - 69.00	n/a	1 d	NR	2.5 c		Peak (1970)
Counting	Control	10	5/5	50.00 - 59.00	n/a	1 d	NR	1.0 c		Peak (1970)
Counting	Control	10	5/5	40.00 - 49.00	n/a	1 d	NR	1.2 c		Peak (1970)
Counting	Control	10	5/5	70.00 - 79.00	n/a	1 d	NR	1.7 c		Peak (1970)

instrument	group	n	m/f	age	intervention	inter	t #1	t #2	note	citation
crossing off	Control (CDR-0)	30	15/15	70.9 (4.6)	n/a	1 y	181.2 (41.3)	181.2 (34.11)	*	Botwinick, et al (1986)
crossing off	DAT (CDR-1)	18	7/11	71.40 (4.40)	n/a	1 y	136.9 (41.8)	124.5 (41.8)	*	Botwinick, et al (1986)
Crossing Out Sign Test	Alcoholic (brief abstin)	27	27/0	43.07	placebo	7 d	41.1 (12.1)	49.1 (21.0)	*	Korsic, et al (1991)
Crossing Out Sign Test	Alcoholic (brief abstin)	27	27/0	40.96	DGAVP	7 d	39.1 (15.6)	46.4 (12.7)	*	Korsic, et al (1991)
Crossing Out Sign Test	Alcoholic (long abstin)	26	26/0	41.40	placebo	7 d	37.7 (15.1)	46.1 (17.8)	*	Korsic, et al (1991)
Crossing Out Sign Test	Alcoholic (long abstin)	23	23/0	46.26	DGAVP	7 d	42.4 (14.6)	50.2 (16.1)	*	Korsic, et al (1991)
Digit Seq Learning Test	Dementia (2° to steroids)	6	6/0	49.67	steriods d/c or reduced	10.9 m	5.8	11.2		Varney, et al (1984)
Digit Seq Learning Test Supraspan	Cardiac	17	12/5	50.00 (10.48)	heart transplant	36.0 m	17.0 (5.6)	17.0 (4.51)		Roman, et al (1997)
Digit Vigil Test (errors)	HIV+ (IVDU)	8	5/3	39.00 (8.00)	MSR or placebo	7 d	7.4 (8.7)	5.0 (5.2)	*	Van Dyck, et al (1997)
Digit Vigil Test (time)	Control	20	10/10	20.00 (2.80)	n/a	1 w	314.6 (57.2)	289.0 (49.1)	AF, *	Kelland, et al (1996)
Digit Vigil Test (time)	HIV+ (IVDU)	8	5/3	39.00 (8.00)	MSR or placebo	7 d	393.6 (73.4)	398.7 (49.1)	*	Van Dyck, et al (1997)
Knox Cube Test	TBI	15	15/0	18.00 - 56.00	n/a	1-1.5 d	12.53 (2.04)	12.50 (2.08)		desRosiers, et al (1987)

instrument	group	n	m/f	age	intervention	inter	t #1	t #2	note	citation
Knox Cube Test	TIA	12	6/6	66.00 (5.30)	LCE	59.8 d	11 (4.1)	12.8 (4.7)		Casey, et al (1989)
Knox Cube Test	TIA	12	6/6	63.40 (6.00)	RCE	60.7 d	10.3 (4.4)	11. (5.4)		Casey, et al (1989)
Knox Cube Test	TIA	12	6/6	59.20 (13.30)	n/a	59.1 d	9.3 (5.7)	9.5 (6.2)		Casey, et al (1989)
Number Connection Test (sec)	Control	11	9/2	31.60 (5.00)	n/a	6 m	63.5 (11.2)	59.0 (10.7)		Di Stefano, et al (1996)
Number Connection Test (sec)	Whiplash	21	8/13	35.50 (10.50)	n/a	6 m	68.7 (14.6)	61.9 (17.5)	*	Di Stefano, et al (1995)
Number Connection Test (sec)	Whiplash	58	26/32	29.60 (8.90)	n/a	6 m	72.0 (15.3)	63.2 (14.2)		Di Stefano, et al (1996)
Number Connection Test (sec)	Whiplash - asx	67	28/36	29.00 (8.50)	n/a	6 m	70.1 (14.5)	61.7 (13.8)		Radanov, et al (1993)
Number Connection Test (sec)	Whiplash - sx	31	9/19	36.50 (10.20)	n/a	6 m	81.3 (19.5)	69.5 (16.0)		Radanov, et al (1993)
Number Connection Test (sec)	Whiplash w/ continuing sx	21	8/13	35.40 (11.00)	n/a	6 m	83.3 (14.8)	71.1 (15.1)	*	Di Stefano, et al (1995)

instrument	group	n	m/f	age	intervention	inter	t #1	t #2	note	citation
Number Connection Test (sec)	Whiplash w/ continuing sx	28	9/19	34.10 (10.20)	n/a	6 m	80.0 (20.7)	68.0 (17.4)		Di Stefano, et al (1996)
serial sevens (errors)	Ocular Disease	50	27/23	42.00 (17.00)	steroid tx	~8 d	1.5 (1.8)	1.9 (2.1)		Naber, et al (1996)
serial sevens (time, sec)	Ocular Disease	50	27/23	42.00 (17.00)	steroid tx	~8 d	25.0 (11.0)	23.0 (12.0)		Naber, et al (1996)
Span of Attention Test	Hypertension	25	17/8	50.10 (14.00)	n/a	7-10 d	320.15 (74.29)	314.53 (70.12)		McCaffrey, et al (1992)
TOVA (comissions)	Homeless	15	9/6	32.80 (6.10)	cognitive remediation	2-3 m	12.40 (7.74)	9.93 (7.48)		Cotman, et al (1997)
TOVA (comissions)	Homeless	9	4/5	27.00 (5.80)	n/a	2-3 m	6.44 (6.89)	9.44 (10.22)		Cotman, et al (1997)
TOVA (omissions)	Homeless	9	4/5	27.00 (5.80)	n/a	2-3 m	0.67 (1.00)	5.78 (16.59)		Cotman, et al (1997)
TOVA (omissions)	Homeless	15	9/6	32.80 (6.10)	cognitive remediation	2-3 m	2.60 (4.60)	11.93 (32.67)		Cotman, et al (1997)
TOVA (time)	Homeless	15	9/6	32.80 (6.10)	cognitive remediation	2-3 m	448.47 (103.5)	401.53 (70.26)		Cotman, et al (1997)
TOVA (time)	Homeless	9	4/5	27.00 (5.80)	n/a	2-3 m	409.22 (94.54)	451.56 (118.5)		Cotman, et al (1997)
TOVA (variability)	Homeless	15	9/6	32.80 (6.10)	cognitive remediation	2-3 m	102.53 (33.25)	107.80 (26.30)		Cotman, et al (1997)
TOVA (variability)	Homeless	9	4/5	27.00 (5.80)	n/a	2-3 m	101.44 (30.55)	102.11 (29.93)		Cotman, et al (1997)

Table 4. Auditory Consonant Trigrams (CCC)

instrument	group	n	m/f	age	intervention	inter	t #1	t #2	note	citation
CCC	Control	59	37/22	68.70 (5.70)	n/a	3.4 y	73.9 (27.3)	71.8 (25.7)		Flicker, et al (1993)
CCC-03 [60]	Myasthenia Gravis	11	7/4	49.00	prednisolone	3-11 m	46.5 (10.7)	48.3 (9.4)		Glennerster, et al (1996)
CCC-05 (errors)	Control	38	18/20	35.70 (10.5)	n/a	54.7 w	3.8 (2.1)	3.1 (2.4)		Tarter, et al (1990)
CCC-05 (errors)	Crohn's Disease	22	9/13	37.30 (10.6)	std tx	62.6 w	3.9 (2.2)	3.6 (2.3)		Tarter, et al (1990)
CCC-05 (errors)	Liver Disease	62	23/39	39.20 (10.5)	liver transplant	60.1 w	6.3 (2.9)	4.9 (2.5)		Tarter, et al (1990)
CCC-09 (errors)	Control	30	14/16	40.63 (2.97)	n/a	1 w	12.0 (2.52)	12.10 (2.85)		Stuss, et al (1988)
CCC-09 (errors)	Control	30	16/14	22.43 (2.67)	n/a	1 w	12.03 (2.24)	12.57 (2.03)		Stuss, et al (1988)
CCC-09 (errors)	Control	30	14/16	61.77 (3.00)	n/a	1 w	11.47 (2.33)	11.70 (2.28)		Stuss, et al (1988)
CCC-09 (errors)	Control	10	5/5	17.30 (0.95)	n/a	1 w	11.8 (1.9)	13.0 (1.4)		Stuss, et al (1987)
CCC-09 (errors)	Control	10	6/4	55.30 (2.98)	n/a	1 w	10.9 (2.5)	11.0 (3.0)		Stuss, et al (1987)
CCC-09 (errors)	Control	10	6/4	23.00 (2.67)	n/a	1 w	12.2 (2.5)	13.0 (2.0)		Stuss, et al (1987)

instrument	group	n	m/f	age	intervention	inter	t #1	t #2	note	citation
CCC-09 (errors)	Control	10	5/5	63.70 (3.13)	n/a	1 w	12.2 (1.6)	12.3 (1.7)		Stuss, et al (1987)
CCC-09 (errors)	Control	10	5/5	33.90 (2.88)	n/a	1 w	12.8 (1.8)	12.6 (3.5)		Stuss, et al (1987)
CCC-09 (errors)	Control	10	6/4	44.20 (3.12)	n/a	1 w	11.0 (2.8)	11.2 (2.5)		Stuss, et al (1987)
CCC-09 (errors)	Control	22	15/7	27.70 (11.6)	n/a	6 d	11.7 (2.9)	13.0 (1.9)	*	Stuss, et al (1989)
CCC-09 (errors)	Control	26	20/6	29.70 (12.4)	n/a	1 w	11.6 (3.0)	12.4 (3.0)	*	Stuss, et al (1989)
CCC-09 (errors)	TBI	22	15/7	29.50 (12.6)	n/a	6 d	10.8 (2.5)	10.3 (3.9)	*	Stuss, et al (1989)
CCC-09 (errors)	TBI	26	20/6	30.90 (11.9)	n/a	1 w	9.8 (2.9)	10.2 (3.2)	*	Stuss, et al (1989)
CCC-15 (errors)	Control	38	18/20	35.70 (10.5)	n/a	54.7 w	5.2 (3.5)	5.3 (3.1)		Tarter, et al (1990)
CCC-15 (errors)	Crohn's Disease	22	9/13	37.30 (10.6)	std tx	62.6 w	6.7 (3.5)	5.1 (3.1)		Tarter, et al (1990)
CCC-15 (errors)	Liver Disease	62	23/39	39.20 (10.5)	liver transplant	60.1 w	9.2 (4.8)	7.5 (4.1)		Tarter, et al (1990)
CCC-18 (errors)	Control	30	14/16	61.77 (3.00)	n/a	1 w	10.23 (2.46)	10.67 (2.92)		Stuss, et al (1988)

instrument	group	n	m/f	age	intervention	inter	t #1	t #2	note	citation
CCC-18 (errors)	Control	30	16/14	22.43 (2.67)	n/a	1 w	11.37 (2.82)	12.27 (2.41)		Stuss, et al (1988)
CCC-18 (errors)	Control	30	14/16	40.63 (2.97)	n/a	1 w	10.5 (3.11)	12.0 (2.59)		Stuss, et al (1988)
CCC-18 (errors)	Control	10	5/5	63.70 (3.13)	n/a	1 w	10.5 (1.7)	11.8 (2.0)		Stuss, et al (1987)
CCC-18 (errors)	Control	10	5/5	17.30 (0.95)	n/a	1 w	11.8 (21.2)	12.2 (2.4)		Stuss, et al (1987)
CCC-18 (errors)	Control	10	6/4	23.00 (2.67)	n/a	1 w	11.7 (2.9)	12.6 (2.6)		Stuss, et al (1987)
CCC-18 (errors)	Control	10	5/5	33.90 (2.88)	n/a	1 w	12.5 (3.0)	12.7 (2.5)		Stuss, et al (1987)
CCC-18 (errors)	Control	10	6/4	55.30 (2.98)	n/a	1 w	9.8 (3.4)	11.1 (2.9)		Stuss, et al (1987)
CCC-18 (errors)	Control	10	6/4	44.20 (3.12)	n/a	1 w	10.0 (2.8)	12.0 (2.2)		Stuss, et al (1987)
CCC-18 (errors)	Control	22	15/7	27.70 (11.6)	n/a	6 d	12.1 (2.7)	13.1 (2.1)	*	Stuss, et al (1989)
CCC-18 (errors)	Control	26	20/6	29.70 (12.4)	n/a	1 w	11.7 (2.0)	12.0 (2.7)	*	Stuss, et al (1989)
CCC-18 (errors)	TBI	22	15/7	29.50 (12.6)	n/a	6 d	9.8 (2.9)	10.8 (2.8)	*	Stuss, et al (1989)

instrument	group	n	m/f	age	intervention	inter	t #1	t #2	note	citation
CCC-18 (errors)	TBI	26	20/6	30.90 (11.9)	n/a	1 w	8.7 (2.7)	8.7 (3.1)	*	Stuss, et al (1989)
CCC-18 [60]	Myasthenia Gravis	11	7/4	49.00	prednisolone	3-11 m	26.8 (9.8)	30.4 (14.4)		Glennerster, et al (1996)
CCC-30 (errors)	Control	38	18/20	35.70 (10.5)	n/a	54.7 w	6.0 (3.7)	6.2 (4.0)		Tarter, et al (1990)
CCC-30 (errors)	Crohn's Disease	22	9/13	37.30 (10.6)	std tx	62.6 w	7.6 (3.4)	7.1 (3.8)		Tarter, et al (1990)
CCC-30 (errors)	Liver Disease	62	23/39	39.20 (10.5)	liver transplant	60.1 w	10.8 (4.40	8.4 (3.6)		Tarter, et al (1990)
CCC-36 (errors)	Control	30	14/16	40.63 (2.97)	n/a	1 w	9.90 (3.04)	11.1 (2.37)		Stuss, et al (1988)
CCC-36 (errors)	Control	30	14/16	61.77 (3.00)	n/a	1 w	8.67 (2.85)	8.57 (3.54)		Stuss, et al (1988)
CCC-36 (errors)	Control	30	16/14	22.43 (2.67)	n/a	1 w	9.43 (2.71)	10.93 (2.88)		Stuss, et al (1988)
CCC-36 (errors)	Control	10	6/4	55.30 (2.98)	n/a	1 w	8.2 (3.1)	8.2 (4.1)		Stuss, et al (1987)
CCC-36 (errors)	Control	10	5/5	17.30 (0.95)	n/a	1 w	9.9 (2.3)	10.0 (3.6)		Stuss, et al (1987)
CCC-36 (errors)	Control	10	6/4	23.00 (2.67)	n/a	1 w	8.7 (3.3)	10.9 (2.3)		Stuss, et al (1987)

instrument	group	n	m/f	age	intervention	inter	t #1	t #2	note	citation
CCC-36 (errors)	Control	10	6/4	44.20 (3.12)	n/a	1 w	8.7 (3.4)	11.0 (2.1)		Stuss, et al (1987)
CCC-36 (errors)	Control	10	5/5	63.70 (3.13)	n/a	1 w	10.0 (1.8)	9.8 (2.4)		Stuss, et al (1987)
CCC-36 (errors)	Control	10	5/5	33.90 (2.88)	n/a	1 w	11.0 (2.5)	11.5 (3.0)		Stuss, et al (1987)
CCC-36 (errors)	Control	26	20/6	29.70 (12.4)	n/a	1 w	10.0 (2.2)	10.5 (3.0)	*	Stuss, et al (1989)
CCC-36 (errors)	Control	22	15/7	27.70 (11.6)	n/a	6 d	10.1 (2.9)	11.1 (3.3)	*	Stuss, et al (1989)
CCC-36 (errors)	TBI	26	20/6	30.90 (11.9)	n/a	1 w	6.7 (3.4)	7.8 (3.7)	*	Stuss, et al (1989)
CCC-36 (errors)	TBI	22	15/7	29.50 (12.6)	n/a	6 d	8.3 (2.7)	8.7 (3.2)	*	Stuss, et al (1989)

Table 5. Bayley Scales of Infant Development (BSID)

instrument	group	n	m/f	age	intervention	inter	t #1	t #2	note	citation
BSID Mental	Anemia	23	n/a	1.00 - 1.50	placebo	4 m	92.4	92.9		Soewondo (1995)
BSID Mental	Anemia	24	n/a	1.00 - 1.50	iron	4 m	88.8	108.1		Soewondo (1995)
BSID Mental	Control	22	n/a	1.00 - 1.50	placebo	4 m	104.7	106.8		Soewondo (1995)

instrument	group	n	m/f	age	intervention	inter	t #1	t #2	note	citation
BSID Mental	Control	35	n/a	1.50	early intervention	~3 m	124.74	140.23		Soewondo (1995)
BSID Mental	Control	34	n/a	1.50	placebo	~3 m	127.76	135.35		Soewondo (1995)
BSID Mental	Control	22	n/a	1.00 - 1.50	iron	4 m	105.4	109.1		Soewondo (1995)
BSID Mental	"at-risk"	80	36/44	0.50	n/a	6 m	40.7 (29.3)	82.3 (33.2)		Cook, et al (1989)
BSID Mental	Iron Deficiency	14	n/a	1.00 - 1.50	placebo	4 m	101.8	109.3		Soewondo (1995)
BSID Mental	Iron Deficiency	14	n/a	1.00 - 1.50	iron	4 m	102.4	107.7		Soewondo (1995)
BSID Motor	Anemia	23	n/a	1.00 - 1.50	placebo	4 m	92.4	97.5		Soewondo (1995)
BSID Motor	Anemia	24	n/a	1.00 - 1.50	iron	4 m	88.5	112		Soewondo (1995)
BSID Motor	Control	22	n/a	1.00 - 1.50	placebo	4 m	105.9	108.3		Soewondo (1995)
BSID Motor	Control	34	n/a	1.50	placebo	~3 m	56.09	58.29		Soewondo (1995)
BSID Motor	Control	35	n/a	1.50	early intervention	~3 m	55.46	65.7		Soewondo (1995)
BSID Motor	Control	22	n/a	1.00 - 1.50	iron	4 m	105.3	108.7		Soewondo (1995)
BSID Motor	"at-risk"	80	36/44	0.50	n/a	6 m	16.7 (11.9)	37.1 (15.7)		Cook, et al (1989)

instrument	group	n	m/f	age	intervention	inter	t #1	t #2	note	citation
BSID Motor	Iron Deficiency	14	n/a	1.00 - 1.50	placebo	4 m	103.5	106.6		Soewondo (1995)
BSID Motor	Iron Deficiency	14	n/a	1.00 - 1.50	iron	4 m	102.9	107.8		Soewondo (1995)

Table 6. Beery Test of Visual Motor Integration (VMI)

instrument	group	n	m/f	age	intervention	inter	t #1	t #2	note	citation
Beery VMI	BMT	25	14/11	~12.0	BMT	8.2 m	100.7 (15.8)	98.3 (13.2)		Phipps, et al (1995)
Beery VMI	Brain Tumor	7	3/4	10.33	surgery	1 m	8.4 (1.4)	10.1 (2.7)		Bordeaux, et al (1988)
Beery VMI	Brain Tumor	7	4/3	9.83	radiotherapy	11 m	8.0 (3.5)	11.0 (9.0)		Bordeaux, et al (1988)
Beery VMI	Down Syndrome	34	20/14	22.0 - 56.0	n/a	1 y	10. (2.76)	9.74 (2.54)	*	Burt, et al (1995)
Beery VMI (age in months)	LD	29	24/5	10.83 (1.40)	methylphen	8 w	110.72 (3.93)	107.88 (4.2)		Gittleman-Klein, et al (1976)

instrument	group	n	m/f	age	intervention	inter	t #1	t #2	note	citation
Beery VMI (age in months)	LD	32	23/9	10.67 (1.30)	placebo	8 w	95.43 (3.93)	95.67 (4.2)		Gittleman-Klein, et al (1976)
Beery VMI (age ratio)	Depression w/ Melancholia	7	5/2	9.50	tricyclic antidepress	3 - 6 m	0.82 (0.21)	0.89 (0.21)		Stanton, et al (1981)
Beery VMI (age ratio)	Depression	4	4/2	11.00	tricyclic antidepress	3 - 6 m	0.80 (0.30)	0.90 (0.42)		Stanton, et al (1981)
Beery VMI (std)	Control	28	16/12	6.50 (0.70)	n/a	1 y	92.8 (14.8)	92.4 (17.9)	*	Brookshire, et al (1995)
Beery VMI (std)	Control	59	n/a	~6.00	n/a	~6 m	NR	1.15 c	*	Neyens, et al (1996)
Beery VMI (std)	Hydroceph (arrested)	11	6/5	6.20 (0.40)	n/a	1 y	88.9 (13.8)	85.8 (14.7)	*	Brookshire, et al (1995)
Beery VMI (std)	Hydroceph (shunted)	26	14/12	6.20 (0.70)	n/a	1 y	72.1 (11.9)	69.6 (12.3)	*	Brookshire, et al (1995)

Table 7. Bender Gestalt

instrument	group	n	m/f	age	intervention	inter	t #1	t #2	note	citation
Bender Gestalt	Alcoholic	100	n/a	40.60	inpt tx	30 d	79.9 (16.7)	69.6 (13.9)		Farmer (1973)
Bender Gestalt	Control (CDR-0)	30	15/15	70.9 (4.6)	n/a	1 y	10.8 (0.9)	10.9 (1.2)	*	Botwinick, et al (1986)
Bender Gestalt	DAT (CDR-1)	18	7/11	71.40 (4.40)	n/a	1 y	8.7 (2.2)	7.7 (3.2)	*	Botwinick, et al (1986)

instrument	group	n	m/f	age	intervention	inter	t #1	t #2	note	citation
Bender Gestalt (errors)	Cardiac	60	35/25	44.30 (9.40)	open heart surgery	10 m	41.25 (19.81)	37.55 (16.97)		Joulasmaa, et al (1981)
Bender Gestalt (errors)	Epilepsy	3	n/a	9.00	barbituate anticonvulsant	7.7 w	6.0	7.0		Willis, et al (1997)
Bender Gestalt (errors)	Epilepsy	8	n/a	9.20	barbituate anticonvulsant	7.7 w	3.9	4.25		Willis, et al (1997)
Bender Gestalt Recall	Cardiac	17	12/5	50.00 (10.48)	heart transplant	36.0 m	2.6 (0.73)	2.9 (0.22)		Roman, et al (1997)

Table 8. Benton Tests

instrument	group	n	m/f	age	intervention	inter	t #1	t #2	note	citation
Benton 3D CP	Depression	9	6/3	50.20 (18.50)	right ECT	2d	23.7	21.9	*	Kronfol, et al (1978)
Benton 3D CP	Depression	9	6/3	48.30 (17.80)	left ECT	2d	23.2	22.2	*	Kronfol, et al (1978)
Benton FRT	DAT (mild)	11	10/1	63.00 (8.00)	n/a	26 m	42.0 (5.0)	42.0 (4.0)		Haxby, et al (1990)
Benton FRT	Dementia	<35	n/a	66.00 (9.60)	n/a	19.0 m	37.2 (14.3)	39.8 (5.9)		Jones, et al (1992)
Benton FRT	Depression	9	6/3	50.20 (18.50)	right ECT	2 d	41.0	39.1	*	Kronfol, et al (1978)
Benton FRT	Depression	9	6/3	48.30 (17.80)	left ECT	2 d	43.3	39.4	*	Kronfol, et al (1978)

instrument	group	n	m/f	age	intervention	inter	t #1	t #2	note	citation
Benton FRT	Epilepsy	40	23/ 17	32.20 (8.20)	n/a	~9 m	45.20 (4.34)	44.77 (5.34)		Hermann, et al (1996)
Benton FRT	Pseudo-dementia	<35	n/a	66.00 (9.60)	n/a	19.0 m	44.3 (3.9)	43.2 (5.4)		Jones, et al (1992)
Benton FRT	Schizophrenia	15	10/5	35.00	neuroleptics	~15 m	44.7 (6.1)	45.3 (4.1)		Goldberg, et al (1993)
Benton FRT	Spinal Cord Injury	67	54/ 13	32.00 (14.70)	n/a	38 w	45.38 (4.7)	44.8 (5.01)		Richards, et al (1988)
Benton FRT (correct)	PD	4	3/1	53.50	fetal tissue implanted	12 m	43.6	41.8		Sass, et al (1995)
Benton FDT	Epilepsy	40	23/ 17	32.20 (8.20)	n/a	~9 m	29.10 (2.57)	28.98 (3.08)		Hermann, et al (1996)
Benton JLOT	Depression	9	6/3	48.30 (17.80)	left ECT	2 d	20.1	18.9	*	Kronfol, et al (1978)
Benton JLOT	Depression	9	6/3	50.20 (18.50)	right ECT	2 d	16.4	18.0	*	Kronfol, et al (1978)
Benton JLOT	Epilepsy	40	23/ 17	32.20 (8.20)	n/a	~9 m	22.30 (4.77)	24.02 (5.22)		Hermann, et al (1996)
Benton JLOT	IVDU	16	13/3	39.50	n/a	10.4 d	20.62 (4.69)	21.88 (5.08)		Richards, et al (1992)
Benton JLOT	Patients	37	n/a	n/a	n/a	6 h - 21 d	23.1	23.5		Benton, et al (1983)
Benton JLOT	PD	4	3/1	53.50	fetal tissue implanted	12 m	21.3	20.5		Sass, et al (1995)

instrument	group	n	m/f	age	intervention	inter	t #1	t #2	note	citation
Benton JLOT	Schizophrenia	15	10/5	35.00	neuroleptics	~15 m	25.1 (4.1)	23.7 (4.0)		Goldberg, et al (1993)
Benton JLOT	Schizophrenia (acute)	39	24/15	28.60 (8.60)	n/a	1 y	22.5 (5.0)	25.5 (3.3)		Sweeney, et al (1991)
Benton JLOT	Spinal Cord Injury	67	54/13	32.00 (14.70)	n/a	38 w	22.96 (4.8)	22.08 (5.2)		Richards, et al (1988)
Benton JLOT (derived)	Schizophrenia	33	n/a	~33.70 (6.30)	clozapine	1 y	11.3 (11.8)	11.8 (11.8)		Buchanan, et al (1994)
Benton JLOT (derived)	Schizophrenia	19	13/6	33.70 (6.30)	clozapine	10 w	11.4 (15.0)	15.6 (20.9)		Buchanan, et al (1994)
Benton JLOT (derived)	Schizophrenia	19	15/4	34.00 (6.90)	haloperidol	10 w	9.9 (6.7)	10.6 (6.4)		Buchanan, et al (1994)
Benton JLOT (std)	Control	28	16/12	6.50 (0.70)	n/a	1 y	98.7 (11.7)	98.4 (13.9)	*	Brookshire, et al (1995)
Benton JLOT (std)	Hydroceph (arrested)	11	6/5	6.20 (0.40)	n/a	1 y	94.1 (14.1)	96.6 (14.9)	*	Brookshire, et al (1995)
Benton JLOT (std)	Hydroceph (shunted)	26	14/12	6.20 (0.70)	n/a	1 y	76.0 (19.6)	84.9 (12.6)	*	Brookshire, et al (1995)
Benton ST (correct DH)	Brain Tumor	7	3/4	10.33	surgery	1 m	8.3 (5.5)	7.0 (6.0)		Bordeaux, et al (1988)
Benton ST (correct DH)	Brain Tumor	7	4/3	9.83	radiotherapy	11 m	0.9 (15.1)	4.9 (9.9)		Bordeaux, et al (1988)
Benton ST (correct NDH)	Brain Tumor	7	4/3	9.83	radiotherapy	11 m	12.9 (0.9)	12.1 (0.4)		Bordeaux, et al (1988)

instrument	group	n	m/f	age	intervention	inter	t #1	t #2	note	citation
Benton ST (correct NDH)	Brain Tumor	7	3/4	10.33	surgery	1 m	4.7 (9.0)	8.5 (2.9)		Bordeaux, et al (1988)
Benton ST (time DH)	Brain Tumor	7	4/3	9.83	radiotherapy	11 m	-1.6 (15.3)	3.3 (13.7)		Bordeaux, et al (1988)
Benton ST (time DH)	Brain Tumor	7	3/4	10.33	surgery	1 m	7.7 (7.3)	9.5 (5.0)		Bordeaux, et al (1988)
Benton ST (time NDH)	Brain Tumor	7	3/4	10.33	surgery	1 m	5.6 (9.1)	10.3 (3.0)		Bordeaux, et al (1988)
Benton ST (time NDH)	Brain Tumor	7	4/3	9.83	radiotherapy	11 m	4.4 (2.8)	11.2 (1.9)		Bordeaux, et al (1988)
Benton TFPT	Control	56	n/a	n/a	n/a	imm	8.98	9.08		Benton, et al (1983)
Benton TOT	Dementia	<35	n/a	66.00 (9.60)	n/a	19.0 m	4.9 (7.2)	15.3 (23.9)		Jones, et al (1992)
Benton TOT	Pseudo-dementia	<35	n/a	66.00 (9.60)	n/a	19.0 m	3.86 (9.3)	3.1 (6.9)		Jones, et al (1992)
Benton TOT [10]	Depression	9	6/3	48.30 (17.80)	left ECT	2 d	8.6	9.2	*	Kronfol, et al (1978)
Benton TOT [10]	Depression	9	6/3	50.20 (18.50)	right ECT	2 d	8.9	9.7	*	Kronfol, et al (1978)
Benton TOT	Breast Cancer	20	3/17	39.28 (9.38)	ABMT	~12 d	0.1 (0.3)	0.2 (0.8)		Ahles, et al (1996)
Benton TOT	Hematologic D/O	14	2/12	39.28 (9.38)	ABMT	~12 d	0.0 (0.0)	0.1 (0.4)		Ahles, et al (1996)
Benton VRT	Schizophrenia Inpts	7	7/0	51.00	placebo	2 m	6.8 (0.9)	6.4 (0.8)	*	de Beaurepaire, et al (1993)

instrument	group	n	m/f	age	intervention	inter	t #1	t #2	note	citation
Benton VRT	Schizophrenia Inpts	9	7/2	51.00	bromocriptine	2 m	7.7 (1.3)	10.2 (1.9)	*	de Beaurepaire, et al (1993)
Benton VRT (% forg)	Control	21	3/18	30.10 (8.20)	n/a	6 m	8.3 (7.4)	4.8 (4.9)		Pulliainen, et al (1994)
Benton VRT (% forg)	Epilepsy	20	9/11	31.50 (11.30)	phenytoin	6 m	12.7 (13.2)	16 (14.5)		Pulliainen, et al (1994)
Benton VRT (% forg)	Epilepsy	23	11/12	26.80 (13.20)	carbamaz	6 m	13 (11.8)	9.9 (10.0)		Pulliainen, et al (1994)
Benton VRT (correct)	AAMI	75	27/48	61.93 (6.05)	n/a	4.6 y	6.48 (1.43)	6.66 (1.85)		Youngjohn, et al (1993)
Benton VRT (correct)	Alcoholic (brief abstin)	27	27/0	43.07	placebo	7 d	5.7 (1.9)	5.8 (1.9)	*	Korsic, et al (1991)
Benton VRT (correct)	Alcoholic (brief abstin)	27	27/0	40.96	DGAVP	7 d	4.7 (2.3)	5.6 (2.0)	*	Korsic, et al (1991)
Benton VRT (correct)	Alcoholic (long abstin)	23	23/0	46.26	DGAVP	7 d	5.4 (2.2)	5.3 (1.8)	*	Korsic, et al (1991)
Benton VRT (correct)	Alcoholic (long abstin)	26	26/0	41.40	placebo	7 d	5.3 (2.2)	5.9 (2.1)	*	Korsic, et al (1991)
Benton VRT (correct)	Alcoholic Inpts	91	91/0	42.20 (10.00)	n/a	12-22 d	5.1 (1.9)	5.7 (1.9)		Eckardt, et al (1979)
Benton VRT (correct)	Bipolar Inpts	18	12/6	45.80 (13.70)	lithium	6 y	6.8 (2.3)	6.5 (1.9)		Engelsmann, et al (1988)
Benton VRT (correct)	Breast Cancer	20	3/17	39.28 (9.38)	ABMT	~12 d	7.6 (1.6)	6.7 (1.3)		Ahles, et al (1996)
Benton VRT (correct)	Cardiac	60	35/25	44.30 (9.40)	open heart surgery	10 m	6.52 (1.97)	6.67 (1.62)		Joulasmaa, et al (1981)

instrument	group	n	m/f	age	intervention	inter	t #1	t #2	note	citation
Benton VRT (correct)	Cardiac	135	120/15	55.40	CABG	3 m	4.9	4.4	*	Klonoff, et al (1989)
Benton VRT (correct)	Control	24	n/a	58.50	n/a	2.1 y	7.0 (1.6)	6.8 (1.5)		La Rue, et al (1995)
Benton VRT (correct)	Control	38	18/20	35.70 (10.50)	n/a	54.7 w	8.2 (1.1)	8.4 (1.2)		Tarter, et al (1990)
Benton VRT (correct)	Control	115	56/59	48.90 (19.30)	n/a	20.9 d	7.05 (1.54)	7.65 (1.62)		Youngjohn, et al (1992)
Benton VRT (correct)	Control (overweight)	24	24/0	40.70 (8.30)	placebo	8 w	8.8 (1.1)	8.8 (1.3)		Hatsukami, et al (1986)
Benton VRT (correct)	Control (overweight)	26	26/0	37.20 (4.80)	naltrexone	8 w	8.7 (1.5)	9.0 (1.2)		Hatsukami, et al (1986)
Benton VRT (correct)	Crohn's Disease	22	9/13	37.30 (10.60)	std tx	62.6 w	8.0 (1.6)	8.3 (1.2)		Tarter, et al (1990)
Benton VRT (correct)	Dementia	<35	n/a	66.00 (9.60)	n/a	19.0 m	3.0 (1.3)	2.3 (1.6)		Jones, et al (1992)
Benton VRT (correct)	Dementia (2° to steroids)	6	6/0	49.67	steriods d/c or reduced	10.9 m	7.0	12.0		Varney, et al (1984)
Benton VRT (correct)	Depression	19	9/10	37.95 (12.70)	amitriptyline	4 d	6.59 (2.29)	7.59 (1.66)		Lamping, et al (1984)
Benton VRT (correct)	Depression	21	12/9	31.19 (6.34)	clovoxamine	4 d	7.47 (1.81)	7.84 (1.89)		Lamping, et al (1984)
Benton VRT (correct)	Epilepsy	18	14/4	28.30	reduction in meds	1 y	4.08	4.75		Ludgate, et al (1985)
Benton VRT (correct)	Hematologic D/O	14	2/12	39.28 (9.38)	ABMT	~12 d	7.9 (1.6)	7.6 (1.4)		Ahles, et al (1996)

instrument	group	n	m/f	age	intervention	inter	t #1	t #2	note	citation
Benton VRT (correct)	Homeless	9	4/5	27.00 (5.80)	n/a	2-3 m	7.17 (3.25)	8.17 (0.75)		Cotman, et al (1997)
Benton VRT (correct)	Homeless	15	9/6	32.80 (6.10)	cognitive remediation	2-3 m	6.00 (1.84)	5.67 (2.02)		Cotman, et al (1997)
Benton VRT (correct)	Liver Disease	62	23/39	39.20 (10.50)	liver transplant	60.1w	6.9 (1.6)	7.4 (1.8)		Tarter, et al (1990)
Benton VRT (correct)	Major Depression	12	n/a	46.80	improved post-ECT	11 d	4.4	4.1	*	Kurland, et al (1976)
Benton VRT (correct)	Major Depression	7	n/a	46.80	unimproved post-ECT	11 d	3.8	3.3	*	Kurland, et al (1976)
Benton VRT (correct)	Medical Inpts	20	20/0	45.60 (11.10)	n/a	12-22 d	5.1 (2.0)	5.2 (1.6)		Eckardt, et al (1979)
Benton VRT (correct)	Myotonic Dystrophy	15	n/a	35.40	n/a	12 y	6.1 (2.2)	6.2 (2.1)		Tuikka, et al (1993)
Benton VRT (correct)	Ocular Disease	50	27/23	42.00 (17.00)	steroid tx	~8 d	4.6 (2.4)	4.9 (2.4)		Naber, et al (1996)
Benton VRT (correct)	Orthopedic	128	38/90	69.00	general anesthesia	1 w	5.1 (2.0)	-0.8 (1.9) c	*	Williams-Russo, et al (1995)
Benton VRT (correct)	Orthopedic	134	39/95	69.00	epidural anesthesia	1 w	5.1 (2.0)	-0.8 (2.0) c	*	Williams-Russo, et al (1995)
Benton VRT (correct)	PD	8	5/3	59.40 (8.30)	apomorphine	15 min	5.0 (2.1)	4.8 (2.0)	C/D	Ruzicka, et al (1994)
Benton VRT (correct)	Pseudo-dementia	<35	n/a	66.00 (9.60)	n/a	19.0 m	4.5 (1.7)	4.8 (2.2)		Jones, et al (1992)
Benton VRT (correct)	early onset DAT relatives	19	n/a	57.10	n/a	4.6 y	7.5 (1.2)	6.6 (1.3)		La Rue, et al (1995)

instrument	group	n	m/f	age	intervention	inter	t #1	t #2	note	citation
Benton VRT (correct)	late onset DAT relatives	21	n/a	55.10	n/a	4.4 y	6.8 (1.4)	6.7 (2.1)		La Rue, et al (1995)
Benton VRT (correct)	Schizophrenia Inpts	35	29/6	23.71 (4.50)	neuroleptics	1-2 y	6.5 (2.2)	6.1 (2.1)		Nopoulos, et al (1994)
Benton VRT (correct) [10]	DAT	11	n/a	71.70 (6.40)	oxiracetam	1 m	1.5 (1.0)	1.8 (1.3)	AF	Green, et al (1992)
Benton VRT (correct) [10]	DAT	13	n/a	71.70 (6.40)	placebo	1 m	1.8 (1.5)	2.2 (1.9)	AF	Green, et al (1992)
Benton VRT (errors)	AAMI	75	27/48	61.93 (6.05)	n/a	4.6 y	5.45 (2.57)	4.73 (3.02)		Youngjohn, et al (1993)
Benton VRT (errors)	Alcoholic (brief abstin)	27	27/0	43.07	placebo	7 d	5.6 (3.2)	6.3 (3.5)	*	Korsic, et al (1991)
Benton VRT (errors)	Alcoholic (brief abstin)	27	27/0	40.96	DGAVP	7 d	8.1 (3.9)	6.6 (3.9)	*	Korsic, et al (1991)
Benton VRT (errors)	Alcoholic (long abstin)	23	23/0	46.26	DGAVP	7 d	7.0 (4.4)	6.9 (3.8)	*	Korsic, et al (1991)
Benton VRT (errors)	Alcoholic (long abstin)	26	26/0	41.40	placebo	7 d	7.3 (4.8)	5.7 (4.1)	*	Korsic, et al (1991)
Benton VRT (errors)	Bipolar Inpts	18	12/6	45.80 (13.70)	lithium	6 y	5.1 (4.9)	4.9 (3.7)		Engelsmann, et al (1988)
Benton VRT (errors)	Cardiac	60	35/25	44.30 (9.40)	open heart surgery	10 m	5.41 (3.48)	3.43 (1.38)		Joulasmaa, et al (1981)
Benton VRT (errors)	Control	42	n/a	59.70 (3.10)	n/a	6.7 y	4.19 (2.96)	5.64 (3.35)	*	Alder, et al (1990)
Benton VRT (errors)	Control	33	n/a	69.70 (3.50)	n/a	6.7 y	5.12 (3.32)	6.79 (4.36)	*	Alder, et al (1990)

instrument	group	n	m/f	age	intervention	inter	t #1	t #2	note	citation
Benton VRT (errors)	Control	101	n/a	49.90 (2.70)	n/a	6.7 y	3.36 (2.47)	3.57 (2.47)	*	Alder, et al (1990)
Benton VRT (errors)	Control	27	n/a	31.20 (3.10)	n/a	6.7 y	2.59 (2.36)	2.00 (2.20)	*	Alder, et al (1990)
Benton VRT (errors)	Control	74	n/a	40.60 (3.00)	n/a	6.7 y	2.77 (2.06)	2.84 (2.35)	*	Alder, et al (1990)
Benton VRT (errors)	Control	54	54/0	52.00 - 57.00	n/a	19.0 y	2.79 (2.29)	3.11 (2.19)		Giambra, et al (1995)
Benton VRT (errors)	Control	73	73/0	46.00 - 51.00	n/a	13.1 y	2.90 (2.29)	2.78 (2.43)		Giambra, et al (1995)
Benton VRT (errors)	Control	22	22/0	76.00 - 81.00	n/a	19.0 y	4.64 (2.31)	6.82 (2.71)		Giambra, et al (1995)
Benton VRT (errors)	Control	98	98/0	58.00 - 63.00	n/a	13.1 y	2.98 (2.33)	3.03 (2.01)		Giambra, et al (1995)
Benton VRT (errors)	Control	30	0/30	58.00 - 63.00	n/a	6.8 y	4.20 (1.85)	4.47 (2.80)		Giambra, et al (1995)
Benton VRT (errors)	Control	42	42/0	70.00 - 75.00	n/a	13.1 y	4.41 (2.87)	5.88 (3.21)		Giambra, et al (1995)
Benton VRT (errors)	Control	90	90/0	52.00 - 57.00	n/a	13.1 y	2.75 (2.19)	2.96 (2.16)		Giambra, et al (1995)
Benton VRT (errors)	Control	73	73/0	58.00 - 63.00	n/a	19.0 y	2.69 (2.25)	2.68 (2.00)		Giambra, et al (1995))
Benton VRT (errors)	Control	69	69/0	64.00 - 69.00	n/a	19.0 y	2.77 (2.09)	3.90 (2.92)		Giambra, et al (1995)
Benton VRT (errors)	Control	54	54/0	70.00 - 75.00	n/a	19.0 y	3.84 (2.49)	4.93 (2.35)		Giambra, et al (1995)

instrument	group	n	m/f	age	intervention	inter	t #1	t #2	note	citation
Benton VRT (errors)	Control	27	27/0	58.00 - 63.00	n/a	25.1 y	2.78 (2.22)	2.96 (2.12)		Giambra, et al (1995)
Benton VRT (errors)	Control	28	28/0	64.00 - 69.00	n/a	25.1 y	2.21 (1.52)	3.83 (2.78)		Giambra, et al (1995)
Benton VRT (errors)	Control	33	33/0	76.00 - 81.00	n/a	6.8 y	5.45 (3.35)	7.55 (3.62)		Giambra, et al (1995)
Benton VRT (errors)	Control	16	0/16	76.00 - 81.00	n/a	6.8 y	5.31 (2.52)	7.50 (3.50)		Giambra, et al (1995)
Benton VRT (errors)	Control	21	21/0	76.00 - 81.00	n/a	13.1 y	4.50 (2.44)	6.61 (3.39)		Giambra, et al (1995)
Benton VRT (errors)	Control	7	7/0	82.00 - 87.00	n/a	13.1 y	6.52 (3.53)	8.52 (4.32)		Giambra, et al (1995)
Benton VRT (errors)	Control	20	20/0	82.00 - 87.00	n/a	6.8 y	7.03 (4.22)	8.49 (4.36)		Giambra, et al (1995)
Benton VRT (errors)	Control	23	23/0	76.00 - 81.00	n/a	25.1 y	3.57 (2.86)	6.26 (3.35)		Giambra, et al (1995)
Benton VRT (errors)	Control	75	75/0	64.00 - 69.00	n/a	13.1 y	3.49 (2.58)	4.24 (3.09)		Giambra, et al (1995)
Benton VRT (errors)	Control	32	32/0	70.00 - 75.00	n/a	25.1 y	2.86 (2.16)	5.37 (2.06)		Giambra, et al (1995)
Benton VRT (errors)	Control	34	34/0	46.00 - 51.00	n/a	19.0 y	2.20 (1.91)	2.37 (1.44)		Giambra, et al (1995)
Benton VRT (errors)	Control	137	137/0	52.00 - 57.00	n/a	6.8 y	3.06 (2.37)	3.24 (2.38)		Giambra, et al (1995)
Benton VRT (errors)	Control	103	103/0	40.00 - 45.00	n/a	6.8 y	3.15 (2.12)	3.05 (2.56)		Giambra, et al (1995)

instrument	group	n	m/f	age	intervention	inter	t #1	t #2	note	citation
Benton VRT (errors)	Control	24	0/24	34.00 - 39.00	n/a	6.8 y	2.92 (2.19)	2.96 (2.10)		Giambra, et al (1995)
Benton VRT (errors)	Control	35	0/35	64.00 - 69.00	n/a	6.8 y	4.22 (2.33)	5.39 (3.31)		Giambra, et al (1995)
Benton VRT (errors)	Control	116	116/0	58.00 - 63.00	n/a	6.8 y	3.54 (2.48)	3.76 (2.61)		Giambra, et al (1995)
Benton VRT (errors)	Control	26	0/26	70.00 - 75.00	n/a	6.8 y	5.11 (2.55)	6.59 (3.05)		Giambra, et al (1995)
Benton VRT (errors)	Control	81	81/0	64.00 - 69.00	n/a	6.8 y	4.04 (2.62)	4.52 (2.82)		Giambra, et al (1995)
Benton VRT (errors)	Control	46	46/0	70.00 - 75.00	n/a	6.8 y	4.67 (2.51)	5.93 (2.96)		Giambra, et al (1995)
Benton VRT (errors)	Control	49	49/0	40.00 - 45.00	n/a	13.1 y	2.06 (1.73)	2.41 (1.84)		Giambra, et al (1995)
Benton VRT (errors)	Control	134	134/0	46.00 - 51.00	n/a	6.8 y	2.72 (2.24)	2.89 (2.44)		Giambra, et al (1995)
Benton VRT (errors)	Control	10	0/10	28.00 - 33.00	n/a	6.8 y	2.22 (1.65)	2.22 (1.93)		Giambra, et al (1995)
Benton VRT (errors)	Control	27	0/27	40.00 - 45.00	n/a	6.8 y	2.19 (1.55)	3.11 (2.28)		Giambra, et al (1995)
Benton VRT (errors)	Control	92	92/0	34.00 - 39.00	n/a	6.8 y	2.46 (2.24)	2.56 (1.94)		Giambra, et al (1995)
Benton VRT (errors)	Control	28	0/28	46.00 - 51.00	n/a	6.8 y	3.04 (2.15)	2.43 (2.23)		Giambra, et al (1995)
Benton VRT (errors)	Control	24	0/24	52.00 - 57.00	n/a	6.8 y	3.32 (2.51)	3.48 (2.02)		Giambra, et al (1995)

instrument	group	n	m/f	age	intervention	inter	t #1	t #2	note	citation
Benton VRT (errors)	Control	9	9/0	71.50 (4.30)	n/a	6-7 m	7.67 (5.00)	7.67 (3.90)		Netherton, et al (1989)
Benton VRT (errors)	Control	12	0/12	71.50 (4.30)	n/a	6-7 m	6.75 (4.14)	7.17 (2.79)		Netherton, et al (1989)
Benton VRT (errors)	Control	115	56/59	48.90 (19.30)	n/a	20.9 d	3.76 (2.13)	3.03 (2.43)		Youngjohn, et al (1992)
Benton VRT (errors)	Control (overweight)	24	24/0	40.70 (8.30)	placebo	8 w	1.5 (1.5)	1.6 (1.6)		Hatsukami, et al (1986)
Benton VRT (errors)	Control (overweight)	26	26/0	37.20 (4.80)	naltrexone	8 w	1.4 (1.7)	1.4 (2.2)		Hatsukami, et al (1986)
Benton VRT (errors)	Dementia	<35	n/a	66.00 (9.60)	n/a	19.0 m	13.5 (4.1)	16.3 (5.7)		Jones, et al (1992)
Benton VRT (errors)	Depression	19	9/10	37.95 (12.70)	amitriptyline	4 d	4.71 (3.90)	3.18 (2.40)		Lamping, et al (1984)
Benton VRT (errors)	Depression	21	12/9	31.19 (6.34)	clovoxamine	4 d	3.79 (3.22)	3.11 (2.77)		Lamping, et al (1984)
Benton VRT (errors)	Epilepsy	18	14/4	28.30	reduction in meds	1 y	8.08	6.83		Ludgate, et al (1985)
Benton VRT (errors)	Homeless	9	4/5	27.00 (5.80)	n/a	2-3 m	4.50 (5.61)	2.33 (1.21)		Cotman, et al (1997)
Benton VRT (errors)	Homeless	15	9/6	32.80 (6.10)	cognitive remediation	2-3 m	6.00 (4.66)	5.42 (2.91)		Cotman, et al (1997)
Benton VRT (errors)	Left AVM	15	10/5	31.00 (11.00)	surgery	4 m	4.3 (2.3)	4.5 (4.2)	*	Stabell, et al (1994)
Benton VRT (errors)	MS & Fatigue	16	4/12	40.00 (6.40)	amantadine hydrochloride	6 w	3.4 (1.1)	4.3 (2.4)		Geisler, et al (1996)

instrument	group	n	m/f	age	intervention	inter	t #1	t #2	note	citation
Benton VRT (errors)	MS & Fatigue	13	4/9	41.00 (6.20)	pemoline	6 w	2.7 (2.0)	3.0 (2.0)		Geisler, et al (1996)
Benton VRT (errors)	MS & Fatigue	16	2/14	40.00 (5.60)	placebo	6 w	2.6 (1.3)	2.8 (1.8)		Geisler, et al (1996)
Benton VRT (errors)	Myotonic Dystrophy	15	n/a	35.40	n/a	12 y	5.6 (3.6)	7.0 (4.6)		Tuikka, et al (1993)
Benton VRT (errors)	PD	12	12/0	65.30 (10.30)	n/a	6-7 m	10.58 (5.88)	12.75 (5.40)		Netherton, et al (1989)
Benton VRT (errors)	PD	6	0/6	65.30 (10.30)	n/a	6-7 m	4.83 (2.22)	8.00 (3.90)		Netherton, et al (1989)
Benton VRT (errors)	PD	8	5/3	59.40 (8.30)	apomorphine	15 min	7.0 (2.7)	8.5 (4.9)	C/D	Ruzicka, et al (1994)
Benton VRT (errors)	Pseudo-dementia	<35	n/a	66.00 (9.60)	n/a	19.0 m	10.1 (4.1)	9.5 (4.3)		Jones, et al (1992)
Benton VRT (errors)	Right AVM	16	5/11	34.00 (13.00)	surgery	4 m	2.7 (2.1)	3.9 (2.3)	*	Stabell, et al (1994)
Benton VRT (errors)	Schizophrenia Inpts	35	29/6	23.71 (4.50)	neuroleptics	1-2 y	5.5 (4.0)	6.1 (3.9)		Nopoulos, et al (1994)
Benton VRT (errors; t)	Lung Cancer	11	n/a	~61.00	cranial irradiation	11 m	32.4	28.3		Komaki, et al (1995)
Benton VRT Copy	Control	22	12/10	65.82 (5.20)	n/a	2 y	9.47 (1.12)	9.76 (0.44)		Rebok, et al (1990)
Benton VRT Copy	Control (CDR-0)	30	15/15	70.9 (4.6)	n/a	1 y	9.4 (0.9)	9.3 (1.2)	*	Botwinick, et al (1986)
Benton VRT Copy	DAT	51	16/35	67.29 (7.94)	n/a	2 y	8.69 (2.55)	4.62 (4.41)		Rebok, et al (1990)

instrument	group	n	m/f	age	intervention	inter	t #1	t #2	note	citation
Benton VRT Copy	DAT (CDR-1)	18	7/11	71.40 (4.40)	n/a	1 y	7.9 (2.9)	6.4 (3.5)	*	Botwinick, et al (1986)
Benton VRT Delay	Control	21	3/18	30.10 (8.20)	n/a	6 m	21.9 (2.4)	23.1 (2.2)		Pulliainen, et al (1994)
Benton VRT Delay	DAT	117	n/a	69.93	n/a	1 y	0.58	0.44 c		Rich, et al (1995)
Benton VRT Delay	DAT	32	n/a	70.70	NSAID	1 y	1.07	0.5 c		Rich, et al (1995)
Benton VRT Delay	Epilepsy	23	11/12	26.80 (13.20)	carbamaz	6 m	19.4 (4.6)	21.3 (3.7)		Pulliainen, et al (1994)
Benton VRT Delay	Epilepsy	20	9/11	31.50 (11.30)	phenytoin	6 m	19.4 (4.8)	19.1 (4.5)		Pulliainen, et al (1994)
Benton VRT-F (correct)	Epilepsy	36	17/19	34.89 (8.38)	vigabatrin 1 g	18 w	11.81 (1.92)	11.94 (2.24)		Dodrill, et al (1995)
Benton VRT-F (correct)	Epilepsy	40	14/26	33.88 (9.77)	placebo	18 w	11.28 (2.32)	11.80 (2.07)		Dodrill, et al (1995)
Benton VRT-F (correct)	Epilepsy	38	21/17	34.26 (9.18)	vigabatrin 3 g	18 w	11.26 (1.77)	12.08 (1.89)		Dodrill, et al (1995)
Benton VRT-F (correct)	Epilepsy	32	17/15	33.72 (9.66)	vigabatrin 6 g	18 w	11.47 (1.93)	11.66 (2.12)		Dodrill, et al (1995)
Benton VRT-G (correct)	Epilepsy	38	21/17	34.26 (9.18)	vigabatrin 3 g	18 w	13.66 (1.34)	13.47 (1.67)		Dodrill, et al (1995)
Benton VRT-G (correct)	Epilepsy	32	17/15	33.72 (9.66)	vigabatrin 6 g	18 w	13.50 (1.92)	13.66 (1.72)		Dodrill, et al (1995)
Benton VRT-G (correct)	Epilepsy	36	17/19	34.89 (8.38)	vigabatrin 1 g	18 w	13.11 (2.49)	13.86 (1.55)		Dodrill, et al (1995)

instrument	group	n	m/f	age	intervention	inter	t #1	t #2	note	citation
Benton VRT-G (correct)	Epilepsy	40	14/26	33.88 (9.77)	placebo	18 w	13.18 (2.17)	13.55 (1.87)		Dodrill, et al (1995)
Benton VRT Imm	Control	21	3/18	30.10 (8.20)	n/a	6 m	23.8 (1.3)	24.1 (1.8)		Pulliainen, et al (1994)
Benton VRT Imm	DAT	117	n/a	69.93	n/a	1 y	4.58	2.68 c		Rich, et al (1995)
Benton VRT Imm	DAT	32	n/a	70.72	NSAID	1 y	6.15	2.00 c		Rich, et al (1995)
Benton VRT Imm	Epilepsy	20	9/11	31.50 (11.30)	phenytoin	6 m	22 .0(3.6)	22.0 (3.1)		Pulliainen, et al (1994)
Benton VRT Imm	Epilepsy	23	11/12	26.80 (13.20)	carbamaz	6 m	22.1 (3.1)	23.5 (2.2)		Pulliainen, et al (1994)
Benton VRT MC Match	CVA/Control	71	n/a	70.70	declined	9-12 m	NR	0.2 (2.1) c		Desmond, et al (1995)
Benton VRT MC Match	CVA/Control	300	n/a	70.70	improved/ stable	9-12 m	NR	0.2 (1.4) c		Desmond, et al (1995)
Benton VRT MC Match	DAT	13	n/a	60.00 - 80.00	acetyl levocarnitine	6 m	7.8 (2.6)	7.8 (3.1)		Sano, et al (1992)
Benton VRT MC Match	DAT	14	n/a	60.00 - 80.00	placebo	6 m	7.5 (2.5)	7.1 (3.6)		Sano, et al (1992)
Benton VRT MC Recog	DAT	14	n/a	60.00 - 80.00	placebo	6 m	5.8 (2.9)	5.5 (2.3)		Sano, et al (1992)
Benton VRT MC Recog	DAT	13	n/a	60.00 - 80.00	acetyl levocarnitine	6 m	5.1 (2.2)	5.3 (2.4)		Sano, et al (1992)
Benton VRT Memory	Spinal Cord Injury	67	54/13	32.00 (14.70)	n/a	38 w	26.0 (4.12)	25.88 (4.49)		Richards, et al (1988)

instrument	group	n	m/f	age	intervention	inter	t #1	t #2	note	citation
Benton VRT Recall	Control	22	12/10	65.82 (5.20)	n/a	2 y	4.82 (2.27)	6.47 (2.29)		Rebok, et al (1990)
Benton VRT Recall	Control (CDR-0)	30	15/15	70.9 (4.6)	n/a	1 y	5.8 (1.4)	6.2 (2.2)	*	Botwinick, et al (1986)
Benton VRT Recall	DAT	51	16/35	67.29 (7.94)	n/a	2 y	1.69 (1.08)	0.56 (0.81)		Rebok, et al (1990)
Benton VRT Recall	DAT (CDR-1)	18	7/11	71.40 (4.40)	n/a	1 y	2.3 (1.8)	2.1 (1.5)	*	Botwinick, et al (1986)
Benton VRT Recog	CVA/Control	300	n/a	70.70	improved/ stable	9-12 m	NR	0.2 (1.7) c		Desmond, et al (1995)
Benton VRT Recog	CVA/Control	71	n/a	70.70	declined	9-12 m	NR	-0.2 (1.8) c		Desmond, et al (1995)
Benton VRT Recog	Orthopedic	128	38/90	69.00	general anesthesia	1 w	7.2 (1.7)	0.1 (1.8) c	*	Williams-Russo, et al (1995)
Benton VRT Recog	Orthopedic	134	39/95	69.00	epidural anesthesia	1 w	7.3 (1.5)	0.1 (1.7) c	*	Williams-Russo, et al (1995)
Benton VRT Recog	Spinal Cord Injury	67	54/13	32.00 (14.70)	n/a	38 w	28.8 (3.38)	29.26 (3.17)		Richards, et al (1988)

Table 9. Bilateral Simultaneous Sensory Stimulation (BSSS)

instrument	group	n	m/f	age	intervention	inter	t #1	t #2	note	citation
BSSS	TBI (sev)	15	13/2	24.80	n/a	11.5 m	22.9	38.7		Drudge, et al (1984)
BSSS (errors)	CAD	17	n/a	57.90 (8.40)	n/a	6 m	13.4	10.6	*	Parker, et al (1986)

instrument	group	n	m/f	age	intervention	inter	t #1	t #2	note	citation
BSSS (errors)	CAD	36	n./a	61.10 (8.30)	CE	6 m	14.3	14.2	*	Parker, et al (1986)
BSSS (errors)	Surgical	26	n/a	55.30 (6.80)	surgery (non-CE)	6 m	8.9	7.3	*	Parker, et al (1986)
BSSS Auditory (t)	ALL	31	16/15	8.38 (3.19)	n/a	2.0 y	49.2 (12.4)	50.1 (9.5)		Berg, et al (1983)
BSSS Auditory (t)	ALL w/ Somnolence	48	27/21	8.63 (3.15)	n/a	2.25 y	49.8 (13.5)	46.1 (14.6)		Berg, et al (1983)
BSSS Auditory LE (errors)	Neuropsych referrals	248	203/45	8.00 (1.70)	n/a	2.65 y	0.34 (0.84)	0.28 (0.77)		Brown, et al (1989)
BSSS Auditory RE (errors)	Neuropsych referrals	248	203/45	8.00 (1.70)	n/a	2.65 y	0.30 (0.88)	0.24 (0.79)		Brown, et al (1989)
BSSS LFH (errors)	Depression	33	14/19	37.40	antidepress	7 w	1.3 (2.3)	0.2 (0.7)		Fromm, et al (1984)
BSSS RFH (errors)	Depression	33	14/19	37.40	antidepress	7 w	1.1 (2.2)	0.2 (0.7)		Fromm, et al (1984)
BSSS Percep (errors)	CAD	17	n/a	57.20 (7.20)	n/a	6 m	16.6	13.6		Parker, et al (1983)
BSSS Percep (errors)	CAD	20	n/a	57.20 (7.20)	CE	6 m	15.4	15.8		Parker, et al (1983)
BSSS Percep (errors)	Surgical	17	n/a	57.20 (7.20)	surgery	6 m	11.2	8.3		Parker, et al (1983)
BSSS Tactile (errors)	TIA/CVA	34	34/0	60.30	CE	8-16 d	2.37	5.00		Cushman, et al (1984)
BSSS Tactile (t)	ALL	31	16/15	8.38 (3.19)	n/a	2.0 y	48.9 (11.1)	49.1 (9.2)		Berg, et al (1983)

instrument	group	n	m/f	age	intervention	inter	t #1	t #2	note	citation
BSSS Tactile (t)	ALL w/ Somnolence	48	27/21	8.63 (3.15)	n/a	2.25 y	53.5 (12.3)	49.7 (13.2)		Berg, et al (1983)
BSSS Visual (errors)	TIA/CVA	34	34/0	60.30	CE	8-16 d	1.22	1.51		Cushman, et al (1984)
BSSS Visual (t)	ALL	31	16/15	8.38 (3.19)	n/a	2.0 y	51.0 (10.1)	50.5 (10.8)		Berg, et al (1983)
BSSS Visual (t)	ALL w/ Somnolence	48	27/21	8.63 (3.15)	n/a	2.25 y	50.1 (10.8)	51.2 (12.2)		Berg, et al (1983)
BSSS Visual LE (errors)	Neuropsych referrals	248	203/ 45	8.00 (1.70)	n/a	2.65 y	3.2 (2.8)	2.0 (2.7)		Brown, et al (1989)
BSSS Visual LE (errors)	Neuropsych referrals	248	203/ 45	8.00 (1.70)	n/a	2.65 y	0.57 (1.6)	0.52 (1.5)		Brown, et al (1989)
BSSS Visual RE (errors)	Neuropsych referrals	248	203/ 45	8.00 (1.70)	n/a	2.65 y	0.64 (2.0)	0.45 (1.3)		Brown, et al (1989)
BSSS Visual RE (errors)	Neuropsych referrals	248	203/ 45	8.00 (1.70)	n/a	2.65 y	3.1 (3.0)	1.8 (2.5)		Brown, et al (1989)

Table 10. Boston Diagnostic Aphasia Examination (BDAE)

instrument	group	n	m/f	age	intervention	inter	t #1	t #2	note	citation
BDAE Animal Naming	Control	21	21/0	31.45 (5.53)	n/a	18 m	24.95 (5.61)	25.90 (6.09)		Saykin, et al (1991)
BDAE Animal Naming	Control	38	18/20	35.70 (10.50)	n/a	54.7w	24.8 (6.0)	25.3 (5.4)		Tarter, et al (1990)
BDAE Animal Naming	Crohn's Disease	22	9/13	37.30 (10.60)	std tx	62.6 w	22.4 (4.2)	24.0 (4.2)		Tarter, et al (1990)

instrument	group	n	m/f	age	intervention	inter	t #1	t #2	note	citation
BDAE Animal Naming	HIV+/ARC	8	8/0	33.57 (6.35)	n/a	18 m	18.86 (3.89)	21.71 (7.43)		Saykin, et al (1991)
BDAE Animal Naming	HIV+/PGL	13	13/0	31.15 (4.91)	n/a	18 m	20.85 (3.67)	23.77 (4.88)		Saykin, et al (1991)
BDAE Animal Naming	Liver Disease	62	23/39	39.20 (10.50)	liver transplant	60.1 w	21.3 (5.4)	23.2 (5.6)		Tarter, et al (1990)
BDAE Complex Ideation	CVA/Control	71	n/a	70.70	declined	9-12 m	NR	-0.3 (1.0) c		Desmond, et al (1995)
BDAE Complex Ideation	CVA/Control	300	n/a	70.70	improved/ stable	9-12 m	NR	0.0 (0.9) c		Desmond, et al (1995)
BDAE Reading	MS w/ Depression	11	n/a	n/a	depressed/ euthymic	7 m	NR	0.30 c		Schiffer, et al (1991)
BDAE Repetition	CVA/Control	71	n/a	70.70	declined	9-12 m	NR	0.0 (0.9) c		Desmond, et al (1995)
BDAE Repetition	CVA/Control	300	n/a	70.70	improved/ stable	9-12 m	NR	0.0 (0.7) c		Desmond, et al (1995)
BDAE Repetition	MS w/ Depression	11	n/a	n/a	depressed/ euthymic	7 m	NR	-0.20 c		Schiffer, et al (1991)

Table 11. Boston Naming Test (BNT)

instrument	group	n	m/f	age	intervention	inter	t #1	t #2	note	citation
BNT	Control (CDR-0)	30	15/ 15	70.9 (4.6)	n/a	1 y	71.5 (9.5)	70.0 (10.8)	*	Botwinick, et al (1986)
BNT	DAT	10	8/2	74.10	placebo	12 w	29.75 (14.60)	27.37 (15.56)		McCaffrey, et al (1987)
BNT	DAT	10	6/4	74.30	suloctidil 450 mg	12 w	28.50 (19.50)	36.66 (15.55)		McCaffrey, et al (1987)
BNT	DAT	10	5/5	74.90	suloctidil 600 mg	12 w	29.77 (19.34)	29.22 (19.24)		McCaffrey, et al (1987)
BNT	DAT (CDR-1)	18	7/11	71.40 (4.40)	n/a	1 y	42.7 (22.4)	31.9 (21.2)	*	Botwinick, et al (1986)
BNT	PD	4	3/1	53.50	fetal tissue implanted	12 m	53.5	54.5		Sass, et al (1995)
BNT	PD	19	13/6	54.30	pergolide	~6 w	74.5 (9.61)	76.8 (9.89)		Stern, et al (1984)
BNT (odd items)	DAT (mild)	11	10/1	63.00 (8.00)	n/a	26 m	35.0 (13.0)	29.0 (11.0)		Haxby, et al (1990)
BNT [15]	CVA/Control	71	n/a	70.70	declined	9-12 m	NR	-0.2 (1.9)c		Desmond, et al (1995)
BNT [15]	CVA/Control	300	n/a	70.70	improved/ stable	9-12 m	NR	0.3 (1.3) c		Desmond, et al (1995)
BNT [15]	DAT	13	n/a	71.70 (6.40)	placebo	1 m	10.8 (3.5)	11.0 (3.7)	AF	Green, et al (1992)

instrument	group	n	m/f	age	intervention	inter	t #1	t #2	note	citation
BNT [15]	DAT	11	n/a	71.70 (6.40)	oxiracetam	1 m	8.0 (3.3)	8.5 (3.9)	AF	Green, et al (1992)
BNT [15]	MS w/ Depression	11	n/a	n/a	depressed/ euthymic	7 m	NR	0.81 c		Schiffer, et al (1991)
BNT [30]	Control	60	26/34	71.24 (5.96)	n/a	12 m	27.02 (3.01)	26.86 (4.55)		Olin, et al (1991)
BNT [30]	Control	22	12/10	65.82 (5.20)	n/a	2 y	28.95 (1.21)	29.36 (0.85)		Rebok, et al (1990)
BNT [30]	DAT	51	16/35	67.29 (7.94)	n/a	2 y	15.73 (8.36)	8.06 (7.98)		Rebok, et al (1990)
BNT [30]	DAT	117	n/a	69.93	n/a	1 y	13.84	4.29 c		Rich, et al (1995)
BNT [30]	DAT	32	n/a	70.72	NSAID	1 y	18.00	3.74 c		Rich, et al (1995)
BNT [30]	Orthopedic	128	38/90	69.00	general anesthesia	1 w	24.8 (4.4)	0.0 (2.5) c	*	Williams-Russo, et al (1995)
BNT [30]	Orthopedic	134	39/95	69.00	epidural anesthesia	1 w	25.1 (4.5)	-0.3 (2.6) c	*	Williams-Russo, et al (1995)
BNT [42]	Control	20	6/14	69.40 (4.20)	n/a	1 y	38.2 (2.9)	38.3 (3.2)	*	Fromm, et al (1991)
BNT [42]	DAT	18	5/13	71.00 (9.40)	n/a	1 y	27.5 (7.2)	23.7 (8.5)	*	Fromm, et al (1991)
BNT [60]	AIDS	10	10/0	41.70 (5.50)	n/a	6.53 m	55.1 (3.8)	56.6 (2.9)		Hinkin, et al (1995)
BNT [60]	Control	31	14/17	63.74 (7.40)	n/a	7-17 d	55.61 (3.41)	56.48 (3.74)		Flanagan, et al (1997)

instrument	group	n	m/f	age	intervention	inter	t #1	t #2	note	citation
BNT [60]	Control	16	4/12	78.30 (2.50)	n/a	1 y	51.2 (7.3)	51.1 (8.6)	*	Mitrushina, et al (1991b)
BNT [60]	Control	47	14/33	72.90 (1.40)	n/a	1 y	53.7 (7.3)	54.6 (5.3)	*	Mitrushina, et al (1991b)
BNT [60]	Control	40	6/34	68.20 (1.20)	n/a	1 y	56.1 (3.1)	55.4 (7.0)	*	Mitrushina, et al (1991b)
BNT [60]	Control	19	2/17	62.20 (2.50)	n/a	1 y	56.0 (3.3)	56.2 (2.8)	*	Mitrushina, et al (1991b)
BNT [60]	Control	16	n/a	78.30 (2.50)	n/a	1 y	51.2 (7.3)	51.1 (8.6)	*	Mitrushina, et al (1995)
BNT [60]	Control	19	n/a	62.60 (2.50)	n/a	1 y	56.0 (3.3)	56.2 (2.8)	*	Mitrushina, et al (1995)
BNT [60]	Control	47	n/a	72.90 (1.40)	n/a	1 y	53.7 (7.3)	54.6 (5.3)	*	Mitrushina, et al (1995)
BNT [60]	Control	122	49/73	70.40 (5.00)	n/a	1 y	54.5 (5.9)	54.7 (6.2)	*	Mitrushina, et al (1995)
BNT [60]	Control	40	n/a	68.20 (1.20)	n/a	1 y	56.1 (3.1)	56.0 (2.9)	*	Mitrushina, et al (1995)
BNT [60]	Control	21	21/0	31.45 (5.53)	n/a	18 m	58.05 (1.84)	58.60 (1.47)		Saykin, et al (1991)
BNT [60]	HIV+/ARC	8	8/0	33.57 (6.35)	n/a	18 m	52.57 (5.53)	54.86 (4.91)		Saykin, et al (1991)

instrument	group	n	m/f	age	intervention	inter	t #1	t #2	note	citation
BNT [60]	HIV+/PGL	13	13/0	31.15 (4.91)	n/a	18 m	56.92 (3.28)	58.31 (2.02)		Saykin, et al (1991)
CERAD BNT	Control	278	89/ 189	68.10 (7.70)	n/a	1 m	14.6 (0.6)	14.7 (0.6)		Morris, et al (1989)
CERAD BNT	Control	47	n/a	~68.00	n/a	1 y	14.5 (0.7)	14.7 (0.6)		Morris, et al (1989)
CERAD BNT	DAT	354	166/ 188	71.50 (8.00)	n/a	1 m	11.3 (3.2)	11.5 (3.3)		Morris, et al (1989)
CERAD BNT	DAT	52	n/a	~71.00	n/a	1 y	11.6 (2.6)	10.7 (3.6)		Morris, et al (1989)
CERAD BNT (high freq)	Control	278	89/ 189	68.10 (7.70)	n/a	1 m	5.0 (0.1)	5.0 (0.1)		Morris, et al (1989)
CERAD BNT (high freq)	DAT	354	166/ 188	71.50 (8.00)	n/a	1 m	4.7 (0.6)	4.7 (0.7)		Morris, et al (1989)
CERAD BNT (low freq)	Control	278	89/ 189	68.10 (7.70)	n/a	1 m	4.7 (0.6)	4.8 (0.4)		Morris, et al (1989)
CERAD BNT (low freq)	DAT	354	166/ 188	71.50 (8.00)	n/a	1 m	2.9 (1.6)	3.1 (1.6)		Morris, et al (1989)
CERAD BNT (med. freq)	Control	278	89/ 189	68.10 (7.70)	n/a	1 m	4.9 (0.3)	4.9 (0.3)		Morris, et al (1989)
CERAD BNT (med. freq)	DAT	354	166/ 188	71.50 (8.00)	n/a	1 m	3.7 (1.4)	3.7 (1.4)		Morris, et al (1989)
CERAD BNT [15]	Control	1017	436/ 581	74.30 (5.40)	n/a	2 y	14.2 (1.0)	14.1 (1.3)		Ganguli, et al (1996)

instrument	group	n	m/f	age	intervention	inter	t #1	t #2	note	citation
CERAD BNT [15]	DAT	430	198/ 232	70.90 (8.00)	n/a	1 y	11.4 (3.1)	-0.6 (2.6) c	*	Morris, et al (1993)
mBNT	IVDU	16	13/3	39.50	n/a	10.4 d	22.56 (3.2)	23.94 (3.34)		Richards, et al (1992)

Table 12. California Verbal Learning Test (CVLT)

instrument	group	n	m/f	age	intervention	inter	t #1	t #2	note	citation
CVLT Cons (%)	Control	151	63/88	69.63 (6.46)	n/a	15.8 m	80.36 (10.43)	80.81 (9.17)		Paolo, et al (1997)
CVLT Cons (%)	Control	30	26/4	29.90 (6.20)	RAVLT admin first	2-4 h	NR	85.2 (10.0)		Crossen, et al (1994)
CVLT Cons (%)	Control	41	10/31	38.60 (20.2)	n/a	8 d	85.6 (9.4)	83.3 (11.4)	AF, CB	Delis, et al (1991)
CVLT Cons (%)	Epilepsy	26	10/16	29.20 (7.80)	LTL	6 m	77.69 (10.47)	77.54 (13.18)		Hermann, et al (1992)
CVLT Cons (%)	Epilepsy	31	13/18	32.90 (11.6)	RTL	6 m	80.61 (8.40)	82.71 (8.17)		Hermann, et al (1992)
CVLT CR Intrus	Control	151	63/88	69.63 (6.46)	n/a	15.8 m	2.11 (2.36)	1.89 (2.44)		Paolo, et al (1997)
CVLT CR Intrus	Control	21	12/9	33.00 (8.82)	n/a	1 y	1.62 (2.0)	1.81 (2.8)		Delis, et al (1987)

instrument	group	n	m/f	age	intervention	inter	t #1	t #2	note	citation
CVLT CR Intrus	Epilepsy	26	10/16	29.20 (7.80)	LTL	6 m	2.35 (2.06)	4.08 (3.54)		Hermann, et al (1992)
CVLT CR Intrus	Epilepsy	31	13/18	32.90 (11.6)	RTL	6 m	2.10 (2.23)	2.03 (3.38)		Hermann, et al (1992)
CVLT Discrim	Control	17	n/a	~39.0	n/a	12 m	98.18	98.65		Hanly, et al (1994)
CVLT Discrim	Control	21	12/9	33.00 (8.82)	n/a	1 y	94.16 (4.5)	95.89 (4.1)		Delis, et al (1987)
CVLT Discrim	Control	151	63/88	69.63 (6.46)	n/a	15.8 m	91.87 (5.65)	93.36 (5.34)		Paolo, et al (1997)
CVLT Discrim	Control	30	26/4	29.90 (6.20)	RAVLT admin first	2-4 h	NR	95.3 (3.8)		Crossen, et al (1994)
CVLT Discrim	Control	41	10/31	38.60 (20.2)	n/a	8 d	94.7 (4.9)	96 (5.3)	AF, CB	Delis, et al (1991)
CVLT Discrim	Control (avg IQ)	23	n/a	~28.8	n/a	2 w	95.39 (4.34)	97.65 (3.07)		Rapport, et al (1997a)
CVLT Discrim	Control (high avg IQ)	21	n/a	~28.8	n/a	2 w	97.10 (3.82)	99.10 (2.05)		Rapport, et al (1997a)
CVLT Discrim	Control (low avg IQ)	20	n/a	~28.8	n/a	2 w	92.5 (6.10)	96.85 (3.00)		Rapport, et al (1997a)
CVLT Discrim	Epilepsy	40	23/17	32.20 (8.20)	n/a	~9 m	88.53 (10.21)	91.45 (6.88)		Hermann, et al (1996)
CVLT Discrim	Epilepsy	31	13/18	32.90 (11.6)	RTL	6 m	91.00 (6.75)	88.77 (9.23)		Hermann, et al (1992)

instrument	group	n	m/f	age	intervention	inter	t #1	t #2	note	citation
CVLT Discrim	Epilepsy	26	10/16	29.20 (7.80)	LTL	6 m	87.39 (10.11)	79.65 (14.93)		Hermann, et al (1992)
CVLT Discrim	Rheumatoid Arthritis	11	n/a	~39.0	n/a	12 m	93.08	94.09		Hanly, et al (1994)
CVLT Discrim	SLE	59	n/a	39.60 (1.30)	n/a	12 m	96.17	97.37		Hanly, et al (1994)
CVLT FP	Control	30	26/4	29.90 (6.20)	RAVLT admin first	2-4 h	NR	0.9 (1.5)		Crossen, et al (1994)
CVLT FP	Control	21	12/9	33.00 (8.82)	n/a	1 y	1.14 (1.3)	1.10 (1.4)		Delis, et al (1987)
CVLT FP	Control	41	10/31	38.60 (20.2)	n/a	8 d	0.6 (0.8)	0.5 (0.8)	AF, CB	Delis, et al (1991)
CVLT FP	Control	151	63/88	69.63 (6.46)	n/a	15.8 m	1.64 (2.0)	1.38 (1.76)		Paolo, et al (1997)
CVLT FP	Control	21	21/0	31.45 (5.53)	n/a	18 m	0.40 (0.68)	0.45 (0.76)		Saykin, et al (1991)
CVLT FP	Epilepsy	26	10/16	29.20 (7.80)	LTL	6 m	3.50 (4.06)	6.04 (5.23)		Hermann, et al (1992)
CVLT FP	Epilepsy	40	23/17	32.20 (8.20)	n/a	~9 m	2.98 (3.41)	2.45 (2.44)		Hermann, et al (1996)
CVLT FP	Epilepsy	31	13/18	32.90 (11.6)	RTL	6 m	1.94 (1.84)	3.42 (4.15)		Hermann, et al (1992)
CVLT FP	HIV+ (asx)	25	n/a	38.20 (9.30)	n/a	15.8 d	0.8 (1.3)	0.4 (0.7)	*	Duff, et al (1999)

instrument	group	n	m/f	age	intervention	inter	t #1	t #2	note	citation
CVLT FP	HIV+ (sx)	18	n/a	37.80 (7.30)	n/a	15.8 d	0.8 (1.5)	0.2 (0.6)	*	Duff, et al (1999)
CVLT FP	HIV+/ARC	8	8/0	33.57 (6.35)	n/a	18 m	0.43 (0.79)	0.71 (1.11)		Saykin, et al (1991)
CVLT FP	HIV+/PGL	13	13/0	31.15 (4.91)	n/a	18 m	0.38 (0.87)	1.54 (3.10)		Saykin, et al (1991)
CVLT FP	HIV- ("At-Risk")	26	n/a	37.60 (11.2)	n/a	15.8 d	0.5 (0.7)	0.3 (0.4)	*	Duff, et al (1999)
CVLT FR Intrus	Control	151	63/88	69.63 (6.46)	n/a	15.8 m	2.32 (2.99)	2.57 (3.13)		Paolo, et al (1997)
CVLT FR Intrus	Control	21	12/9	33.00 (8.82)	n/a	1 y	2.57 (4.0)	2.14 (3.3)		Delis, et al (1987)
CVLT FR Intrus	Epilepsy	31	13/18	32.90 (11.6)	RTL	6 m	2.87 (2.78)	2.97 (3.91)		Hermann, et al (1992)
CVLT FR Intrus	Epilepsy	26	10/16	29.20 (7.80)	LTL	6 m	2.69 (2.94)	5.54 (5.35)		Hermann, et al (1992)
CVLT Hits	Control	21	21/0	31.45 (5.53)	n/a	18 m	15.45 (1.10)	15.40 (0.99)		Saykin, et al (1991)
CVLT Hits	Control	30	26/4	29.90 (6.20)	RAVLT admin first	2-4 h	NR	14.9 (1.2)		Crossen, et al (1994)
CVLT Hits	Control	41	10/31	38.60 (20.2)	n/a	8 d	14.5 (1.6)	15.0 (1.2)	AF, CB	Delis, et al (1991)

instrument	group	n	m/f	age	intervention	inter	t #1	t #2	note	citation
CVLT Hits	Control	21	12/9	33.00 (8.82)	n/a	1 y	14.57 (1.4)	15.29 (1.3)		Delis, et al (1987)
CVLT Hits	Control	151	63/88	69.63 (6.46)	n/a	15.8 m	14.09 (1.66)	14.48 (1.67)		Paolo, et al (1997)
CVLT Hits	Epilepsy	31	13/18	32.90 (11.6)	RTL	6 m	13.97 (2.39)	14.48 (1.34)		Hermann, et al (1992)
CVLT Hits	Epilepsy	26	10/16	29.20 (7.80)	LTL	6 m	13.96 (2.55)	13.08 (3.03)		Hermann, et al (1992)
CVLT Hits	Epilepsy	40	23/17	32.20 (8.20)	n/a	~9 m	13.92 (2.09)	14.70 (1.54)		Hermann, et al (1996)
CVLT Hits	HIV+ (asx)	25	n/a	38.20 (9.30)	n/a	15.8 d	14.3 (1.6)	15.2 (1.2)	*	Duff, et al (1999)
CVLT Hits	HIV+ (sx)	18	n/a	37.80 (7.30)	n/a	15.8 d	14.2 (1.8)	14.6 (2.8)	*	Duff, et al (1999)
CVLT Hits	HIV+/ARC	8	8/0	33.57 (6.35)	n/a	18 m	14.86 (1.07)	14.71 (1.25)		Saykin, et al (1991)
CVLT Hits	HIV+/PGL	13	13/0	31.15 (4.91)	n/a	18 m	15.38 (1.12)	15.31 (0.95)		Saykin, et al (1991)
CVLT Hits	HIV- ("At-Risk")	26	n/a	37.60 (11.2)	n/a	15.8 d	15.2 (1.3)	15.6 (0.7)	*	Duff, et al (1999)
CVLT Hits	Whiplash	21	8/13	35.50 (10.5)	n/a	6 m	15.4 (0.9)	15.4 (1.1)		Di Stefano, et al (1995)
CVLT Hits	Whiplash w/ continuing sx	21	8/13	35.40 (11.0)	n/a	6 m	14.7 (1.4)	15.5 (1.0)		Di Stefano, et al (1995)

instrument	group	n	m/f	age	intervention	inter	t #1	t #2	note	citation
CVLT Hits (%)	Control	11	9/2	31.60 (5.00)	n/a	6 m	98.3 (2.9)	99.4 (1.9)		Di Stefano, et al (1996)
CVLT Hits (%)	Whiplash	58	26/32	29.60 (8.90)	n/a	6 m	95.4 (6.8)	97.1 (5.4)		Di Stefano, et al (1996)
CVLT Hits (%)	Whiplash w/ continuing sx	28	9/19	34.10 (10.2)	n/a	6 m	94.2 (7.8)	97.5 (5.5)		Di Stefano, et al (1996)
CVLT Intrus	Control	151	63/88	69.63 (6.46)	n/a	15.8 m	4.43 (4.95)	4.46 (5.12)		Paolo, et al (1997)
CVLT Intrus	Control	21	21/0	31.45 (5.53)	n/a	18 m	2.30 (3.63)	3.60 (5.03)		Saykin, et al (1991)
CVLT Intrus	Control	41	10/31	38.60 (20.2)	n/a	8 d	1.1 (1.2)	1.0 (1.0)	AF, CB	Delis, et al (1991)
CVLT Intrus	Control	30	26/4	29.90 (6.20)	RAVLT admin first	2-4 h	NR	3.7 (3.7)		Crossen, et al (1994)
CVLT Intrus	HIV+/ARC	8	8/0	33.57 (6.35)	n/a	18 m	4.00 (3.92)	2.00 (2.45)		Saykin, et al (1991)
CVLT Intrus	HIV+/PGL	13	13/0	31.15 (4.91)	n/a	18 m	2.00 (3.54)	3.46 (3.41)		Saykin, et al (1991)
CVLT LDCR	Control	17	n/a	~39.0	n/a	12 m	13.18	14.24		Hanly, et al (1994)
CVLT LDCR	Control	21	21/0	31.45 (5.53)	n/a	18 m	14.25 (1.83)	14.15 (1.57)		Saykin, et al (1991)

instrument	group	n	m/f	age	intervention	inter	t #1	t #2	note	citation
CVLT LDCR	Control	41	10/31	38.60 (20.2)	n/a	8 d	12.2 (3.1)	12.9 (2.9)	AF, CB	Delis, et al (1991)
CVLT LDCR	Control	21	12/9	33.00 (8.82)	n/a	1 y	11.71 (2.8)	12.71 (2.0)		Delis, et al (1987)
CVLT LDCR	Control	151	63/88	69.63 (6.46)	n/a	15.8 m	10.57 (2.59)	11.02 (2.66)		Paolo, et al (1997)
CVLT LDCR	Control	30	26/4	29.90 (6.20)	RAVLT admin first	2-4 h	NR	12.7 (2.1)		Crossen, et al (1994)
CVLT LDCR	Epilepsy	26	10/16	29.20 (7.80)	LTL	6 m	8.00 (3.48)	7.15 (3.51)		Hermann, et al (1992)
CVLT LDCR	Epilepsy	31	13/18	32.90 (11.6)	RTL	6 m	10.32 (2.69)	10.84 (3.38)		Hermann, et al (1992)
CVLT LDCR	HIV+ (asx)	25	n/a	38.20 (9.30)	n/a	15.8 d	12.0 (2.9)	13.5 (2.7)	*	Duff, et al (1999)
CVLT LDCR	HIV+ (sx)	18	n/a	37.80 (7.30)	n/a	15.8 d	11.5 (2.6)	13.8 (1.7)	*	Duff, et al (1999)
CVLT LDCR	HIV+/ARC	8	8/0	33.57 (6.35)	n/a	18 m	13.00 (0.82)	12.96 (1.68)		Saykin, et al (1991)
CVLT LDCR	HIV+/PGL	13	13/0	31.15 (4.91)	n/a	18 m	14.54 (1.71)	13.46 (1.98)		Saykin, et al (1991)
CVLT LDCR	HIV- ("At-Risk")	26	n/a	37.60 (11.2)	n/a	15.8 d	13.0 (2.0)	14.8 (1.4)	*	Duff, et al (1999)

instrument	group	n	m/f	age	intervention	inter	t #1	t #2	note	citation
CVLT LDCR	Rheumatoid Arthritis	11	n/a	~39.0	n/a	12 m	12.00	12.36		Hanly, et al (1994)
CVLT LDCR	SLE	59	n/a	39.60 (1.30)	n/a	12 m	12.59	13.24		Hanly, et al (1994)
CVLT LDCR	Whiplash	21	8/13	35.50 (10.5)	n/a	6 m	13.8 (2.4)	14.5 (1.8)		Di Stefano, et al (1995)
CVLT LDCR	Whiplash w/ continuing sx	21	8/13	35.40 (11.0)	n/a	6 m	11.7 (2.9)	12.8 (2.9)		Di Stefano, et al (1995)
CVLT LDCR (% of best trial)	Control	11	9/2	31.60 (5.00)	n/a	6 m	92.4 (14.7)	101.4 (6.4)		Di Stefano, et al (1996)
CVLT LDCR (% of best trial)	Whiplash	58	26/32	29.60 (8.90)	n/a	6 m	95.5 (15.6)	96.7 (7.7)		Di Stefano, et al (1996)
CVLT LDCR (% of best trial)	Whiplash w/ continuing sx	28	9/19	34.10 (10.2)	n/a	6 m	90 (13.9)	93.5 (9.7)		Di Stefano, et al (1996)
CVLT LDFR	Control	21	21/0	31.45 (5.53)	n/a	18 m	13.80 (1.96)	14.00 (1.78)		Saykin, et al (1991)
CVLT LDFR	Control	17	n/a	~39.0	n/a	12 m	12.65	13.76		Hanly, et al (1994)
CVLT LDFR	Control	21	12/9	33.00 (8.82)	n/a	1 y	11.05 (2.9)	12.00 (2.3)		Delis, et al (1987)
CVLT LDFR	Control	30	26/4	29.90 (6.20)	RAVLT admin first	2-4 h	NR	12.4 (2.2)		Crossen, et al (1994)
CVLT LDFR	Control	41	10/31	38.60 (20.2)	n/a	8 d	11.8 (3.4)	12.6 (2.8)	AF, CB	Delis, et al (1991)
CVLT LDFR	Control	151	63/88	69.63 (6.46)	n/a	15.8 m	9.65 (2.85)	10.25 (2.84)		Paolo, et al (1997)

instrument	group	n	m/f	age	intervention	inter	t #1	t #2	note	citation
CVLT LDFR	Control (avg IQ)	23	n/a	~28.8	n/a	2 w	12.35 (2.71)	13.96 (2.42)		Rapport, et al (1997a)
CVLT LDFR	Control (high avg IQ)	21	n/a	~28.8	n/a	2 w	12.81 (2.11)	15.05 (1.12)		Rapport, et al (1997a)
CVLT LDFR	Control (low avg IQ)	20	n/a	~28.8	n/a	2 w	10.85 (2.74)	13.20 (2.24)		Rapport, et al (1997a)
CVLT LDFR	Epilepsy	40	23/17	32.20 (8.20)	n/a	~9 m	9.53 (3.20)	11.08 (3.80)		Hermann, et al (1996)
CVLT LDFR	Epilepsy	26	10/16	29.20 (7.80)	LTL	6 m	7.46 (3.42)	6.58 (3.33)		Hermann, et al (1992)
CVLT LDFR	Epilepsy	31	13/18	32.90 (11.6)	RTL	6 m	9.81 (2.92)	10.52 (3.31)		Hermann, et al (1992)
CVLT LDFR	HIV+ (asx)	25	n/a	38.20 (9.30)	n/a	15.8 d	11.6 (3.0)	13.0 (2.9)	*	Duff, et al (1999)
CVLT LDFR	HIV+ (sx)	18	n/a	37.80 (7.30)	n/a	15.8 d	11.5 (2.6)	13.8 (1.7)	*	Duff, et al (1999)
CVLT LDFR	HIV+/ARC	8	8/0	33.57 (6.35)	n/a	18 m	12.29 (1.11)	11.71 (2.14)		Saykin, et al (1991)
CVLT LDFR	HIV+/PGL	13	13/0	31.15 (4.91)	n/a	18 m	14.31 (2.29)	13.38 (2.14)		Saykin, et al (1991)
CVLT LDFR	HIV- ("At-Risk")	26	n/a	37.60 (11.2)	n/a	15.8 d	12.3 (2.5)	14.2 (1.7)	*	Duff, et al (1999)
CVLT LDFR	Rheumatoid Arthritis	11	n/a	~39.0	n/a	12 m	11.09	12.18		Hanly, et al (1994)
CVLT LDFR	SLE	59	n/a	39.60 (1.30)	n/a	12 m	11.76	12.66		Hanly, et al (1994)

instrument	group	n	m/f	age	intervention	inter	t #1	t #2	note	citation
CVLT LDFR	Whiplash	21	8/13	35.50 (10.5)	n/a	6,18 m	9.6 (1.8)	10.3 (1.7)		Di Stefano, et al (1995)
CVLT LDFR	Whiplash w/ continuing sx	21	8/13	35.40 (11.0)	n/a	6 m	8.6 (2.0)	9.3 (2.0)		Di Stefano, et al (1995)
CVLT LDFR (% of best trial)	Control	11	9/2	31.60 (5.00)	n/a	6 m	95.0 (14.9)	98.9 (6.5)		Di Stefano, et al (1996)
CVLT LDFR (% of best trial)	Whiplash	58	26/32	29.60 (8.90)	n/a	6 m	93 (12.1)	95.6 (9.0)		Di Stefano, et al (1996)
CVLT LDFR (% of best trial)	Whiplash w/ continuing sx	28	9/19	34.10 (10.2)	n/a	6 m	91.1 (11.8)	91.8 (10.4)		Di Stefano, et al (1996)
CVLT List B	Control	21	12/9	33.00 (8.82)	n/a	1 y	6.14 (2.4)	6.52 (1.6)		Delis, et al (1987)
CVLT List B	Control	30	26/4	29.90 (6.20)	RAVLT admin first	2-4 h	NR	8.0 (2.1)		Crossen, et al (1994)
CVLT List B	Control	41	10/31	38.60 (20.2)	n/a	8 d	7.3 (2.1)	6.8 (2.6)	AF, CB	Delis, et al (1991)
CVLT List B	Control	21	21/0	31.45 (5.53)	n/a	18 m	9.55 (2.28)	8.65 (2.72)		Saykin, et al (1991)
CVLT List B	Control	151	63/88	69.63 (6.46)	n/a	15.8 m	5.78 (2.18)	5.90 (1.74)		Paolo, et al (1997)
CVLT List B	Control	17	n/a	~39.0	n/a	12 m	9.06	8.76		Hanly, et al (1994)
CVLT List B	Epilepsy	26	10/16	29.20 (7.80)	LTL	6 m	4.31 (1.91)	3.89 (1.63)		Hermann, et al (1992)
CVLT List B	Epilepsy	31	13/18	32.90 (11.6)	RTL	6 m	5.39 (2.01)	5.61 (1.75)		Hermann, et al (1992)

instrument	group	n	m/f	age	intervention	inter	t #1	t #2	note	citation
CVLT List B	HIV+ (asx)	25	n/a	38.20 (9.30)	n/a	15.8 d	6.2 (1.8)	6.8 (1.9)	*	Duff, et al (1999)
CVLT List B	HIV+ (sx)	18	n/a	37.80 (7.30)	n/a	15.8 d	5.8 (1.3)	7.0 (1.3)	*	Duff, et al (1999)
CVLT List B	HIV+/ARC	8	8/0	33.57 (6.35)	n/a	18 m	6.57 (1.40)	6.57 (2.30)		Saykin, et al (1991)
CVLT List B	HIV+/PGL	13	13/0	31.15 (4.91)	n/a	18 m	7.23 (2.05)	6.62 (2.22)		Saykin, et al (1991)
CVLT List B	HIV- ("At-Risk")	26	n/a	37.60 (11.2)	n/a	15.8 d	6.9 (2.1)	8.1 (1.8)	*	Duff, et al (1999)
CVLT List B	Rheumatoid Arthritis	11	n/a	~39.0	n/a	12 m	7.27	7.36		Hanly, et al (1994)
CVLT List B	SLE	59	n/a	39.60 (1.30)	n/a	12 m	7.42	7.63		Hanly, et al (1994)
CVLT List B	Whiplash	21	8/13	35.50 (10.5)	n/a	6 m	5.0 (2.2)	4.4 (2.1)		Di Stefano, et al (1995)
CVLT List B	Whiplash w/ continuing sx	21	8/13	35.40 (11.0)	n/a	6 m	4.4 (1.8)	4.5 (1.9)		Di Stefano, et al (1995)
CVLT List B (% of Trial 1)	Control	11	9/2	31.60 (5.00)	n/a	6 m	86.5 (27.9)	96.0 (42.1)		Di Stefano, et al (1996)
CVLT List B (% of Trial 1)	Whiplash	58	26/32	29.60 (8.90)	n/a	6 m	107.6 (44.3)	79.9 (29.2)		Di Stefano, et al (1996)
CVLT List B (% of Trial 1)	Whiplash w/ continuing sx	28	9/19	34.10 (10.2)	n/a	6 m	94.7 (22.3)	83.6 (39.1)		Di Stefano, et al (1996)

instrument	group	n	m/f	age	intervention	inter	t #1	t #2	note	citation
CVLT Middle (%)	Control	30	26/4	29.90 (6.20)	RAVLT admin first	2-4 h	NR	45.3 (4.1)		Crossen, et al (1994)
CVLT Middle (%)	Control	21	12/9	33.00 (8.82)	n/a	1 y	43.60 (6.8)	45.87 (6.5)		Delis, et al (1987)
CVLT Middle (%)	Control	151	63/88	69.63 (6.46)	n/a	15.8 m	40.08 (7.82)	42.23 (7.66)		Paolo, et al (1997)
CVLT Middle (%)	Epilepsy	26	10/16	29.20 (7.80)	LTL	6 m	38.12 (8.33)	34.15 (7.89)		Hermann, et al (1992)
CVLT Middle (%)	Epilepsy	31	13/18	32.90 (11.6)	RTL	6 m	41.58 (7.85)	45.23 (8.57)		Hermann, et al (1992)
CVLT Persev	Control	30	26/4	29.90 (6.20)	RAVLT admin first	2-4 h	NR	8.1 (6.8)		Crossen, et al (1994)
CVLT Persev	Control	21	12/9	33.00 (8.82)	n/a	1 y	6.95 (4.4)	6.90 (5.7)		Delis, et al (1987)
CVLT Persev	Control	151	63/88	69.63 (6.46)	n/a	15.8 m	4.97 (5.0)	5.01 (4.98)		Paolo, et al (1997)
CVLT Persev	Control	21	21/0	31.45 (5.53)	n/a	18 m	6.50 (3.72)	4.05 (3.63)		Saykin, et al (1991)
CVLT Persev	Control	41	10/31	38.60 (20.2)	n/a	8 d	4.0 (4.0)	4.7 (4.1)	AF, CB	Delis, et al (1991)
CVLT Persev	Epilepsy	26	10/16	29.20 (7.80)	LTL	6 m	4.15 (3.30)	4.50 (4.21)		Hermann, et al (1992)

instrument	group	n	m/f	age	intervention	inter	t #1	t #2	note	citation
CVLT Persev	Epilepsy	31	13/18	32.90 (11.6)	RTL	6 m	6.87 (5.64)	5.16 (1.75)		Hermann, et al (1992)
CVLT Persev	HIV+/ARC	8	8/0	33.57 (6.35)	n/a	18 m	5.00 (6.40)	6.00 (4.47)		Saykin, et al (1991)
CVLT Persev	HIV+/PGL	13	13/0	31.15 (4.91)	n/a	18 m	5.31 (6.06)	6.08 (5.09)		Saykin, et al (1991)
CVLT Primacy (%)	Control	41	10/31	38.60 (20.2)	n/a	8 d	28.4 (4.2)	29.3 (4.8)	AF, CB	Delis, et al (1991)
CVLT Primacy (%)	Control	151	63/88	69.63 (6.46)	n/a	15.8 m	29.9 (6.54)	28.36 (5.71)		Paolo, et al (1997)
CVLT Primacy (%)	Control	30	26/4	29.90 (6.20)	RAVLT admin first	2-4 h	NR	28.1 (4.0)		Crossen, et al (1994)
CVLT Primacy (%)	Control	21	12/9	33.00 (8.82)	n/a	1 y	28.31 (4.2)	27.60 (5.5)		Delis, et al (1987)
CVLT Primacy (%)	Epilepsy	26	10/16	29.20 (7.80)	LTL	6 m	31.26 (7.96)	31.96 (7.62)		Hermann, et al (1992)
CVLT Primacy (%)	Epilepsy	31	13/18	32.90 (11.6)	RTL	6 m	30.03 (6.25)	29.84 (5.37)		Hermann, et al (1992)
CVLT Recency (%)	Control	21	12/9	33.00 (8.82)	n/a	1 y	28.09 (6.1)	26.54 (6.1)		Delis, et al (1987)
CVLT Recency (%)	Control	41	10/31	38.60 (20.2)	n/a	8 d	27.8 (5.0)	26.6 (5.8)	AF, CB	Delis, et al (1991)
CVLT Recency (%)	Control	30	26/4	29.90 (6.20)	RAVLT admin first	2-4 h	NR	26.4 (3.7)		Crossen, et al (1994)

instrument	group	n	m/f	age	intervention	inter	t #1	t #2	note	citation
CVLT Recency (%)	Control	151	63/88	69.63 (6.46)	n/a	15.8 m	29.72 (7.95)	29.47 (6.10)		Paolo, et al (1997)
CVLT Recency (%)	Epilepsy	31	13/18	32.90 (11.6)	RTL	6 m	28.26 (7.52)	24.81 (7.26)		Hermann, et al (1992)
CVLT Recency (%)	Epilepsy	26	10/16	29.20 (7.80)	LTL	6 m	30.35 (5.52)	33.81 (9.67)		Hermann, et al (1992)
CVLT RB	Control	41	10/31	38.60 (20.2)	n/a	8 d	-0.06 (0.33)	-0.04 (0.27)	AF, CB	Delis, et al (1991)
CVLT RB	Control	30	26/4	29.90 (6.20)	RAVLT admin first	2-4 h	NR	-0.02 (0.3)		Crossen, et al (1994)
CVLT RB	Epilepsy	31	13/18	32.90 (11.6)	RTL	6 m	0.14 (0.97)	0.14 (0.42)		Hermann, et al (1992)
CVLT RB	Epilepsy	26	10/16	29.20 (7.80)	LTL	6 m	0.14 (0.43)	0.22 (0.45)		Hermann, et al (1992)
CVLT SDCR	Control	21	12/9	33.00 (8.82)	n/a	1 y	11.62 (2.6)	12.62 (1.8)		Delis, et al (1987)
CVLT SDCR	Control	41	10/31	38.60 (20.2)	n/a	8 d	12.0 (3.1)	12.8 (2.8)	AF, CB	Delis, et al (1991)
CVLT SDCR	Control	17	n/a	~39.0	n/a	12 m	13.00	14.18		Hanly, et al (1994)
CVLT SDCR	Control	21	21/0	31.45 (5.53)	n/a	18 m	0.85 (1.76)	14.25 (1.68)		Saykin, et al (1991)
CVLT SDCR	Control	151	63/88	69.63 (6.46)	n/a	15.8 m	10.71 (2.57)	11.01 (2.57)		Paolo, et al (1997)
CVLT SDCR	Control	30	26/4	29.90 (6.20)	RAVLT admin first	2-4 h	NR	13.0 (2.2)		Crossen, et al (1994)

instrument	group	n	m/f	age	intervention	inter	t #1	t #2	note	citation
CVLT SDCR	Epilepsy	31	13/18	32.90 (11.6)	RTL	6 m	10.03 (2.51)	11.07 (2.45)		Hermann, et al (1992)
CVLT SDCR	Epilepsy	26	10/16	29.20 (7.80)	LTL	6 m	8.15 (3.34)	7.35 (3.15)		Hermann, et al (1992)
CVLT SDCR	HIV+ (asx)	25	n/a	38.20 (9.30)	n/a	15.8d	11.8 (2.8)	13.5 (2.6)	*	Duff, et al (1999)
CVLT SDCR	HIV+ (sx)	18	n/a	37.80 (7.30)	n/a	15.8 d	11.8 (2.2)	14.1 (1.4)	*	Duff, et al (1999)
CVLT SDCR	HIV+/ARC	8	8/0	33.57 (6.35)	n/a	18 m	12.57 (1.51)	12.57 (1.40)		Saykin, et al (1991)
CVLT SDCR	HIV+/PGL	13	13/0	31.15 (4.91)	n/a	18 m	0.23 (1.64)	13.31 (1.38)		Saykin, et al (1991)
CVLT SDCR	HIV- ("At-Risk")	26	n/a	37.60 (11.2)	n/a	15.8d	13.1 (1.7)	15.0 (1.2)	*	Duff, et al (1999)
CVLT SDCR	Rheumatoid Arthritis	11	n/a	~39.0	n/a	12 m	11.55	11.64		Hanly, et al (1994)
CVLT SDCR	SLE	59	n/a	39.60 (1.30)	n/a	12 m	12.39	13.15		Hanly, et al (1994)
CVLT SDCR	Whiplash	21	8/13	35.50 (10.5)	n/a	6 m	13.8 (2.0)	14.5 (1.7)		Di Stefano, et al (1995)
CVLT SDCR	Whiplash w/ continuing sx	21	8/13	35.40 (11.0)	n/a	6 m	11.4 (2.9)	12.5 (2.6)		Di Stefano, et al (1995)
CVLT SDCR (% of best trial)	Control	11	9/2	31.60 (5.00)	n/a	6 m	89.1 (15)	97.1 (11.7)		Di Stefano, et al (1996)

instrument	group	n	m/f	age	intervention	inter	t #1	t #2	note	citation
CVLT SDCR (% of best trial)	Whiplash	58	26/32	29.60 (8.90)	n/a	6 m	94.8 (18.2)	94.3 (11)		Di Stefano, et al (1996)
CVLT SDCR (% of best trial)	Whiplash w/ continuing sx	28	9/19	34.10 (10.2)	n/a	6 m	89.3 (13.5)	93.3 (14.8)		Di Stefano, et al (1996)
CVLT SDFR	Control	17	n/a	~39.0	n/a	12 m	12.71	13.29		Hanly, et al (1994)
CVLT SDFR	Control	30	26/4	29.90 (6.20)	RAVLT admin first	2-4 h	NR	12.0 (2.1)		Crossen, et al (1994)
CVLT SDFR	Control	151	63/88	69.63 (6.46)	n/a	15.8 m	9.24 (2.86)	9.7 (3.01)		Paolo, et al (1997)
CVLT SDFR	Control	21	21/0	31.45 (5.53)	n/a	18 m	13.65 (1.90)	13.85 (1.57)		Saykin, et al (1991)
CVLT SDFR	Control	41	10/31	38.60 (20.2)	n/a	8 d	11.4 (3.9)	12.0 (3.6)	AF, CB	Delis, et al (1991)
CVLT SDFR	Control	21	12/9	33.00 (8.82)	n/a	1 y	10.38 (2.5)	11.38 (2.4)		Delis, et al (1987)
CVLT SDFR	Epilepsy	26	10/16	29.20 (7.80)	LTL	6 m	7.42 (3.37)	6.77 (3.46)		Hermann, et al (1992)
CVLT SDFR	Epilepsy	31	13/18	32.90 (11.6)	RTL	6 m	9.74 (2.86)	10.71 (2.67)		Hermann, et al (1992)
CVLT SDFR	Epilepsy	40	23/17	32.20 (8.20)	n/a	~9 m	9.12 (3.43)	10.40 (3.50)		Hermann, et al (1996)
CVLT SDFR	HIV+ (asx)	25	n/a	38.20 (9.30)	n/a	15.8d	10.4 (2.7)	12.5 (2.9)	*	Duff, et al (1999)
CVLT SDFR	HIV+ (sx)	18	n/a	37.80 (7.30)	n/a	15.8d	10.0 (2.7)	12.7 (2.3)	*	Duff, et al (1999)

instrument	group	n	m/f	age	intervention	inter	t #1	t #2	note	citation
CVLT SDFR	HIV+/ARC	8	8/0	33.57 (6.35)	n/a	18 m	11.86 (2.12)	11.86 (2.04)		Saykin, et al (1991)
CVLT SDFR	HIV+/PGL	13	13/0	31.15 (4.91)	n/a	18 m	13.62 (1.56)	12.46 (2.44)		Saykin, et al (1991)
CVLT SDFR	HIV- ("At-Risk")	26	n/a	37.60 (11.2)	n/a	15.8d	11.6 (2.6)	14.0 (2.2)	*	Duff, et al (1999)
CVLT SDFR	Rheumatoid Arthritis	11	n/a	~39.0	n/a	12 m	10.73	11.45		Hanly, et al (1994)
CVLT SDFR	SLE	59	n/a	39.60 (1.30)	n/a	12 m	11.29	12.46		Hanly, et al (1994)
CVLT SDFR	Whiplash	21	8/13	35.50 (10.5)	n/a	6 m	9.4 (1.9)	10.0 (2.1)		Di Stefano, et al (1995)
CVLT SDFR	Whiplash w/ continuing sx	21	8/13	35.40 (11.0)	n/a	6 m	8.2 (2.1)	8.5 (2.0)		Di Stefano, et al (1995)
CVLT SDFR (% of best trial)	Control	11	9/2	31.60 (5.00)	n/a	6 m	91.8 (12)	96.6 (8.9)		Di Stefano, et al (1996)
CVLT SDFR (% of best trial)	Whiplash	58	26/32	29.60 (8.90)	n/a	6 m	90.2 (11.4)	93.9 (9.2)		Di Stefano, et al (1996)
CVLT SDFR (% of best trial)	Whiplash w/ continuing sx	28	9/19	34.10 (10.2)	n/a	6 m	88.4 (11.5)	88.6 (13.5)		Di Stefano, et al (1996)
CVLT Sem Cluster	Control	30	26/4	29.90 (6.20)	RAVLT admin first	2-4 h	NR	2.3 (0.9)		Crossen, et al (1994)
CVLT Sem Cluster	Control	41	10/31	38.60 (20.2)	n/a	8 d	2.4 (1.0)	2.1 (1.1)	AF, CB	Delis, et al (1991)
CVLT Sem Cluster	Control	151	63/88	69.63 (6.46)	n/a	15.8 m	1.79 (0.85)	2.07 (0.88)		Paolo, et al (1997)

instrument	group	n	m/f	age	intervention	inter	t #1	t #2	note	citation
CVLT Sem Cluster	Control	21	12/9	33.00 (8.82)	n/a	1 y	1.84 (0.7)	2.39 (0.8)		Delis, et al (1987)
CVLT Sem Cluster	Epilepsy	26	10/16	29.20 (7.80)	LTL	6 m	1.44 (0.62)	1.34 (0.68)		Hermann, et al (1992)
CVLT Sem Cluster	Epilepsy	31	13/18	32.90 (11.6)	RTL	6 m	1.74 (0.62)	2.04 (0.78)		Hermann, et al (1992)
CVLT Ser Cluster	Control	30	26/4	29.90 (6.20)	RAVLT admin first	2-4 h	NR	2.3 (2.0)		Crossen, et al (1994)
CVLT Ser Cluster	Control	21	12/9	33.00 (8.82)	n/a	1 y	2.65 (1.7)	1.80 (1.2)		Delis, et al (1987)
CVLT Ser Cluster	Control	151	63/88	69.63 (6.46)	n/a	15.8 m	2.22 (1.8)	1.92 (1.55)		Paolo, et al (1997)
CVLT Ser Cluster	Epilepsy	31	13/18	32.90 (11.6)	RTL	6 m	2.56 (1.46)	2.2 (1.52)		Hermann, et al (1992)
CVLT Ser Cluster	Epilepsy	26	10/16	29.20 (7.80)	LTL	6 m	2.10 (1.69)	3.19 (2.27)		Hermann, et al (1992)
CVLT Slope	Control	30	26/4	29.90 (6.20)	RAVLT admin first	2-4 h	NR	1.2 (0.5)		Crossen, et al (1994)
CVLT Slope	Control	41	10/31	38.60 (20.2)	n/a	8 d	1.3 (0.5)	1.5 (0.5)	AF, CB	Delis, et al (1991)
CVLT Slope	Control	151	63/88	69.63 (6.46)	n/a	15.8 m	1.25 (0.5)	1.17 (0.54)		Paolo, et al (1997)
CVLT Slope	Control	21	12/9	33.00 (8.82)	n/a	1 y	1.14 (0.5)	1.05 (0.5)		Delis, et al (1987)
CVLT Slope	Control (avg IQ)	23	n/a	~28.8	n/a	2 w	1.56 (0.52)	0.80 (0.45)		Rapport, et al (1997a)

instrument	group	n	m/f	age	intervention	inter	t #1	t #2	note	citation
CVLT Slope	Control (high avg IQ)	21	n/a	~28.8	n/a	2 w	1.43 (0.48)	0.93 (0.42)		Rapport, et al (1997a)
CVLT Slope	Control (low avg IQ)	20	n/a	~28.8	n/a	2 w	0.92 (0.40)	0.84 (0.43)		Rapport, et al (1997a)
CVLT Slope	Homeless	15	9/6	32.80 (6.10)	cognitive remediation	2-3 m	1.47 (0.55)	1.21 (0.50)		Cotman, et al (1997)
CVLT Slope	Homeless	9	4/5	27.00 (5.80)	n/a	2-3 m	1.23 (0.43)	2.12 (0.68)		Cotman, et al (1997)
CVLT Total	Control	21	21/0	31.45 (5.53)	n/a	18 m	64.50 (7.34)	63.35 (8.80)		Saykin, et al (1991)
CVLT Total	Control	151	63/88	69.63 (6.46)	n/a	15.8 m	45.72 (9.79)	47.72 (10.17)		Paolo, et al (1997)
CVLT Total	Control	21	12/9	33.00 (8.82)	n/a	1 y	52.81 (7.2)	54.95 (8.40)		Delis, et al (1987)
CVLT Total	Control	41	10/31	38.60 (20.2)	n/a	8 d	55.8 (9.3)	53.8 (11.2)	AF, CB	Delis, et al (1991)
CVLT Total	Control	30	26/4	29.90 (6.20)	RAVLT admin first	2-4 h	NR	55.8 (8.5)		Crossen, et al (1994)
CVLT Total	Control	17	n/a	~39.0	n/a	12 m	59.82	63.82		Hanly, et al (1994)
CVLT Total	Control (avg IQ)	23	n/a	~28.8	n/a	2 w	53.65 (8.23)	65.83 (9.83)		Rapport, et al (1997a)
CVLT Total	Control (high avg IQ)	21	n/a	~28.8	n/a	2 w	56.38 (7.88)	69.38 (7.21)		Rapport, et al (1997a)

instrument	group	n	m/f	age	intervention	inter	t #1	t #2	note	citation
CVLT Total	Control (low avg IQ)	20	n/a	~28.8	n/a	2 w	48.75 (9.44)	59.30 (10.62)		Rapport, et al (1997a)
CVLT Total	Epilepsy	31	13/18	32.90 (11.6)	RTL	6 m	45.68 (8.00)	48.26 (8.86)		Hermann, et al (1992)
CVLT Total	Epilepsy	40	23/17	32.20 (8.20)	n/a	~9 m	46.10 (8.78)	48.28 (10.81)		Hermann, et al (1996)
CVLT Total	Epilepsy	26	10/16	29.20 (7.80)	LTL	6 m	37.19 (10.10)	36.92 (10.01)		Hermann, et al (1992)
CVLT Total	HIV+ (asx)	25	n/a	38.20 (9.30)	n/a	15.8d	50.6 (10.0)	61.5 (11.4)	*	Duff, et al (1999)
CVLT Total	HIV+ (sx)	18	n/a	37.80 (7.30)	n/a	15.8d	47.7 (8.2)	59.5 (9.3)	*	Duff, et al (1999)
CVLT Total	HIV+/ARC	8	8/0	33.57 (6.35)	n/a	18 m	57.86 (6.89)	52.00 (8.33)		Saykin, et al (1991)
CVLT Total	HIV+/PGL	13	13/0	31.15 (4.91)	n/a	18 m	61.38 (6.01)	59.38 (8.02)		Saykin, et al (1991)
CVLT Total	HIV- ("At-Risk")	26	n/a	37.60 (11.2)	n/a	15.8d	55.8 (8.7)	67.5 (10.1)	*	Duff, et al (1999)
CVLT Total	Homeless	9	4/5	27.00 (5.80)	n/a	2-3 m	52.56 (11.59)	37.50 (8.57)		Cotman, et al (1997)
CVLT Total	Homeless	15	9/6	32.80 (6.10)	cognitive remediation	2-3 m	38.40 (12.47)	29.75 (13.54)		Cotman, et al (1997)

instrument	group	n	m/f	age	intervention	inter	t #1	t #2	note	citation
CVLT Total	Rheumatoid Arthritis	11	n/a	~39.0	n/a	12 m	53.82	57.45		Hanly, et al (1994)
CVLT Total	SLE	59	n/a	39.60 (1.30)	n/a	12 m	57.53	59.85		Hanly, et al (1994)
CVLT Total (t)	HIV+ (asx)	20	15/5	36.70 (9.90)	n/a	7-10 d	35.5 (12.9)	53.8 (14.4)		McCaffrey, et al (1995)
CVLT Total (t)	HIV+ (sx)	12	11/1	37.20 (6.40)	n/a	7-10 d	39.4 (11.0)	57.7 (16.9)		McCaffrey, et al (1995)
CVLT Total (t)	HIV- ("At-Risk")	12	12/0	40.40 (13.0)	n/a	7-10 d	48.7 (10.7)	61.4 (11.1)		McCaffrey, et al (1995)
CVLT Trial 1	Control	17	n/a	~39.0	n/a	12 m	8.71	8.88		Hanly, et al (1994)
CVLT Trial 1	Control	30	26/4	29.90 (6.20)	RAVLT admin first	2-4 h	NR	7.9 (1.8)		Crossen, et al (1994)
CVLT Trial 1	Control	151	63/88	69.63 (6.46)	n/a	15.8 m	5.89 (1.82)	6.46 (1.91)		Paolo, et al (1997)
CVLT Trial 1	Control	41	10/31	38.60 (20.2)	n/a	8 d	7.5 (1.9)	6.9 (2.0)	AF, CB	Delis, et al (1991)
CVLT Trial 1	Control	21	21/0	31.45 (5.53)	n/a	18 m	9.25 (1.94)	8.95 (2.37)		Saykin, et al (1991)
CVLT Trial 1	Epilepsy	26	10/16	29.20 (7.80)	LTL	6 m	4.54 (1.68)	4.54 (1.75)		Hermann, et al (1992)
CVLT Trial 1	Epilepsy	31	13/18	32.90 (11.6)	RTL	6 m	5.55 (1.52)	6.13 (1.63)		Hermann, et al (1992)
CVLT Trial 1	Epilepsy	40	23/17	32.20 (8.20)	n/a	~9 m	5.95 (2.06)	6.57 (1.81)		Hermann, et al (1996)

instrument	group	n	m/f	age	intervention	inter	t #1	t #2	note	citation
CVLT Trial 1	HIV+ (asx)	25	n/a	38.20 (9.30)	n/a	15.8d	7.0 (2.1)	10.4 (2.7)	*	Duff, et al (1999)
CVLT Trial 1	HIV+ (sx)	18	n/a	37.80 (7.30)	n/a	15.8d	6.5 (1.5)	9.5 (2.4)	*	Duff, et al (1999)
CVLT Trial 1	HIV+/ARC	8	8/0	33.57 (6.35)	n/a	18 m	8.29 (1.98)	6.57 (1.62)		Saykin, et al (1991)
CVLT Trial 1	HIV+/PGL	13	13/0	31.15 (4.91)	n/a	18 m	8.92 (1.61)	7.92 (1.80)		Saykin, et al (1991)
CVLT Trial 1	HIV- ("At-Risk")	26	n/a	37.60 (11.2)	n/a	15.8d	7.8 (1.6)	11.9 (2.9)	*	Duff, et al (1999)
CVLT Trial 1	Rheumatoid Arthritis	11	n/a	~39.0	n/a	12 m	7.91	8.36		Hanly, et al (1994)
CVLT Trial 1	SLE	59	n/a	39.60 (1.30)	n/a	12 m	8.17	8.73		Hanly, et al (1994)
CVLT Trial 1	Whiplash	21	8/13	35.50 (10.5)	n/a	6 m	4.6 (1.3)	5.8 (2.5)		Di Stefano, et al (1995)
CVLT Trial 1	Whiplash w/ continuing sx	21	8/13	35.40 (11.0)	n/a	6 m	4.6 (1.2)	5.8 (1.7)		Di Stefano, et al (1995)
CVLT Trial 1 (% of 16)	Control	11	9/2	31.60 (5.00)	n/a	6 m	53.4 (11.7)	50.6 (13.8)		Di Stefano, et al (1996)
CVLT Trial 1 (% of 16)	Whiplash	58	26/32	29.60 (8.90)	n/a	6 m	43.9 (13.5)	55 (17.4)		Di Stefano, et al (1996)
CVLT Trial 1 (% of 16)	Whiplash w/ continuing sx	28	9/19	34.10 (10.2)	n/a	6 m	44.6 (9.7)	54 (14)		Di Stefano, et al (1996)
CVLT Trial 2	Control	21	21/0	31.45 (5.53)	n/a	18 m	12.95 (1.76)	11.95 (2.58)		Saykin, et al (1991)

instrument	group	n	m/f	age	intervention	inter	t #1	t #2	note	citation
CVLT Trial 2	Control	30	26/4	29.90 (6.20)	RAVLT admin first	2-4 h	NR	10.7 (2.2)		Crossen, et al (1994)
CVLT Trial 2	Epilepsy	40	23/17	32.20 (8.20)	n/a	~9 m	8.33 (2.15)	9.30 (2.44)		Hermann, et al (1996)
CVLT Trial 2	HIV+/ARC	8	8/0	33.57 (6.35)	n/a	18 m	10.71 (1.38)	9.43 (2.44)		Saykin, et al (1991)
CVLT Trial 2	HIV+/PGL	13	13/0	31.15 (4.91)	n/a	18 m	11.46 (1.90)	11.31 (2.10)		Saykin, et al (1991)
CVLT Trial 2	Whiplash	21	8/13	35.50 (10.5)	n/a	6 m	8.1 (1.6)	8.6 (2.4)		Di Stefano, et al (1995)
CVLT Trial 2	Whiplash w/ continuing sx	21	8/13	35.40 (11.0)	n/a	6 m	7.0 (1.9)	7.6 (1.7)		Di Stefano, et al (1995)
CVLT Trial 2 (% of 16)	Control	11	9/2	31.60 (5.00)	n/a	6 m	71.0 (8.0)	74.4 (15.4)		Di Stefano, et al (1996)
CVLT Trial 2 (% of 16)	Whiplash	58	26/32	29.60 (8.90)	n/a	6 m	65.9 (14.9)	78.2 (16.5)		Di Stefano, et al (1996)
CVLT Trial 2 (% of 16)	Whiplash w/ continuing sx	28	9/19	34.10 (10.2)	n/a	6 m	64.7 (15.7)	73.4 (15.9)		Di Stefano, et al (1996)
CVLT Trial 3	Control	21	21/0	31.45 (5.53)	n/a	18 m	13.70 (2.03)	13.70 (1.81)		Saykin, et al (1991)
CVLT Trial 3	Control	30	26/4	29.90 (6.20)	RAVLT admin first	2-4 h	NR	11.8 (2.2)		Crossen, et al (1994)
CVLT Trial 3	Epilepsy	40	23/17	32.20 (8.20)	n/a	~9 m	9.67 (2.16)	10.33 (2.56)		Hermann, et al (1996)
CVLT Trial 3	HIV+/ARC	8	8/0	33.57 (6.35)	n/a	18 m	12.29 (1.50)	11.57 (2.07)		Saykin, et al (1991)

instrument	group	n	m/f	age	intervention	inter	t #1	t #2	note	citation
CVLT Trial 3	HIV+/PGL	13	13/0	31.15 (4.91)	n/a	18 m	13.08 (1.85)	13.08 (1.80)		Saykin, et al (1991)
CVLT Trial 3	Whiplash	21	8/13	35.50 (10.5)	n/a	6 m	9.0 (1.5)	10.0 (1.5)		Di Stefano, et al (1995)
CVLT Trial 3	Whiplash w/ continuing sx	21	8/13	35.40 (11.0)	n/a	6 m	8.4 (1.7)	8.5 (2.0)		Di Stefano, et al (1995)
CVLT Trial 3 (% of 16)	Control	11	9/2	31.60 (5.00)	n/a	6 m	73.3 (10.7)	86.4 (11.8)		Di Stefano, et al (1996)
CVLT Trial 3 (% of 16)	Whiplash	58	26/32	29.60 (8.90)	n/a	6 m	75.1 (14.4)	84.8 (14.7)		Di Stefano, et al (1996)
CVLT Trial 3 (% of 16)	Whiplash w/ continuing sx	28	9/19	34.10 (10.2)	n/a	6 m	76.1 (12.6)	80.4 (15.8)		Di Stefano, et al (1996)
CVLT Trial 4	Control	21	21/0	31.45 (5.53)	n/a	18 m	14.40 (1.73)	14.35 (1.69)		Saykin, et al (1991)
CVLT Trial 4	Control	30	26/4	29.90 (6.20)	RAVLT admin first	2-4 h	NR	12.5 (2.0)		Crossen, et al (1994)
CVLT Trial 4	Epilepsy	40	23/17	32.20 (8.20)	n/a	~9 m	10.88 (2.14)	11.20 (2.73)		Hermann, et al (1996)
CVLT Trial 4	HIV+/ARC	8	8/0	33.57 (6.35)	n/a	18 m	12.29 (1.25)	11.57 (1.72)		Saykin, et al (1991)
CVLT Trial 4	HIV+/PGL	13	13/0	31.15 (4.91)	n/a	18 m	13.69 (1.38)	13.46 (1.98)		Saykin, et al (1991)
CVLT Trial 4	Whiplash	21	8/13	35.50 (10.5)	n/a	6 m	9.5 (1.2)	10.6 (1.7)		Di Stefano, et al (1995)
CVLT Trial 4	Whiplash w/ continuing sx	21	8/13	35.40 (11.0)	n/a	6 m	8.6 (1.8)	9.1 (1.6)		Di Stefano, et al (1995)

instrument	group	n	m/f	age	intervention	inter	t #1	t #2	note	citation
CVLT Trial 4 (% of 16)	Control	11	9/2	31.60 (5.00)	n/a	6 m	81.3 (6.3)	90.9 (6.5)		Di Stefano, et al (1996)
CVLT Trial 4 (% of 16)	Whiplash	58	26/32	29.60 (8.90)	n/a	6 m	82 (12.7)	88.6 (12.5)		Di Stefano, et al (1996)
CVLT Trial 4 (% of 16)	Whiplash w/ continuing sx	28	9/19	34.10 (10.2)	n/a	6 m	77 (14.5)	84.6 (14.4)		Di Stefano, et al (1996)
CVLT Trial 5	Control	151	63/88	69.63 (6.46)	n/a	15.8 m	11.07 (2.49)	11.36 (2.45)		Paolo, et al (1997)
CVLT Trial 5	Control	30	26/4	29.90 (6.20)	RAVLT admin first	2-4 h	NR	12.9 (1.8)		Crossen, et al (1994)
CVLT Trial 5	Control	21	21/0	31.45 (5.53)	n/a	18 m	14.20 (1.51)	14.40 (1.73)		Saykin, et al (1991)
CVLT Trial 5	Control	41	10/31	38.60 (20.2)	n/a	8 d	13.1 (2.1)	13 (2.7)	AF, CB	Delis, et al (1991)
CVLT Trial 5	Control	17	n/a	~39.0	n/a	12 m	13.35	14.06		Hanly, et al (1994)
CVLT Trial 5	Epilepsy	40	23/17	32.20 (8.20)	n/a	~9 m	11.27 (2.51)	11.88 (2.76)		Hermann, et al (1996)
CVLT Trial 5	Epilepsy	26	10/16	29.20 (7.80)	LTL	6 m	9.27 (2.86)	9.27 (2.52)		Hermann, et al (1992)
CVLT Trial 5	Epilepsy	31	13/18	32.90 (11.6)	RTL	6 m	11.39 (1.82)	11.65 (2.18)		Hermann, et al (1992)
CVLT Trial 5	HIV+ (asx)	25	n/a	38.20 (9.30)	n/a	15.8d	12.1 (2.4)	13.0 (2.6)	*	Duff, et al (1999)
CVLT Trial 5	HIV+ (sx)	18	n/a	37.80 (7.30)	n/a	15.8d	10.8 (2.5)	12.9 (2.1)	*	Duff, et al (1999)

instrument	group	n	m/f	age	intervention	inter	t #1	t #2	note	citation
CVLT Trial 5	HIV+/ARC	8	8/0	33.57 (6.35)	n/a	18 m	14.29 (1.60)	12.86 (1.68)		Saykin, et al (1991)
CVLT Trial 5	HIV+/PGL	13	13/0	31.15 (4.91)	n/a	18 m	14.23 (1.36)	13.62 (1.98)		Saykin, et al (1991)
CVLT Trial 5	HIV- ("At-Risk")	26	n/a	37.60 (11.2)	n/a	15.8d	13.0 (2.2)	14.5 (1.8)	*	Duff, et al (1999)
CVLT Trial 5	Rheumatoid Arthritis	11	n/a	~39.0	n/a	12 m	12.64	12.91		Hanly, et al (1994)
CVLT Trial 5	SLE	59	n/a	39.60 (1.30)	n/a	12 m	13.25	13.76		Hanly, et al (1994)
CVLT Trial 5	Whiplash	21	8/13	35.50 (10.5)	n/a	6 m	10.3 (1.4)	10.9 (1.3)		Di Stefano, et al (1995)
CVLT Trial 5	Whiplash w/ continuing sx	21	8/13	35.40 (11.0)	n/a	6 m	9.4 (1.8)	9.5 (1.7)		Di Stefano, et al (1995)
CVLT Trial 5 (% of 16)	Control	11	9/2	31.60 (5.00)	n/a	6 m	84.1 (6.5)	96 (4.2)		Di Stefano, et al (1996)
CVLT Trial 5 (% of 16)	Whiplash	58	26/32	29.60 (8.90)	n/a	6 m	85.5 (13.4)	91.2 (11.3)		Di Stefano, et al (1996)
CVLT Trial 5 (% of 16)	Whiplash w/ continuing sx	28	9/19	34.10 (10.2)	n/a	6 m	81.5 (13.7)	87.1 (13.9)		Di Stefano, et al (1996)

Table 13. Cambridge Automated Neuropsychological Test Assessment Battery (CANTAB)

instrument	group	n	m/f	age	intervention	inter	t #1	t #2	note	citation
CANTAB Choice RT	Control	16	n/a	46.00 (3.10)	n/a	1 m	625.0 (64.0)	614.0 (73.0)		Jalan, et al (1995)
CANTAB Choice RT	Variceal Hemorr	29	19/10	54.30 (5.60)	TIPSS	1 m	836.0 (168.0)	840.0 (223.0)	*	Jalan, et al (1995)
CANTAB Choice RT	Variceal Hemorr & Cirrhosis	12	7/5	53.10 (7.10)	variceal band ligation	1 m	865.0 (245.0)	878.0 (221.0)	*	Jalan, et al (1995)
CANTAB Complex RT	Control	10	8/2	31.10 (7.50)	flumazenil	1 w	571.8 (57.1)	582.6 (89.1)		Gooday, et al (1995)
CANTAB Complex RT	Control	10	8/2	31.10 (7.50)	saline	1 w	571.8 (86.7)	567 (87.4)		Gooday, et al (1995)
CANTAB Complex RT	Liver Disease	10	8/2	53.90 (7.40)	saline	1 w	748.5 (106)	842.6 (291.3)		Gooday, et al (1995)
CANTAB Complex RT	Liver Disease	10	8/2	53.90 (7.40)	flumazenil	1 w	762.3 (162.3)	733.5 (139.5)		Gooday, et al (1995)
CANTAB DMtS	Control	16	n/a	46.00 (3.10)	n/a	1 m	35.8 (2.5)	36.7 (3.8)		Jalan, et al (1995)
CANTAB DMtS	Variceal Hemorr	29	19/10	54.30 (5.60)	TIPSS	1 m	32.9 (4.2)	31.8 (3.6)	*	Jalan, et al (1995)

instrument	group	n	m/f	age	intervention	inter	t #1	t #2	note	citation
CANTAB DMtS	Variceal Hemorr & Cirrhosis	12	7/5	53.10 (7.10)	variceal band ligation	1 m	30.1 (5.1)	30.9 (6.0)	*	Jalan, et al (1995)
CANTAB Simple RT	Control	10	8/2	31.10 (7.50)	saline	1 w	503.3 (69.7)	521.9 (78.5)		Gooday, et al (1995)
CANTAB Simple RT	Control	10	8/2	31.10 (7.50)	flumazenil	1 w	515.5 (63.5)	526.7 (100.7)		Gooday et al (1995)
CANTAB Simple RT	Control	16	n/a	46.00 (3.10)	n/a	1 m	586.0 (83.0)	584.0 (83.0)		Jalan, et al (1995)
CANTAB Simple RT	Liver Disease	10	8/2	53.90 (7.40)	flumazenil	1 w	834.8 (269.9)	700 (141.1)		Gooday, et al (1995)
CANTAB Simple RT	Liver Disease	10	8/2	53.90 (7.40)	saline	1 w	770 (232.9)	760.2 (122.4)		Gooday, et al (1995)
CANTAB Simple RT	Variceal Hemorr	29	19/10	54.30 (5.60)	TIPSS	1 m	885.0 (256.0)	824.0 (282.0)	*	Jalan, et al (1995)
CANTAB Simple RT	Variceal Hemorr & Cirrhosis	12	7/5	53.10 (7.10)	variceal band ligation	1 m	861.0 (257.0)	872.0 (229.0)	*	Jalan, et al (1995)

Table 14. Cancellation Tests

instrument	group	n	m/f	age	intervention	inter	t #1	t #2	note	citation
B-W DCT (error/rows)	Control	21	3/18	30.10 (8.20)	n/a	6 m	0.55 (0.36)	0.3 (0.27)		Pulliainen, et al (1994)
B-W DCT (error/rows)	Epilepsy	23	11/12	26.80 (13.20)	carbamaz	6 m	0.41 (0.35)	0.33 (0.31)		Pulliainen, et al (1994)
B-W DCT (error/rows)	Epilepsy	20	9/11	31.50 (11.30)	phenytoin	6 m	0.49 (0.52)	0.44 (0.47)		Pulliainen, et al (1994)
B-W DCT (errors)	Control	21	3/18	30.10 (8.20)	n/a	6 m	20.3 (15.4)	11.9 (12)		Pulliainen, et al (1994)
B-W DCT (errors)	Epilepsy	23	11/12	26.80 (13.20)	carbamaz	6 m	14.3 (13.4)	11.9 (12.4)		Pulliainen, et al (1994)
B-W DCT (errors)	Epilepsy	20	9/11	31.50 (11.30)	phenytoin	6 m	16.9 (17.8)	15.6 (16.3)		Pulliainen, et al (1994)
B-W DCT (rows)	Control	21	3/18	30.10 (8.20)	n/a	6 m	36.0 (4.8)	37.8 (5.3)		Pulliainen, et al (1994)
B-W DCT (rows)	Epilepsy	23	11/12	26.80 (13.20)	carbamaz	6 m	33.7 (4.6)	34.2 (4.7)		Pulliainen, et al (1994)
B-W DCT (rows)	Epilepsy	20	9/11	31.50 (11.30)	phenytoin	6 m	34.5 (6.5)	35.8 (6.2)		Pulliainen, et al (1994)
Bourdon-Vos (time/line)	Control	63	8/55	56.22 (11.00)	n/a	~6 m	NR	-0.7 (0.9)c		Bruggemans, et al (1997)

instrument	group	n	m/f	age	intervention	inter	t #1	t #2	note	citation
cancell task	Control (mental work)	34	n/a	51.20	n/a	4 y	556.0	9% c		Suvanto, et al (1991)
cancell task	Control (physical work)	28	n/a	51.20	n/a	4 y	456.0	-4% c		Suvanto, et al (1991)
cancell task	Control (mental/ physical)	21	n/a	51.20	n/a	4 y	429.0	-5% c		Suvanto, et al (1991)
cancell task (omiss)	DAT	13	n/a	60.00 - 80.00	acetyl levocarnitine	6 m	4.2 (7.5)	3.1 (7.5)		Sano, et al (1992)
cancell task (omiss)	DAT	14	n/a	60.00 - 80.00	placebo	6 m	4.3 (7.7)	4.3 (5.9)		Sano, et al (1992)
cancell task (sec)	DAT	13	n/a	60.00 - 80.00	acetyl levocarnitine	6 m	227.8 (73.6)	235.0 (85.8)		Sano, et al (1992)
cancell task (sec)	DAT	14	n/a	60.00 - 80.00	placebo	6 m	233.8 (80.6)	299.2 (110.3)		Sano, et al (1992)
cancell task - designs	Control	15	8/7	41.00 (12.00)	n/a	29 d	47.0 (8.0)	49.5 (8.0)		Trichard, et al (1995)
cancell task - designs	Major Depression	23	12/11	47.00 (14.00)	n/a	29 d	38.0 (10.0)	40.5 (12.0)		Trichard, et al (1995)
cancell task - digits (comiss)	Control	216	106/ 110	7.91 (0.47)	n/a	2-3 y	0.07 (0.35)	0.22 (2.81)		Rebok, et al (1997)
cancell task - digits (time)	Control	216	106/ 110	7.91 (0.47)	n/a	2-3 y	73.3 (19.08)	55.77 (14.34)		Rebok, et al (1997)
cancell task - digits (omiss)	Control	216	106/ 110	7.91 (0.47)	n/a	2-3 y	3.5 (3.11)	2.32 (1.99)		Rebok, et al (1997)

instrument	group	n	m/f	age	intervention	inter	t #1	t #2	note	citation
cancell task - digits (correct)	Epilepsy	38	21/17	34.26 (9.18)	vigabatrin 3 g	18 w	147.45 (49.20)	141.58 (55.39)		Dodrill, et al (1995)
cancell task - digits (correct)	Epilepsy	32	17/15	33.72 (9.66)	vigabatrin 6 g	18 w	163.58 (53.18)	150.48 (43.03)		Dodrill, et al (1995)
cancell task - digits (correct)	Epilepsy	40	14/26	33.88 (9.77)	placebo	18 w	140.82 (48.77)	175.44 (59.18)		Dodrill, et al (1995)
cancell task - digits (correct)	Epilepsy	36	17/19	34.89 (8.38)	vigabatrin 1 g	18 w	153.06 (53.18)	161.94 (59.19)		Dodrill, et al (1995)
cancell task - digits (hits)[50]	DAT	34	16/18	62.76 (6.30)	n/a	7.72 m	19.98 (10.94)	17.49 (10.94)		Della Sala, et al (1992)
cancell task - digits (omiss)	Epilepsy	40	14/26	33.88 (9.77)	placebo	18 w	3.54 (3.69)	2.67 (4.02)		Dodrill, et al (1995)
cancell task - digits (omiss)	Epilepsy	36	17/19	34.89 (8.38)	vigabatrin 1 g	18 w	4.50 (5.39)	2.86 (4.33)		Dodrill, et al (1995)
cancell task - digits (omiss)	Epilepsy	38	21/17	34.26 (9.18)	vigabatrin 3 g	18 w	2.79 (4.10)	4.16 (4.77)		Dodrill, et al (1995)
cancell task - digits (omiss)	Epilepsy	32	17/15	33.72 (9.66)	vigabatrin 6 g	18 w	3.94 (9.43)	9.58 (21.22)		Dodrill, et al (1995)
cancell task - letters	Control	10	n/a	27.00	trazadone 100 mg	2 h	465.2	481.9		Curran, et al (1988)
cancell task - letters	Control	10	n/a	27.00	viloxazine 200 mg	2 h	449.7	473.0		Curran, et al (1988)
cancell task - letters	Control	10	n/a	27.00	trazadone 200 mg	2 h	588.9	539.3		Curran, et al (1988)
cancell task - letters	Control	10	n/a	27.00	protriptyline 10 mg	2 h	451.0	511.4		Curran, et al (1988)

instrument	group	n	m/f	age	intervention	inter	t #1	t #2	note	citation
cancell task - letters	Control	10	n/a	27.00	placebo	2 h	510.8	511.5		Curran, et al (1988)
cancell task - letters	Control	10	n/a	27.00	viloxazine 100 mg	2 h	490.3	529.3		Curran, et al (1988)
cancell task - letters	Control	10	n/a	27.00	protriptyline 20 mg	2 h	439.3	535.9		Curran, et al (1988)
cancell task - letters	Control	10	n/a	27.00	amitriptyline 75 mg	2 h	465.2	389.2		Curran, et al (1988)
cancell task - letters	Control	10	n/a	27.00	amitriptyline 37.5 mg	2 h	439.0	488.9		Curran, et al (1988)
cancell task - letters	Control	20	0/20	29.10 (4.70)	n/a	1 m	132.0 (32.1)	126.4 (26.0	*	Harris, et al (1996)
cancell task - letters	Pregnant	20	0/20	29.00 (4.60)	normal delivery	1 m	141.0 (30.5)	139.7 (29.8)	*	Harris, et al (1996)
cancell task - letters (correct)	Control	8	8/0	24.00	metoprolol	3 w	NR	7.0 c		Brooks, et al (1988)
cancell task - letters (correct)	Control	8	8/0	24.00	propranolol	3 w	NR	8.0 c		Brooks, et al (1988)
cancell task - letters (correct)	Control	8	8/0	24.00	atenolol	3 w	NR	2.5 c		Brooks, et al (1988)
cancell task - letters (correct)	Control	8	8/0	24.00	placebo	3 w	NR	4.5 c		Brooks, et al (1988)
cancell task - letters (omiss)	Control	8	8/0	24.00	atenolol	3 w	NR	-0.5 c		Brooks, et al (1988)
cancell task - letters (omiss)	Control	8	8/0	24.00	placebo	3 w	NR	-0.5 c		Brooks, et al (1988)

instrument	group	n	m/f	age	intervention	inter	t #1	t #2	note	citation
cancell task - letters (omiss)	Control	8	8/0	24.00	propranolol	3 w	NR	-5.0 c		Brooks, et al (1988)
cancell task - letters (omiss)	Control	8	8/0	24.00	metoprolol	3 w	NR	-3.0 c		Brooks, et al (1988)
cancell task I	TBI	42	40/2	33.20 (11.20)	n/a	9 m	114.1 (85.44)	76.6 (55.3)		Mukundan, et al (1987)
cancell task II	TBI	42	40/2	33.20 (11.20)	n/a	9 m	435.8 (216.3)	265.41 (29.1)		Mukundan, et al (1987)
Letter Triad Cancell (omiss)	IVDU	16	13/3	39.50	n/a	10.4 d	1.13 (2.53)	1.25 (2.52)		Richards, et al (1992)
Letter Triad Cancell (time)	IVDU	16	13/3	39.50	n/a	10.4 d	58.62 (18.72)	56.75 (17.92)		Richards, et al (1992)
Mesulam Cancell Test – Designs (omiss)	Psychotic	15	n/a	38.00 (13.00)	unmedicated	36.0 d	3.0 (0.8)	2.9 (0.6)		Tomer, et al (1989)
Mesulam Cancell Test - Letters (omiss)	Psychotic	15	n/a	38.00 (13.00)	unmedicated	36.0 d	5.8 (1.2)	5.1 (1.1)		Tomer, et al (1989)
Shape Cancell (omiss)	IVDU	16	13/3	39.50	n/a	10.4 d	2.19 (2.17)	2.38 (1.78)		Richards, et al (1992)
Shape Cancell (time)	IVDU	16	13/3	39.50	n/a	10.4 d	48.0 (10.03)	46.62 (13.77)		Richards, et al (1992)

Table 15. Category Test

instrument	group	n	m/f	age	intervention	inter	t #1	t #2	note	citation
Booklet Category Test	Control	21	21/0	31.45 (5.53)	n/a	18 m	22.90 (11.43)	14.75 (7.09)		Saykin, et al (1991)
Booklet Category Test	HIV+/ARC	8	8/0	33.57 (6.35)	n/a	18 m	42.71 (21.56)	34.57 (19.71)		Saykin, et al (1991)
Booklet Category Test	HIV+/PGL	13	13/0	31.15 (4.91)	n/a	18 m	34.85 (26.78)	21.00 (10.42)		Saykin, et al (1991)
Category Test	Alcoholic	4	4/0	48.75	min alcohol use	18.75 m	83.5	50.2		Johnson-Greene, et al (1997)
Category Test	Alcoholic	2	2/0	48.50	excessive alcohol use	18.5 m	32.5	26.0		Johnson-Greene, et al (1997)
Category Test	Alcoholic (1 yr abstin)	23	23/0	36.80 (6.30)	n/a	1 y	36.3	33.1		Adams, et al (1980)
Category Test	Alcoholic (2.5 yrs abstin)	25	25/0	36.50 (6.30)	n/a	1 y	34.9	22.8		Adams, et al (1980)
Category Test	Alcoholic (detoxed)	17	n/a	44.47	abstin	1 y	63.29 (32.5)	40.12 (24.8)		Long, et al (1974)
Category Test	Alcoholic Inpts	91	91/0	42.20 (10.00)	n/a	16.8 d	75.2 (28)	50.3 (27.1)		Eckardt, et al (1981)
Category Test	Alcoholic Inpts	91	91/0	42.20 (10.00)	n/a	12-22 d	75.2 (28.0)	49.9 (27.0)		Eckardt, et al (1979)

instrument	group	n	m/f	age	intervention	inter	t #1	t #2	note	citation
Category Test	Alcoholic Inpts	27	27/0	50.40 (6.22)	n/a	14 m	52.9 (26.11)	-9.4 (31.1)c		Schau, et al (1980)
Category Test	CAD	20	n/a	57.20 (7.20)	CE	6 m	85.7	74.6		Parker, et al (1983)
Category Test	CAD	17	n/a	57.20 (7.20)	n/a	6 m	86.2	76.6		Parker, et al (1983)
Category Test	CAD	17	n/a	57.90 (8.40)	n/a	6 m	82.9	76.7	*	Parker, et al (1986)
Category Test	CAD	36	n./a	61.10 (8.30)	CE	6 m	84.6	75.4	*	Parker, et al (1986)
Category Test	CVD	17	15/2	62.00	CE	20w	76.27 (33.07)	70.13 (23.41)		Matarazzo, et al (1979)
Category Test	CVD	16	n/a	60.00	n/a	12w	82.38 (18.16)	83.63 (17.09)		Matarazzo, et al (1979)
Category Test	Control	21	21/0	36.90 (5.90)	n/a	1 y	36.4	26.0		Adams, et al (1980)
Category Test	Control	23	9/14	32.30 (10.30)	n/a	3 w	46.7 (25.3)	23.8 (19.0)		Bornstein, et al (1987)
Category Test	Control	102	65/37	24.52	n/a	12 m	23.0	13.0	*	Dikmen, et al (1990)
Category Test	Control	9	4/5	53.10 (7.30)	n/a	5.8 y	32.0 (16.1)	35.9 (14.5)		Elias, et al (1989)
Category Test	Control	18	8/10	48.50 (10.10)	n/a	5.6 y	35.3 (21.9)	35.5 (22.1)		Elias, et al (1989)
Category Test	Control	102	~69/33	~26.00	n/a	12 m	23.0	13.0		Fraser, et al (1988)

instrument	group	n	m/f	age	intervention	inter	t #1	t #2	note	citation
Category Test	Control	29	29/0	24.00	n/a	20w	22.83 (19.15)	11.21 (9.32)		Matarazzo, et al (1979)
Category Test	Control	27	27/0	49.50	n/a	14 m	35.2 (18.7)	-5.8 (16.9) c		Schau, et al (1980)
Category Test	Control	174	174/0	24.00 - 85.00	n/a	2 y	45.33	32.01	*	Schludermann, et al (1983)
Category Test	Control	86	86/0	24.00 - 85.00	n/a	2 y	48.24	31.28	*	Schludermann, et al (1983)
Category Test	Depression	33	14/19	37.40	antidepress	7 w	72.7 (32.6)	51.3 (35.8)		Fromm, et al (1984)
Category Test	Epilepsy	17	7/10	27.44 (6.04)	meds	6-12 m	61.71 (30.69)	51.59 (33.36)	*	Dodrill, et al (1975)
Category Test	Epilepsy	21	n/a	22.30 (7.60)	improved WAIS on re-test	20.5 m	66.4 (27.0)	49.6 (26.7)		Seidenberg, et al (1981)
Category Test	Epilepsy	19	n/a	20.30 (4.30)	min. improved WAIS on re-test	20.1 m	63.2 (29.8)	49.5 (35.3)		Seidenberg, et al (1981)
Category Test	Epilepsy	18	n/a	20.30 (5.40)	stable WAIS on re-test	21.6 m	73.2 (25.1)	58.8 (23.3)		Seidenberg, et al (1981)
Category Test	Epilepsy (sz continued)	26	n/a	~21.00	n/a	20.7 m	70.96 (27.26)	55.62 (32.17)		Seidenberg, et al (1981)
Category Test	Epilepsy (sz remitted)	24	n/a	~21.00	n/a	20.7 m	64.12 (29.39)	49.54 (27.15)		Seidenberg, et al (1981)
Category Test	HIV+ (IVDU)	18	10/8	29.80 (5.40)	drug tx	17.7 m	49.1 (18.9)	40.1 (21.8)		Hestad, et al (1996)
Category Test	HIV- (IVDU)	30	16/14	27.90 (4.90)	drug tx	14.9 m	47.0 (18.4)	36.2 (20.3)		Hestad, et al (1996)

instrument	group	n	m/f	age	intervention	inter	t #1	t #2	note	citation
Category Test	Hypertension	19	8/11	46.80 (9.60)	n/a	5.6 y	44.7 (24.3)	38.0 (23.7)		Elias, et al (1989)
Category Test	Hypertension	10	6/4	52.20 (3.10)	n/a	5.7 y	53.6 (27.6)	45.7 (27.0)		Elias, et al (1989)
Category Test	Medical Inpts	20	20/0	45.60 (11.10)	n/a	22.9 d	72.6 (26.8)	21.6 (12.4)		Eckardt, et al (1981)
Category Test	Medical Inpts	20	20/0	45.60 (11.10)	n/a	12-22 d	72.6 (26.8)	52.2 (31.1)		Eckardt, et al (1979)
Category Test	Neurology/ Rehab Inpts	23	23/0	n/a	n/a	1-2 d	98.87 (37.13)	82.04 (39.08)		Choca, et al (1992)
Category Test	Neurology/ Rehab Inpts	23	23/0	n/a	n/a	1-2 d	88.39 (34.78)	81.57 (48.83)		Choca, et al (1992)
Category Test	Psychiatric Inpts	231	83/ 148	30.70	ECT	4 - 5 w	78.25 (31.0)	68.8 (34.3)		Malloy, et al (1982)
Category Test	Schizophrenia	15	10/5	35.00	neuroleptics	~15 m	43.4 (14.2)	42.5 (15.5)		Goldberg, et al (1993)
Category Test	Schizophrenia (chronic)	35	n/a	47.00	n/a	52 w	81.83 (25.61)	60.14 (28.12)		Matarazzo, et al (1979)
Category Test	Spinal Cord Injury	67	54/13	32.00 (14.70)	n/a	38 w	61.38 (31.01)	45.46 (27.61)		Richards, et al (1988)
Category Test	Substance Abuse	15	8/7	21.10 (4.50)	outpt tx	4 w	65.9 (33.8)	48.1 (19.4)		Cosgrove, et al (1991)
Category Test	Substance Abuse (PCP)	15	8/7	21.10 (4.50)	outpt tx	4 w	71.8 (26.7)	51.0 (30.2)		Cosgrove, et al (1991)
Category Test	Surgical	17	n/a	57.20 (7.20)	surgery	6 m	66.8	48.0		Parker, et al (1983)

instrument	group	n	m/f	age	intervention	inter	t #1	t #2	note	citation
Category Test	Surgical	26	n/a	55.30 (6.80)	surgery (non-CE)	6 m	65.3	50.6	*	Parker, et al (1986)
Category Test	TBI	31	20/11	24.16	n/a	12 m	108.0	25.0	*	Dikmen, et al (1990)
Category Test	TBI	27	23/4	24.62	n/a	12 m	43.51	33.78		Dikmen, et al (1983)
Category Test	TBI (did not return to work)	13	3/10	24.00	n/a	12 m	76.0	24.0		Fraser, et al (1988)
Category Test	TBI (did return to work)	35	26/9	29.00	n/a	12 m	46.0	21.0		Fraser, et al (1988)
Category Test	TBI (in litigation)	20	14/6	41.85 (10.19)	n/a	14.45 m	65.80 (27.13)	80.20 (33.57)		Reitan, et al (1996)
Category Test	TBI (not in litigation)	20	17/3	29.65 (14.91)	n/a	12.00 m	45.95 (27.88)	35.90 (27.45)		Reitan, et al (1996)
Category Test	TBI (sev)	15	13/2	24.80	n/a	11.5 m	89.3	55.1		Drudge, et al (1984)
Category Test (error ratio)	Depression w/ Melancholia	7	5/2	9.50	tricyclic antidepress	3 - 6 m	0.38 (0.15)	0.28 (0.12)		Stanton, et al (1981)
Category Test (error ratio)	Depression w/o Melancholia	4	4/2	11.00	tricyclic antidepress	3 - 6 m	0.31 (0.29)	0.29 (0.31)		Stanton, et al (1981)
Category Test (Imp Rating)	Control	10	n/a	48.60 (8.20)	n/a	5.6 y	0.70 (0.67)	0.70 (0.67)	*	Elias, et al (1986)
Category Test (Imp Rating)	Hypertension	11	n/a	51.20 (4.50)	n/a	5.7 y	1.45 (1.29)	1.36 (1.03)	*	Elias, et al (1986)

instrument	group	n	m/f	age	intervention	inter	t #1	t #2	note	citation
Category Test (short form [80])	LD	35	n/a	10.00	n/a	15 y	59.8 (25.3)	23.3 (14.4)		Sarazin, et al (1986)
Category Test (short form [80])	LD (brain damage)	67	n/a	10.00	n/a	15 y	65.7 (19.1)	28.7 (13.6)		Sarazin, et al (1986)
Category Test (short form [80])	LD (min brain dysfunction)	73	n/a	10.00	n/a	15 y	55.4 (21.0)	32.4 (14.4)		Sarazin, et al (1986)
Category Test (short form)	Alcoholic	16	16/0	37.50 (11.10)	inpt tx	3-4 w	43.4 (8.3)	35.9 (12.4)		Unkenstein, et al (1991)
Category Test (short form)	Cardiac	135	120/ 15	55.40	CABG	3 m	32.9	24.1	*	Klonoff, et al (1989)
Category Test I	Psychiatric Inpts	231	83/ 148	30.70	ECT	4 - 5 w	0.2 (0.6)	0.1 (0.3)		Malloy, et al (1982)
Category Test II	Psychiatric Inpts	231	83/ 148	30.70	ECT	4 - 5 w	1.0 (1.6)	0.6 (1.0)		Malloy, et al (1982)
Category Test III	Psychiatric Inpts	231	83/ 148	30.70	ECT	4 - 5 w	20.6 (11.3)	18.6 (12.5)		Malloy, et al (1982)
Category Test IV	Psychiatric Inpts	231	83/ 148	30.70	ECT	4 - 5 w	19.1 (10.9)	15.4 (12.0)		Malloy, et al (1982)
Category Test V	Psychiatric Inpts	231	83/ 148	30.70	ECT	4 - 5 w	18.0 (7.2)	16.3 (7.1)		Malloy, et al (1982)
Category Test VI	Psychiatric Inpts	231	83/ 148	30.70	ECT	4 - 5 w	13.4 (7.7)	12.1 (7.5)		Malloy, et al (1982)

instrument	group	n	m/f	age	intervention	inter	t #1	t #2	note	citation
Category Test VII	Psychiatric Inpts	231	83/148	30.70	ECT	4 - 5 w	6.4 (3.5)	5.8 (3.4)		Malloy, et al (1982)

Table 16. Cognitive Drug Research Test (CDRT)

instrument	group	n	m/f	age	intervention	inter	t #1	t #2	note	citation
CDRT Delay Word Recog	DAT	102	40/62	74.70 (9.00)	cycloserine 15 mg	26 w	0.279	0.295		Fakouhi, et al (1995)
CDRT Delay Word Recog	DAT	99	47/52	74.80 (7.50)	cycloserine 50 mg	26 w	0.298	0.346		Fakouhi, et al (1995)
CDRT Delay Word Recog	DAT	102	45/57	73.00 (8.10)	cycloserine 5 mg	26 w	0.360	0.270		Fakouhi, et al (1995)
CDRT Delay Word Recog	DAT	107	57/50	72.00 (7.20)	placebo	26 w	0.307	0.344		Fakouhi, et al (1995)
CDRT Face Recog	DAT	107	57/50	72.00 (7.20)	placebo	26 w	0.315	0.267		Fakouhi, et al (1995)
CDRT Face Recog	DAT	99	47/52	74.80 (7.50)	cycloserine 50 mg	26 w	0.312	0.258		Fakouhi, et al (1995)
CDRT Face Recog	DAT	102	40/62	74.70 (9.00)	cycloserine 15 mg	26 w	0.290	0.263		Fakouhi, et al (1995)
CDRT Face Recog	DAT	102	45/57	73.00 (8.10)	cycloserine 5 mg	26 w	0.293	0.257		Fakouhi, et al (1995)
CDRT Imm Word Recog	DAT	99	47/52	74.80 (7.50)	cycloserine 50 mg	26 w	0.416	0.395		Fakouhi, et al (1995)
CDRT Imm Word Recog	DAT	107	57/50	72.00 (7.20)	placebo	26 w	0.462	0.450		Fakouhi, et al (1995)

instrument	group	n	m/f	age	intervention	inter	t #1	t #2	note	citation
CDRT Imm Word Recog	DAT	102	40/62	74.70 (9.00)	cycloserine 15 mg	26 w	0.405	0.427		Fakouhi, et al (1995)
CDRT Imm Word Recog	DAT	102	45/57	73.00 (8.10)	cycloserine 5 mg	26 w	0.441	0.410		Fakouhi, et al (1995)
CDRT Memory Scanning	DAT	107	57/50	72.00 (7.20)	placebo	26 w	0.704	0.701		Fakouhi, et al (1995)
CDRT Memory Scanning	DAT	102	45/57	73.00 (8.10)	cycloserine 5 mg	26 w	0.747	0.737		Fakouhi, et al (1995)
CDRT Memory Scanning	DAT	102	40/62	74.70 (9.00)	cycloserine 15 mg	26 w	0.747	0.777		Fakouhi, et al (1995)
CDRT Memory Scanning	DAT	99	47/52	74.80 (7.50)	cycloserine 50 mg	26 w	0.737	0.722		Fakouhi, et al (1995)
CDRT Picture Recog	DAT	99	47/52	74.80 (7.50)	cycloserine 50 mg	26 w	0.469	0.376		Fakouhi, et al (1995)
CDRT Picture Recog	DAT	107	57/50	72.00 (7.20)	placebo	26 w	0.455	0.382		Fakouhi, et al (1995)
CDRT Picture Recog	DAT	102	40/62	74.70 (9.00)	cycloserine 15 mg	26 w	0.386	0.425		Fakouhi, et al (1995)
CDRT Picture Recog	DAT	102	45/57	73.00 (8.10)	cycloserine 5 mg	26 w	0.453	0.378		Fakouhi, et al (1995)

Table 17. Complex Figure Test (CFT)

instrument	group	n	m/f	age	intervention	inter	t #1	t #2	note	citation
CFT Delay	Epilepsy	14	8/6	41.20 (10.5)	sabeluzole	12 w	20.7 (4.8)	21.9 (5.6)		Aldenkamp, et al (1995)
CFT Delay	Epilepsy	19	11/8	40.00 (8.00)	placebo	12 w	15.5 (5.6)	21.5 (6.5)		Aldenkamp, et al (1995)
ROCFT	DAT/MID	30	15/15	71.70 (1.30)	oxiracetam	3 m	8.9 (1.0)	9.8 (1.0)	*	Villardita, et al (1992)
ROCFT	DAT/MID	30	21/9	67.80 (1.50)	placebo	3 m	8.4 (1.0)	8.1 (0.8)	*	Villardita, et al (1992)
ROCFT	DAT/MID	29	14/15	71.50 (1.30)	oxiracetam	6 m	9.3 (1.0)	9.1 (1.1)	*	Villardita, et al (1992)
ROCFT Copy	AIDS	10	10/0	41.70 (5.50)	n/a	6.53 m	28.9 (6.2)	27.3 (5.2)		Hinkin, et al (1995)
ROCFT Copy	Alcoholic (1 yr abstin)	23	23/0	36.80 (6.30)	n/a	1 y	34.0	32.4		Adams, et al (1980)
ROCFT Copy	Alcoholic (2.5 yrs abstin)	25	25/0	36.50 (6.30)	n/a	1 y	32.4	33.0		Adams, et al (1980)
ROCFT Copy	Boxers	20	20/0	20.50	n/a	15-18 m	34.9	35.9		Porter, et al (1996)
ROCFT Copy	Control	21	21/0	36.90 (5.90)	n/a	1 y	32.2	32.7		Adams, et al (1980)

instrument	group	n	m/f	age	intervention	inter	t #1	t #2	note	citation
ROCFT Copy	Control	42	n/a	45.80	n/a	1m	33.8 (2.1)	33.6 (2.2)	Rey/ Taylor	Delaney, et al (1992)
ROCFT Copy	Control	4	0/4	67.30	placebo	60 min	34.5 (0.58)	34.8 (2.61)	Rey/ Taylor	Kirkby, et al (1995)
ROCFT Copy	Control	5	1/4	68.40	lorazepam	60 min	34.4 (2.07)	34.4 (2.61)	Rey/ Taylor	Kirkby, et al (1995)
ROCFT Copy	Control	9	4/5	26.40	lorazepam	60 min	34.2 (1.97)	33.9 (2.8)	Rey/ Taylor	Kirkby, et al (1995)
ROCFT Copy	Control	8	4/4	21.80	placebo	60 min	34.9 (1.73)	34.9 (1.64)	Rey/ Taylor	Kirkby, et al (1995)
ROCFT Copy	Control	21	5/16	34.00	carbamaz/ phenytoin cb	1 m	34.0 (2.0)	35.0 (1.0)	*	Meador, et al (1991)
ROCFT Copy	Control	40	6/34	68.20 (1.20)	n/a	1 y	33.5 (2.9)	33.9 (2.3)	*	Mitrushina, et al (1991b)
ROCFT Copy	Control	19	2/17	62.20 (2.50)	n/a	1 y	32.8 (3.6)	32.8 (4.0)	*	Mitrushina, et al (1991b)
ROCFT Copy	Control	16	4/12	78.30 (2.50)	n/a	1 y	31.7 (5.2)	31.0 (4.6)	*	Mitrushina, et al (1991b)
ROCFT Copy	Control	47	14/33	72.90 (1.40)	n/a	1 y	32.1 (3.5)	33.0 (3.8)	*	Mitrushina, et al (1991b)
ROCFT Copy	Control	37	n/a	~6.00	n/a	~6 m	NR	2.50 c	*	Neyens, et al (1996)
ROCFT Copy	Control	20	20/0	20.50	n/a	15-18 m	35.2	36.0		Porter, et al (1996)
ROCFT Copy	Control	72	67/5	44.50 (12.4)	n/a	6 m	34.3 (4.1)	33.6 (2.1)		Prevey, et al (1996)

instrument	group	n	m/f	age	intervention	inter	t #1	t #2	note	citation
ROCFT Copy	Control	38	18/20	35.70 (10.5)	n/a	54.7 w	35.3 (1.3)	36.7 (0.9)		Tarter, et al (1990)
ROCFT Copy	Control	18	12/6	37.20 (9.70)	n/a	76.5 d	30.58 (3.27)	30.24 (4.51)		Verdoux, et al (1995)
ROCFT Copy	Crohn's Disease	22	9/13	37.30 (10.6)	std tx	62.6 w	35.5 (0.9)	35.8 (0.7)		Tarter, et al (1990)
ROCFT Copy	DAT	11	n/a	71.70 (6.40)	oxiracetam	1 m	22.2 (9.9)	21.5 (13.0)		Green, et al (1992)
ROCFT Copy	DAT	13	n/a	71.70 (6.40)	placebo	1 m	22.9 (12.4)	21.1 (12.4)		Green, et al (1992)
ROCFT Copy	Depression	33	14/19	37.40	antidepress	7 w	34.5 (2.9)	32.8 (2.4)		Fromm, et al (1984)
ROCFT Copy	elderly	41	n/a	~65.0	n/a	1 y	32.6 (2.4)	31.6 (2.8)		Berry, et al (1991)
ROCFT Copy	Epilepsy	39	36/3	44.30 (14.2)	valproate	6 m	32.5 (5.0)	32.0 (4.5)		Prevey, et al (1996)
ROCFT Copy	Epilepsy	26	24/2	43.50 (17.1)	carbamaz	6 m	33.8 (2.7)	32.8 (3.1)		Prevey, et al (1996)
ROCFT Copy	HIV+	69	51/18	34.70 (6.30)	n/a	6 m	29.8 (4.6)	28.5 (6.1)	*	Selnes, et al (1992)
ROCFT Copy	HIV-	37	27/10	35.60 (7.10)	n/a	6 m	30.4 (5.4)	30.1 (5.3)	*	Selnes, et al (1992)
ROCFT Copy	Liver Disease	62	23/39	39.20 (10.5)	liver transplant	60.1 w	34.4 (3.1)	35.1 (2.8)		Tarter, et al (1990)
ROCFT Copy	Myotonic Dystrophy	15	n/a	35.40	n/a	12 y	31.4 (4.0)	25.1 (8.9)		Tuikka, et al (1993)

instrument	group	n	m/f	age	intervention	inter	t #1	t #2	note	citation
ROCFT Copy	Schizophrenia	38	25/13	30.90 (8.73)	n/a	6 m	32.87 (5.35)	34.05 (4.32)		Addington, et al (1991)
ROCFT Copy	Schizophrenia	11	11/0	52.50 (11.5)	neuroleptic reduction	29.3 w	26.5 (7.4)	28.0 (6.6)		Seidman, et al (1993)
ROCFT Copy	Schizophrenia	18	12/6	37.90 (10.8)	n/a	84.3 d	30.08 (3.12)	30.65 (2.12)		Verdoux, et al (1995)
ROCFT Copy	Substance Abuse	15	8/7	21.10 (4.50)	outpt tx	4 w	34.5 (1.9)	34.7 (1.8)		Cosgrove, et al (1991)
ROCFT Copy	Substance Abuse (PCP)	15	8/7	21.10 (4.50)	outpt tx	4 w	32.7 (3.3)	33.3 (2.1)		Cosgrove, et al (1991)
ROCFT Delay	AIDS	10	10/0	41.70 (5.50)	n/a	6.53 m	13.4 (5.4)	14.1 (17.2)		Hinkin, et al (1995)
ROCFT Delay	Alcoholic (1 yr abstin)	23	23/0	36.80 (6.30)	n/a	1 y	19.5	19.0		Adams, et al (1980)
ROCFT Delay	Alcoholic (2.5 yrs abstin)	25	25/0	36.50 (6.30)	n/a	1 y	18.7	24.1		Adams, et al (1980)
ROCFT Delay	Boxers	20	20/0	20.50	n/a	15-18 m	22.1	23.2		Porter, et al (1996)
ROCFT Delay	Control	21	21/0	36.90 (5.90)	n/a	1 y	21.0	23.7		Adams, et al (1980)
ROCFT Delay	Control	42	n/a	45.80	n/a	1m	20.8 (8.0)	25.7 (7.2)	Rey/ Taylor	Delaney, et al (1992)
ROCFT Delay	Control	21	5/16	34.00	carbamaz/ phenytoin cb	1 m	28.0 (4.0)	29.0 (5.0)	*	Meador, et al (1991)
ROCFT Delay	Control	40	6/34	68.20 (1.20)	n/a	1 y	15.1 (7.0)	16.0 (6.0)	*	Mitrushina, et al (1991b)

instrument	group	n	m/f	age	intervention	inter	t #1	t #2	note	citation
ROCFT Delay	Control	47	14/33	72.90 (1.40)	n/a	1 y	11.3 (6.6)	14.3 (7.9)	*	Mitrushina, et al (1991b)
ROCFT Delay	Control	16	4/12	78.30 (2.50)	n/a	1 y	11.4 (5.5)	11.3 (7.7)	*	Mitrushina, et al (1991b)
ROCFT Delay	Control	19	2/17	62.20 (2.50)	n/a	1 y	13.1 (7.1)	15.8 (6.9)	*	Mitrushina, et al (1991b)
ROCFT Delay	Control	20	20/0	20.50	n/a	15-18 m	22.5	23.3		Porter, et al (1996)
ROCFT Delay	Control	72	67/5	44.50 (12.4)	n/a	6 m	21.9 (7.8)	25.7 (6.4)		Prevey, et al (1996)
ROCFT Delay	Control	38	18/20	35.70 (10.5)	n/a	54.7 w	20.0 (6.6)	24.0 (7.6)		Tarter, et al (1990)
ROCFT Delay	Control	18	12/6	37.20 (9.70)	n/a	76.5 d	17.89 (7.0)	22.53 (5.3)		Verdoux, et al (1995)
ROCFT Delay	Crohn's Disease	22	9/13	37.30 (10.6)	std tx	62.6 w	20.3 (5.5)	24.2 (5.4)		Tarter, et al (1990)
ROCFT Delay	Depression	33	14/19	37.40	antidepress	7 w	18.7 (8.7)	28.0 (13.8)		Fromm, et al (1984)
ROCFT Delay	elderly	41	n/a	~65.0	n/a	1 y	17.2 (5.1)	17.9 (5.0)		Berry, et al (1991)
ROCFT Delay	Epilepsy	12	12/0	~30.0	RTL	12 m	13.4 (4.7)	13.0 (4.0)		McGlone (1994)
ROCFT Delay	Epilepsy	13	0/13	~30.0	RTL	12 m	12.7 (4.8)	14.2 (6.7)		McGlone (1994)
ROCFT Delay	Epilepsy	7	0/7	~32.0	LTL	12 m	9.9 (5.7)	13.6 (4.0)		McGlone (1994)

instrument	group	n	m/f	age	intervention	inter	t #1	t #2	note	citation
ROCFT Delay	Epilepsy	9	9/0	~32.0	LTL	12 m	18.5 (5.2)	20.1 (5.5)		McGlone (1994)
ROCFT Delay	Epilepsy	39	36/3	44.30 (14.2)	valproate	6 m	18.6 (6.8)	22.5 (7.6)		Prevey, et al (1996)
ROCFT Delay	Epilepsy	26	24/2	43.50 (17.1)	carbamaz	6 m	18.0 (6.3)	22.4 (6.9)		Prevey, et al (1996)
ROCFT Delay	Epilepsy	12	n/a	29.20 (7.70)	LTL	1.2 y	14.2 (7.4)	14.3 (6.8)		Rausch, et al (1993)
ROCFT Delay	Epilepsy	13	n/a	29.20 (7.70)	RTL	1.2 y	15.9 (5.5)	19.0 (3.8)		Rausch, et al (1993)
ROCFT Delay	HIV+	69	51/18	34.70 (6.30)	n/a	6 m	13.4 (5.8)	14.2 (6.6)	*	Selnes, et al (1992)
ROCFT Delay	HIV-	37	27/10	35.60 (7.10)	n/a	6 m	13.3 (5.7)	15.8 (6.9)	*	Selnes, et al (1992)
ROCFT Delay	Liver Disease	62	23/39	39.20 (10.5)	liver transplant	60.1 w	18.5 (6.3)	20.8 (7.6)		Tarter, et al (1990)
ROCFT Delay	Schizophrenia	38	25/13	30.90 (8.73)	n/a	6 m	14.69 (8.47)	17.41 (8.69)		Addington, et al (1991)
ROCFT Delay	Schizophrenia	11	11/0	52.50 (11.5)	neuroleptic reduction	29.3 w	14.7 (9.4)	13.3 (9.3)		Seidman, et al (1993)
ROCFT Delay	Schizophrenia	18	12/6	37.90 (10.8)	n/a	84.3 d	13.86 (5.89)	15.73 (6.71)		Verdoux, et al (1995)
ROCFT Delay	Substance Abuse	15	8/7	21.10 (4.50)	outpt tx	4 w	22.7 (8.5)	28.1 (6.8)		Cosgrove, et al (1991)
ROCFT Delay	Substance Abuse (PCP)	15	8/7	21.10 (4.50)	outpt tx	4 w	17.7 (5.7)	26.1 (6.5)		Cosgrove, et al (1991)

instrument	group	n	m/f	age	intervention	inter	t #1	t #2	note	citation
ROCFT Delay (% ret)	Alcoholic	10	10/0	33.05 (7.09)	lorazepam	1 h	64.4	41.7	Taylor CB	Mallick, et al (1993)
ROCFT Delay (% ret)	Alcoholic	10	10/0	33.05 (7.09)	placebo	1 h	65.9	65.3	Taylor CB	Mallick, et al (1993)
ROCFT Delay (% ret)	Control	10	10/0	31.30 (6.14)	lorazepam	1 h	75.1	50.4	Taylor CB	Mallick, et al (1993)
ROCFT Delay (% ret)	Control	10	10/0	31.30 (6.14)	placebo	1 h	79.9	79.6	Taylor CB	Mallick, et al (1993)
ROCFT Delay (% ret)	Epilepsy	30	21/9	26.30 (10.8)	RTL	4 w	59.96 (16.00)	58.23 (19.6)		Powell, et al (1985)
ROCFT Delay (% ret)	Epilepsy	29	13/16	24.70 (8.30)	LTL	4 w	53.74 (20.07)	57.71 (19.4)		Powell, et al (1985)
ROCFT Delay (%ile)	Epilepsy	4	2/2	23.00	lamotrigine/ placebo	12 w	26.7	25.8	*	Banks, et al (1991)
ROCFT Delay (%ile)	Epilepsy	4	2/2	23.00	lamotrigine/ placebo	12 w	15.0	20.0	*	Banks, et al (1991)
ROCFT Delay (3')	Control	5	1/4	68.40 (6.10)	lorazepam	60 min	19.4 (4.78)	9.8 (6.06)	Rey/ Taylor	Kirkby, et al (1995)
ROCFT Delay (3')	Control	8	4/4	21.80 (4.20)	placebo	60 min	26.8 (6.71)	22.5 (8.07)	Rey/ Taylor	Kirkby, et al (1995)
ROCFT Delay (3')	Control	4	0/4	67.30 (0.50)	placebo	60 min	18.3 (5.52)	17.8 (4.99)	Rey/ Taylor	Kirkby, et al (1995)
ROCFT Delay (3')	Control	9	4/5	26.40 (7.70)	lorazepam	60 min	24.3 (3.91)	23.3 (12.6)	Rey/ Taylor	Kirkby, et al (1995)
ROCFT Imm	Control	42	n/a	45.80	n/a	1m	21.0 (7.8)	26.1 (6.4)	Rey/ Taylor	Delaney, et al (1992)

instrument	group	n	m/f	age	intervention	inter	t #1	t #2	note	citation
ROCFT Imm	Control	21	5/16	34.00	carbamaz/ phenytoin CB	1 m	28.0 (4.0)	30.0 (4.0)	*	Meador, et al (1991)
ROCFT Imm	Control	72	67/5	44.50 (12.4)	n/a	6 m	22.3 (7.7)	26.0 (6.1)		Prevey, et al (1996)
ROCFT Imm	Depression	33	14/19	37.40	antidepress	7 w	18.9 (8.7)	26.4 (7.1)		Fromm, et al (1984)
ROCFT Imm	elderly	41	n/a	~65.0	n/a	1 y	17.8 (5.1)	17.5 (5.1)		Berry, (1991)
ROCFT Imm	Epilepsy	39	36/3	44.30 (14.2)	valproate	6 m	18.9 (6.8)	23.2 (6.3)		Prevey, et al (1996)
ROCFT Imm	Epilepsy	26	24/2	43.50 (17.1)	carbamaz	6 m	17.9 (6.0)	23.4 (6.3)		Prevey, et al (1996)
ROCFT Imm	HIV+	69	51/18	34.70 (6.30)	n/a	6 m	13.1 (6.1)	14.3 (6.6)	*	Selnes, et al (1992)
ROCFT Imm	HIV-	37	27/10	35.60 (7.10)	n/a	6 m	13.3 (6.1)	15.2 (7.1)	*	Selnes, et al (1992)
ROCFT Imm	Schizophrenia	11	11/0	52.50 (11.5)	neuroleptic reduction	29.3 w	12.7 (8.2)	14.9 (9.1)		Seidman, et al (1993)
ROCFT Recall	Control	37	n/a	~6.00	n/a	~6 m	NR	2.93 c	*	Neyens, et al (1996)
ROCFT Recall/Copy	Control	37	n/a	~6.00	n/a	~6 m	NR	0.03 c	*	Neyens, et al (1996)
Taylor CFT	Control	29	n/a	~80.0	n/a	1 w	12.2 (6.2)	18.7 (6.7)		Freides, et al (1996)
Taylor CFT	Control	40	n/a	~20.0	n/a	1 w	22.1 (4.4)	29.9 (4.3)		Freides, et al (1996)

instrument	group	n	m/f	age	intervention	inter	t #1	t #2	note	citation
Taylor CFT	Control	51	n/a	~70.0	n/a	1 w	17.1 (6.0)	22.5 (6.5)		Freides, et al (1996)
Taylor CFT	Control	28	n/a	~60.0	n/a	1 w	19.1 (4.4)	24.4 (6.1)		Freides, et al (1996)

Table 18. Consortium to Establish a Registry for the Assessment of Dementia (CERAD)

instrument	group	n	m/f	age	intervention	inter	t #1	t #2	note	citation
CERAD BNT	Control	47	n/a	~68.00	n/a	1 y	14.5 (0.7)	14.7 (0.6)		Morris, et al (1989)
CERAD BNT	Control	278	89/ 189	68.10 (7.70)	n/a	1 m	14.6 (0.6)	14.7 (0.6)		Morris, et al (1989)
CERAD BNT	DAT	52	n/a	~71.00	n/a	1 y	11.6 (2.6)	10.7 (3.6)		Morris, et al (1989)
CERAD BNT	DAT	354	166/ 188	71.50 (8.00)	n/a	1 m	11.3 (3.2)	11.5 (3.3)		Morris, et al (1989)
CERAD BNT (high freq)	Control	278	89/ 189	68.10 (7.70)	n/a	1 m	5.0 (0.1)	5.0 (0.1)		Morris, et al (1989)
CERAD BNT (high freq)	DAT	354	166/ 188	71.50 (8.00)	n/a	1 m	4.7 (0.6)	4.7 (0.7)		Morris, et al (1989)
CERAD BNT (low freq)	Control	278	89/18 9	68.10 (7.70)	n/a	1 m	4.7 (0.6)	4.8 (0.4)		Morris, et al (1989)

instrument	group	n	m/f	age	intervention	inter	t #1	t #2	note	citation
CERAD BNT (low freq)	DAT	354	166/ 188	71.50 (8.00)	n/a	1 m	2.9 (1.6)	3.1 (1.6)		Morris, et al (1989)
CERAD BNT (med freq)	Control	278	89/ 189	68.10 (7.70)	n/a	1 m	4.9 (0.3)	4.9 (0.3)		Morris, et al (1989)
CERAD BNT (med freq)	DAT	354	166/ 188	71.50 (8.00)	n/a	1 m	3.7 (1.4)	3.7 (1.4)		Morris, et al (1989)
CERAD BNT [15]	Control	1017	436/ 581	74.30 (5.40)	n/a	2 y	14.2 (1.0)	14.1 (1.3)		Ganguli, et al (1996)
CERAD BNT [15]	DAT	430	198/ 232	70.90 (8.00)	n/a	1 y	11.4 (3.1)	-0.6 (2.6) c	*	Morris, et al (1993)
CERAD Construction Praxis	Control	1017	436/ 581	74.30 (5.40)	n/a	2 y	10.7 (1.3)	9.4 (1.5)		Ganguli, et al (1996)
CERAD Construction Praxis	Control	47	n/a	~68.00	n/a	1 y	10.6 (0.9)	10.3 (1.2)		Morris, et al (1989)
CERAD Construction Praxis	DAT	52	n/a	~71.00	n/a	1 y	7.6 (2.7)	6.9 (2.6)		Morris, et al (1989)
CERAD Construction Praxis	Schizophrenia	10	8/2	71.00	risperidone	4 w	7.3 (2.2)	8.6 (2.2)		Berman, et al (1996)
CERAD Construction Praxis	DAT	430	198/ 232	70.90 (8.00)	n/a	1 y	7.3 (2.7)	-0.9 (2.3) c	*	Morris, et al (1993)

instrument	group	n	m/f	age	intervention	inter	t #1	t #2	note	citation
CERAD Draw-a-Clock	Control	1017	436/581	74.30 (5.40)	n/a	2 y	7.4 (0.9)	7.1 (1.1)		Ganguli, et al (1996)
CERAD Word List (loss)	Control	1017	436/581	74.30 (5.40)	n/a	2 y	1.6 (1.4)	1.5 (1.3)		Ganguli, et al (1996)
CERAD Word List Learning	Control	1017	436/581	74.30 (5.40)	n/a	2 y	19.5 (3.7)	19.1 (4.0)		Ganguli, et al (1996)
CERAD Word List Learning	Control	278	89/189	68.10 (7.70)	n/a	1 m	21.1 (3.7)	21.4 (3.8)		Morris, et al (1989)
CERAD Word List Learning	Control	47	n/a	~68.00	n/a	1 y	20.4 (4.1)	22.3 (3.7)		Morris, et al (1989)
CERAD Word List Learning	DAT	430	198/232	70.90 (8.00)	n/a	1 y	8.0 (4.2)	-1.8 (3.1) c	*	Morris, et al (1993)
CERAD Word List Learning	DAT	354	166/188	71.50 (8.00)	n/a	1 m	7.9 (4.3)	8.6 (4.5)		Morris, et al (1989)
CERAD Word List Learning & Delayed Recall	Schizophrenia	10	8/2	71.00	risperidone	4 w	12.9 (4.7)	16.7 (6.3)		Berman, et al (1996)
CERAD Word List Recall	Control	1017	436/581	74.30 (5.40)	n/a	2 y	6.4 (2.0)	6.4 (2.0)		Ganguli, et al (1996)
CERAD Word List Recall	Control	47	n/a	~68.00	n/a	1 y	7.2 (1.9)	7.9 (1.7)		Morris, et al (1989)
CERAD Word List Recall	DAT	430	198/232	70.90 (8.00)	n/a	1 y	0.8 (1.2)	-0.3 (1.1) c	*	Morris, et al (1993)
CERAD Word List Recall	DAT	52	n/a	~71.00	n/a	1 y	0.8 (1.4)	0.4 (0.9)		Morris, et al (1989)

instrument	group	n	m/f	age	intervention	inter	t #1	t #2	note	citation
CERAD Word List Recog	Control	47	n/a	~68.00	n/a	1 y	9.4 (1.1)	9.7 (0.7)		Morris, et al (1989)
CERAD Word List Recog	DAT	430	198/ 232	70.90 (8.00)	n/a	1 y	4.4 (2.8)	-1.1 (2.9) c	*	Morris, et al (1993)
CERAD Word List Recog	DAT	52	n/a	~71.00	n/a	1 y	4.7 (2.8)	3.7 (2.5)		Morris, et al (1989)
CERAD Word List Recog (correct "no")	Control	1017	436/ 581	74.30 (5.40)	n/a	2 y	9.9 (0.4)	9.9 (0.5)		Ganguli, et al (1996)
CERAD Word List Recog (correct "yes")	Control	1017	436/ 581	74.30 (5.40)	n/a	2 y	9.5 (1.0)	9.5 (1.1)		Ganguli, et al (1996)
CERAD Word List Trial 1	Control	278	89/ 189	68.10 (7.70)	n/a	1 m	5.4 (1.6)	5.6 (1.6)		Morris, et al (1989)
CERAD Word List Trial 1	DAT	354	166/ 188	71.50 (8.00)	n/a	1 m	1.7 (1.4)	2.2 (1.5)		Morris, et al (1989)
CERAD Word List Trial 2	Control	278	89/ 189	68.10 (7.70)	n/a	1 m	7.4 (1.5)	7.5 (1.5)		Morris, et al (1989)
CERAD Word List Trial 2	DAT	354	166/ 188	71.50 (8.00)	n/a	1 m	3.0 (1.7)	3.0 (1.7)		Morris, et al (1989)
CERAD Word List Trial 3	Control	278	89/ 189	68.10 (7.70)	n/a	1 m	8.3 (1.3)	8.3 (1.4)		Morris, et al (1989)
CERAD Word List Trial 3	DAT	354	166/ 188	71.50 (8.00)	n/a	1 m	3.2 (1.8)	3.4 (1.8)		Morris, et al (1989)

Table 19. Continuous Performance Test (CPT)

instrument	group	n	m/f	age	intervention	inter	t #1	t #2	note	citation
CPT (comissions)	LD	29	24/5	10.83 (1.40)	methylphen	8 w	0.75 (0.78)	0.08 (0.79)		Gittleman-Klein, et al (1976)
CPT (comissions)	LD	32	23/9	10.67 (1.30)	placebo	8 w	1.12 (0.69)	2.3 (0.77)		Gittleman-Klein, et al (1976)
CPT (comissions)	Schizophrenia Inpts	35	29/6	23.71 (4.50)	neuroleptics	1-2 y	2.9 (3.1)	2.9 (5.0)		Nopoulos, et al (1994)
CPT (correct)	Orthopedic Injury	25	14/11	10.03 (2.00)	n/a	4 m	26.8 (14.5)	26.6 (15.9)		Chadwick, et al (1981)
CPT (correct)	TBI	25	14/11	10.12 (2.60)	n/a	4 m	13.1 (19.9)	20.7 (16.1)		Chadwick, et al (1981)
CPT (msec)	Control	76	76/0	32.20	n/a	8 h	364.9 (4.1)	359.3 (4.9)	*	Eisen, et al (1988)
CPT (omissions)	LD	32	23/9	10.67 (1.30)	placebo	8 w	0.45 (0.18)	0.37 (0.18)		Gittleman-Klein, et al (1976)
CPT (omissions)	LD	29	24/5	10.83 (1.40)	methylphen	8 w	0.33 (0.21)	0.28 (0.19)		Gittleman-Klein, et al (1976)
CPT (omissions)	Schizophrenia Inpts	35	29/6	23.71 (4.50)	neuroleptics	1-2 y	4.6 (3.5)	3.1 (2.8)		Nopoulos, et al (1994)
CPT-A	DAT/MID	30	15/15	71.70 (1.30)	oxiracetam	3 m	17.2 (0.9)	21.6 (1.0)	*	Villardita, et al (1992)
CPT-A	DAT/MID	30	21/9	67.80 (1.50)	placebo	3 m	18.5 (0.8)	17.3 (0.7)	*	Villardita, et al (1992)

instrument	group	n	m/f	age	intervention	inter	t #1	t #2	note	citation
CPT-A	DAT/MID	29	14/15	71.50 (1.30)	oxiracetam	6 m	17.0 (0.9)	19.5 (0.9)	*	Villardita, et al (1992)
CPT-A	Schizophrenia	12	10/2	28.70 (6.50)	n/a	3 y	27.8 (2.5)	27.6 (4.1)		Seidman, et al (1991)
CPT-A	Schizophrenia	10	10/0	52.00 (11.90)	neuroleptic reduction	6 m	28.2 (4.7)	28.6 (3.0)		Seidman, et al (1991)
CPT-A (comissions)	Asthma	9	n/a	6.00 - 12.00	theophylline/ placebo	2 w	1.33	0.33		Rappaport, et al (1989)
CPT-A (comissions)	Asthma	9	n/a	6.00 - 12.00	theophylline/ placebo	2 w	0.77	0.22		Rappaport, et al (1989)
CPT-A (comissions)	Asthma	8	n/a	6.00 - 12.00	placebo/ theophylline	2 w	1.5	0.62		Rappaport, et al (1989)
CPT-A (comissions)	Asthma	8	n/a	6.00 - 12.00	placebo/ theophylline	2 w	0.87	0.25		Rappaport, et al (1989)
CPT-A (comissions)	Control	216	106/ 110	7.91 (0.47)	n/a	2-3 y	19.28 (18.01)	10.06 (20.08)		Rebok, et al (1997)
CPT-A (hits)	Schizophrenia	11	11/0	52.50 (11.50)	neuroleptic reduction	29.3 w	28 (4.5)	27.0 (5.1)		Seidman, et al (1993)
CPT-A (mean RT)	Control	216	106/ 110	7.91 (0.47)	n/a	2-3 y	508.66 (70.1)	477.21 (73.93)		Rebok, et al (1997)
CPT-A (omissions)	Asthma	9	n/a	6.00 - 12.00	theophylline/ placebo	2 w	2.55	2.0		Rappaport, et al (1989)

instrument	group	n	m/f	age	intervention	inter	t #1	t #2	note	citation
CPT-A (omissions)	Asthma	9	n/a	6.00 - 12.00	theophylline/ placebo	2 w	2.44	1.77		Rappaport, et al (1989)
CPT-A (omissions)	Asthma	8	n/a	6.00 - 12.00	placebo/ theophylline	2 w	2.25	0.62		Rappaport, et al (1989)
CPT-A (omissions)	Asthma	8	n/a	6.00 - 12.00	placebo/ theophylline	2 w	1.5	1.0		Rappaport, et al (1989)
CPT-A (omissions)	Control	216	106/ 110	7.91 (0.47)	n/a	2-3 y	14.78 (11.8)	11.3 (13.09)		Rebok, et al (1997)
CPT-A (total errors)	Schizophrenia	11	11/0	52.50 (11.50)	neuroleptic reduction	29.3 w	2.4 (4.5)	2.2 (3.0)		Seidman, et al (1993)
CPT-V	DAT/MID	29	14/15	71.50 (1.30)	oxiracetam	6 m	42.1 (2.4)	40.9 (2.2)	*	Villardita, et al (1992)
CPT-V	DAT/MID	30	15/15	71.70 (1.30)	oxiracetam	3 m	42.0 (2.3)	42.8 (2.4)	*	Villardita, et al (1992)
CPT-V	DAT/MID	30	21/9	67.80 (1.50)	placebo	3 m	40.3 (2.1)	38.8 (2.2)	*	Villardita, et al (1992)
CPT-V (msec)	TBI (mild - mod)	7	7/0	25.00	CDP-choline	1 m	1527.0	1225.0		Levin (1991)
CPT-V X (comissions)	Control	216	106/ 110	7.91 (0.47)	n/a	2-3 y	4.84 (4.48)	3.91 (7.45)		Rebok, et al (1997)
CPT-V X (mean RT)	Control	216	106/ 110	7.91 (0.47)	n/a	2-3 y	615.2 (51.3)	527.45 (55.26)		Rebok, et al (1997)
CPT-V X (omissions)	Control	216	106/ 110	7.91 (0.47)	n/a	2-3 y	7.31 (6.79)	3.23 (4.28)		Rebok, et al (1997)

instrument	group	n	m/f	age	intervention	inter	t #1	t #2	note	citation
CPT-Visual (msec)	TBI (mild - mod)	7	7/0	20.00	placebo	1 m	1444.0	1108.0		Levin (1991)
NES CPT	Control	16	16/0	25.00	placebo	1 h	NR	0.92 %c	*	Golden, et al (1994)
NES CPT	Control	16	16/0	25.00	adinazolam + probenecid	1 h	NR	8.31 %c	*	Golden, et al (1994)
NES CPT	Control	16	16/0	25.00	adinazolam	1 h	NR	9.45 %c	*	Golden, et al (1994)
NES CPT	Control	16	16/0	25.00	probenecid	1 h	NR	-1.50 %c	*	Golden, et al (1994)

Table 20. Continuous Recognition Memory Test (CRMT)

instrument	group	n	m/f	age	intervention	inter	t #1	t #2	note	citation
CRMT (correct)	TBI (mild - mod)	8	4/4	14.60 (0.70)	n/a	1 y	85.0 (12.6)	90.9 (6.2)		Levin, et al (1988)
CRMT (correct)	TBI (mild - mod)	9	9/0	11.40 (1.20)	n/a	1 y	86.1 (4.9)	89.7 (9.3)		Levin, et al (1988)
CRMT (correct)	TBI (mild - mod)	10	7/3	7.80 (0.90)	n/a/	1 y	82.2 (10.0)	89.1 (7.4)		Levin, et al (1988)
CRMT (correct)	TBI (sev)	8	6/2	14.70 (0.60)	n/a	1 y	75.6 (8.0)	80.1 (7.8)		Levin, et al (1988)
CRMT (correct)	TBI (sev)	5	1/4	10.70 (1.30)	n/a	1 y	84.2 (8.3)	84.0 (10.5)		Levin, et al (1988)
CRMT (correct)	TBI (sev)	6	2/4	7.40 (0.60)	n/a	1 y	76.8 (9.7)	79.0 (10.6)		Levin, et al (1988)

instrument	group	n	m/f	age	intervention	inter	t #1	t #2	note	citation
CRMT (d')	TBI (mild - mod)	8	4/4	14.60 (0.70)	n/a	1 y	2.7 (1.0)	3.2 (1.0)		Levin, et al (1988)
CRMT (d')	TBI (mild - mod)	9	9/0	11.40 (1.20)	n/a	1 y	2.5 (0.6)	3.0 (0.8)		Levin, et al (1988)
CRMT (d')	TBI (mild - mod)	10	7/3	7.80 (0.90)	n/a/	1 y	2.4 (0.7)	2.9 (0.8)		Levin, et al (1988)
CRMT (d')	TBI (sev)	8	6/2	14.70 (0.60)	n/a	1 y	1.6 (0.7)	2.2 (0.6)		Levin, et al (1988)
CRMT (d')	TBI (sev)	5	1/4	10.70 (1.30)	n/a	1 y	2.1 (0.7)	2.3 (1.0)		Levin, et al (1988)
CRMT (d')	TBI (sev)	6	2/4	7.40 (0.60)	n/a	1 y	1.9 (0.6)	2.0 (0.8)		Levin, et al (1988)

Table 21. Corsi Blocks

instrument	group	n	m/f	age	intervention	inter	t #1	t #2	note	citation
Corsi Blocks	Control	70	26/44	29.30 (1.15)	n/a	4 y	4.92 (1.0)	4.86 (1.0)		Amato, et al (1995)
Corsi Blocks	Control	10	n/a	27.00	amitriptyline 75 mg	2 h	7.4	6.4		Curran, et al (1988)
Corsi Blocks	Control	10	n/a	27.00	amitriptyline 37.5 mg	2 h	7.7	7.3		Curran, et al (1988)
Corsi Blocks	Control	10	n/a	27.00	placebo	2 h	7.2	6.9		Curran, et al (1988)

instrument	group	n	m/f	age	intervention	inter	t #1	t #2	note	citation
Corsi Blocks	Control	10	n/a	27.00	protriptyline 20 mg	2 h	6.9	6.7		Curran, et al (1988)
Corsi Blocks	Control	10	n/a	27.00	protriptyline 10 mg	2 h	7.4	7.4		Curran, et al (1988)
Corsi Blocks	Control	10	n/a	27.00	trazadone 200 mg	2 h	7.2	6.3		Curran, et al (1988)
Corsi Blocks	Control	10	n/a	27.00	trazadone 100 mg	2 h	6.9	6.3		Curran, et al (1988)
Corsi Blocks	Control	10	n/a	27.00	viloxazine 100 mg	2 h	8.1	7.7		Curran, et al (1988)
Corsi Blocks	Control	10	n/a	27.00	viloxazine 200 mg	2 h	6.9	6.9		Curran, et al (1988)
Corsi Blocks	Control	11	9/2	31.60 (5.00)	n/a	6 m	11.5 (1.4)	11.6 (2.1)		Di Stefano, et al (1996)
Corsi Blocks	Control	21	3/18	30.10 (8.20)	n/a	6 m	5.4 (1.0)	5.4 (1.0)		Pulliainen, et al (1994)
Corsi Blocks	DAT/MID	30	15/15	71.70 (1.30)	oxiracetam	3 m	3.4 (0.5)	4.3 (0.3)	*	Villardita, et al (1992)
Corsi Blocks	DAT/MID	30	21/9	67.80 (1.50)	placebo	3 m	3.2 (0.2)	2.7 (0.2)	*	Villardita, et al (1992)
Corsi Blocks	DAT/MID	29	14/15	71.50 (1.30)	oxiracetam	6 m	2.9 (0.2)	3.8 (0.3)	*	Villardita, et al (1992)

instrument	group	n	m/f	age	intervention	inter	t #1	t #2	note	citation
Corsi Blocks	Epilepsy	20	9/11	31.50 (11.30)	phenytoin	6 m	5.2 (1.0)	5.3 (1.1)		Pulliainen, et al (1994)
Corsi Blocks	Epilepsy	23	11/12	26.80 (13.20)	carbamaz	6 m	5.0 (1.2)	5.2 (1.0)		Pulliainen, et al (1994)
Corsi Blocks	HIV+ (IVDU)	42	31/11	27.00 (5.30)	n/a	12 m	5.5 (1.1)	5.6 (1.0)		Bono, et al (1996)
Corsi Blocks	HIV+ (stage 2/3)	14	14/0	31.40 (8.54)	n/a	12.8 m	6.9 (2.4)	6.7 (2.0)		Burgess, et al (1994)
Corsi Blocks	HIV+ (stage 4)	6	6/0	36.20 (7.60)	n/a	12.8 m	6.2 (1.2)	4.8 (1.0)		Burgess, et al (1994)
Corsi Blocks	HIV-	41	41/0	31.50 (9.32)	n/a	12.8 m	7.2 (1.8)	6.6 (1.9)		Burgess, et al (1994)
Corsi Blocks	HIV- (IVDU)	39	30/9	28.60 (4.90)	n/a	12 m	5.4 (1.0)	5.6 (0.9)		Bono, et al (1996)
Corsi Blocks	MS	50	18/32	29.90 (8.48)	n/a	4 y	4.54 (1.4)	4.73 (1.6)		Amato, et al (1995)
Corsi Blocks	Whiplash	21	8/13	35.50 (10.50)	n/a	6 m	11.2 (1.3)	11.5 (1.4)	*	Di Stefano, et al (1995)
Corsi Blocks	Whiplash	58	26/32	29.60 (8.90)	n/a	6 m	11.3 (1.4)	11.9 (1.5)		Di Stefano, et al (1996)
Corsi Blocks	Whiplash (asx at 6 mos)	67	28/36	29.00 (8.50)	n/a	6 m	11.3 (1.4)	11.8 (1.5)		Radanov, et al (1993)

instrument	group	n	m/f	age	intervention	inter	t #1	t #2	note	citation
Corsi Blocks	Whiplash (sx at 6 mos)	31	9/19	36.50 (10.20)	n/a	6 m	10.8 (1.7)	11.0 (1.5)		Radanov, et al (1993)
Corsi Blocks	Whiplash w/ continuing sx	21	8/13	35.40 (11.00)	n/a	6 m	10.6 (2.0)	11.0 (1.7)	*	Di Stefano, et al (1995)
Corsi Blocks	Whiplash w/ continuing sx	28	9/19	34.10 (10.20)	n/a	6 m	10.9 (1.7)	11.3 (1.8)		Di Stefano, et al (1996)
Corsi Blocks (longest span;t)	Epilepsy	13	8/5	23.07 (8.90)	carbamaz	3 m	48.83 (8.0)	49.73 (5.8)	*	Gallassi, et al (1988)
Corsi Blocks (longest span;t)	Epilepsy	12	6/6	28.50 (7.00)	phenytoin	3 m	45.74 (6.8)	44.13 (7.5)	*	Gallassi, et al (1988)

Table 22. Design Fluency

instrument	group	n	m/f	age	intervention	inter	t #1	t #2	note	citation
Design Fluency	Control	10	0/10	22.00	hypnosis induction	~15 min	34.9 (10.6)	42.6 (12.0)		Gruzelier, et al (1993)
Design Fluency	Control (highly hypnotizable)	10	0/10	22.00	hypnosis induction	~15 min	31.4 (9.4)	36.3 (14.8)		Gruzelier, et al (1993)
Design Fluency	Schizophrenia	38	25/13	30.90(8.73)	n/a	6 m	13.15 (9.85)	26.13 (15.98)		Addington, et al (1991)
Design Fluency-Fixed	TBI (mild - mod)	7	7/0	25.00	CDP-choline	1 m	14.0	11.0		Levin (1991)

instrument	group	n	m/f	age	intervention	inter	t #1	t #2	note	citation
Design Fluency-Fixed	TBI (mild - mod)	7	7/0	20.00	placebo	1 m	13.0	20.0		Levin (1991)
Design Fluency-Free	TBI (mild - mod)	7	7/0	25.00	CDP-choline	1 m	18.0	16.0		Levin (1991)
Design Fluency-Free	TBI (mild - mod)	7	7/0	20.00	placebo	1 m	13.0	20.0		Levin (1991)

Table 23. Dichotic Listening Tests

instrument	group	n	m/f	age	intervention	inter	t #1	t #2	note	citation
dichotic digits LE (accuracy)	Schizophrenia	11	11/0	52.50 (11.5)	neuroleptic reduction	29.3 w	79.8 (15.3)	89.9 (18.4)		Seidman, et al (1993)
dichotic digits RE (accuracy)	Schizophrenia	11	11/0	52.50 (11.5)	neuroleptic reduction	29.3 w	93.1 (18.4)	95.3 (18.9)		Seidman, et al (1993)
dichotic digits Total (accuracy)	Schizophrenia	11	11/0	52.50 (11.5)	neuroleptic reduction	29.3 w	172.9 (31.2)	185.2 (35.1)		Seidman, et al (1993)
dichotic numbers LE (correct)	Control	38	18/20	35.70 (10.5)	n/a	54.7 w	31.2 (5.1)	32.0 (3.7)		Tarter, et al (1990)

instrument	group	n	m/f	age	intervention	inter	t #1	t #2	note	citation
dichotic numbers LE (correct)	Crohn's Disease	22	9/13	37.30 (10.6)	std tx	62.6 w	28.8 (5.2)	27.1 (6.4)		Tarter, et al (1990)
dichotic numbers LE (correct)	Liver Disease	62	23/39	39.20 (10.5)	liver transplant	60.1 w	25.8 (6.5)	26.8 (9.1)		Tarter, et al (1990)
dichotic numbers RE (correct)	Control	38	18/20	35.70 (10.5)	n/a	54.7 w	28.4 (6.1)	27.3 (4.9)		Tarter, et al (1990)
dichotic numbers RE (correct)	Crohn's Disease	22	9/13	37.30 (10.6)	std tx	62.6 w	27.1 (5.7)	28.2 (4.4)		Tarter, et al (1990)
dichotic numbers RE (correct)	Liver Disease	62	23/39	39.20 (10.5)	liver transplant	60.1 w	24.5 (7.0)	26.0 (7.4)		Tarter, et al (1990)

Table 24. Digit Span Tests

instrument	group	n	m/f	age	intervention	inter	t #1	t #2	note	citation
digit span	DAT	7	n/a	n/a	placebo	~35 min	2.86 (1.22)	3.19 (0.94)		Reisberg, et al (1983)
digit span	DAT	7	n/a	n/a	naloxone	~35 min	2.91 (0.85)	4.67 (0.94)		Reisberg, et al (1983)
digit span	Depression	21	n/a	n/a	fluoxetine	3 w	10.6 (1.6)	11.1 (2.0)	*	Fudge, et al (1990)

instrument	group	n	m/f	age	intervention	inter	t #1	t #2	note	citation
digit span	Depression	17	n/a	n/a	trazodone	3 w	12.2 (2.4)	11.6 (2.4)	*	Fudge, et al (1990)
digit span backward	Control	8	8/0	24.0	propranolol	3 w	NR	-1.0 c		Brooks, et al (1988)
digit span backward	Control	8	8/0	24.0	placebo	3 w	NR	0.0 c		Brooks, et al (1988)
digit span backward	Control	8	8/0	24.0	metoprolol	3 w	NR	1.0 c		Brooks, et al (1988)
digit span backward	Control	8	8/0	24.0	atenolol	3 w	NR	1.5 c		Brooks, et al (1988)
digit span backward	Control	10	8/2	31.1 (7.5)	saline	1 w	6.4 (1.4)	6.7 (1.4)		Gooday, et al (1995)
digit span backward	Control	10	8/2	31.1 (7.5)	flumazenil	1 w	6.5 (1.3)	6.0 (1.6)		Gooday, et al (1995)
digit span backward	Control	21	3/18	30.1 (8.2)	n/a	6 m	4.8 (0.8)	4.8 (0.8)		Pulliainen, et al (1994)
digit span backward	Epilepsy	23	11/12	26.8 (13.2)	carbamaz	6 m	4.9 (1.0)	4.8 (0.7)		Pulliainen, et al (1994)
digit span backward	Epilepsy	20	9/11	31.5 (11.3)	phenytoin	6 m	4.6 (0.9)	4.7 (1.0)		Pulliainen, et al (1994)
digit span backward	Liver Disease	10	8/2	53.9 (7.4)	saline	1 w	3.9 (1.5)	4.3 (1.4)		Gooday, et al (1995)
digit span backward	Liver Disease	10	8/2	53.9 (7.4)	flumazenil	1 w	4.9 (1.5)	5.0 (1.6)		Gooday, et al (1995)
digit span backward	PD	8	5/3	59.4 (8.3)	apomorphine	15 min	3.5 (0.9)	4.1 (1.8)		Ruzicka, et al (1994)

instrument	group	n	m/f	age	intervention	inter	t #1	t #2	note	citation
digit span backward	subjective memory problems	12	6/6	72.0	methylphen	45 min	3.75	3.62		Crook, et al (1977)
digit span forward	Control	8	8/0	24.0	metoprolol	3 w	NR	0.0 c		Brooks, et al (1988)
digit span forward	Control	8	8/0	24.0	placebo	3 w	NR	0.0 c		Brooks, et al (1988)
digit span forward	Control	8	8/0	24.0	propranolol	3 w	NR	0.0 c		Brooks, et al (1988)
digit span forward	Control	8	8/0	24.0	atenolol	3 w	NR	0.0 c		Brooks, et al (1988)
digit span forward	Control	10	n/a	27.0	viloxazine 200 mg	2 h	7.3	7.4		Curran, et al (1988)
digit span forward	Control	10	n/a	27.0	viloxazine 100 mg	2 h	7.9	8.0		Curran, et al (1988)
digit span forward	Control	10	n/a	27.0	trazadone 100 mg	2 h	7.6	7.4		Curran, et al (1988)
digit span forward	Control	10	n/a	27.0	protriptyline 10 mg	2 h	8.1	8.0		Curran, et al (1988)
digit span forward	Control	10	n/a	27.0	protriptyline 20 mg	2 h	7.2	6.8		Curran, et al (1988)
digit span forward	Control	10	n/a	27.0	placebo	2 h	7.2	7.5		Curran, et al (1988)

instrument	group	n	m/f	age	intervention	inter	t #1	t #2	note	citation
digit span forward	Control	10	n/a	27.0	amitriptyline 37.5 mg	2 h	8.0	8.0		Curran, et al (1988)
digit span forward	Control	10	n/a	27.0	amitriptyline 75 mg	2 h	8.1	7.3		Curran, et al (1988)
digit span forward	Control	10	n/a	27.0	trazadone 200 mg	2 h	7.7	6.9		Curran, et al (1988)
digit span forward	Control	10	8/2	31.1 (7.5)	flumazenil	1 w	7.7 (1.3)	7.9 (0.9)		Gooday, et al (1995)
digit span forward	Control	10	8/2	31.1 (7.5)	saline	1 w	7.8 (1.1)	7.7 (1.4)		Gooday, et al (1995)
digit span forward	Control	21	3/18	30.1 (8.2)	n/a	6 m	5.9 (0.7)	6.1 (0.7)		Pulliainen, et al (1994)
digit span forward	Epilepsy	23	11/12	26.8 (13.2)	carbamaz	6 m	6.0 (1.0)	6.0 (1.0)		Pulliainen, et al (1994)
digit span forward	Epilepsy	20	9/11	31.5 (11.3)	phenytoin	6 m	5.8 (1.0)	6.1 (1.2)		Pulliainen, et al (1994)
digit span forward	Liver Disease	10	8/2	53.9 (7.4)	saline	1 w	6.5 (1.3)	6.6 (1.7)		Gooday, et al (1995)
digit span forward	Liver Disease	10	8/2	53.9 (7.4)	flumazenil	1 w	6.2 (1.7)	6.4 (1.5)		Gooday, et al (1995)
digit span forward	PD	8	5/3	59.4 (8.3)	apomorphine	15 min	5.9 (0.8)	6.3 (1.0)		Ruzicka, et al (1994)
digit span forward	subjective memory problems	12	6/6	72.0	methylphen	45 min	6.00	6.00		Crook, et al (1977)

instrument	group	n	m/f	age	intervention	inter	t #1	t #2	note	citation
digit span, longest span (t)	Epilepsy	13	8/5	23.07 (8.9)	carbamaz	3 m	51.73 (8.1)	51.55 (12.7)	*	Gallassi, et al (1988)
digit span, longest span (t)	Epilepsy	12	6/6	28.5 (7.0)	phenytoin	3 m	47.24 (9.0)	44.69 (8.3)	*	Gallassi, et al (1988)
Digit-Span Supra-Span	DAT	14	n/a	53.0 - 81.0	lithium carbonate	7 d	19.3 (1.6)	17.6 (2.5)	*	Brinkman, et al (1984)
NES D Span Backward	Control	16	16/0	25.0	adinazolam + probenecid	1 h	NR	4.70 %c	*	Golden, et al (1994)
NES D Span Backward	Control	16	16/0	25.0	placebo	1 h	NR	-8.44 %c	*	Golden, et al (1994)
NES D Span Backward	Control	16	16/0	25.0	adinazolam	1 h	NR	10.8 %c	*	Golden, et al (1994)
NES D Span Backward	Control	16	16/0	25.0	probenecid	1 h	NR	-4.32 %c	*	Golden, et al (1994)
NES D Span Forward	Control	16	16/0	25.0	probenecid	1 h	NR	-0.69 %c	*	Golden, et al (1994)
NES D Span Forward	Control	16	16/0	25.0	adinazolam + probenecid	1 h	NR	6.36 %c	*	Golden, et al (1994)
NES D Span Forward	Control	16	16/0	25.0	placebo	1 h	NR	0.65 %c	*	Golden, et al (1994)
NES D Span Forward	Control	16	16/0	25.0	adinazolam	1 h	NR	2.78 %c	*	Golden, et al (1994)
RCPMB D Span	Epilepsy	36	n/a	n/a	carbamaz	3 w	10.44	10.33		Rennick, et al (1974)
Serial Digit Learning Task	Control	21	3/18	30.1 (8.2)	n/a	6 m	17.0 (3.0)	18.0 (3.9)		Pulliainen, et al (1994)

instrument	group	n	m/f	age	intervention	inter	t #1	t #2	note	citation
Serial Digit Learning Task	Epilepsy	23	11/12	26.8 (13.2)	carbamaz	6 m	13.9 (7.7)	15.5 (5.6)		Pulliainen, et al (1994)
Serial Digit Learning Task	Epilepsy	20	9/11	31.5 (11.3)	phenytoin	6 m	13.5 (7.8)	13.4 (7.9)		Pulliainen, et al (1994)
Serial Digit Learning Task (%ile)	Anorexia	18	0/18	n/a	refeeding tx	69.8 d	50.6 (31)	64.2 (32.9)		Szmukler, et al (1992)
Serial Digit Learning Task (%ile)	Control	18	0/18	n/a	n/a	108.4 d	67.3 (20.4)	74.3 (23.5)		Szmukler, et al (1992)

Table 25. Digit Symbol Tests

instrument	group	n	m/f	age	intervention	inter	t #1	t #2	note	citation
digit symbol	Control	10	n/a	27.0	viloxazine 100 mg	2 h	73.2	75.6		Curran, et al (1988)
digit symbol	Control	10	n/a	27.0	viloxazine 200 mg	2 h	70.0	71.2		Curran, et al (1988)
digit symbol	Control	10	n/a	27.0	trazadone 100 mg	2 h	66.0	64.7		Curran, et al (1988)
digit symbol	Control	10	n/a	27.0	trazadone 200 mg	2 h	68.4	61.7		Curran, et al (1988)
digit symbol	Control	10	n/a	27.0	protriptyline 10 mg	2 h	66.0	67.4		Curran, et al (1988)
digit symbol	Control	10	n/a	27.0	protriptyline 20 mg	2 h	67.4	69.9		Curran, et al (1988)

instrument	group	n	m/f	age	intervention	inter	t #1	t #2	note	citation
digit symbol	Control	10	n/a	27.0	placebo	2 h	64.8	64.9		Curran, et al (1988)
digit symbol	Control	10	n/a	27.0	amitriptyline 37.5 mg	2 h	72.0	70.7		Curran, et al (1988)
digit symbol	Control	10	n/a	27.0	amitriptyline 75 mg	2 h	64.1	56.6		Curran, et al (1988)
digit symbol	Schizophrenia	10	10/0	34.8 (8.7)	clonidine	6 w	33.4 (12.08)	34.8 (8.79)		Fields, et al (1988)
digit symbol	TIA/CVA	34	34/0	60.3	CE	8-16 d	23.87	23.71		Cushman, et al (1984)
digit symbol substitution test	DAT	7	n/a	n/a	placebo	~35 min	4.19 (6.30)	4.33 (5.38)		Reisberg, et al (1983)
digit symbol substitution test	DAT	7	n/a	n/a	naloxone	~35 min	2.43 (4.42)	8.52 (6.73)		Reisberg, et al (1983)
mD Sym (time per correct response)	Control	76	76/0	32.2	n/a	8 h	2.96 (0.08)	2.76 (0.08)	*	Eisen, et al (1988)
NES D Sym	Control	16	16/0	25.0	adinazolam + probenecid	1h	NR	11.1 %c	*	Golden, et al (1994)
NES D Sym	Control	16	16/0	25.0	adinazolam	1 h	NR	11.1 %c	*	Golden, et al (1994)
NES D Sym	Control	16	16/0	25.0	probenecid	1 h	NR	-1.13 %c	*	Golden, et al (1994)
NES D Sym	Control	16	16/0	25.0	placebo	1 h	NR	0.31 %c	*	Golden, et al (1994)
RCPMB D Sym	Alcoholic	11	8/3	50.6	abstin	4 w	38.4	46.3		Goldman, et al (1983)

instrument	group	n	m/f	age	intervention	inter	t #1	t #2	note	citation
RCPMB D Sym	Alcoholic	10	9/1	35.2	abstin	4 w	49.2	59.0		Goldman, et al (1983)
RCPMB D Sym	Alcoholic	10	7/3	25.5	abstin	4 w	49.2	53.1		Goldman, et al (1983)
RCPMB D Sym	Boxers	20	20/0	20.5	n/a	15-18 m	73.6	74.0		Porter, et al (1996)
RCPMB D Sym	Control	15	15/0	47.5	n/a	4 w	55.7	59.6		Goldman, et al (1983)
RCPMB D Sym	Control	15	9/6	26.4	n/a	4 w	60.7	69.5		Goldman, et al (1983)
RCPMB D Sym	Control	20	20/0	20.5	n/a	15-18 m	71.1	72.1		Porter, et al (1996)
RCPMB D Sym	Epilepsy	71	n/a	n/a	anticonvulsant	n/a	7.5	7.97		Clifford, et al (1976)
RCPMB D Sym	Epilepsy	36	n/a	n/a	carbamaz	3 w	8.50	8.53		Rennick, et al (1974)
symbol digit	Control	38	18/20	35.7 (10.5)	n/a	54.7 w	55.6 (8.9)	58.8 (9.6)		Tarter, et al (1990)
symbol digit	Crohn's Disease	22	9/13	37.3 (10.6)	std tx	62.6 w	54.0 (10.3)	55.6 (12.8)		Tarter, et al (1990)
symbol digit	Liver Disease	62	23/39	39.2 (10.5)	liver transplant	60.1 w	39.9 (11.0)	45.8 (9.4)		Tarter, et al (1990)

symbol digit substitution test (% correct)	Control	12	12/0	26.0	methanol	~1 h	98.7	97.9		Cook, et al (1991)
symbol digit substitution test (% correct)	Control	12	12/0	26.0	placebo	~1 h	98.1	98.3		Cook, et al (1991)
symbol digit substitution test (avg RT)	Control	12	12/0	26.0	methanol	~1 h	1.67 (0.57)	1.69 (0.53)		Cook, et al (1991)
symbol digit substitution test (avg RT)	Control	12	12/0	26.0	placebo	~1 h	1.58 (0.43)	1.68 (0.47)		Cook, et al (1991)

Table 26. Embedded Figure Tests (EFT)

instrument	group	n	m/f	age	intervention	inter	t #1	t #2	note	citation
Children's EFT (correct)	Seizure D/O	45	n/a	10.8	carbamaz	4-6 m	9.5 (5.8)	13.0 (5.8)		Schain, et al (1977)
EFT	mild Toxic Enceph	14	n/a	40.1 (6.0)	unimproved at retest	15.9 m	7.2 (2.1)	8.1 (1.1)		Morrow, et al (1991)
EFT	mild Toxic Enceph	13	n/a	36.4 (10.3)	improved at retest	18.1 m	8.0 (1.3)	7.5 (1.7)		Morrow, et al (1991)
EFT (sec)	Control	26	13/13	28.8 (8.2)	n/a	4 w	72.8 (55.5)	52.8 (53.5)		Killian, et al (1984)
EFT (sec)	Depression	6	4/2	26.3 (6.3)	std meds	4 w	48.0 (29.6)	45.7 (31.1)		Killian, et al (1984)

instrument	group	n	m/f	age	intervention	inter	t #1	t #2	note	citation
EFT (sec)	Depression	26	12/4	37.1 (12.7)	no meds	4 w	82.3 (46.4)	56.2 (49.2)		Killian, et al (1984)
EFT (sec)	Schizophrenia	34	17/17	24.3 (6.4)	d/c meds	4 w	118.2 (52.6)	96.6 (64.0)		Killian, et al (1984)
EFT (sec)	Schizophrenia	13	8/5	24.1 (3.1)	std meds	4 w	107.2 (60.5)	98.1 (66.6)		Killian, et al (1984)
EFT (time)	mild Toxic Enceph	14	n/a	40.1 (6.0)	unimproved at retest	15.9 m	12.2 (6.0)	10.5 (4.2)		Morrow, et al (1991)
EFT (time)	mild Toxic Enceph	13	n/a	36.4 (10.3)	improved at retest	18.1 m	10.4 (3.6)	6.8 (2.1)		Morrow, et al (1991)
Group EFT	Control	65	27/38	26.3	n/a	10 d	9.14 (5.39)	11.85 (5.23)		Kepner, et al (1984)
Group EFT	Control	43	2/41	20.1	n/a	imm	9.14 (4.49)	13.42 (4.58)		Kepner, et al (1984)
Group EFT	Control	75	27/48	25.4	n/a	imm	8.05 (5.38)	11.65 (5.00)		Kepner, et al (1984)

Table 27. Finger Naming Test

instrument	group	n	m/f	age	intervention	inter	t #1	t #2	note	citation
Finger Naming LH (errors)	Cardiac	90	77/13	59.0 (10.6)	CABG/CPB	8 d	1.3 (3.7)	8.5 (9.2)	*	Townes, et al (1989)
Finger Naming LH (errors)	Control	47	35/12	59.0 (9.8)	n/a	8 d	0.6 (1.6)	0.5 (1.5)	*	Townes, et al (1989)
Finger Naming LH (t)	ALL	31	16/15	8.38 (3.2)	n/a	2.0 y	48.9 (11.1)	49.8 (8.7)		Berg, et al (1983)

instrument	group	n	m/f	age	intervention	inter	t #1	t #2	note	citation
Finger Naming LH (t)	ALL w/ Somnolence	48	27/21	8.63 (3.1)	n/a	2.25 y	50.5 (10.0)	47.2 (13.2)		Berg, et al (1983)
Finger Naming RH (errors)	Cardiac	90	77/13	59.0 (10.6)	CABG/CPB	8 d	1.3 (3.6)	8.3 (9.2)	*	Townes, et al (1989)
Finger Naming RH (errors)	Control	47	35/12	59.0 (9.8)	n/a	8 d	0.8 (1.8)	0.5 (1.1)	*	Townes, et al (1989)
Finger Naming RH (t)	ALL	31	16/15	8.38 (3.2)	n/a	2.0 y	46.8 (12.2)	50.2 (9.8)		Berg, et al (1983)
Finger Naming RH (t)	ALL w/ Somnolence	48	27/21	8.6 (3.1)	n/a	2.25 y	53.2 (9.8)	52.1 (12.4)		Berg, et al (1983)

Table 28. Finger Tapping Test (FTT)

instrument	group	n	m/f	age	intervention	inter	t #1	t #2	note	citation
finger tapping	DAT	7	n/a	n/a	naloxone	~35 min	21.06 (15.11)	40.66 (16.74)		Reisberg, et al (1983)
finger tapping	DAT	7	n/a	n/a	placebo	~35 min	20.67 (16.85)	25.36 (21.88)		Reisberg, et al (1983)
finger tapping (15 sec)	Control	50	n/a	71.90 (0.90)	n/a	2 y	71.8 (2.5)	68.1 (2.5)		Flicker, et al (1993)
finger tapping (15 sec)	Control	59	37/22	68.70 (5.70)	n/a	3.4 y	73.8 (12.7)	71.8 (12.8)		Flicker, et al (1993)
finger tapping (15 sec)	DAT (advanced)	39	n/a	72.20 (1.20)	n/a	2 y	40.5 (7.1)	37.0 (8.8)		Flicker, et al (1993)
finger tapping (15 sec)	DAT (early)	47	n/a	69.80 (1.20)	n/a	2 y	64.3 (4.2)	63.1 (4.9)		Flicker, et al (1993)

instrument	group	n	m/f	age	intervention	inter	t #1	t #2	note	citation
finger tapping (20 sec)	Orthopedic Injury	25	14/11	10.03 (2.00)	n/a	4 m	72.7 (19.5)	74.4 (16.9)		Chadwick, et al (1981)
finger tapping (20 sec)	TBI	25	14/11	10.12 (2.60)	n/a	4 m	50.7 (22.7)	55.7 (20.6)		Chadwick, et al (1981)
finger tapping (t)	Epilepsy	12	6/6	28.50 (7.00)	phenytoin	3 m	46.20 (10.3)	52.27 (10.6)	*	Gallassi, et al (1988)
finger tapping (t)	Epilepsy	13	8/5	23.07 (8.90)	carbamaz	3 m	51.50 (7.4)	52.00 (7.5)	*	Gallassi, et al (1988)
finger tapping DH	Control	21	3/18	30.10 (8.20)	n/a	6 m	48.6 (4.6)	48.7 (4.5)		Pulliainen, et al (1994)
finger tapping DH	Epilepsy	20	9/11	31.50 (11.3)	phenytoin	6 m	45.8 (6.2)	45.6 (6.8)		Pulliainen, et al (1994)
finger tapping DH	Epilepsy	23	11/12	26.80 (13.2)	carbamaz	6 m	47.6 (7.3)	46.9 (7.6)		Pulliainen, et al (1994)
finger tapping DH (15 sec)	subjective memory impairment	12	6/6	72.00	methylphen	45 min	80.13	73.63		Crook, et al (1977)
finger tapping LH	Cardiac	60	35/25	44.30 (9.40)	open heart surgery	10 m	38.47 (6.19)	38.29 (6.58)		Joulasmaa, et al (1981)
finger tapping LH	Control	10	0/10	22.00	hypnosis induction	~15 min	42.4 (4.3)	43.6 (3.6)		Gruzelier, et al (1993)
finger tapping LH	Control (highly hypnotizable)	10	0/10	22.00	hypnosis induction	~15 min	43.7 (4.5)	42.7 (5.5)		Gruzelier, et al (1993)
finger tapping NDH	Control	21	3/18	30.10 (8.20)	n/a	6 m	44.5 (5.2)	46.0 (5.3)		Pulliainen, et al (1994)

instrument	group	n	m/f	age	intervention	inter	t #1	t #2	note	citation
finger tapping NDH	Epilepsy	23	11/12	26.80 (13.2)	carbamaz	6 m	41.5 (7.5)	42.2 (6.7)		Pulliainen, et al (1994)
finger tapping NDH	Epilepsy	20	9/11	31.50 (11.3)	phenytoin	6 m	40.6 (5.7)	40.5 (6.3)		Pulliainen, et al (1994)
finger tapping NDH (15 sec)	subjective memory impairment	12	6/6	72.00	methylphen	45 min	63.50	62.75		Crook, et al (1977)
finger tapping RH	Cardiac	60	35/25	44.30 (9.40)	open heart surgery	10 m	41.91 (6.85)	41.80 (7.64)		Joulasmaa, et al (1981)
finger tapping RH	Control	10	0/10	22.00	hypnosis induction	~15 min	48.1 (4.4)	49.0 (4.8)		Gruzelier, et al (1993)
finger tapping RH	Control (highly hypnotizable)	10	0/10	22.00	hypnosis induction	~15 min	47.6 (7.6)	45.7 (8.1)		Gruzelier, et al (1993)
FTT	Control	21	5/16	34.00	carbamaz/ phenytoin CB	1 m	42.0 (6.0)	43.0 (6.0)	*	Meador, et al (1991)
FTT	Control	86	86/0	24.0 - 85.0	n/a	2 y	51.32	52.19	*	Schludermann, et al (1983)
FTT	Control	174	174/0	24.0 - 85.0	n/a	2 y	51.98	51.02	*	Schludermann, et al (1983)
FTT	Control	38	18/20	35.70 (10.5)	n/a	54.7 w	90.3 (12.0)	94.2 (11.1)		Tarter, et al (1990)

instrument	group	n	m/f	age	intervention	inter	t #1	t #2	note	citation
FTT	Crohn's Disease	22	9/13	37.30 (10.6)	std tx	62.6 w	87.6 (14.0)	94.4 (13.2)		Tarter, et al (1990)
FTT	Epilepsy	19	n/a	20.30 (4.30)	slightly improved WAIS re-test	20.1 m	43.5 (5.3)	45.5 (5.4)		Seidenberg, et al (1981)
FTT	Epilepsy	21	n/a	22.30 (7.60)	improved WAIS re-test	20.5 m	39.9 (7.7)	43.3 (7.0)		Seidenberg, et al (1981)
FTT	Epilepsy	18	n/a	20.30 (5.40)	stable WAIS re-test	21.6 m	38.2 (8.0)	41.2 (6.2)		Seidenberg, et al (1981)
FTT	Epilepsy (sz continued)	26	n/a	~21.0	n/a	20.7 m	39.98 (6.92)	42.17 (6.72)		Seidenberg, et al (1981)
FTT	Epilepsy (sz remitted)	24	n/a	~21.0	n/a	20.7 m	40.68 (8.74)	43.95 (6.83)		Seidenberg, et al (1981)
FTT	HD (at risk, + genetic marker)	8	1/7	26.20 (2.70)	n/a	2 y	45.5	44.3	*	Giordani, et al (1995)
FTT	HD (at risk, - genetic marker)	8	1/7	28.40 (5.20)	n/a	2 y	45.3	46.1	*	Giordani, et al (1995)
FTT	Liver Disease	62	23/39	39.20 (10.5)	liver transplant	60.1 w	84.7 (15.8)	93.6 (14.5)		Tarter, et al (1990)
FTT	Schizophrenia	8	n/a	21.0 - 61.0	chlorpromaz	4 h	93.63	91.38		Serafetinides, et al (1973)
FTT	Schizophrenia	8	n/a	21.0 - 61.0	drug-free	4 h	58.25	52.38		Serafetinides, et al (1973)
FTT	Schizophrenia	13	n/a	21.0 - 61.0	drug-free	4 h	65.25	64.92		Serafetinides, et al (1973)

instrument	group	n	m/f	age	intervention	inter	t #1	t #2	note	citation
FTT	Schizophrenia	9	n/a	21.0 - 61.0	drug-free	4 h	63.00	61.89		Serafetinides, et al (1973)
FTT	Schizophrenia	11	n/a	21.0 - 61.0	placebo	4 h	98.00	107.00		Serafetinides, et al (1973)
FTT	Schizophrenia	11	n/a	21.0 - 61.0	drug-free	4 h	107.89	104.56		Serafetinides, et al (1973)
FTT	Schizophrenia	9	n/a	21.0 - 61.0	clopenthixol	4 h	83.11	80.78		Serafetinides, et al (1973)
FTT	Schizophrenia	13	n/a	21.0 - 61.0	haloperidol	4 h	69.42	76.00		Serafetinides, et al (1973)
FTT LH	Alcoholic (acute)	13	13/0	39.90	inpt tx	8 w	44 .0 (7.9)	47.5 (7.7)		Tarter, et al (1971)
FTT LH	Alcoholic (chronic)	13	13/0	43.80	inpt tx	8 w	39.2 (5.9)	40.4 (6.2)		Tarter, et al (1971)
FTT RH	Alcoholic (acute)	13	13/0	39.90	inpt tx	8 w	50.0 (6.4)	54.5 (9.2)		Tarter, et al (1971)
FTT RH	Alcoholic (chronic)	13	13/0	43.80	inpt tx	8 w	45.4 (10.3)	45.4 (10.3)		Tarter, et al (1971)
FTT (Imp Rating)	Control	10	n/a	48.60 (8.20)	n/a	5.6 y	1.00 (0.94)	1.30 (0.83)	*	Elias, et al (1986)
FTT (Imp Rating)	Hypertension	11	n/a	51.20 (4.50)	n/a	5.7 y	0.82 (0.75)	1.55 (0.69)	*	Elias, et al (1986)
FTT DH	Alcoholic	2	2/0	48.50	excessive alcohol use	18 5 m	49.8	50.3		Johnson-Greene, et al (1997)
FTT DH	Alcoholic	4	4/0	48.75	minimal alcohol use	18.75 m	42.8	45.6		Johnson-Greene, et al (1997)

instrument	group	n	m/f	age	intervention	inter	t #1	t #2	note	citation
FTT DH	Alcoholic (1 yr abstin)	23	23/0	36.80 (6.30)	n/a	1 y	50.9	50.4		Adams, et al (1980)
FTT DH	Alcoholic (2.5 yrs abstin)	25	25/0	36.50 (6.30)	n/a	1 y	51.9	51.9		Adams, et al (1980)
FTT DH	Alcoholic Inpts	25	25/0	44.84	n/a	4 w	49.85 (7.33)	54.70 (6.51)		Claiborn, et al (1981)
FTT DH	Alcoholic Inpts	91	91/0	42.20 (10.0)	n/a	16.8 d	44.3 (8.0)	48.5 (7.61)		Eckardt, et al (1981)
FTT DH	Alcoholic Inpts	91	91/0	42.20 (10.0)	n/a	12-22 d	44.3 (8.0)	48.6 (7.6)		Eckardt, et al (1979)
FTT DH	Brain Tumor	7	4/3	9.83	radiotherapy	11 m	5.4 (4.8)	4.3 (5.8)		Bordeaux, et al (1988)
FTT DH	Brain Tumor	7	3/4	10.33	surgery	1 m	7.2 (2.5)	8.3 (3.8)		Bordeaux, et al (1988)
FTT DH	Cardiac	22	10/12	47.30 (14.0)	open heart surgery	8.4 d	56.8 (14.6)	60.0 (7.6)	*	Heyer, et al (1995)
FTT DH	Cardiac	33	19/14	73.10 (5.50)	open heart surgery	8.4 d	53.6 (1.0)	49.5 (7.8)	*	Heyer, et al (1995)
FTT DH	Cardiac	135	120/15	55.40	CABG	3 m	46.3	48.7	*	Klonoff, et al (1989)
FTT DH	Cardiac	90	77/13	59.00 (10.6)	CABG/CPB	8 d	46.4 (7.3)	41.6 (14.0)	*	Townes, et al (1989)
FTT DH	CAD	17	n/a	57.20 (7.20)	n/a	6 m	38.4	40.8		Parker, et al (1983)
FTT DH	CAD	20	n/a	57.20 (7.20)	CE	6 m	40.9	42.3		Parker, et al (1983)

instrument	group	n	m/f	age	intervention	inter	t #1	t #2	note	citation
FTT DH	CAD	36	n./a	61.10 (8.30)	CE	6 m	41.8	42.9	*	Parker, et al (1986)
FTT DH	CAD	17	n/a	57.90 (8.40)	n/a	6 m	40.0	41.9	*	Parker, et al (1986)
FTT DH	CVD	16	n/a	60.00	n/a	12w	34.12 (5.38)	34.00 (5.10)		Matarazzo, et al (1979)
FTT DH	CVD	17	15/2	62.00	CE	20w	42.67 (8.72)	42.67 (9.32)		Matarazzo, et al (1979)
FTT DH	Control	21	21/0	36.90 (5.90)	n/a	1 y	51.3	51.8		Adams, et al (1980)
FTT DH	Control	23	9/14	32.30 (10.3)	n/a	3 w	44.8 (6.3)	43.5 (7.1)		Bornstein, et al (1987)
FTT DH	Control	25	25/0	28.68	n/a	4 w	53.87 (6.37)	54.22 (4.64)		Claiborn, et al (1981)
FTT DH	Control	102	65/37	24.52	n/a	12 m	51.0	52.0	*	Dikmen, et al (1990)
FTT DH	Control	88	55/33	24.50 (8.30)	n/a	1 y	50.24	51.04		Haaland, et al (1994)
FTT DH	Control	29	29/0	24.00	n/a	20w	54.12 (4.35)	54.2 (5.3)		Matarazzo, et al (1979)
FTT DH	Control	47	35/12	59.00 (9.81)	n/a	8 d	47.8 (7.4)	48.4 (6.4)	*	Townes, et al (1989)
FTT DH	Control (Clinic/ Volunteer)	15	5/10	33.90 (8.40)	n/a	20.7 d	49.4 (8.6)	49.6 (6.0)		Goulet Fisher, et al (1986)
FTT DH	Depression	33	14/19	37.40	antidepress	7 w	40.8 (12.2)	44.2 (9.6)		Fromm, et al (1984)

instrument	group	n	m/f	age	intervention	inter	t #1	t #2	note	citation
FTT DH	Depression	15	6/9	28.50 (10.6)	inpt tx	19.5 d	44.2 (12.1)	47.3 (10.3)		Goulet Fisher, et al (1986)
FTT DH	Epilepsy	17	7/10	27.44 (6.04)	meds	6-12 m	44.94 (6.22)	43.53 (7.91)	*	Dodrill, et al (1975)
FTT DH	HIV+	46	n/a	~33.0	n/a	7.4 m	46.0 (6.0)	48.0 (6.0)		McKegney, et al (1990)
FTT DH	HIV+	69	51/18	34.70 (6.30)	n/a	6 m	42.3 (7.8)	45.1 (6.6)	*	Selnes, et al (1992)
FTT DH	HIV+ (asx)	19	10/19	30.30	n/a	4y	47.6 (6.5)	44.1 (6.8)		Silberstein, et al (1993)
FTT DH	HIV+ (IVDU)	42	31/11	27.00 (5.30)	n/a	12 m	42.1 (7.6)	42.0 (7.4)		Bono, et al (1996)
FTT DH	HIV+ (IVDU)	8	5/3	39.00 (8.00)	MSR/placebo	7 d	51.9 (8.6)	57.2 (10.4)	*	Van Dyck, et al (1997)
FTT DH	HIV+ (sx)	21	9/12	28.50	n/a	4y	45.3 (7.8)	45.0 (7.5)		Silberstein, et al (1993)
FTT DH	HIV-	45	n/a	~33.0	n/a	7.4 m	48.0 (6.0)	47.0 (9.0)		McKegney, et al (1990)
FTT DH	HIV-	37	27/10	35.60 (7.10)	n/a	6 m	42.5 (7.5)	43.9 (7.7)	*	Selnes, et al (1992)
FTT DH	HIV-	81	45/36	29.70	n/a	4 y	48.7 (6.5)	48.0 (6.7)		Silberstein, et al (1993)

instrument	group	n	m/f	age	intervention	inter	t #1	t #2	note	citation
FTT DH	HIV- (IVDU)	39	30/9	28.60 (4.90)	n/a	12 m	43.7 (8.9)	44.1 (8.7)		Bono, et al (1996)
FTT DH	Hydroceph (control pressure)	14	9/5	66.00 (14.2)	extracranial shunting	27.37 w	25.33 (17.55)	22.0 (18.69)		Stambrook, et al (1988)
FTT DH	Hypertension	25	17/8	50.10 (14.0)	n/a	7-10 d	54.67 (11.55)	55.94 (10.50)		McCaffrey, et al (1992)
FTT DH	Left AVM	15	10/5	31.00 (11.0)	surgery	4, 8 m	53.5 (7.2)	51.4 (6.2)	*	Stabell, et al (1994)
FTT DH	Medical Inpts	20	20/0	45.60 (11.1)	n/a	22.9 d	42.1 (9.4)	43.6 (10.4)		Eckardt, et al (1981)
FTT DH	Medical Inpts	20	20/0	45.60 (11.1)	n/a	12-22 d	41.6 (9.8)	43.6 (10.4)		Eckardt, et al (1979)
FTT DH	MS & Fatigue	16	2/14	40.00 (5.60)	placebo	6 w	50.4 (7.8)	57.2 (9.5)		Geisler, et al (1996)
FTT DH	MS & Fatigue	13	4/9	41.00 (6.20)	pemoline	6 w	44.6 (11.8)	45.8 (12.6)		Geisler, et al (1996)
FTT DH	MS & Fatigue	16	4/12	40.00 (6.40)	amantadine hydrochloride	6 w	52.4 (14.5)	56.6 (14.9)		Geisler, et al (1996)
FTT DH	Psychiatric Inpts	12	12/0	40.17	n/a	4 w	44.72 (10.01)	48.78 (7.65)		Claiborn, et al (1981)
FTT DH	Right AVM	16	5/11	34.00 (13.0)	surgery	4 m	52.9 (5.8)	53.1 (5.0)	*	Stabell, et al (1994)
FTT DH	Schizophrenia (acute)	39	24/15	28.60 (8.60)	n/a	1 y	45.9 (8.5)	48.0 (8.8)		Sweeney, et al (1991)

instrument	group	n	m/f	age	intervention	inter	t #1	t #2	note	citation
FTT DH	Schizophrenia (chronic)	35	n/a	47.00	n/a	52w	40.71 (9.24)	45.37 (8.42)		Matarazzo, et al (1979)
FTT DH	Substance Abuse	15	8/7	21.10 (4.50)	outpt tx	4 w	48.9 (5.4)	47.6 (4.0)		Cosgrove, et al (1991)
FTT DH	Substance Abuse (PCP)	15	8/7	21.10 (4.50)	outpt tx	4 w	49.8 (4.3)	49.5 (4.8)		Cosgrove, et al (1991)
FTT DH	Surgical	13	11/2	74.20 (6.70)	major surgery	6 d	55.1 (9.6)	54.7 (7.6)	*	Heyer, et al (1995)
FTT DH	Surgical	17	n/a	57.20 (7.20)	surgery	6 m	44.2	46.2		Parker, et al (1983)
FTT DH	Surgical	26	n/a	55.30 (6.80)	surgery (non-CE)	6 m	45.7	45.8	*	Parker, et al (1986)
FTT DH	TBI	31	20/11	24.16	n/a	12 m	39.0	45.0	*	Dikmen, et al (1990)
FTT DH	TBI	27	23/4	24.62	n/a	12 m	48.56	48.83		Dikmen, et al (1983)
FTT DH	TBI	40	24/16	24.70 (6.40)	n/a	1 y	44.44	47.4		Haaland, et al (1994)
FTT DH	TBI	18	15/3	26.10 (8.30)	rehab	7.5 m	42.6	44.2		Prigatano, et al (1984)
FTT DH	TBI	17	15/2	23.50 (5.10)	n/a	12.6 m	36.2	36.8		Prigatano, et al (1984)
FTT DH	TBI (sev)	15	13/2	24.80	n/a	11.5 m	32.8	41.2		Drudge, et al (1984)
FTT DH (t)	ALL	31	16/15	8.38 (3.19)	n/a	2.0 y	37.6 (18.6)	32.1 (11.7)		Berg, et al (1983)
FTT DH (t)	ALL w/ Somnolence	48	27/21	8.63 (3.15)	n/a	2.25 y	50.8 (17.2)	43.5 (12.4)		Berg, et al (1983)

instrument	group	n	m/f	age	intervention	inter	t #1	t #2	note	citation
FTT DH + NDH	AIDS	10	10/0	41.70 (5.50)	n/a	6.53 m	75.5 (18.7)	82.9 (11.7)		Hinkin, et al (1995)
FTT DH Trial 1	Control	88	55/33	24.50 (8.30)	n/a	1 y	49.9 (2.6)	49.9 (2.3)		Haaland, et al (1994)
FTT DH Trial 1	TBI	40	24/16	24.70 (6.40)	n/a	1 y	43.3 (2.9)	46.9 (2.2)		Haaland, et al (1994)
FTT DH Trial 2	Control	88	55/33	24.50 (8.30)	n/a	1 y	48.8 (2.5)	50.1 (2.3)		Haaland, et al (1994)
FTT DH Trial 2	TBI	40	24/16	24.70 (6.40)	n/a	1 y	43.9 (2.6)	46.9 (2.2)		Haaland, et al (1994)
FTT DH Trial 3	Control	88	55/33	24.50 (8.30)	n/a	1 y	49.6 (2.5)	49.3 (2.3)		Haaland, et al (1994)
FTT DH Trial 3	TBI	40	24/16	24.70 (6.40)	n/a	1 y	43.4 (2.6)	46.3 (2.1)		Haaland, et al (1994)
FTT DH Trial 4	Control	88	55/33	24.50 (8.30)	n/a	1 y	52.0 (2.4)	53.2 (2.3)		Haaland, et al (1994)
FTT DH Trial 4	TBI	40	24/16	24.70 (6.40)	n/a	1 y	46.3 (2.8)	49.5 (2.2)		Haaland, et al (1994)
FTT DH Trial 5	Control	88	55/33	24.50 (8.30)	n/a	1 y	50.9 (2.3)	52.7 (2.4)		Haaland, et al (1994)
FTT DH Trial 5	TBI	40	24/16	24.70 (6.40)	n/a	1 y	45.3 (2.7)	47.4 (2.4)		Haaland, et al (1994)
FTT LH	Alcoholic (detoxed)	17	n/a	44.47	abstin	1 y	33.64 (6.13)	42.61 (4.43)		Long, et al (1974)
FTT LH	CVD	15	n/a	59.76 (3.74)	n/a	2 w	33.92 (9.45)	37.39 (7.77)		Greiffenstein, et al (1988)

instrument	group	n	m/f	age	intervention	inter	t #1	t #2	note	citation
FTT LH	CVD	15	n/a	60.00 (4.57)	LCE	2-3 m	32.92 (7.12)	34.61 (8.18)		Greiffenstein, et al (1988)
FTT LH	CVD	15	n/a	60.32 (4.02)	RCE	2-3 m	38.69 (6.12)	40.46 (6.51)		Greiffenstein, et al (1988)
FTT LH	Control	23	11/12	25.00	diphenhydram	2 d	48.0 (1.2)	46.0 (1.2)		Oken, et al (1995)
FTT LH	Control	23	11/12	25.00	methylphen	2 d	49.0 (1.1)	48.0 (1.0)		Oken, et al (1995)
FTT LH	Control	23	11/12	25.00	placebo	2 d	48.0 (1.2)	47.0 (1.1)		Oken, et al (1995)
FTT LH	Control	14	6/8	11.20	n/a	4-6 h	61.5 (13.2)	65.8 (14.9)		Reich, et al (1990)
FTT LH	Control	21	21/0	31.45 (5.53)	n/a	18 m	51.04 (4.64)	49.74 (4.12)		Saykin, et al (1991)
FTT LH	Control (mental work)	34	n/a	51.20	n/a	4 y	45.0	-3.0 %c		Suvanto, et al (1991)
FTT LH	Control (physical work)	28	n/a	51.20	n/a	4 y	43.0	-7.0 %c		Suvanto, et al (1991)
FTT LH	Control (physical/ mental)	21	n/a	51.20	n/a	4 y	43.0	-2.0 %c		Suvanto, et al (1991)
FTT LH	Diabetes	14	6/8	10.50	mild hypoglycemia	4-6 h	51.9 (9.5)	52.2 (8.0)		Reich, et al (1990)

instrument	group	n	m/f	age	intervention	inter	t #1	t #2	note	citation
FTT LH	Diabetes	10	5/5	12.20	hypoglycemia	4-6 h	59.4 (12)	61.0 (13.1)		Reich, et al (1990)
FTT LH	HIV+/ARC	8	8/0	33.57 (6.35)	n/a	18 m	44.74 (4.78)	47.54 (3.96)		Saykin, et al (1991)
FTT LH	HIV+/PGL	13	13/0	31.15 (4.91)	n/a	18 m	48.56 (6.49)	48.22 (7.95)		Saykin, et al (1991)
FTT LH	Mountain climbers	6	6/0	21.0 - 31.0	progressive decompression	~43 d	44.29 (4.79)	44.50 (6.47)		Hornbein, et al (1989)
FTT LH	Mountain climbers	35	34/1	24.0 - 45.0	Climb of 5,000- 8,000 meters	~1 m	48.91 (5.39)	46.06 (7.24)		Hornbein, et al (1989)
FTT LH	Myotonic Dystrophy	15	n/a	35.40	n/a	12 y	33.0 (5.4)	30.6 (6.9)		Tuikka, et al (1993)
FTT LH	Neuropsych referrals	248	203/ 45	8.00 (1.70)	n/a	2.65 y	25.0 (6.3)	31.3 (7.5)		Brown, et al (1989)
FTT LH	PVD	20	18/2	56.80	major surgery	10 w	49.33	50.33		Van Den Burg, et al (1985)
FTT LH	Psychiatric Inpts	231	83/ 148	30.70	ECT	4 - 5 w	38.0 (8.6)	38.5 (8.1)		Malloy, et al (1982)
FTT LH	Schizophrenia	11	11/0	52.50 (11.5)	neuroleptic reduction	29.3 w	40.5 (9.6)	42.6 (7.7)		Seidman, et al (1993)
FTT LH	Schizophrenia Inpts	35	29/6	23.71 (4.50)	neuroleptics	1-2 y	50.1 (7.4)	51.3 (9.8)		Nopoulos, et al (1994)

instrument	group	n	m/f	age	intervention	inter	t #1	t #2	note	citation
FTT LH	TIA	12	6/6	59.20 (13.3)	n/a	59.1 d	38.2 (7.4)	37.5 (8.3)		Casey, et al (1989)
FTT LH	TIA	12	6/6	63.40 (6.00)	RCE	60.7 d	41.6 (6.7)	41.1 (7.6)		Casey, et al (1989)
FTT LH	TIA	12	6/6	66.00 (5.30)	LCE	59.8 d	41.1 (5.6)	42.6 (5.7)		Casey, et al (1989)
FTT LH	TIA	20	13/7	59.60	CE	10 w	44.67	44.0		Van Den Burg, et al (1985)
FTT NDH	Alcoholic (1 yr abstin)	23	23/0	36.80 (6.30)	n/a	1 y	46.0	45.1		Adams, et al (1980)
FTT NDH	Alcoholic (2.5 yrs abstin)	25	25/0	36.50 (6.30)	n/a	1 y	47.1	48.9		Adams, et al (1980)
FTT NDH	Alcoholic Inpts	25	25/0	44.84	n/a	4 w	44.92 (6.15)	47.58 (5.29)		Claiborn, et al (1981)
FTT NDH	Alcoholic Inpts	91	91/0	42.20 (10.0)	n/a	12-22 d	40.8 (7.4)	43.7 (7.0)		Eckardt, et al (1979)
FTT NDH	Brain Tumor	7	3/4	10.33	surgery	1 m	5.6 (4.3)	7.9 (6.4)		Bordeaux, et al (1988)
FTT NDH	Brain Tumor	7	4/3	9.83	radiotherapy	11 m	8.6 (5.7)	6.8 (5.5)		Bordeaux, et al (1988)
FTT NDH	Cardiac	33	19/14	73.10 (5.50)	open heart surgery	8.4 d	49.1 (7.3)	49.3 (8.2)	*	Heyer, et al (1995)

instrument	group	n	m/f	age	intervention	inter	t #1	t #2	note	citation
FTT NDH	Cardiac	22	10/12	47.30 (14.0)	open heart surgery	8.4 d	55.6 (8.3)	55.6 (8.7)	*	Heyer, et al (1995)
FTT NDH	Cardiac	135	120/15	55.40	CABG	3 m	42.3	43.5	*	Klonoff, et al (1989)
FTT NDH	Cardiac	90	77/13	59.00 (10.6)	CABG/CPB	8 d	41.8 (6.0)	37.2 (13.8)	*	Townes, et al (1989)
FTT NDH	Control	21	21/0	36.90 (5.90)	n/a	1 y	47.4	48.2		Adams, et al (1980)
FTT NDH	Control	23	9/14	32.30 (10.3)	n/a	3 w	42.5 (6.7)	43.0 (7.1)		Bornstein, et al (1987)
FTT NDH	Control	25	25/0	28.68	n/a	4 w	47.56 (5.76)	48.56 (4.91)		Claiborn, et al (1981)
FTT NDH	Control	102	65/37	24.52	n/a	12 m	46.0	50.0	*	Dikmen, et al (1990)
FTT NDH	Control	88	55/33	24.50 (8.30)	n/a	1 y	47.06	47.7		Haaland, et al (1994)
FTT NDH	Control	47	35/12	59.00 (9.81)	n/a	8 d	43.5 (6.6)	43.1 (5.6)	*	Townes, et al (1989)
FTT NDH	Control (Clinic/ Volunteer)	15	5/10	33.90 (8.40)	n/a	20.7 d	41.2 (7.3)	44.0 (6.5)		Goulet Fisher, et al (1986)
FTT NDH	Depression	33	14/19	37.40	antidepress	7 w	36.4 (9.7)	40.1 (7.6)		Fromm, et al (1984)
FTT NDH	Depression	15	6/9	28.50 (10.6)	inpt tx	19.5 d	40.1 (11.6)	42.8 (8.7)		Goulet Fisher, et al (1986)

instrument	group	n	m/f	age	intervention	inter	t #1	t #2	note	citation
FTT NDH	HIV+	46	n/a	~33.0	n/a	7.4 m	43.0 (5.0)	45.0 (7.0)		McKegney, et al (1990)
FTT NDH	HIV+	69	51/18	34.70 (6.30)	n/a	6 m	39.4 (7.2)	40.8 (6.7)	*	Selnes, et al (1992)
FTT NDH	HIV+ (asx)	19	10/19	30.30	n/a	4y	45.8 (7.5)	42.8 (7.1)		Silberstein, et al (1993)
FTT NDH	HIV+ (IVDU)	8	5/3	39.00 (8.00)	MSR/placebo	7 d	45.9 (7.9)	52.0 (7.2)	*	Van Dyck, et al (1997)
FTT NDH	HIV+ (sx)	21	9/12	28.50	n/a	4y	41.4 (6.0)	42.3 (5.8)		Silberstein, et al (1993)
FTT NDH	HIV-	45	n/a	~33.0	n/a	7.4 m	44.0 (5.0)	44.0 (8.0)		McKegney, et al (1990)
FTT NDH	HIV-	37	27/10	35.60 (7.10)	n/a	6 m	38.5 (6.5)	40.0 (6.0)	*	Selnes, et al (1992)
FTT NDH	HIV-	81	45/36	29.70	n/a	4 y	44.8 (5.6)	44.8 (6.2)		Silberstein, et al (1993)
FTT NDH	Hydroceph (control pressure)	14	9/5	66.00 (14.2)	extracranial shunting	27.37 w	25.0 (10.86)	27.0 (12.46)		Stambrook, et al (1988)
FTT NDH	Hypertension	25	17/8	50.10 (14.0)	n/a	7-10 d	50.35 (10.95)	49.78 (10.22)		McCaffrey, et al (1992)
FTT NDH	Left AVM	15	10/5	31.00 (11.0)	surgery	4 m	49.1 (6.9)	47.5 (5.0)	*	Stabell, et al (1994)
FTT NDH	Medical Inpts	20	20/0	45.60 (11.1)	n/a	12-22 d	39.3 (9.7)	40.2 (9.3)		Eckardt, et al (1979)

instrument	group	n	m/f	age	intervention	inter	t #1	t #2	note	citation
FTT NDH	Psychiatric Inpts	12	12/0	40.17	n/a	4 w	41.23 (6.82)	43.75 (6.90)		Claiborn, et al (1981)
FTT NDH	Renal Disease	20	n/a	46.50 (11.3)	long-term hemodialysis	1 d	41.3 (7.5)	43.0 (7.5)	*	Ratner, et al (1983)
FTT NDH	Right AVM	16	5/11	34.00 (13.0)	surgery	4 m	48.8 (5.2)	48.3 (5.2)	*	Stabell, et al (1994)
FTT NDH	Schizophrenia (acute)	39	24/15	28.60 (8.60)	n/a	1 y	42.4 (7.4)	44.2 (7.6)		Sweeney, et al (1991)
FTT NDH	Surgical	13	11/2	74.20 (6.70)	major surgery	6 d	51.3 (9.5)	50.2 (5.5)	*	Heyer, et al (1995)
FTT NDH	TBI	31	20/11	24.16	n/a	12 m	36.0	42.0	*	Dikmen, et al (1990)
FTT NDH	TBI	27	23/4	24.62	n/a	12 m	42.43	45.13		Dikmen, et al (1983)
FTT NDH	TBI	40	24/16	24.70 (6.40)	n/a	1 y	41.58	43.52		Haaland, et al (1994)
FTT NDH	TBI	18	15/3	26.10 (8.30)	rehab	7.5 m	39.0	42.2		Prigatano, et al (1984)
FTT NDH	TBI	17	15/2	23.50 (5.10)	n/a	12.6 m	36.8	38.3		Prigatano, et al (1984)
FTT NDH	TBI (sev)	15	13/2	24.80	n/a	11.5 m	29.4	37.3		Drudge, et al (1984)
FTT NDH (t)	ALL	31	16/15	8.38 (3.19)	n/a	2.0 y	35.0 (21.7)	32.9 (15.0)		Berg, et al (1983)

instrument	group	n	m/f	age	intervention	inter	t #1	t #2	note	citation
FTT NDH (t)	ALL w/ Somnolence	48	27/21	8.63 (3.15)	n/a	2.25 y	50.0 (18.9)	44.8 (15.4)		Berg, et al (1983)
FTT NDH Trial 1	Control	88	55/33	24.50 (8.30)	n/a	1 y	47.4 (2.3)	47.8 (2.4)		Haaland, et al (1994)
FTT NDH Trial 1	TBI	40	24/16	24.70 (6.40)	n/a	1 y	41.2 (2.6)	43.4 (2.3)		Haaland, et al (1994)
FTT NDH Trial 2	Control	88	55/33	24.50 (8.30)	n/a	1 y	45.7 (2.3)	46.5 (2.4)		Haaland, et al (1994)
FTT NDH Trial 2	TBI	40	24/16	24.70 (6.40)	n/a	1 y	40.3 (2.7)	42.2 (2.2)		Haaland, et al (1994)
FTT NDH Trial 3	Control	88	55/33	24.50 (8.30)	n/a	1 y	46.1 (2.4)	46.5 (2.4)		Haaland, et al (1994)
FTT NDH Trial 3	TBI	40	24/16	24.70 (6.40)	n/a	1 y	41.3 (2.6)	42.7 (2.2)		Haaland, et al (1994)
FTT NDH Trial 4	Control	88	55/33	24.50 (8.30)	n/a	1 y	48.6 (2.4)	49.7 (2.3)		Haaland, et al (1994)
FTT NDH Trial 4	TBI	40	24/16	24.70 (6.40)	n/a	1 y	42.9 (2.6)	45.9 (2.3)		Haaland, et al (1994)
FTT NDH Trial 5	Control	88	55/33	24.50 (8.30)	n/a	1 y	47.5 (2.4)	48.0 (2.5)		Haaland, et al (1994)
FTT NDH Trial 5	TBI	40	24/16	24.70 (6.40)	n/a	1 y	42.2 (2.6)	43.4 (2.3)		Haaland, et al (1994)
FTT RH	Alcoholic (detoxed)	17	n/a	44.47	abstin	1 y	39.11 (6.97)	46.25 (6.85)		Long, et al (1974)

instrument	group	n	m/f	age	intervention	inter	t #1	t #2	note	citation
FTT RH	CVD	15	n/a	60.00 (4.57)	LCE	2-3 m	40.15 (7.78)	41.23 (8.41)		Greiffenstein, et al (1988)
FTT RH	CVD	15	n/a	59.76 (3.74)	n/a	2 w	38.07 (14.07)	37.84 (12.10)		Greiffenstein, et al (1988)
FTT RH	CVD	15	n/a	60.32 (4.02)	RCE	2-3 m	40.15 (7.78)	44.23 (8.15)		Greiffenstein, et al (1988)
FTT RH	Control	23	11/12	25.00	methylphen	2 d	52.0 (1.4)	52.0 (1.1)		Oken, et al (1995)
FTT RH	Control	23	11/12	25.00	placebo	2 d	52 (1.1)	52 (0.9)		Oken, et al (1995)
FTT RH	Control	23	11/12	25.00	diphenhydram	2 d	52 (1.1)	51 (1.2)		Oken, et al (1995)
FTT RH	Control	14	6/8	11.20	n/a	4-6 h	61.7 (11.6)	64 (13.2)		Reich, et al (1990)
FTT RH	Control	21	21/0	31.45 (5.53)	n/a	18 m	54.16 (4.91)	53.80 (4.74)		Saykin, et al (1991)
FTT RH	Control (mental work)	34	n/a	51.20	n/a	4 y	50.0	-3.0 %c		Suvanto, et al (1991)
FTT RH	Control (physical work)	28	n/a	51.20	n/a	4 y	47.0	-2.0 %c		Suvanto, et al (1991)
FTT RH	Control (physical/ mental work)	21	n/a	51.20	n/a	4 y	48.0	2.0 %c		Suvanto, et al (1991)
FTT RH	Diabetes	14	6/8	10.50	mild hypoglycemia	4-6 h	48.3 (13.6)	50.7 (12.9)		Reich, et al (1990)

instrument	group	n	m/f	age	intervention	inter	t #1	t #2	note	citation
FTT RH	Diabetes	10	5/5	12.20	hypoglycemia	4-6 h	65.6 (13.1)	67.8 (16.6)		Reich, et al (1990)
FTT RH	HIV+/ARC	8	8/0	33.57 (6.35)	n/a	18 m	51.06 (2.20)	51.94 (4.04)		Saykin, et al (1991)
FTT RH	HIV+/PGL	13	13/0	31.15 (4.91)	n/a	18 m	54.02 (5.43)	53.44 (6.44)		Saykin, et al (1991)
FTT RH	Mountain climbers	6	6/0	21.0 - 31.0	progressive decompression	~43 d	51.57 (2.70)	46.67 (6.53)		Hornbein, et al (1989)
FTT RH	Mountain climbers	35	34/1	24.0 - 45.0	Climb of 5,000-8,000 meters	~1 m	55.88 (4.60)	50.18 (7.75)		Hornbein, et al (1989)
FTT RH	Myotonic Dystrophy	15	n/a	35.40	n/a	12 y	35.7 (6.8)	34.1 (7.0)		Tuikka, et al (1993)
FTT RH	Neuropsych referrals	248	203/45	8.00 (1.70)	n/a	2.65 y	26.3 (6.4)	33.3 (7.5)		Brown, et al (1989)
FTT RH	PVD	20	18/2	56.80	major surgery	10 w	54.0	55.67		Van Den Burg, et al (1985)
FTT RH	Psychiatric Inpts	231	83/148	30.70	ECT	4 - 5 w	40.6 (9.1)	42.2 (8.3)		Malloy, et al (1982)
FTT RH	Schizophrenia	11	11/0	52.50 (11.5)	neuroleptic reduction	29.3 w	44.1 (10.9)	45.9 (8.8)		Seidman, et al (1993)
FTT RH	Schizophrenia Inpts	35	29/6	23.71 (4.50)	neuroleptics	1-2 y	56.4 (8.7)	56.6 (9.4)		Nopoulos, et al (1994)
FTT RH	TIA	12	6/6	63.40 (6.00)	RCE	60.7 d	42.1 (7.7)	43.2 (6.4)		Casey, et al (1989)
FTT RH	TIA	12	6/6	66.00 (5.30)	LCE	59.8 d	42.7 (7.2)	44.5 (7.0)		Casey, et al (1989)

instrument	group	n	m/f	age	intervention	inter	t #1	t #2	note	citation
FTT RH	TIA	12	6/6	59.20 (13.3)	n/a	59.1 d	43.7 (10.6)	42.4 (7.1)		Casey, et al (1989)
FTT RH	TIA	20	13/7	59.60	CE	10 w	47.67	49.0		Van Den Burg, et al (1985)
FTT RH + LH	TIA/CVA	34	34/0	60.30	CE	8-16 d	73.15	74.50		Cushman, et al (1984)
Foot Tap LF	Neuropsych referrals	248	203/45	8.00 (1.70)	n/a	2.65 y	21.5 (5.9)	26.9 (7.5)		Brown, et al (1989)
Foot Tap RF	Neuropsych referrals	248	203/45	8.00 (1.70)	n/a	2.65 y	22.8 (6.2)	28.0 (7.9)		Brown, et al (1989)
hand tapping LH	Cardiac	60	35/25	44.30 (9.40)	open heart surgery	10 m	55.31 (7.58)	54.53 (8.56)		Joulasmaa, et al (1981)
hand tapping RH	Cardiac	60	35/25	44.30 (9.40)	open heart surgery	10 m	60.47 (8.64)	59.59 (8.97)		Joulasmaa, et al (1981)

Table 29. Fingertip Number Writing Test (FNWT)

instrument	group	n	m/f	age	intervention	inter	t #1	t #2	note	citation
FNWT (errors; t)	Epilepsy	13	8/5	23.1 (8.9)	carbamaz	3 m	47.44 (7.7)	51.04 (11.9)	*	Gallassi, et al (1988)
FNWT (errors; t)	Epilepsy	12	6/6	28.5 (7.0)	phenytoin	3 m	46.61 (12.7)	49.81 (9.0)	*	Gallassi, et al (1988)
FNWT LH (errors)	Cardiac	90	77/13	59.0 (10.6)	CABG/CPB	8 d	2.7 (4.2)	10.0 (8.7)	*	Townes, et al (1989)
FNWT LH (errors)	Control	47	35/12	59.0 (9.81)	n/a	8 d	1.8 (2.6)	1.6 (2.1)	*	Townes, et al (1989)

instrument	group	n	m/f	age	intervention	inter	t #1	t #2	note	citation
FNWT LH (t)	ALL	31	16/15	8.38 (3.19)	n/a	2.0 y	50.4 (10.8)	49.9 (11.1)		Berg, et al (1983)
FNWT LH (t)	ALL w/ Somnolence	48	27/21	8.63 (3.15)	n/a	2.25 y	51.2 (8.9)	50.7 (11.6)		Berg, et al (1983)
FNWT RH (errors)	Cardiac	90	77/13	59.0 (10.6)	CABG/CPB	8 d	3.0 (4.0)	10.1 (8.5)	*	Townes, et al (1989)
FNWT RH (errors)	Control	47	35/12	59.0 (9.81)	n/a	8 d	2.4 (2.3)	1.8 (1.7)	*	Townes, et al (1989)
FNWT RH (t)	ALL	31	16/15	8.38 (3.19)	n/a	2.0 y	50.3 (10.1)	50.1 (9.9)		Berg, et al (1983)
FNWT RH (t)	ALL w/ Somnolence	48	27/21	8.63 (3.15)	n/a	2.25 y	50.1 (11.2)	51.1 (12.2)		Berg, et al (1983)

Table 30. Grip Strength

instrument	group	n	m/f	age	intervention	inter	t #1	t #2	note	citation
Grip Strength	HD (at risk, + genetic marker)	8	1/7	26.20 (2.70)	n/a	2 y	28.0	28.2	*	Giordani, et al (1995)
Grip Strength	HD (at risk, - genetic marker)	8	1/7	28.40 (5.20)	n/a	2 y	31.8	34.1	*	Giordani, et al (1995)
Grip Strength DH	Cardiac	135	120/15	55.40	CABG	3 m	44.7	43.4	*	Klonoff, et al (1989)
Grip Strength DH	CVD	16	n/a	60.00	n/a	12w	30.42 (4.76)	29.87 (4.11)		Matarazzo, et al (1979)
Grip Strength DH	CVD	17	15/2	62.00	CE	20w	35.93 (9.27)	31.2 (7.83)		Matarazzo, et al (1979)

instrument	group	n	m/f	age	intervention	inter	t #1	t #2	note	citation
Grip Strength DH	Control	23	9/14	32.30 (10.3)	n/a	3 w	35.5 (13.0)	6.6 (13.9)		Bornstein, et al (1987)
Grip Strength DH	Control	29	29/0	24.00	n/a	20w	56.84 (7.66)	55.16 (8.48)		Matarazzo, et al (1979)
Grip Strength DH	Depression	33	14/19	37.40	antidepress	7 w	31.7 (10.6)	33.8 (10.4)		Fromm, et al (1984)
Grip Strength DH	Epilepsy	17	7/10	27.44 (6.04)	meds	6-12 m	41.24 (13.43)	40.62 (15.16)	*	Dodrill, et al (1975)
Grip Strength DH	Epilepsy	21	n/a	22.30 (7.60)	improved WAIS re-test	20.5 m	30.4 (8.6)	33.2 (8.3)		Seidenberg, et al (1981)
Grip Strength DH	Epilepsy	19	n/a	20.30 (4.30)	slightly improved WAIS re-test	20.1 m	40.4 (12.2)	42.1 (11.1)		Seidenberg, et al (1981)
Grip Strength DH	Epilepsy	18	n/a	20.30 (5.40)	stable WAIS on re-test	21.6 m	33.5 (11.7)	31.7 (13.4)		Seidenberg, et al (1981)
Grip Strength DH	Epilepsy (sz continued)	26	n/a	~21.0	n/a	20.7 m	35.65 (12.65)	36.22 (12.84)		Seidenberg, et al (1981)
Grip Strength DH	Epilepsy (sz remitted)	24	n/a	~21.0	n/a	20.7 m	35.54 (11.64)	37.29 (11.01)		Seidenberg, et al (1981)
Grip Strength DH	TBI	27	23/4	24.62	n/a	12 m	47.50	54.85		Dikmen, et al (1983)
Grip Strength DH	TBI (severe)	15	13/2	24.80	n/a	11.5 m	34.0	42.9		Drudge, et al (1984)
Grip Strength LH	Alcoholic (1 yr abstin)	23	23/0	36.80 (6.30)	n/a	1 y	45.8	45.2		Adams, et al (1980)

instrument	group	n	m/f	age	intervention	inter	t #1	t #2	note	citation
Grip Strength LH	Alcoholic (2.5 yrs abstin)	25	25/0	36.50 (6.30)	n/a	1 y	52.3	53.9		Adams, et al (1980)
Grip Strength LH	Alcoholic (acute)	13	13/0	39.90	inpt tx	8 w	45.2 (10.2)	46.5 (9.9)		Tarter, et al (1971)
Grip Strength LH	Alcoholic (chronic)	13	13/0	43.80	inpt tx	8 w	42.1 (7.7)	44.8 (7.9)		Tarter, et al (1971)
Grip Strength LH	Control	21	21/0	36.90 (5.90)	n/a	1 y	54.1	54.3		Adams, et al (1980)
Grip Strength LH	Control	50	0/50	67.92 (4.89)	n/a	~3 m	22.63 (4.16)	23.48 (5.03)		Anstey, et al (1997)
Grip Strength LH	LD	35	n/a	10.00	n/a	15 y	12.0 (4.2)	35.3 (16)		Sarazin, et al (1986)
Grip Strength LH	LD (brain damage)	67	n/a	10.00	n/a	15 y	11.1 (4.9)	32.0 (13.8)		Sarazin, et al (1986)
Grip Strength LH	LD (min brain dysfunction)	73	n/a	10.00	n/a	15 y	13.4 (3.8)	35.0 (13)		Sarazin, et al (1986)
Grip Strength LH	Neuropsych referrals	248	203/45	8.00 (1.70)	n/a	2.65 y	9.3 (4.4)	14.9 (7.4)		Brown, et al (1989)
Grip Strength NDH	Cardiac	135	120/15	55.40	CABG	3 m	42.5	40.7	*	Klonoff, et al (1989)
Grip Strength NDH	CVD	16	n/a	60.00	n/a	12w	29.67 (5.8)	29.2 (4.76)		Matarazzo, et al (1979)
Grip Strength NDH	CVD	17	15/2	62.00	CE	20w	32.3 (8.89)	30.43 (6.75)		Matarazzo, et al (1979)

instrument	group	n	m/f	age	intervention	inter	t #1	t #2	note	citation
Grip Strength NDH	Control	23	9/14	32.30 (10.3)	n/a	3 w	31.4 (12.7)	33.7 (13.0)		Bornstein, et al (1987)
Grip Strength NDH	Control	29	29/0	24.00	n/a	20w	53.59 (6.14)	51.74 (7.2)		Matarazzo, et al (1979)
Grip Strength NDH	Depression	33	14/19	37.40	antidepress	7 w	29.3 (10.5)	31.5 (11.2)		Fromm, et al (1984)
Grip Strength NDH	Epilepsy	18	n/a	20.30 (5.40)	stable WAIS on re-test	21.6 m	29.0 (10.2)	30.3 (9.4)		Seidenberg, et al (1981)
Grip Strength NDH	Epilepsy	21	n/a	22.30 (7.60)	improved WAIS re-test	20.5 m	27.2 (8.8)	29.4 (9.0)		Seidenberg, et al (1981)
Grip Strength NDH	Epilepsy	19	n/a	20.30 (4.30)	slightly improved WAIS re-test	20.1 m	35.5 (14.3)	36.6 (13.3)		Seidenberg, et al (1981)
Grip Strength NDH	Epilepsy (sz continued)	26	n/a	~21.0	n/a	20.7 m	30.72 (13.84)	30.50 (12.75)		Seidenberg, et al (1981)
Grip Strength NDH	Epilepsy (sz remitted)	24	n/a	~21.0	n/a	20.7 m	31.93 (10.63)	34.84 (10.21)		Seidenberg, et al (1981)
Grip Strength NDH	TBI	27	23/4	24.62	n/a	12, 6 m	46.95	51.15		Dikmen, et al (1983)
Grip Strength NDH	TBI (sev)	15	13/2	24.80	n/a	11.5 m	26.1	38.7		Drudge, et al (1984)
Grip Strength RH	Alcoholic (1 yr abstin)	23	23/0	36.80 (6.30)	n/a	1 y	51.9	53.1		Adams, et al (1980)
Grip Strength RH	Alcoholic (2.5 yrs abstin)	25	25/0	36.50 (6.30)	n/a	1 y	57.4	57.1		Adams, et al (1980)

instrument	group	n	m/f	age	intervention	inter	t #1	t #2	note	citation
Grip Strength RH	Alcoholic (acute)	13	13/0	39.90	inpt tx	8 w	48.7 (8.3)	50.9 (8.8)		Tarter, et al (1971)
Grip Strength RH	Alcoholic (chronic)	13	13/0	43.80	inpt tx	8 w	47.5 (7.2)	50.5 (7.2)		Tarter, et al (1971)
Grip Strength RH	Control	21	21/0	36.90 (5.90)	n/a	1 y	60.6	59.2		Adams, et al (1980)
Grip Strength RH	Control	50	0/50	67.92 (4.89)	n/a	~3 m	25.52 (4.55)	26.15 (5.91)		Anstey, et al 1997)
Grip Strength RH	LD	35	n/a	10.00	n/a	15 y	13.1 (3.7)	38.0 (14.6)		Sarazin, et al (1986)
Grip Strength RH	LD (brain damage)	67	n/a	10.00	n/a	15 y	12.1 (4.5)	35.1 (14.3)		Sarazin, et al (1986)
Grip Strength RH	LD (min brain dysfunction)	73	n/a	10.00	n/a	15 y	14.0 (3.5)	35.8 (13.)		Sarazin, et al (1986)
Grip Strength RH	Neuropsych referrals	248	203/45	8.00 (1.70)	n/a	2.65 y	9.9 (4.7)	16.0 (7.9)		Brown, et al (1989)
RCPMB Grip Strength DH	Epilepsy	36	n/a	n/a	carbamaz	3 w	36.24	35.36		Rennick, et al (1974)

Table 31. Guild Memory Test (GMT)

instrument	group	n	m/f	age	intervention	inter	t #1	t #2	note	citation
GMT Design Recall	Control	59	37/22	68.70 (5.70)	n/a	3.4 y	4.6 (2.2)	5.3 (2.2)		Flicker, et al (1993)
GMT Paired Associates	Control	59	37/22	68.70 (5.70)	n/a	3.4 y	2.8 (1.7)	3.7 (2.2)		Flicker, et al (1993)

instrument	group	n	m/f	age	intervention	inter	t #1	t #2	note	citation
GMT Paragraph Delay	subjective memory impairment	12	6/6	72.00	methylphen	45 min	1.38	3.50		Crook, et al (1977)
GMT Paragraph Imm	subjective memory impairment	12	6/6	72.00	methylphen	45 min	1.75	0.12		Crook, et al (1977)
GMT Paragraph Recall	Control	59	37/22	68.70 (5.70)	n/a	3.4 y	7.9 (2.3)	8.4 (3.2)		Flicker, et al (1993)
GMT Paragraph Recall	Control	50	n/a	71.90 (0.90)	n/a	2 y	8.8 (0.6)	8.2 (0.6)		Flicker, et al (1993)
GMT Paragraph Recall	DAT (advanced)	39	n/a	72.20 (1.20)	n/a	2 y	1.1 (0.4)	0.5 (0.3)		Flicker, et al (1993)
GMT Paragraph Recall	DAT (early)	47	n/a	69.80 (1.20)	n/a	2 y	3.6 (0.4)	2.0 (0.4)		Flicker, et al (1993)

Table 32. Language Tests

instrument	group	n	m/f	age	intervention	inter	t #1	t #2	note	citation
AAT Comp	CVA	36	n/a	~68.0	placebo	12 w	NR	6.5 %c	*	Enderby, et al (1994)
AAT Comp	CVA	30	n/a	~64.0	piracetam	12 w	NR	9.8 %c	*	Enderby, et al (1994)

instrument	group	n	m/f	age	intervention	inter	t #1	t #2	note	citation
AAT Confrontation Naming	CVA	36	n/a	~68.0	placebo	12 w	NR	9.03 %c	*	Enderby, et al (1994)
AAT Confrontation Naming	CVA	30	n/a	~64.0	piracetam	12 w	NR	9.9 %c	*	Enderby, et al (1994)
AAT Repetition	CVA	30	n/a	~64.0	piracetam	12 w	NR	10.53 %c	*	Enderby, et al (1994)
AAT Repetition	CVA	36	n/a	~68.0	placebo	12 w	NR	5.64 %c	*	Enderby, et al (1994)
AAT Token Test	CVA	30	n/a	~64.0	piracetam	12 w	NR	8.6 %c	*	Enderby, et al (1994)
AAT Token Test	CVA	36	n/a	~68.0	placebo	12 w	NR	ᴼ ᴼ7 %c	*	Enderby, et al (1994)
AAT Written Language	CVA	30	n/a	~64.0	piracetam	12 w	NR	9.6 %c	*	Enderby, et al (1994)
AAT Written Language	CVA	36	n/a	~68.0	placebo	12 w	NR	4.76 %c	*	Enderby, et al (1994)
Alphabet	Control	10	5/5	40.0 - 49.0	n/a	1 d	NR	1.4 c		Peak (1970)
Alphabet	Control	10	5/5	50.0 - 59.0	n/a	1 d	NR	0.7 c		Peak (1970)
Alphabet	Control	10	5/5	70.0 - 79.0	n/a	1 d	NR	-0.1 c		Peak (1970)

instrument	group	n	m/f	age	intervention	inter	t #1	t #2	note	citation
Alphabet	Control	10	5/5	60.0 - 69.0	n/a	1 d	NR	2.9 c		Peak (1970)
Anomalous Sentences Repetition Test	Hypertension	34	n/a	76.10	captopril	24 w	10.2 (7.7)	10.4 (9.4)		Starr, et al (1996)
Anomalous Sentences Repetition Test	Hypertension	35	n/a	76.10	bendrofluazide	24 w	10.5 (9.7)	10.2 (7.6)		Starr, et al (1996)
comp of commands	Epilepsy	18	n/a	28.10 (6.70)	LTL	1 y	3.9 (0.3)	3.8 (0.4)		Loring, et al (1994)
comp of commands	Epilepsy	12	n/a	29.00 (6.40)	LTL	1 w	3.8 (0.6)	2.9 (1.3)		Loring, et al (1994)
comp of commands	Epilepsy	16	n/a	25.70 (6.40)	RTL	1 y	3.9 (0.2)	4.0 (0.0)		Loring, et al (1994)
comp of commands	Epilepsy	11	n/a	25.90 (7.00)	RTL	1 w	3.9 (0.3)	3.9 (0.3)		Loring, et al (1994)
confrontational naming	PD	20	9/11	57.90	posteroventral pallidotomy	3 m	21.5	22.0		Scott, et al (1998)
CVS	Control	25	n/a	6.50 - 12.50	n/a	3 m	48.3 (15.2)	50.7 (16.8)	*	Raven, et al (1977)
CVS	Disturbed Children	29	n/a	6.50 - 12.50	n/a	3 m	42.0 (14.7)	39.9 (15)	*	Raven, et al (1977)
descriptive naming	Epilepsy	18	n/a	28.10 (6.70)	LTL	1 y	5.4 (1.1)	5.3 (1.5)		Loring, et al (1994)

instrument	group	n	m/f	age	intervention	inter	t #1	t #2	note	citation
descriptive naming	Epilepsy	16	n/a	25.70 (6.40)	RTL	1 y	5.6 (0.9)	5.8 (0.8)		Loring, et al (1994)
descriptive naming	Epilepsy	12	n/a	29.00 (6.40)	LTL	1 w	4.9 (1.0)	2.5 (2.2)		Loring, et al (1994)
descriptive naming	Epilepsy	11	n/a	25.90 (7.00)	RTL	1 w	5.8 (0.6)	5.7 (0.6)		Loring, et al (1994)
Gorham Proverbs Test	CAD	35	23/12	62.30 (8.30)	CE	50.9 d	11.91 (3.88)	11.14 (4.25)		Kelly, et al (1980)
Gorham Proverbs Test	PVD	17	14/3	61.40 (7.90)	PVD surgery	51.5 d	12.35 (2.94)	12.59 (3.32)		Kelly, et al (1980)
MHV	Control	106	106/0	40.0 - 50.0	n/a	n/a	31.0 (9.0)	34.0 (12.2)		Raven, et al (1977)
MHV	Control	77	77/0	50.0+	n/a	n/a	31.0 (12.1)	31.0 (13.2)		Raven, et al (1977)
MHV	Control	104	104/0	30.0 - 40.0	n/a	n/a	33.0 (8.9)	33.0 (11.3)		Raven, et al (1977)
MHV	Control	263	n/a	12.50	n/a	n/a	31.0 (8.6)	34.0 (8.7)		Raven, et al (1977)
MHV	Control	44	44/0	20.0 - 30.0	n/a	n/a	41.0 (15.7)	40.0 (15.1)		Raven, et al (1977)
MHV (IQ)	Schizophrenia	28	n/a	n/a	n/a	12 m	88.27 (6.77)	88.12 (10.22)		Scottish Schizophrenia Research Group (1988)
MHV Synonyms	DAT	23	n/a	77.30 (5.60)	n/a	1 y	12.07 (3.41)	10.00 (4.75)		O'Carroll, et al (1987)

Practitioner's Guide to Evaluating Change with Neuropsychological Assessment Instruments   177

instrument	group	n	m/f	age	intervention	inter	t #1	t #2	note	citation
Object Naming	Control	50	n/a	71.90 (0.90)	n/a	2 y	17.0 (0.6)	16.6 (0.7)		Flicker, et al (1993)
Object Naming	DAT (advanced)	39	n/a	72.20 (1.20)	n/a	2 y	3.8 (1.4)	1.1 (0.5)		Flicker, et al (1993)
Object Naming	DAT (early)	47	n/a	69.80 (1.20)	n/a	2 y	11.5 (1.1)	8.9 (1.2)		Flicker, et al (1993)
Object Naming (sec)	Orthopedic Injury	25	14/11	10.03 (2.00)	n/a	4 m	1.31 (0.25)	1.25 (0.21)		Chadwick, et al (1981)
Object Naming (sec)	TBI	25	14/11	10.12 (2.60)	n/a	4 m	1.61 (0.35)	1.48 (0.40)		Chadwick, et al (1981)
rapid naming	Brain Tumor	7	3/4	10.33	surgery	1 m	11.9 (2.9)	12.5 (0.7)		Bordeaux, et al (1988)
rapid naming	Brain Tumor	7	4/3	9.83	radiotherapy	11 m	7.1 (5.6)	9.9 (3.4)		Bordeaux, et al (1988)
Reading Comp Battery for Aphasia [100]	Control	31	14/17	63.74 (7.40)	n/a	7-17 d	97.32 (2.72)	97.97 (2.11)		Flanagan, et al (1997)
reading simple sentences	Epilepsy	11	n/a	25.90 (7.00)	RTL	1 w	3.9 (0.3)	3.8 (0.4)		Loring, et al (1994)
reading simple sentences	Epilepsy	18	n/a	28.10 (6.70)	LTL	1 y	3.5 (0.6)	3.7 (0.6)		Loring, et al (1994)
reading simple sentences	Epilepsy	16	n/a	25.70 (6.40)	RTL	1 y	3.9 (0.3)	3.9 (0.5)		Loring, et al (1994)
reading simple sentences	Epilepsy	12	n/a	29.00 (6.40)	LTL	1 w	3.8 (0.6)	3.0 (1.2)		Loring, et al (1994)

instrument	group	n	m/f	age	intervention	inter	t #1	t #2	note	citation
repetition of sentences	Epilepsy	11	n/a	25.90 (7.00)	RTL	1 w	2.9 (0.3)	2.7 (0.6)		Loring, et al (1994)
repetition of sentences	Epilepsy	18	n/a	28.10 (6.70)	LTL	1 y	2.7 (0.6)	2.7 (0.7)		Loring, et al (1994)
repetition of sentences	Epilepsy	12	n/a	29.00 (6.40)	LTL	1 w	3.0 (0.4)	2.2 (0.7)		Loring, et al (1994)
repetition of sentences	Epilepsy	16	n/a	25.70 (6.40)	RTL	1 y	2.9 (0.3)	2.9 (0.5)		Loring, et al (1994)
Responsive Naming Test	DAT	32	n/a	70.72	NSAID	1 y	10.31	1.13 c		Rich, et al (1995)
Responsive Naming Test	DAT	117	n/a	69.93	n/a	1 y	8.72	1.68 c		Rich, et al (1995)
Responsive Naming Test [15]	Control	22	12/10	65.82 (5.20)	n/a	2 y	14.78 (0.43)	15.00 (0.00)		Rebok, et al (1990)
Responsive Naming Test [15]	DAT	51	16/35	67.29 (7.94)	n/a	2 y	11.60 (3.07)	8.93 (4.67)		Rebok, et al (1990)
Sentence Repetition (correct) [22]	LD	35	n/a	10.00	n/a	15 y	11.9 (2.1)	15.0 (3.3)		Sarazin, et al (1986)
Sentence Repetition (correct) [22]	LD (brain damage)	67	n/a	10.00	n/a	15 y	10.4 (2.7)	13.9 (2.6)		Sarazin, et al (1986)

instrument	group	n	m/f	age	intervention	inter	t #1	t #2	note	citation
Sentence Repetition (correct) [22]	LD (min brain dysfunction)	73	n/a	10.00	n/a	15 y	11.3 (2.0)	14.8 (1.9)		Sarazin, et al (1986)
visual naming	Epilepsy	18	n/a	28.10 (6.70)	LTL	1 y	5.8 (0.5)	5.8 (0.7)		Loring, et al (1994)
visual naming	Epilepsy	16	n/a	25.70 (6.40)	RTL	1 y	5.9 (0.2)	6.0 (0.0)		Loring, et al (1994)
visual naming	Epilepsy	12	n/a	29.00 (6.40)	LTL	1 w	5.4 (0.7)	4.0 (2.0)		Loring, et al (1994)
visual naming	Epilepsy	11	n/a	25.90 (7.00)	RTL	1 w	6.0 (0.0)	6.0 (0.0)		Loring, et al (1994)
Woodcock Language Profiency Battery: Broad Language Cluster	Control	147	84/63	18.60 (2.60)	n/a	2 y	537.9 (15.4)	539.2 (15.3)		Farnill, et al (1995)
writing-to-dictation	Epilepsy	12	n/a	29.00 (6.40)	LTL	1 w	3.4 (1.0)	2.2 (1.3)		Loring, et al (1994)
writing-to-dictation	Epilepsy	18	n/a	28.10 (6.70)	LTL	1 y	3.5 (0.9)	3.5 (0.7)		Loring, et al (1994)
writing-to-dictation	Epilepsy	11	n/a	25.90 (7.00)	RTL	1 w	3.5 (0.8)	3.4 (1.4)		Loring, et al (1994)
writing-to-dictation	Epilepsy	16	n/a	25.70 (6.40)	RTL	1 y	3.8 (0.8)	3.8 (0.5)		Loring, et al (1994)

Table 33. Lateral Dominance Tests

instrument	group	n	m/f	age	intervention	inter	t #1	t #2	note	citation
Eye Preference Right	Control	36	24/12	32.50 (15.0)	n/a	5 y	1.39 (0.87)	1.36 (0.87)		Dodrill, et al (1993)
Eye Preference Right	Epilepsy	126	67/59	28.45 (10.4)	n/a	5 y	1.39 (0.83)	1.37 (0.83)		Dodrill, et al (1993)
Foot Preference Right	Control	36	24/12	32.50 (15.0)	n/a	5 y	1.69 (0.62)	1.78 (0.59)		Dodrill, et al (1993)
Foot Preference Right	Epilepsy	126	67/59	28.45 (10.4)	n/a	5 y	1.70 (0.65)	1.762 (0.65)		Dodrill, et al (1993)
Hand Preference Right	Control	36	24/12	32.50 (15.0)	n/a	5 y	6.17 (2.04)	6.28 (1.80)		Dodrill, et al (1993)
Hand Preference Right	Epilepsy	126	67/59	28.45 (10.4)	n/a	5 y	6.20 (2.06)	6.22 (1.97)		Dodrill, et al (1993)
LDE (# R side responses) [14]	LD	35	n/a	10.00	n/a	15 y	11.0 (3.4)	11.5 (3.3)		Sarazin, et al (1986)
LDE (# R side responses) [14]	LD (brain damage)	67	n/a	10.00	n/a	15 y	10.8 (2.9)	11.6 (3.0)		Sarazin, et al (1986)
LDE (# R side responses) [14]	LD (min brain dysfunction)	73	n/a	10.00	n/a	15 y	11.5 (4.0)	12.0 (4.3)		Sarazin, et al (1986)

instrument	group	n	m/f	age	intervention	inter	t #1	t #2	note	citation
Miles ABC Test of Ocular Dominance	Control	36	24/12	32.50 (15.0)	n/a	5 y	5.43 (4.82)	5.74 (4.77)		Dodrill, et al (1993)
Miles ABC Test of Ocular Dominance	Epilepsy	126	67/59	28.45 (10.4)	n/a	5 y	6.72 (9.24)	6.12 (4.67)		Dodrill, et al (1993)
Right-Left Discrimination Test	CAD	35	23/12	62.30 (8.30)	CE	50.9 d	11.97 (0.17)	12.00 (0.0)		Kelly, et al (1980)
Right-Left Discrimination Test	PVD	17	14/3	61.40 (7.90)	PVD surgery	51.5 d	11.88 (0.33)	12.00 (0.0)		Kelly, et al (1980)

Table 34. Luria Tests

instrument	group	n	m/f	age	intervention	inter	t #1	t #2	note	citation
LNNB Arithmetic	Diffuse Brain D/Os	27	14/13	35.30 (11.2)	n/a	167.0 d	84.7 (33.6)	83.5 (32.0)		Golden, et al (1982)
LNNB Arithmetic	Psychiatric	30	16/14	31.80 (12.7)	std inpt tx	8.1 m	17.2 (14.0)	16.3 (14.0)		Plaisted, et al (1982)
LNNB Expressive	Diffuse Brain D/Os	27	14/13	35.30 (11.2)	n/a	167.0 d	67.5 (24.7)	66.7 (24.3)		Golden, et al (1982)
LNNB Expressive	Psychiatric	30	16/14	31.80 (12.7)	std inpt tx	8.1 m	27.9 (19.6)	26.9 (19.2)		Plaisted, et al (1982)

instrument	group	n	m/f	age	intervention	inter	t #1	t #2	note	citation
LNNB Intelligence	Diffuse Brain D/Os	27	14/13	35.30 (11.2)	n/a	167.0 d	78.8 (17.4)	75.5 (17.9)		Golden, et al (1982)
LNNB Intelligence	Psychiatric	30	16/14	31.80 (12.7)	std inpt tx	8.1 m	39.1 (15.8)	35.1 (15.3)		Plaisted, et al (1982)
LNNB Left Hemisphere	Diffuse Brain D/Os	27	14/13	35.30 (11.2)	n/a	167.0 d	54.9 (19.0)	53.9 (16.2)		Golden, et al (1982)
LNNB Left Hemisphere	Psychiatric	30	16/14	31.80 (12.7)	std inpt tx	8.1 m	11.9 (10.5)	11.3 (10.0)		Plaisted, et al (1982)
LNNB Memory	Diffuse Brain D/Os	27	14/13	35.30 (11.2)	n/a	167.0 d	70.4 (13.4)	70.2 (16.0)		Golden, et al (1982)
LNNB Memory	Psychiatric	30	16/14	31.80 (12.7)	std inpt tx	8.1 m	15.6 (6.2)	15.9 (6.4)		Plaisted, et al (1982)
LNNB Motor	Diffuse Brain D/Os	27	14/13	35.30 (11.2)	n/a	167.0 d	62.2 (20.9)	60.8 (21.9)		Golden, et al (1982)
LNNB Motor	Psychiatric	30	16/14	31.80 (12.7)	std inpt tx	8.1 m	33.3 (19.0)	33.7 (21.3)		Plaisted, et al (1982)
LNNB Pathognomonic	Control (Clinic/ Volunteer)	15	5/10	33.90 (8.40)	n/a	20.7 d	6.7 (3.7)	5.6 (3.8)		Goulet Fisher, et al (1986)
LNNB Pathognomonic	Depression	15	6/9	28.50 (10.6)	inpt tx	19.5 d	12.9 (4.5)	9.3 (3.5)		Goulet Fisher, et al (1986)
LNNB Pathognomonic	Psychiatric	30	16/14	31.80 (12.7)	std inpt tx	8.1 m	25.5 (11.6)	23.9 (13.4)		Plaisted, et al (1982)
LNNB Reading	Diffuse Brain D/Os	27	14/13	35.30 (11.2)	n/a	167.0 d	63.3 (16.0)	63.2 (16.0)		Golden, et al (1982)

instrument	group	n	m/f	age	intervention	inter	t #1	t #2	note	citation
LNNB Reading	Psychiatric	30	16/14	31.80 (12.7)	std inpt tx	8.1 m	10.3 (7.1)	10.4 (7.0)		Plaisted, et al (1982)
LNNB Receptive	Diffuse Brain D/Os	27	14/13	35.30 (11.2)	n/a	167.0 d	68.5 (17.5)	67.8 (19.7)		Golden, et al (1982)
LNNB Receptive	Psychiatric	30	16/14	31.80 (12.7)	std inpt tx	8.1 m	17.8 (12.3)	18.1 (13.4)		Plaisted, et al (1982)
LNNB Rhythm	Diffuse Brain D/Os	27	14/13	35.30 (11.2)	n/a	167.0 d	68.5 (20.6)	66.3 (19.4)		Golden, et al (1982)
LNNB Rhythm	Psychiatric	30	16/14	31.80 (12.7)	std inpt tx	8.1 m	12.3 (6.6)	12.7 (6.9)		Plaisted, et al (1982)
LNNB Right Hemisphere	Diffuse Brain D/Os	27	14/13	35.30 (11.2)	n/a	167.0 d	53.7 (19.6)	50.6 (14.0)		Golden, et al (1982)
LNNB Right Hemisphere	Psychiatric	30	16/14	31.80 (12.7)	std inpt tx	8.1 m	11.9 (10.1)	11.7 (10.1)		Plaisted, et al (1982)
LNNB Tactile	Diffuse Brain D/Os	27	14/13	35.30 (11.2)	n/a	167.0 d	60.6 (16.1)	57.0 (12.4)		Golden, et al (1982)
LNNB Tactile	Psychiatric	30	16/14	31.80 (12.7)	std inpt tx	8.1 m	13.9 (11.2)	11.3 (11.3)		Plaisted, et al (1982)
LNNB Visual	Diffuse Brain D/Os	27	14/13	35.30 (11.2)	n/a	167.0 d	65.0 (12.8)	61.8 (11.3)		Golden, et al (1982)
LNNB Visual	Psychiatric	30	16/14	31.80 (12.7)	std inpt tx	8.1 m	13.4 (5.0)	13.2 (5.4)		Plaisted, et al (1982)
LNNB Writing	Diffuse Brain D/Os	27	14/13	35.30 (11.2)	n/a	167.0 d	66.7 (15.9)	67.5 (14.7)		Golden, et al (1982)
LNNB Writing	Psychiatric	30	16/14	31.8 (12.7)	std inpt tx	8.1 m	13.5 (6.9)	13.1 (6.6)		Plaisted, et al (1982)

instrument	group	n	m/f	age	intervention	inter	t #1	t #2	note	citation
Luria Alternating Series	DAT/MID	30	15/15	71.7 (1.3)	oxiracetam	3 m	4.6 (0.5)	6.6 (0.6)	*	Villardita, et al (1992)
Luria Alternating Series	DAT/MID	29	14/15	71.5 (1.3)	oxiracetam	6 m	4.4 (0.5)	7.1 (0.5)	*	Villardita, et al (1992)
Luria Alternating Series	DAT/MID	30	21/9	67.8 (1.5)	placebo	3 m	4.2 (0.5)	4.2 (0.4)	*	Villardita, et al (1992)

Table 35. Mattis Dementia Rating Scale (DRS)

instrument	group	n	m/f	age	intervention	inter	t #1	t #2	note	citation
DRS Attention	BMT pts	61	34/27	37.50	BMT	12 d	36.5 (0.7)	36.3 (0.71)	*	Meyers, et al (1994)
DRS Attention	DAT	30	n/a	n/a	n/a	1 wk	79.54 (33.98)	83.18 (30.60)		Coblentz, et al (1973)
DRS Attention	DAT	30	n/a	58.0 - 71.0	n/a	1 w	23.55 (9.91)	24.16 (6.80)		Mattis (1988)
DRS Concept	BMT pts	61	34/27	37.50	BMT	12 d	36.3 (2.02)	36.8 (2.0)	*	Meyers, et al (1994)
DRS Concept	DAT	30	n/a	n/a	n/a	1 wk	21.18 (10.58)	21.91 (9.28)		Coblentz, et al (1973)
DRS Concept	DAT	30	n/a	58.0 - 71.0	n/a	1 w	21.18 (10.58)	21.91 (9.28)		Mattis (1988)

instrument	group	n	m/f	age	intervention	inter	t #1	t #2	note	citation
DRS Construction	BMT pts	61	34/27	37.50	BMT	12 d	5.97 (0.18)	5.98 (0.14)	*	Meyers, et al (1994)
DRS Construction	DAT	30	n/a	n/a	n/a	1 wk	2.54 (1.81)	2.91 (1.70)		Coblentz, et al (1973)
DRS Construction	DAT	30	n/a	58.0 - 71.0	n/a	1 w	2.55 (1.81)	2.91 (1.70)		Mattis (1988)
DRS Identities and Oddities	CVA/Control	300	n/a	70.70	improved/ stable	9-12 m	NR	0.2 (1.7) c		Desmond, et al (1995)
DRS Identities and Oddities	CVA/Control	71	n/a	70.70	declined	9-12 m	NR	-0.6 (2.4) c		Desmond, et al (1995)
DRS Initiation/ Preseveration	DAT	30	n/a	58.0 - 71.0	n/a	1 w	21.36 (9.78)	22.00 (7.34)		Mattis (1988)
DRS Memory	BMT pts	61	34/27	37.50	BMT	12 d	24.3 (0.96)	24.2 (1.17)	*	Meyers, et al (1994)
DRS Memory	DAT	30	n/a	n/a	n/a	1 wk	10.91 (6.58)	12.20 (6.00)		Coblentz, et al (1973)
DRS Memory	DAT	30	n/a	58.0 - 71.0	n/a	1 w	10.91 (6.58)	12.20 (6.00)		Mattis (1988)
DRS Perseveration	DAT	30	n/a	n/a	n/a	1 wk	23.55 (9.91)	24.16 (6.80)		Coblentz, et al (1973)
DRS Preseveration	BMT pts	61	34/27	37.50	BMT	12 d	36.0 (2.3)	36.5 (1.41)	*	Meyers, et al (1994)
DRS Total	BMT pts	61	34/27	37.50	BMT	12 d	139.0 (3.97)	139.8 (3.13)	*	Meyers, et al (1994)

instrument	group	n	m/f	age	intervention	inter	t #1	t #2	note	citation
DRS Total	Control	40	20/20	73.0 (7.70)	n/a	1 y	140.9 (2.7)	140.6 (2.7)	*	Taylor, et al (1996)
DRS Total	DAT	30	n/a	58.0 - 71.0	n/a	1 w	79.55 (33.98)	83.18 (30.60)		Mattis (1988)
DRS Total	DAT	40	20/20	73.0 (7.60)	n/a	1 y	110.6 (13 4)	100.8 (22.4)	*	Taylor, et al (1996)
DRS Total	DAT (mild)	11	10/1	63.0 (8.00)	n/a	26 m	132.0 (6.0)	124.0 (11.0)		Haxby, et al (1990)
DRS Verbal Fluency	DAT/MID	29	14/15	71.50 (1.30)	oxiracetam	6 m	6.4 (0.4)	7.9 (0.6)	*	Villardita, et al (1992)
DRS Verbal Fluency	DAT/MID	30	21/9	67.80 (1.50)	placebo	3 m	6.3 (0.5)	6.4 (0.4)	*	Villardita, et al (1992)
DRS Verbal Fluency	DAT/MID	30	15/15	71.70 (1.30)	oxiracetam	3 m	6.5 (0.4)	8.8 (0.5)	*	Villardita, et al (1992)

Table 36. Maze Tests

instrument	group	n	m/f	age	intervention	inter	t #1	t #2	note	citation
Austin Maze Test	Alcoholic	16	16/0	37.50 (11.1)	inpt tx	3-4 w	87.6 (43.2)	80.5 (65.0)		Unkenstein, et al (1991)
Austin Maze Test (errors)	Anorexia	18	0/18	n/a	refeeding tx	69.8 d	64.4 (30.1)	39.0 (20.5)		Szmukler, et al (1992)
Austin Maze Test (errors)	Control	18	0/18	n/a	n/a	108.4 d	40.9 (15.3)	37.9 (20.0)		Szmukler, et al (1992)

instrument	group	n	m/f	age	intervention	inter	t #1	t #2	note	citation
Austin Maze Test (trials)	Anorexia	18	0/18	n/a	refeeding tx	69.8 d	14.3 (4.9)	10.2 (5.0)		Szmukler, et al (1992)
Austin Maze Test (trials)	Control	18	0/18	n/a	n/a	108.4 d	12.1 (4.6)	11.3 (5.2)		Szmukler, et al (1992)
Maze Counter LH (errors)	Neuropsych referrals	248	203/ 45	8.00 (1.70)	n/a	2.65 y	87.1 (38.1)	60.7 (41.5)		Brown, et al (1989)
Maze Counter RH (errors)	Neuropsych referrals	248	203/ 45	8.00 (1.70)	n/a	2.65 y	70.3 (42.2)	40.0 (34.3)		Brown, et al (1989)
Maze Speed LH (sec)	Neuropsych referrals	248	203/ 45	8.00 (1.70)	n/a	2.65 y	98.4 (28.6)	105.5 (35.1)		Brown, et al (1989)
Maze Speed RH (sec)	Neuropsych referrals	248	203/ 45	8.00 (1.70)	n/a	2.65 y	100.7 (30.4)	108.9 (34.2)		Brown, et al (1989)
Maze Test LH (errors)	Control	14	6/8	11.20	n/a	4-6 h	66.1 (4.8)	67.8 (5.9)		Reich, et al (1990)
Maze Test LH (errors)	Diabetes	10	5/5	12.20	hypoglycemia	4-6 h	66.1 (4.0)	64.3 (7.2)		Reich, et al (1990)
Maze Test LH (errors)	Diabetes	14	6/8	10.50	mild hypoglycemia	4-6 h	62.4 (7.2)	64.3 (6.4)		Reich, et al (1990)
Maze Test LH (sec)	Control	14	6/8	11.20	n/a	4-6 h	62.5 (3.7)	64.5 (3.3)		Reich, et al (1990)
Maze Test LH (sec)	Diabetes	14	6/8	10.50	mild hypoglycemia	4-6 h	60.2 (5.9)	62.4 (5.3)		Reich, et al (1990)
Maze Test LH (sec)	Diabetes	10	5/5	12.20	hypoglycemia	4-6 h	63.3 (3.1)	62.2 (5.10		Reich, et al (1990)

instrument	group	n	m/f	age	intervention	inter	t #1	t #2	note	citation
Maze Test RH (errors)	Control	14	6/8	11.20	n/a	4-6 h	64.0 (4.3)	65.9 (2.0)		Reich, et al (1990)
Maze Test RH (errors)	Diabetes	10	5/5	12.20	hypoglycemia	4-6 h	63.6 (3.8)	65.5 (4.7)		Reich, et al (1990)
Maze Test RH (errors)	Diabetes	14	6/8	10.50	mild hypoglycemia	4-6 h	58.6 (6.8)	63.4 (3.5)		Reich, et al (1990)
Maze Test RH (sec)	Control	14	6/8	11.20	n/a	4-6 h	60.1 (3.4)	62.1 (1.0)		Reich, et al (1990)
Maze Test RH (sec)	Diabetes	10	5/5	12.20	hypoglycemia	4-6 h	60.8 (3.2)	61.0 (4.0)		Reich, et al (1990)
Maze Test RH (sec)	Diabetes	14	6/8	10.50	mild hypoglycemia	4-6 h	54.7 (6.1)	59.6 (2.4)		Reich, et al (1990)
Maze Time LH (sec)	Neuropsych referrals	248	203/ 45	8.00 (1.70)	n/a	2.65 y	19.3 (12.4)	12.4 (11.2)		Brown, et al (1989)
Maze Time RH (sec)	Neuropsych referrals	248	203/ 45	8.00 (1.70)	n/a	2.65 y	13.9 (10.9)	7.4 (7.7)		Brown, et al (1989)
MKMSB Maze Counter DH	HIV+ (IVDU)	18	10/8	29.80 (5.40)	drug tx	17.7 m	4.6 (6.2)	2.1 (2.7)		Hestad, et al (1996)
MKMSB Maze Counter DH	HIV- (IVDU)	30	16/14	27.90 (4.90)	drug tx	14.9 m	3.6 (3.5)	2.9 (4.1)		Hestad, et al (1996)
MKMSB Maze Time DH	HIV+ (IVDU)	18	10/8	29.80 (5.40)	drug tx	17.7 m	0.46 (0.5)	0.23 (0.4)		Hestad, et al (1996)
MKMSB Maze Time DH	HIV- (IVDU)	30	16/14	27.90 (4.90)	drug tx	14.9 m	0.42 (0.5)	0.32 (0.5)		Hestad, et al (1996)

instrument	group	n	m/f	age	intervention	inter	t #1	t #2	note	citation
Porteus Mazes	Depression w/ Melancholia	7	5/2	9.50	tricyclic antidepress	3 - 6 m	109.6 (14.5)	105.9 (19.8)		Stanton, et al (1981)
Porteus Mazes	Depression w/o Melancholia	4	4/2	11.00	tricyclic antidepress	3 - 6 m	93.5 (17.7)	101.0 (26.1)		Stanton, et al (1981)
Porteus Mazes	Schizophrenia Inpts	9	7/2	51.00	bromocriptine	2 m	9.6 (1.6)	9.6 (1.3)	*	de Beaurepaire, et al (1993)
Porteus Mazes	Schizophrenia Inpts	7	7/0	51.00	placebo	2 m	8.8 (1.4)	9.2 (1.0)	*	de Beaurepaire, et al (1993)
Porteus Mazes (blind alleys)	Control	16	n/a	24.50 (7.70)	n/a	1 d	1.28 (0.93)	1.02 (0.60)	*	Ewert, et al (1989)
Porteus Mazes (blind alleys)	TBI & PTA	16	n/a	24.50 (7.70)	n/a	1 d	2.91 (1.16)	2.01 (1.03)	*	Ewert, et al (1989)
Porteus Mazes (IQ)	LD	32	23/9	10.67 (1.30)	placebo	8 w	106.8 (2.52)	108.12 (3.22)		Gittleman-Klein, et al (1976)
Porteus Mazes (IQ)	LD	29	24/5	10.83 (1.40)	methylphen	8 w	123.29 (2.65)	125.94 (3.39)		Gittleman-Klein, et al (1976)
Porteus Mazes (IQ)	Schizophrenia	11	11/0	52.50 (11.5)	neuroleptic reduction	29.3 w	108.8 (21.7)	104.8 (27.7)		Seidman, et al (1993)
Porteus Mazes (lines crossed)	Control	16	n/a	24.50 (7.70)	n/a	1 d	0.67 (0.74)	0.52 (0.54)	*	Ewert, et al (1989)
Porteus Mazes (lines crossed)	TBI & PTA	16	n/a	24.50 (7.70)	n/a	1 d	3.57 (3.40)	2.76 (2.55)	*	Ewert, et al (1989)
Porteus Mazes (sec)	Control	16	n/a	24.50 (7.70)	n/a	1 d	13.95 (5.15)	12.29 (4.35)	*	Ewert, et al (1989)

instrument	group	n	m/f	age	intervention	inter	t #1	t #2	note	citation
Porteus Mazes (sec)	TBI & PTA	16	n/a	24.50 (7.70)	n/a	1 d	42.31 (21.00)	36.30 (18.48)	*	Ewert, et al (1989)
Porteus Mazes (test age)	Asthma	9	n/a	6.00 - 12.00	theophylline	2 w	11.27	13.05		Rappaport, et al (1989)
Porteus Mazes (test age)	Asthma	8	n/a	6.00 - 12.00	placebo	2 w	13.37	14.37		Rappaport, et al (1989)
Porteus Mazes (test age)	DAT (mild)	11	10/1	63.00 (8.00)	n/a	26 m	12.8 (3.9)	11.6 (3.3)		Haxby, et al (1990)
Porteus Mazes (test age)	Seizure D/O	45	n/a	10.80	carbamaz	4-6 m	10.2 (3.4)	11.6 (3.4)		Schain, et al (1977)
Porteus Mazes (TQ)	Hyperactivity	18	18/0	7.90	pemoline	~8 w	99.33	111.44		Conners, et al (1980)
Porteus Mazes (TQ)	Hyperactivity	20	19/1	7.90	placebo	~8 w	98.6	103.65		Conners, et al (1980)
Porteus Mazes (TQ)	Hyperactivity	20	18/2	7.90	methylphen	~8 w	105.55	114.00		Conners, et al (1980)
Porteus Mazes (unsuccessful trials)	Asthma	8	n/a	6.00 - 12.00	placebo	2 w	6.12	5.25		Rappaport, et al (1989)
Porteus Mazes (unsuccessful trials)	Asthma	9	n/a	6.00 - 12.00	theophylline	2 w	10.0	6.55		Rappaport, et al (1989)

Table 37. McCarthy Scales of Children's Abilities (MSCA)

instrument	group	n	m/f	age	intervention	inter	t #1	t #2	note	citation
MSCA Blocks	Down Syndrome	34	20/14	22.0-56.0	n/a	1 y	9.63 (1.04)	9.56 (0.89)	*	Burt, et al (1995)
MSCA Fluency	Down Syndrome	34	20/14	22.0-56.0	n/a	1 y	15.58 (8.62)	14.81 (7.10)	*	Burt, et al (1995)
MSCA GCI	Brain Tumor (post-surgery)	8	n/a	2.0 -5.0	radiation tx	6 m	99.0	97.3		Mulhern, et al (1985)
MSCA GCI	Control	43	n/a	5.60	n/a	12.3 m	129.3 (28.5)	164.1 (26.5)		Davis, et al (1976)
MSCA GCI	Control	43	n/a	5.60	n/a	12.3 m	88.7 (18.9)	92.7 (15.9)		Davis, et al (1976)
MSCA GCI	Control	40	24/16	5.40 (0.2)	n/a	2 w	116.05 (15.00)	119.48 (16.65)		Harrington, et al (1986)
MSCA GCI	Control (Mexican-American)	42	n/a	4.78 (0.3)	n/a	1 y	91.7 (11.1)	94.0 (15.2)		Valencia (1983)
MSCA GCI	Control (Mexican-American)	42	n/a	4.78 (0.3)	n/a	1 y	98.9 (15.5)	100.2 (21.0)		Valencia (1983)
MSCA GCI (raw)	Control	38	20/18	6.00	n/a	24 d	174.1 (20.5)	176.1 (18.7)		Bryant, et al (1978)
MSCA GCI (scaled)	Control	38	20/18	6.00	n/a	24 d	114.5 (15.3)	114.4 (14.2)		Bryant, et al (1978)
MSCA Memory	Brain Tumor (post-surgery)	8	n/a	2.0 -5.0	radiation tx	6 m	46.3	43.0		Mulhern, et al (1985)

instrument	group	n	m/f	age	intervention	inter	t #1	t #2	note	citation
MSCA Memory	Control (Mexican-American)	42	n/a	4.78 (0.3)	n/a	1 y	48.0 (9.8)	47.8 (11.2)		Valencia (1983)
MSCA Memory	Control (Mexican-American)	42	n/a	4.78 (0.3)	n/a	1 y	42.5 (7.5)	41.3 (11.6)		Valencia (1983)
MSCA Memory	Down Syndrome	34	20/14	22.0-56.0	n/a	1 y	22.90 (9.74)	23.52 (10.09)	*	Burt, et al (1995)
MSCA Memory (raw)	Control	38	20/18	6.00	n/a	24 d	42.6 (8.1)	43.5 (7.2)		Bryant, et al (1978)
MSCA Memory (raw)	Control	43	n/a	5.60	n/a	12.3 m	29.3 (9.4)	37.1 (8.6)		Davis, et al (1976)
MSCA Memory (scaled)	Control	38	20/18	6.00	n/a	24 d	55.8 (10.2)	56.2 (9.4)		Bryant, et al (1978)
MSCA Memory (std)	Control	43	n/a	5.60	n/a	12.3 m	41.1 (12.2)	43.3 (10.8)		Davis, et al (1976)
MSCA Motor (raw)	Control	43	n/a	5.60	n/a	12.3 m	42.2 (7.0)	51.8 (5.8)		Davis, et al (1976)
MSCA Motor (std)	Control	43	n/a	5.60	n/a	12.3 m	46.0 (8.7)	48.3 (9.2)		Davis, et al (1976)
MSCA Percep-Perform	Brain Tumor (post-surgery)	8	n/a	2.0 - 5.0	radiation tx	6 m	48.5	46.9		Mulhern, et al (1985)
MSCA Percep-Perform	Control (Mexican-American)	42	n/a	4.78 (0.3)	n/a	1 y	51.5 (9.6)	53.9 (11.4)		Valencia (1983)

instrument	group	n	m/f	age	intervention	inter	t #1	t #2	note	citation
MSCA Percep-Perform	Control (Mexican-American)	42	n/a	4.78 (0.3)	n/a	1 y	48.5 (8.2)	55.5 (9.3)		Valencia (1983)
MSCA Percep-Perform (raw)	Control	38	20/18	6.00	n/a	24 d	66.1 (7.9)	66.8 (6.7)		Bryant, et al (1978)
MSCA Percep-Perform (raw)	Control	43	n/a	5.60	n/a	12.3 m	56.6 (9.4)	69.8 (6.2)		Davis, et al (1976)
MSCA Percep-Perform (scaled)	Control	38	20/18	6.00	n/a	24 d	60.1 (8.7)	60.2 (7.7)		Bryant, et al (1978)
MSCA Percep-Perform (std)	Control	28	16/12	6.50 (0.7)	n/a	1 y	104.6 (12.9)	108.8 (15.4)	*	Brookshire, et al (1995)
MSCA Percep-Perform (std)	Hydroceph (arrested)	11	6/5	6.20 (0.4)	n/a	1 y	102.1 (15.6)	103.6 (16.3)	*	Brookshire, et al (1995)
MSCA Percep-Perform (std)	Hydroceph (shunted)	26	14/12	6.20 (0.7)	n/a	1 y	82.8 (17.2)	85.6 (17.3)	*	Brookshire, et al (1995)
MSCA Percep-Perform (std)	Control	43	n/a	5.60	n/a	12.3 m	51.7 (10.1)	56.3 (9.5)		Davis, et al (1976)
MSCA Puzzles	Down Syndrome	34	20/14	22.0-56.0	n/a	1 y	6.74 (3.50)	7.11 (3.17)	*	Burt, et al (1995)
MSCA Quantitative	Brain Tumor (post-surgery)	8	n/a	2.0 -5.0	radiation tx	6 m	45.6	49.8		Mulhern, et al (1985)
MSCA Quantitative	Control (Mexican-American)	42	n/a	4.78 (0.3)	n/a	1 y	44.3 (7.3)	43.6 (7.7)		Valencia (1983)

instrument	group	n	m/f	age	intervention	inter	t #1	t #2	note	citation
MSCA Quantitative	Control (Mexican-American)	42	n/a	4.78 (0.3)	n/a	1 y	47.6 (8.4)	47.2 (9.7)		Valencia (1983)
MSCA Quantitative (raw)	Control	38	20/18	6.00	n/a	24 d	32.1 (6.5)	31.7 (7.0)		Bryant, et al (1978)
MSCA Quantitative (raw)	Control	43	n/a	5.60	n/a	12.3 m	22.7 (7.0)	29.7 (7.7)		Davis, et al (1976)
MSCA Quantitative (scaled)	Control	38	20/18	6.00	n/a	24 d	54.3 (8.4)	52.9 (9.5)		Bryant, et al (1978)
MSCA Quantitative (std)	Control	43	n/a	5.60	n/a	12.3 m	43.5 (11.5)	43.5 (10.7)		Davis, et al (1976)
MSCA Verbal	Brain Tumor (post-surgery)	8	n/a	2.0 - 5.0	radiation tx	6 m	52.1	49.3		Mulhern, et al (1985)
MSCA Verbal	Control (Mexican-American)	42	n/a	4.78 (0.3)	n/a	1 y	49.1 (11.5)	48.7 (14.2)		Valencia (1983)
MSCA Verbal	Control (Mexican-American)	42	n/a	4.78 (0.3)	n/a	1 y	43.7 (8.7)	41.7 (9.0)		Valencia (1983)
MSCA Verbal (raw)	Control	38	20/18	6.00	n/a	24 d	75.8 (10.1)	77.7 (9.2)		Bryant, et al (1978)

instrument	group	n	m/f	age	intervention	inter	t #1	t #2	note	citation
MSCA Verbal (raw)	Control	43	n/a	5.60	n/a	12.3 m	50.4 (17.8)	64.8 (14.0)		Davis, et al (1976)
MSCA Verbal (scaled)	Control	38	20/18	6.00	n/a	24 d	56.6 (9.8)	57.3 (8.9)		Bryant, et al (1978)
MSCA Verbal (std)	Control	28	16/12	6.50 (0.7)	n/a	1 y	98.4 (12.8)	103 (14.7)	*	Brookshire, et al (1995)
MSCA Verbal (std)	Control	43	n/a	5.60	n/a	12.3 m	38.1 (11.6)	41.5 (9.8)		Davis, et al (1976)
MSCA Verbal (std)	Hydroceph (arrested)	11	6/5	6.20 (0.4)	n/a	1 y	99.2 (19.4)	96.7 (18.1)	*	Brookshire, et al (1995)
MSCA Verbal (std)	Hydroceph (shunted)	26	14/12	6.20 (0.7)	n/a	1 y	92.2 (17.4)	93.4 (18.1)	*	Brookshire, et al (1995)

Table 38. Memory Tests (Non-verbal)

instrument	group	n	m/f	age	intervention	inter	t #1	t #2	note	citation
continuous recog-designs	TBI (mild - mod)	7	7/0	25.00	CDP-choline	1 m	25.0	38.0		Levin (1991)
continuous recog-designs	TBI (mild - mod)	7	7/0	20.00	placebo	1 m	40.0	45.0		Levin (1991)
CVMT (d')	Control	92	30/62	69.02 (5.79)	n/a	13.5 m	1.77 (0.46)	2.06 (0.60)		Paolo, et al (1998)
CVMT Delayed Recog	Control	92	30/62	69.02 (5.79)	n/a	13.5 m	3.63 (1.43)	4.11 (1.36)		Paolo, et al (1998)
CVMT Total	Control	92	30/62	69.02 (5.79)	n/a	13.5 m	73.17 (6.62)	74.12 (7.13)		Paolo, et al (1998)

instrument	group	n	m/f	age	intervention	inter	t #1	t #2	note	citation
design recall delay (10')	TBI	42	40/2	33.20 (11.2)	n/a	9 m	7.2 (6.4)	11.6 (5.4)		Mukundan, et al (1987)
design recall trial I	TBI	42	40/2	33.20 (11.2)	n/a	9 m	4.5 (3.8)	7.0 (3.4)		Mukundan, et al (1987)
design recall trial II	TBI	42	40/2	33.20 (11.2)	n/a	9 m	5.7 (5.4)	7.5 (4.1)		Mukundan, et al (1987)
design recall trial III	TBI	42	40/2	33.20 (11.2)	n/a	9 m	6.9 (6.0)	10.6 (5.1)		Mukundan, et al (1987)
figure recall delay [24]	Control	20	6/14	69.40 (4.20)	n/a	1 y	18.8 (3.9)	19.1 (4.8)	*	Fromm, et al (1991)
figure recall delay [24]	DAT	18	5/13	71.00 (9.40)	n/a	1 y	5.2 (4.3)	2.4 (2.3)	*	Fromm, et al (1991)
figure recall imm [24]	Control	20	6/14	69.40 (4.20)	n/a	1 y	19.7 (3.4)	19.7 (4.2)	*	Fromm, et al (1991)
figure recall imm [24]	DAT	18	5/13	71.00 (9.40)	n/a	1 y	7.2 (4.3)	4.6 (3.1)	*	Fromm, et al (1991)
Heaton Figure Memory Test - Learning	HIV+ (IVDU)	8	5/3	39.00 (8.00)	MSR/placebo	7 d	4.5 (1.7)	11.0 (5.8)	*	Van Dyck, et al (1997)
Heaton Figure Memory Test - Recall	HIV+ (IVDU)	8	5/3	39.00 (8.00)	MSR/placebo	7 d	4.1 (3.4)	0.5 (13.3)	*	Van Dyck, et al (1997)
Memory-For-Designs (x/45)	Depression	33	14/19	37.40	antidepress	7 w	41.6 (4.7)	42.5 (4.9)		Fromm, et al (1984)
MFFT	Asthma	9	n/a	6.00 - 12.00	theophylline	2 w	8.22	7.66		Rappaport, et al (1989)

instrument	group	n	m/f	age	intervention	inter	t #1	t #2	note	citation
MFFT	Asthma	8	n/a	6.00 - 12.00	placebo	2 w	7.0	7.75		Rappaport, et al (1989)
MFFT (errors)	Seizure D/O	45	n/a	10.80	carbamaz	4-6 m	14.9 (8.1)	10.9 (7.2)		Schain, et al (1977)
MFFT (latency)	Asthma	8	n/a	6.00 - 12.00	placebo	2 w	15.88	13.05		Rappaport, et al (1989)
MFFT (latency)	Asthma	9	n/a	6.00 - 12.00	theophylline	2 w	13.42	11.56		Rappaport, et al (1989)
MFFT (sec)	Seizure D/O	45	n/a	10.80	carbamaz	4-6 m	9.5 (4.3)	13.0 (5.8)		Schain, et al (1977)
Milner Face Recog (correct) [12]	PD/Tremor	12	7/5	56.00	left thalamotomy	~6 d	9.0	8.3	AF	Vilkki, et al (1974)
Milner Face Recog (correct) [12]	PD/Tremor	13	8/5	56.00	right thalamotomy	~6 d	8.9	8.8	AF	Vilkki, et al (1974)
Misplaced Objects (trial 1)	Control	16	10/6	64.00 (1.70)	n/a	1 w	11.9 (0.9)	13.6 (0.8)	*	Claus, et al (1991)
Misplaced Objects (trial 1)	DAT	17	7/1	64.00 (1.70)	n/a	1 w	3.4 (0.6)	3.0 (0.4)	*	Claus, et al (1991)
Misplaced Objects (trial 2)	Control	16	10/6	64.00 (1.70)	n/a	1 w	15.6 (0.7)	16.4 (0.7)	*	Claus, et al (1991)
Misplaced Objects (trial 2)	DAT	17	7/1	64.00 (1.70)	n/a	1 w	5.3 (0.8)	5.0 (0.6)	*	Claus, et al (1991)
Moss Spatial Scan	Naphtha Exposure	185	n/a	36.00	n/a	1 y	11.46 (2.56)	12.10 (2.22)		White, et al (1994)

instrument	group	n	m/f	age	intervention	inter	t #1	t #2	note	citation
Moss Spatial Span	Naphtha Exposure	185	n/a	36.00	n/a	1 y	12.74 (1.50)	13.16 (1.04)		White, et al (1994)
Object Memory Retrieval	Control	24	n/a	58.50	n/a	2.1 y	46.8 (2.0)	47.0 (2.8)		La Rue, et al (1995)
Object Memory Retrieval	early onset DAT relatives	19	n/a	57.10	n/a	4.6 y	47.2 (2.4)	45.7 (3.1)		La Rue, et al (1995)
Object Memory Retrieval	late onset DAT relatives	21	n/a	55.10	n/a	4.4 y	44.6 (4.1)	45.1 (4.1)		La Rue, et al (1995)
Recurring Faces Test	Control	20	12/8	56.40	n/a	10 w	51.2 (5.4)	53.8 (3.7)		Van Den Burg, et al (1985)
Recurring Faces Test	PVD	20	18/2	56.80	major surgery	10 w	49.4 (5.3)	51.7 (4.4)		Van Den Burg, et al (1985)
Recurring Faces Test	TIA	20	13/7	59.60	CE	10 w	49.9 (4.9)	51.9 (5.8)		Van Den Burg, et al (1985)
Recurring Figures-Asymmetrical [28]	Depression	33	14/19	37.40	antidepress	7 w	8.3 (6.5)	14.8 (6.3)		Fromm, et al (1984)
Recurring Figures-Geometric [28]	Depression	33	14/19	37.40	antidepress	7 w	22.1 (6.5)	25.8 (3.7)		Fromm, et al (1984)

instrument	group	n	m/f	age	intervention	inter	t #1	t #2	note	citation
Recurring Figures-Total [56]	Depression	33	14/19	37.40	antidepress	7 w	30.4 (11.10)	40.5 (8.8)		Fromm, et al (1984)
Spatial Delayed Recog Span Test	Control	22	12/10	65.82 (5.20)	n/a	2 y	9.52 (1.41)	10.32 (2.21)		Rebok, et al (1990)
Spatial Delayed Recog Span Test	DAT	51	16/35	67.29 (7.94)	n/a	2 y	4.10 (2.27)	2.25 (2.07)		Rebok, et al (1990)
Target Test (correct)	Neuropsych referrals	248	203/45	8.00 (1.70)	n/a	2.65 y	9.4 (5.2)	13.0 (4.9)		Brown, et al (1989)
Time Sense Memory	Control	174	174/0	24.0 - 85.0	n/a	2 y	391.49	319.79	*	Schludermann, et al (1983)
Time Sense Memory	Control	86	86/0	24.0 - 85.0	n/a	2 y	436.59	341.48	*	Schludermann, et al (1983)
Time Sense Visual	Control	174	174/0	24.0 - 85.0	n/a	2 y	29.79	27.13	*	Schludermann, et al (1983)
Time Sense Visual	Control	86	86/0	24.0 - 85.0	n/a	2 y	31.75	27.58	*	Schludermann, et al (1983)
Tonal Memory (correct)	Epilepsy	21	n/a	22.30 (7.60)	improved WAIS re-test	20.5 m	12.9 (4.9)	15.6 (7.2)		Seidenberg, et al (1981)
Tonal Memory (correct)	Epilepsy	19	n/a	20.30 (4.30)	slightly improved WAIS re-test	20.1 m	17.1 (5.8)	16.4 (5.9)		Seidenberg, et al (1981)

instrument	group	n	m/f	age	intervention	inter	t #1	t #2	note	citation
Tonal Memory (correct)	Epilepsy	18	n/a	20.30 (5.40)	stable WAIS on re-test	21.6 m	13.3 (7.5)	14.6 (6.5)		Seidenberg, et al (1981)
Tonal Memory (correct)	Epilepsy (sz continued)	26	n/a	~21.0	n/a	20.7 m	14.61 (6.83)	15.42 (6.36)		Seidenberg, et al (1981)
Tonal Memory (correct)	Epilepsy (sz remitted)	24	n/a	~21.0	n/a	20.7 m	14.50 (6.44)	14.59 (6.09)		Seidenberg, et al (1981)
Visual Sequential Memory Test	LD	32	23/9	10.67 (1.30)	placebo	8 w	22.3 (0.84)	23.63 (0.92)		Gittleman-Klein, et al (1976)
Visual Sequential Memory Test	LD	29	24/5	10.83 (1.40)	methylphen	8 w	25.61 (0.92)	26.38 (0.98)		Gittleman-Klein, et al (1976)
Visual Spatial Learning Test DDEL%	Epilepsy	20	8/12	34.60 (9.80)	LTL	4.1 m	98.6	98.9		Ivnik, et al (1993)
Visual Spatial Learning Test DDEL%	Epilepsy	20	12/8	29.90 (10.1)	RTL	3.8 m	100.9	96.6		Ivnik, et al (1993)
Visual Spatial Learning Test DPLI%	Epilepsy	20	12/8	29.90 (10.1)	RTL	3.8 m	95.7	99.6		Ivnik, et al (1993)
Visual Spatial Learning Test DPLI%	Epilepsy	20	8/12	34.60 (9.80)	LTL	4.1 m	92.1	99.1		Ivnik, et al (1993)

instrument	group	n	m/f	age	intervention	inter	t #1	t #2	note	citation
Visual Spatial Learning Test DSUM	Epilepsy	20	12/8	29.90 (10.1)	RTL	3.8 m	27.2	29.2		Ivnik, et al (1993)
Visual Spatial Learning Test DSUM	Epilepsy	20	8/12	34.60 (9.80)	LTL	4.1 m	27.4	28.1		Ivnik, et al (1993)
Visual Spatial Learning Test PLI	Epilepsy	20	8/12	34.60 (9.80)	LTL	4.1 m	37.2	36.5		Ivnik, et al (1993)
Visual Spatial Learning Test PLI	Epilepsy	20	12/8	29.90 (10.1)	RTL	3.8 m	38.9	42.4		Ivnik, et al (1993)

Table 39. Memory Tests (Verbal)

instrument	group	n	m/f	age	intervention	inter	t #1	t #2	note	citation
Babcock-Levy Story Recall	Control	51	n/a	~70.0	n/a	1 w	9.0 (3.3)	14.0 (4.0)		Freides, et al (1996)
Babcock-Levy Story Recall	Control	28	n/a	~60.0	n/a	1 w	10.5 (3.4)	15.7 (3.2)		Freides, et al (1996)
Babcock-Levy Story Recall	Control	40	n/a	~20.0	n/a	1 w	12.8 (3.5)	19.0 (2.4)		Freides, et al (1996)
Babcock-Levy Story Recall	Control	29	n/a	~80.0	n/a	1 w	8.0 (3.6)	12.8 (4.3)		Freides, et al (1996)

instrument	group	n	m/f	age	intervention	inter	t #1	t #2	note	citation
Category Retrieval-easy	DAT	7	n/a	n/a	placebo	~35 min	1.67 (1.68)	3.28 (3.39)		Reisberg, et al (1983)
Category Retrieval-easy	DAT	7	n/a	n/a	naloxone	~35 min	1.43 (1.90)	4.14 (2.40)		Reisberg, et al (1983)
Category Retrieval-hard	DAT	7	n/a	n/a	naloxone	~35 min	0.19 (0.50)	1.76 (1.57)		Reisberg, et al (1983)
Category Retrieval-hard	DAT	7	n/a	n/a	placebo	~35 min	0.43 (0.88)	0.67 (1.35)		Reisberg, et al (1983)
Double Task Test	Control	10	5/5	70.0 - 79.0	n/a	1 d	NR	10.6 c		Peak (1970)
Double Task Test	Control	10	5/5	60.0 - 69.0	n/a	1 d	NR	7.9 c		Peak (1970)
Double Task Test	Control	10	5/5	50.0 - 59.0	n/a	1 d	NR	5.4 c		Peak (1970)
Double Task Test	Control	10	5/5	40.0 - 49.0	n/a	1 d	NR	20.7 c		Peak (1970)
First-Last Names Task	Control	59	37/22	68.70 (5.70)	n/a	3.4 y	1.6 (0.4)	2.6 (1.0)		Flicker, et al (1993)
Heaton Story Memory Test - Learning	HIV+ (IVDU)	8	5/3	39.00 (8.00)	MSR/placebo	7 d	5.5 (1.9)	11.0 (6.1)	*	Van Dyck, et al (1997)
Heaton Story Memory Test - Recall	HIV+ (IVDU)	8	5/3	39.00 (8.00)	MSR/placebo	7 d	21.7 (21.7)	23.7 (15.4)	*	Van Dyck, et al (1997)

instrument	group	n	m/f	age	intervention	inter	t #1	t #2	note	citation
HVLT FP (errors)	Control	45	n/a	68.80 (6.00)	n/a	9 m	0.33 (0.7)	0.24 (0.5)		Rasmusson, et al (1995)
HVLT Learning Across Trials	Control	45	n/a	68.80 (6.00)	n/a	9 m	3.47 (1.7)	3.80 (1.8)		Rasmusson, et al (1995)
HVLT Total Recall	Control	45	n/a	68.80 (6.00)	n/a	9 m	26.36 (4.4)	24.36 (4.9)		Rasmusson, et al (1995)
HVLT True-Positive Recog	Control	45	n/a	68.80 (6.00)	n/a	9 m	11.69 (0.7)	11.73 (0.8)		Rasmusson, et al (1995)
list learning test: delayed recall [10]	HD	26	12/14	39.00 (10.4)	n/a	12 m	4.9 (0.6)	5.0 (0.5)		Bamford, et al (1995)
list learning test: delayed recall [10]	HD	40	18/22	40.00 (10.3)	n/a	12 m	5.2 (0.4)	4.9 (0.4)		Bamford, et al (1995)
list learning test: delayed recog [20]	HD	40	18/22	40.00 (10.3)	n/a	12 m	17.5 (0.4)	17.6 (0.4)		Bamford, et al (1995)
list learning test: delayed recog [20]	HD	26	12/14	39.00 (10.4)	n/a	12 m	17.2 (0.5)	17.2 (0.6)		Bamford, et al (1995)
Mattis-Kovner Verbal Recall (best % recalled)	Orthopedic	134	39/95	69.00	epidural anesthesia	1w	57.2 (15.8)	-5.6 (16.0)c	*	Williams-Russo, et al (1995)

instrument	group	n	m/f	age	intervention	inter	t #1	t #2	note	citation
Mattis-Kovner Verbal Recall (best % recalled)	Orthopedic	128	38/90	69.00	general anesthesia	1w	55.9 (16.7)	-5.7 (16.5)c	*	Williams-Russo, et al (1995)
Mattis-Kovner Verbal Recog (d')	Orthopedic	134	39/95	69.00	epidural anesthesia	1w	2.88 (0.75)	-0.49 (0.77)c	*	Williams-Russo, et al (1995)
Mattis-Kovner Verbal Recog (d')	Orthopedic	128	38/90	69.00	general anesthesia	1w	2.80 (0.73)	-0.45 (0.77)c	*	Williams-Russo, et al (1995)
Moss 15" Verbal Recall	Naphtha Exposure	185	n/a	36.00	n/a	1 y	5.87 (1.58)	7.10 (2.25)		White, et al (1994)
Moss 2' Verbal Recall	Naphtha Exposure	185	n/a	36.00	n/a	1 y	5.00 (1.74)	6.13 (2.17)		White, et al (1994)
Remote Memory Questionnaire	Control	50	n/a	71.90 (0.90)	n/a	2 y	15.2 (0.5)	15.5 (0.7)		Flicker, et al (1993)
Remote Memory Questionnaire	DAT (advanced)	39	n/a	72.20 (1.20)	n/a	2 y	6.9 (1.0)	3.8 (0.6)		Flicker, et al (1993)
Remote Memory Questionnaire	DAT (early)	47	n/a	69.80 (1.20)	n/a	2 y	11.2 (0.9)	9.7 (0.8)		Flicker, et al (1993)
RPAB (std)	CVA	30	n/a	~64.0	piracetam	12 w	NR	5.7 (5.2) c	*	Enderby, et al (1994)

instrument	group	n	m/f	age	intervention	inter	t #1	t #2	note	citation
RPAB (std)	CVA	36	n/a	~68.0	placebo	12 w	NR	5.0 (5.7) c	*	Enderby, et al (1994)
Sentence Memory (correct)	Neuropsych referrals	248	203/ 45	8.00 (1.70)	n/a	2.65 y	8.4 (3.3)	11.0 (3.3)		Brown, et al (1989)
Shopping List	Control	50	n/a	71.90 (0.90)	n/a	2 y	38.2 (1.4)	39.8 (1.6)		Flicker, et al (1993)
Shopping List	DAT (advanced)	39	n/a	72.20 (1.20)	n/a	2 y	4.5 (2.8)	1.8 (1.8)		Flicker, et al (1993)
Shopping List	DAT (early)	47	n/a	69.80 (1.20)	n/a	2 y	17.3 (1.8)	9.9 (1.6)		Flicker, et al (1993)
Shopping List Task	DAT (early)	47	n/a	69.80 (1.20)	n/a	2 y	17.3 (1.8)	9.9 (1.6)		Flicker, et al (1993)
story recall	TIA	13	13/0	63.39	n/a	8 m	6.15 (3.44)	7.00 (4.22)		de Leo, et al (1987)
story recall	TIA	25	25/0	63.32	CE	8 m	6.72 (2.59)	7.68 (2.90)		de Leo, et al (1987)
story recall (loss)	Control	1017	436/ 581	74.30 (5.40)	n/a	2 y	0.7 (1.3)	0.7 (1.4)		Ganguli, et al (1996)
story recall delay	Alcoholic (1yr abstin)	23	23/0	36.80 (6.30)	n/a	1 y	5.9	5.6		Adams, et al (1980)
story recall delay	Alcoholic (2.5 yrs abstin)	25	25/0	36.50 (6.30)	n/a	1 y	5.9	7.0		Adams, et al (1980)
story recall delay	Control	21	21/0	36.90 (5.90)	n/a	1 y	5.2	6.5		Adams, et al (1980)

instrument	group	n	m/f	age	intervention	inter	t #1	t #2	note	citation
story recall delay	Control	1017	436/ 581	74.30 (5.40)	n/a	2 y	5.4 (3.0)	5.4 (3.0)		Ganguli, et al (1996)
Story Recall Delay	Control	10	5/5	50.0 - 59.0	n/a	1 d	NR	-2.7 c	Bab/ Term	Peak (1970)
Story Recall Delay	Control	10	5/5	60.0 - 69.0	n/a	1 d	NR	-2.3 c	Bab/ Term	Peak (1970)
Story Recall Delay	Control	10	5/5	40.0 - 49.0	n/a	1 d	NR	-0.6 c	Bab/ Term	Peak (1970)
Story Recall Delay	Control	10	5/5	70.0 - 79.0	n/a	1 d	NR	0.8 c	Bab/ Term	Peak (1970)
story recall delay (10')	TBI	42	40/2	33.20 (11.2)	n/a	9 m	11.9 (8.6)	15.2 (6.48)		Mukundan, et al (1987)
story recall delay [18]	Control	20	6/14	69.40 (4.20)	n/a	1 y	7.2 (2.7)	7.9 (2.7)	*	Fromm, et al (1991)
story recall delay [18]	DAT	18	5/13	71.00 (9.40)	n/a	1 y	0.9 (1.8)	0.2 (0.5)	*	Fromm, et al (1991)
story recall imm	Alcoholic (1yr abstin)	23	23/0	36.80 (6.30)	n/a	1 y	6.7	7.2		Adams, et al (1980)
story recall imm	Alcoholic (2.5 yrs abstin)	25	25/0	36.50 (6.30)	n/a	1 y	7.6	9.2		Adams, et al (1980)
story recall imm	Control	21	21/0	36.90 (5.90)	n/a	1 y	6.7	7.8		Adams, et al (1980)
story recall imm	Control	1017	436/ 581	74.30 (5.40)	n/a	2 y	6.2 (2.9)	6.1 (2.8)		Ganguli, et al (1996)
Story Recall Imm	Control	10	5/5	50.0 - 59.0	n/a	1 d	NR	0.1 c	Bab/ Term	Peak (1970)

instrument	group	n	m/f	age	intervention	inter	t #1	t #2	note	citation
Story Recall Imm	Control	10	5/5	60.0 - 69.0	n/a	1 d	NR	2.3 c	Bab/ Term	Peak (1970)
Story Recall Imm	Control	10	5/5	70.0 - 79.0	n/a	1 d	NR	1.4 c	Bab/ Term	Peak (1970)
Story Recall Imm	Control	10	5/5	40.0 - 49.0	n/a	1 d	NR	2.0 c	Bab/ Term	Peak (1970)
story recall imm [18]	Control	20	6/14	69.40 (4.20)	n/a	1 y	7.2 (2.7)	7.9 (2.7)	*	Fromm, et al (1991)
story recall imm [18]	DAT	18	5/13	71.00 (9.40)	n/a	1 y	2.1 (1.7)	2.0 (1.3)	*	Fromm, et al (1991)
story recall trial I	TBI	42	40/2	33.20 (11.2)	n/a	9 m	8.0 (6.5)	12.0 (6.3)		Mukundan, et al (1987)
story recall trial II	TBI	42	40/2	33.20 (11.2)	n/a	9 m	10.8 (7.4)	14.1 (5.8)		Mukundan, et al (1987)
story recall trial III	TBI	42	40/2	33.20 (11.2)	n/a	9 m	12.3 (7.7)	14.7 (6.0)		Mukundan, et al (1987)
Word Pairs	TIA	25	25/0	63.32	CE	8 m	4.56 (2.42)	5.80 (2.27)		de Leo, et al (1987)
Word Pairs	TIA	13	13/0	63.39	n/a	8 m	5.08 (1.98)	5.31 (1.89)		de Leo, et al (1987)

Table 40. Mini Mental State Examination (MMSE)

instrument	group	n	m/f	age	intervention	inter	t #1	t #2	note	citation
mMMSE	DAT	13	n/a	60.0-80.0	acetyl levocarnitine	6 m	35.5 (5.4)	34.3 (6.3)		Sano, et al (1992)
mMMSE	DAT	14	n/a	60.0-80.0	placebo	6 m	35.3 (7.2)	32.4 (9.3)		Sano, et al (1992)
mMMSE	IVDU	16	13/3	39.5	n/a	10.4 d	51.06 (4.09)	51.12 (5.36)		Richards, et al (1992)
mMMSE	PD	19	13/6	54.3	pergolide	~6 w	52.7 (3.95)	52.9 (4.53)		Stern, et al (1984)
MMSE	Affective D/O	12	3/9	58.9	treatment	51 d	25.5 (5.0)	27.2 (3.7)		Folstein, et al (1975)
MMSE	Age Related Cognitive Decline	24	13/11	62.2 (8.8)	n/a	2.0 y	27.7 (2.0)	28.2 (1.8)		Celsis, et al (1997)
MMSE	AIDS	10	10/0	41.7 (5.5)	n/a	6.53 m	27.1 (2.6)	28.1 (2.0)		Hinkin, et al (1995)
MMSE	CVD	48	34/14	62.0	CABG w/ complications	8-10 d	NR	-0.36 c		Malheiros, et al (1995)
MMSE	CVD	33	23/10	64.0	CABG	8-10 d	NR	-0.20 c		Malheiros, et al (1995)
MMSE	Control	70	28/42	62.5 (6.9)	n/a	1 y	27.8 (1.4)	29.0 (1.3)		Becker, et al (1988)
MMSE	Control	101	101/0	78.5 (7.2)	n/a	2.6 y	27.1	28.1		Frank, et al (1996)

instrument	group	n	m/f	age	intervention	inter	t #1	t #2	note	citation
MMSE	Control	141	0/141	78.5 (6.6)	n/a	2.7 y	27.4	28.5		Frank, et al (1996)
MMSE	Control	20	6/14	69.4 (4.2)	n/a	1 y	29.0 (1.0)	29.0 (0.9)	*	Fromm, et al (1991)
MMSE	Control	1017	436/581	74.3 (5.4)	n/a	2 y	27.7 (2.0)	27.0 (2.2)		Ganguli, et al (1996)
MMSE	Control	44	n/a	81.4 (3.2)	n/a	6 m	28.55 (1.44)	28.36 (1.77)	*	Hopp, et al (1997)
MMSE	Control	47	n/a	~68.0	n/a	1 y	29.2 (1.1)	29.1 (1.3)		Morris, et al (1989)
MMSE	Control	45	n/a	68.80 (6.00)	n/a	9 m	28.62 (1.1)	28.84 (0.9)		Rasmusson, et al (1993)
MMSE	Control	14	n/a	60.0+	scopolamine	1 d	28.0	26.0		Richardson, et al (1985)
MMSE	Control	16	n/a	60.0+	placebo	1 d	28.0	28.0		Richardson, et al (1985)
MMSE	Control	247	106/141	73.40 (5.40)	n/a	1 y	27.6 (2.3)	26.5 (3.0)		Schmand, et al (1995)
MMSE	Control	40	20/20	73.00 (7.70)	n/a	1 y	29.5 (0.8)	29.3 (0.9)	*	Taylor, et al (1996)
MMSE	Control w/ APOE-E4	20	5/15	80.35 (4.75)	n/a	3.32 y	28.2 (1.85)	27.6 (2.39)		Small, et al (1998)
MMSE	Control w/o APOE-E4	54	16/38	82.04 (5.26)	n/a	3.21 y	27.93 (1.53)	27.65 (1.96)		Small, et al (1998)

instrument	group	n	m/f	age	intervention	inter	t #1	t #2	note	citation
MMSE	DAT	44	21/23	67.00 (9.40)	n/a	1 y	23.7 (4.2)	21.9 (5.0)		Becker, et al (1988)
MMSE	DAT	18	11/7	65.30 (6.00)	n/a	3.0 y	26.5 (1.3)	21.5 (1.7)		Celsis, et al (1997)
MMSE	DAT	103	n/a	70.30	tacrine	6 w	16.1	16.0		Davis, et al (1992)
MMSE	DAT	112	n/a	70.50	placebo	6 w	16.3	15.3		Davis, et al (1992)
MMSE	DAT	65	35/30	66.70	placebo	13 w	17.42 (0.66)	16.26 (0.68)		Eagger, et al (1992)
MMSE	DAT	65	35/30	66.70	tacrine	13 w	17.5 (0.61)	18.69 (0.68)		Eagger, et al (1992)
MMSE	DAT	14	6/8	81.40	treatment	29 d	10.5 (6.6)	11.1 (5.7)		Folstein, et al (1975)
MMSE	DAT	34	34/0	83.90 (4.30)	n/a	2.1 y	24.5	24.3		Frank, et al (1996)
MMSE	DAT	34	34/0	83.90 (4.30)	n/a	2.1 y	23.5	21.2		Frank, et al (1996)
MMSE	DAT	18	5/13	71.00 (9.40)	n/a	1 y	22.7 (2.3)	19.4 (5.5)	*	Fromm, et al (1991)
MMSE	DAT	14	8/6	66.50	tacrine	3 m	16.6 (6.8)	16.8 (6.6)	*	Maltby, et al (1994)
MMSE	DAT	18	9/9	71.10	placebo	3 m	17.3 (6.7)	17.2 (6.8)	*	Maltby, et al (1994)
MMSE	DAT	430	198/232	70.90 (8.00)	n/a	1 y	18.7 (4.5)	-3.6 (4.4) c	*	Morris, et al (1993)

instrument	group	n	m/f	age	intervention	inter	t #1	t #2	note	citation
MMSE	DAT	52	n/a	~71.0	n/a	1 y	19.4 (4.8)	17.3 (6.0)		Morris, et al (1989)
MMSE	DAT	7	3/4	70.70 (3.30)	acetyl-l-carnitine	6 m	18.4 (1.3)	19.6 (1.5)	*	Pettegrew, et al (1995)
MMSE	DAT	5	1/4	64.20 (2.60)	placebo	6 m	18.5 (0.9)	12.0 (1.9)	*	Pettegrew, et al (1995)
MMSE	DAT	177	n/a	69.90	n/a	1 y	14.10	4.76 c		Rich, et al (1995)
MMSE	DAT	32	n/a	70.70	NSAID	1 y	17.53	3.93 c		Rich, et al (1995)
MMSE	DAT	40	20/20	73.00 (7.60)	n/a	1 y	21.1 (4.5)	17.7 (6.4)	*	Taylor, et al (1996)
MMSE	DAT	40	n/a	50.0 - 90.0	n/a	1 w	16.92 (4.71)	17.42 (4.22)	*	Thal, et al (1986)
MMSE	DAT (at risk)	50	0/50	84.10 (5.10)	n/a	2.3 y	25.8	27.0		Frank, et al (1996)
MMSE	DAT (at risk)	32	32/0	83.30 (6.70)	n/a	2.0 y	25.0	25.8		Frank, et al (1996)
MMSE	DAT (P1 wave absent)	17	8/9	73.88 (7.83)	n/a	56 w	19.74 (2.94)	-3.21 c		Green, et al (1995)
MMSE	DAT (P1 wave present)	18	8/10	74.56 (6.31)	n/a	56 w	19.61 (3.52)	-3.01 c		Green, et al (1995)
MMSE	DAT/MID	29	14/15	71.50 (1.30)	oxiracetam	6 m	15.6 (0.7)	17.9 (1.0)	*	Villardita, et al (1992)
MMSE	DAT/MID	30	21/9	67.80 (1.50)	placebo	3 m	16.7 (0.8)	15.6 (0.8)	*	Villardita, et al (1992)

instrument	group	n	m/f	age	intervention	inter	t #1	t #2	note	citation
MMSE	DAT/MID	30	15/15	71.70 (1.30)	oxiracetam	3 m	15.5 (0.7)	19.2 (0.9)	*	Villardita, et al (1992)
MMSE	Dementia	87	39/48	76.10	nimodipine	90 d	17.6 (5.47)	21.0 (5.14)		Ban, et al (1990)
MMSE	Dementia	88	34/54	74.30	placebo	90 d	18.4 (5.57)	19.2 (5.74)		Ban, et al (1990)
MMSE	Dementia (mod - sev)	57	25/32	80.40 (7.50)	n/a	8 w	9.2 (7.1)	7.8 (7.1)		Lloyd, et al (1995)
MMSE	Depression w/ Cognitive Impairment	7	5/2	75.0	treatment	36 d	18.3 (5.0)	23.4 (2.4)		Folstein, et al (1975)
MMSE	Hydroceph (control pressure)	14	9/5	66.0 (14.2)	extracranial shunting	27.37 w	15.2 (7.51)	19.8 (8.23)		Stambrook, et al (1988)
MMSE	nursing home residents	64	18/46	82.60 (7.70)	antipsychotic meds d/c	6.7 m	11.73	0.47 c		Thapa, et al (1994)
MMSE	nursing home residents	207	54/ 153	78.90 (7.20)	antipsychotic meds	6.7 m	13.64	0.43 c		Thapa, et al (1994)
MMSE	Psychiatric Inpts	22	3/19	41.20	n/a	1 d	24.2 (7.1)	25.3 (7.0)		Folstein, et al (1975)
MMSE	Psychiatric Inpts	23	6/17	74.10	n/a	28 d	19.3 (10.0)	19.2 (9.2)		Folstein, et al (1975)
MMSE	Psychiatric Inpts	19	7/12	45.60	n/a	1 d	23.9 (4.7)	25.2 (5.1)		Folstein, et al (1975)

instrument	group	n	m/f	age	intervention	inter	t #1	t #2	note	citation
MMSE	Schizophrenia	10	8/2	71.00	risperidone	4 w	22.4 (3.9)	25.5 (3.2)		Berman, et al (1996)
MMSE Attention	Control	44	n/a	81.39 (3.17)	n/a	6 m	4.72 (1.03)	4.63 (1.16)	*	Hopp, et al (1997)
MMSE Attention	Control	60	26/34	71.24 (5.96)	n/a	12 m	4.38 (0.83)	4.42 (0.95)		Olin, et al (1991)
MMSE Language	Control	44	n/a	81.39 (3.17)	n/a	6 m	8.91 (0.29)	8.89 (0.32)		Hopp, et al (1997)
MMSE Language	Control	60	26/34	71.24 (5.96)	n/a	12 m	8.78 (0.47)	8.56 (0.68)		Olin, et al (1991)
MMSE Orientation	Control	44	n/a	81.39 (3.17)	n/a	6 m	9.91 (0.29)	9.77 (0.68)	*	Hopp, et al (1997)
MMSE Orientation	Control	60	26/34	71.24 (5.96)	n/a	12 m	9.78 (0.47)	9.84 (0.42)		Olin, et al (1991)
MMSE Orientation	CVA/Control	300	n/a	70.70	improved/ stable	9-12 m	NR	0.1 (1.0) c		Desmond, et al (1995)
MMSE Orientation	CVA/Control	71	n/a	70.70	declined	9-12 m	NR	-0.6 (1.8) c		Desmond, et al (1995)
MMSE Recall	Control	44	n/a	81.39 (3.17)	n/a	6 m	1.80 (1.07)	1.93 (1.04)	*	Hopp, et al (1997)
MMSE Recall	Control	60	26/34	71.24 (5.96)	n/a	12 m	2.14 (1.03)	1.86 (1.11)		Olin, et al (1991)
MMSE Registration	Control	44	n/a	81.39 (3.17)	n/a	6 m	3.00 (0.0)	3.00 (0.0)	*	Hopp, et al (1997)

instrument	group	n	m/f	age	intervention	inter	t #1	t #2	note	citation
MMSE Registration	Control	60	26/34	71.24 (5.96)	n/a	12 m	3.00 (0.00)	3.00 (0.00)		Olin, et al (1991)
MMSE Total	Control	60	26/34	71.24 (5.96)	n/a	12 m	28.08 (1.70)	27.68 (1.87)		Olin, et al (1991)

Table 41. Multilingual Aphasia Examination (MAE)

instrument	group	n	m/f	age	intervention	inter	t #1	t #2	note	citation
MAE Aural Comp	Epilepsy	40	23/17	32.20 (8.20)	n/a	~9 m	16.93 (1.37)	17.20 (1.14)		Hermann, et al (1996)
MAE COWAT	Dementia (2° to steriods)	6	6/0	49.67	steriods d/c or reduced	10.9 m	6.0	12.5		Varney, et al (1984)
MAE COWAT	Depression	9	6/3	48.30 (17.8)	left ECT	2 d	37.9	37.0	*	Kronfol, et al (1978)
MAE COWAT	Depression	9	6/3	50.20 (18.5)	right ECT	2 d	32.8	28.7	*	Kronfol, et al (1978)
MAE COWAT	Epilepsy	40	23/17	32.20 (8.20)	n/a	~9 m	33.00 (11.10)	32.00 (7.51)		Hermann, et al (1996)
MAE COWAT (t)	Lung Cancer	11	n/a	~61.0	cranial irradiation	11 m	38.6	38.4		Komaki, et al (1995)
MAE Oral Spelling	Epilepsy	40	23/17	32.20 (8.20)	n/a	~9 m	9.25 (2.16)	9.27 (2.04)		Hermann, et al (1996)
MAE Reading Comp	Epilepsy	40	23/17	32.20 (8.20)	n/a	~9 m	17.20 (1.32)	17.27 (1.18)		Hermann, et al (1996)

instrument	group	n	m/f	age	intervention	inter	t #1	t #2	note	citation
MAE Sentence Repetition	Brain Tumor (post-surgery)	12	5/7	31.80 (8.60)	radiation tx	3 m	14.8 (1.6)	15.1 (1.5)	*	Armstrong, et al (1995)
MAE Sentence Repetition	Depression	9	6/3	48.30 (17.8)	left ECT	2 d	12.3	12.2	*	Kronfol, et al (1978)
MAE Sentence Repetition	Depression	9	6/3	50.20 (18.5)	right ECT	2 d	12.4	12.3	*	Kronfol, et al (1978)
MAE Sentence Repetition	Epilepsy	40	23/17	32.20 (8.20)	n/a	~9 m	11.00 (2.14)	10.60 (2.23)		Hermann, et al (1996)
MAE Token Test	Depression	9	6/3	50.20 (18.5)	right ECT	2 d	40.2	40.7	*	Kronfol, et al (1978)
MAE Token Test	Depression	9	6/3	48.30 (17.8)	left ECT	2 d	41.0	40.3	*	Kronfol, et al (1978)
MAE Token Test	Epilepsy	40	23/17	32.20 (8.20)	n/a	~9 m	41.85 (2.48)	41.62 (3.59)		Hermann, et al (1996)
MAE Token Test (t)	Lung Cancer	11	n/a	~61.0	cranial irradiation	11 m	44.3	46.7		Komaki, et al (1995)
MAE Visual Naming	Epilepsy	40	23/17	32.20 (8.20)	n/a	~9 m	48.50 (8.15)	48.05 (7.81)		Hermann, et al (1996)

Table 42. Name Writing Tests

instrument	group	n	m/f	age	intervention	inter	t #1	t #2	note	citation
Name Writing LH (sec)	Control	14	6/8	11.2	n/a	4-6 h	52.9 (7.8)	55.0 (4.5)		Reich, et al (1990)
Name Writing LH (sec)	Diabetes	14	6/8	10.5	mild hypoglycemia	4-6 h	49.3 (9.0)	50.4 (9.8)		Reich, et al (1990)
Name Writing LH (sec)	Diabetes	10	5/5	12.2	hypoglycemia	4-6 h	42.3 (15.7)	45.6 (12.0)		Reich, et al (1990)
Name Writing LH (sec)	Neuropsych referrals	248	203/ 45	8.00 (1.7)	n/a	2.65 y	32.6 (20.3)	29.4 (17.6)		Brown, et al (1989)
Name Writing RH (sec)	Control	14	6/8	11.2	n/a	4-6 h	55.3 (3.7)	57.5 (4.3)		Reich, et al (1990)
Name Writing RH (sec)	Diabetes	14	6/8	10.5	mild hypoglycemia	4-6 h	50.6 (6.1)	51.8 (6.4)		Reich, et al (1990)
Name Writing RH (sec)	Diabetes	10	5/5	12.2	hypoglycemia	4-6 h	48.0 (8.8)	40.6 (32.0)		Reich, et al (1990)
Name Writing RH (sec)	Neuropsych referrals	248	203/ 45	8.00 (1.7)	n/a	2.65 y	23.6 (15.4)	20.9 (15)		Brown, et al (1989)
signature writing (sec)	ALS	3	n/a	52.3 (8.1)	placebo	5 d	7.3 (1.5)	6.0 (1.0)	*	Poutiainen, et al (1994)
signature writing (sec)	ALS	12	n/a	49.4 (11.8)	high dose interferon	5 d	8.7 (6.3)	12.6 (6.6)	*	Poutiainen, et al (1994)

Table 43. Neurobehavioral Evaluation System (NES)

instrument	group	n	m/f	age	intervention	inter	t #1	t #2	note	citation
NES CPT	Control	16	16/0	25.00	adinazolam + probenecid	1 h	NR	8.31 %c	*	Golden, et al (1994)
NES CPT	Control	16	16/0	25.00	adinazolam	1 h	NR	9.45 %c	*	Golden, et al (1994)
NES CPT	Control	16	16/0	25.00	probenecid	1 h	NR	-1.50 %c	*	Golden, et al (1994)
NES CPT	Control	16	16/0	25.00	placebo	1 h	NR	0.92 %c	*	Golden, et al (1994)
NES D Span Backward	Control	16	16/0	25.00	adinazolam	1 h	NR	10.8 %c	*	Golden, et al (1994)
NES D Span Backward	Control	16	16/0	25.00	placebo	1 h	NR	-8.44 %c	*	Golden, et al (1994)
NES D Span Backward	Control	16	16/0	25.00	adinazolam + probenecid	1 h	NR	4.70 %c	*	Golden, et al (1994)
NES D Span Backward	Control	16	16/0	25.00	probenecid	1 h	NR	-4.32 %c	*	Golden, et al (1994)
NES D Span Forward	Control	16	16/0	25.00	adinazolam	1 h	NR	2.78 %c	*	Golden, et al (1994)
NES D Span Forward	Control	16	16/0	25.00	probenecid	1 h	NR	-0.69 %c	*	Golden, et al (1994)
NES D Span Forward	Control	16	16/0	25.00	adinazolam + probenecid	1 h	NR	6.36 %c	*	Golden, et al (1994)
NES D Span Forward	Control	16	16/0	25.00	placebo	1 h	NR	0.65 %c	*	Golden, et al (1994)

instrument	group	n	m/f	age	intervention	inter	t #1	t #2	note	citation
NES D Sym	Control	16	16/0	25.00	adinazolam	1 h	NR	11.1 %c	*	Golden, et al (1994)
NES D Sym	Control	16	16/0	25.00	placebo	1 h	NR	0.31 %c	*	Golden, et al (1994)
NES D Sym	Control	16	16/0	25.00	probenecid	1 h	NR	-1.13 %c	*	Golden, et al (1994)
NES D Sym	Control	16	16/0	25.00	adinazolam + probenecid	1 h	NR	11.1 %c	*	Golden, et al (1994)
NES Pattern Memory (% correct)	Naphtha Exposure	185	n/a	36.00	n/a	1 y	80.6 (11.9)	79.9 (11.4)		White, et al (1994)
NES Pattern Memory (sec)	Naphtha Exposure	185	n/a	36.00	n/a	1 y	9.11 (2.46)	8.10 (2.73)		White, et al (1994)
NES Sym Dig (% correct)	Naphtha Exposure	185	n/a	36.00	n/a	1 y	99.2 (2.7)	99.0 (3.1)		White, et al (1994)
NES Sym Dig (sec)	Naphtha Exposure	185	n/a	36.00	n/a	1 y	23.61 (6.22)	22.58 (4.82)		White, et al (1994)

Table 44. North American Reading Tests (NART)

instrument	group	n	m/f	age	intervention	inter	t #1	t #2	note	citation
AMNART (errors)	Control	40	20/20	73.00 (7.70)	n/a	1 y	11.0 (5.6)	10.6 (5.5)	*	Taylor, et al (1996)
AMNART (errors)	DAT	40	20/20	73.00 (7.60)	n/a	1 y	16.0 (8.3)	18.5 (9.1)	*	Taylor, et al (1996)

instrument	group	n	m/f	age	intervention	inter	t #1	t #2	note	citation
NART (errors)	Control	61	n/a	37.10 (12.20)	n/a	10 d	17.98 (10.8)	17.26		Crawford, et al (1989a)
NART (errors)	Control	20	6/14	69.40 (4.20)	n/a	1 y	19.3 (6.1)	19.4 (6.4)	*	Fromm, et al (1991)
NART (errors)	DAT	18	5/13	71.00 (9.40)	n/a	1 y	13.2 (5.4)	12.3 (6.2)	*	Fromm, et al (1991)
NART (errors)	DAT	23	n/a	77.30 (5.60)	n/a	1 y	16.62 (9.69)	15.1 (12.3)		O'Carroll, et al (1987)
NART (IQ)	Renal Failure	8	3/5	67.50	n/a	19.3 w	101.9 (5.2)	102.7 (4.9)		Temple, et al (1995)
NART (IQ)	Renal Failure	9	4/5	65.00	rHuEpo	22.8 w	104.0 (5.8)	104.3 (6.2)		Temple, et al (1995)

Table 45. Paced Auditory Serial Addition Tests (PASAT)

instrument	group	n	m/f	age	intervention	inter	t #1	t #2	note	citation
CHIPASAT-1.2	Control	13	n/a	13.00 - 14.00	n/a	25 d	18.8 (8.1)	22.3 (6.7)		Dyche, et al (1991)
CHIPASAT-1.2	Control	11	n/a	12.00 - 13.00	n/a	25 d	19.1 (7.8)	23.1 (10.3)		Dyche, et al (1991)
CHIPASAT-1.2	Control	13	n/a	11.00 - 12.00	n/a	25 d	18.6 (7.2)	22.5 (6.1)		Dyche, et al (1991)
CHIPASAT-1.2	Control	8	n/a	10.00 - 11.00	n/a	25 d	20.0 (4.2)	24.9 (10.6)		Dyche, et al (1991)

instrument	group	n	m/f	age	intervention	inter	t #1	t #2	note	citation
CHIPASAT-1.2	Control	13	n/a	9.00 - 10.00	n/a	25 d	18.4 (7.5)	21.1 (7.4)		Dyche, et al (1991)
CHIPASAT-1.2	Control	12	n/a	14.00 - 15.00	n/a	25 d	22.4 (8.1)	26.8 (10.8)		Dyche, et al (1991)
CHIPASAT-1.6	Control	13	n/a	9.00 - 10.00	n/a	25 d	26.2 (9.4)	31.0 (10.3)		Dyche, et al (1991)
CHIPASAT-1.6	Control	12	n/a	14.00 - 15.00	n/a	25 d	31.7 (9.9)	39.3 (11.7)		Dyche, et al (1991)
CHIPASAT-1.6	Control	13	n/a	13.00 - 14.00	n/a	25 d	27.0 (5.5)	34.2 (9.5)		Dyche, et al (1991)
CHIPASAT-1.6	Control	11	n/a	12.00 - 13.00	n/a	25 d	29.7 (8.1)	35.3 (8.4)		Dyche, et al (1991)
CHIPASAT-1.6	Control	13	n/a	11.00 - 12.00	n/a	25 d	26.6 (7.5)	33.3 (8.6)		Dyche, et al (1991)
CHIPASAT-1.6	Control	8	n/a	10.00 - 11.00	n/a	25 d	29.4 (9.0)	34.1 (10.2)		Dyche, et al (1991)
CHIPASAT-2.0	Control	13	n/a	9.00 - 10.00	n/a	25 d	30.7 (10.8)	38.2 (11.0)		Dyche, et al (1991)
CHIPASAT-2.0	Control	8	n/a	10.00 - 11.00	n/a	25 d	36.4 (9.3)	41.5 (10.0)		Dyche, et al (1991)
CHIPASAT-2.0	Control	13	n/a	11.00 - 12.00	n/a	25 d	32.9 (7.7)	39.2 (8.2)		Dyche, et al (1991)
CHIPASAT-2.0	Control	11	n/a	12.00 - 13.00	n/a	25 d	33.6 (7.7)	39.1 (7.3)		Dyche, et al (1991)

instrument	group	n	m/f	age	intervention	inter	t #1	t #2	note	citation
CHIPASAT-2.0	Control	12	n/a	14.00 - 15.00	n/a	25 d	36.2 (9.6)	42.5 (10.2)		Dyche, et al (1991)
CHIPASAT-2.0	Control	13	n/a	13.00 - 14.00	n/a	25 d	35.3 (5.9)	40.8 (7.8)		Dyche, et al (1991)
CHIPASAT-2.4	Control	13	n/a	9.00 - 10.00	n/a	25 d	36.2 (10.8)	42.0 (10.7)		Dyche, et al (1991)
CHIPASAT-2.4	Control	12	n/a	14.00 - 15.00	n/a	25 d	38.8 (9.2)	47.6 (8.2)		Dyche, et al (1991)
CHIPASAT-2.4	Control	13	n/a	13.00 - 14.00	n/a	25 d	39.6 (7.1)	46.9 (6.1)		Dyche, et al (1991)
CHIPASAT-2.4	Control	11	n/a	12.00 - 13.00	n/a	25 d	38.7 (7.2)	44.9 (7.5)		Dyche, et al (1991)
CHIPASAT-2.4	Control	13	n/a	11.00 - 12.00	n/a	25 d	35.3 (11.2)	43.5 (8.6)		Dyche, et al (1991)
CHIPASAT-2.4	Control	8	n/a	10.00 - 11.00	n/a	25 d	39.4 (5.6)	47.0 (7.7)		Dyche, et al (1991)
PASAT	Control	110	110/0	19.30 (1.30)	n/a	~3 m	299.5 (50.1)	339.3 (40.0)		Macciocchi (1990)
PASAT	Control	21	5/16	34.00	carbamaz/ phenytoin CB	1 m	30.0 (9.0)	32.0 (8.0)	*	Meador, et al (1991)
PASAT	HIV+ (IVDU)	8	5/3	39.00 (8.00)	MSR/placebo	7 d	76.6 (35.9)	80.9 (53.1)	*	Van Dyck, et al (1997)
PASAT (avg error score)	Control	11	9/2	31.60 (5.00)	n/a	6 m	10.5 (8.1)	8.6 (6.3)		Di Stefano, et al (1996)

instrument	group	n	m/f	age	intervention	inter	t #1	t #2	note	citation
PASAT (avg error score)	Whiplash	21	8/13	35.50 (10.5)	n/a	6 m	13.9 (6.0)	7.1 (4.7)		Di Stefano, et al (1996)
PASAT (avg error score)	Whiplash	58	26/32	29.60 (8.90)	n/a	6 m	16.3 (8.6)	9.4 (7.6)		Di Stefano, et al (1996)
PASAT (avg error score)	Whiplash (asx at 6 mos)	67	28/36	29.00 (8.50)	n/a	6 m	15.0 (8.0)	8.5 (7.3)		Radanov, et al (1993)
PASAT (avg error score)	Whiplash (sx at 6 mos)	31	9/19	36.50 (10.2)	n/a	6 m	19.4 (10.0)	13.0 (7.4)		Radanov, et al (1993)
PASAT (avg error score)	Whiplash w/ continuing sx	21	8/13	35.40 (11.0)	n/a	6 m	20.6 (11.3)	14.4 (8.4)	*	Di Stefano, et al (1995)
PASAT (avg error score)	Whiplash w/ continuing sx	28	9/19	34.10 (10.2)	n/a	6 m	18.1 (10.2)	13.5 (7.4)		Di Stefano, et al (1996)
PASAT (correct/time)	TBI (mild – mod)	7	7/0	25.00	CDP-choline	1 m	0.315	0.344		Levin (1991)
PASAT (correct/time)	TBI (mild – mod)	7	7/0	20.00	placebo	1 m	0.398	0.479		Levin (1991)
PASAT (errors)	Alcoholic	16	16/0	37.50 (11.1)	inpt tx	3-4 w	72.8 (16.3)	57.8 (19.6)		Unkenstein, et al (1991)
PASAT (time/correct)	HIV+ (asx)	20	15/5	36.70 (9.90)	n/a	7-10 d	3.9 (1.4)	3.2 (1.2)		McCaffrey, et al (1995)
PASAT (time/correct)	HIV+ (sx)	12	11/1	37.20 (6.40)	n/a	7-10 d	3.8 (1.2)	3.2 (1.2)		McCaffrey, et al (1995)
PASAT (time/correct)	HIV- ("At-Risk")	12	12/0	40.40 (13.0)	n/a	7-10 d	3.5 (1.1)	3.1 (1.0)		McCaffrey, et al (1995)

instrument	group	n	m/f	age	intervention	inter	t #1	t #2	note	citation
PASAT 1.2	Control	30	16/14	22.43 (2.67)	n/a	1 w	27.4 (9.86)	31.2 (10.24)		Stuss, et al (1988)
PASAT 1.2	Control	30	14/16	40.63 (2.97)	n/a	1 w	24.63 (10.55)	31.6 (10.12)		Stuss, et al (1988)
PASAT 1.2	Control	30	14/16	61.77 (3.00)	n/a	1 w	21.2 (14.44)	27.27 (13.5)		Stuss, et al (1988)
PASAT 1.2	Control	10	5/5	17.30 (0.95)	n/a	1 w	24.0 (9.6)	28.7 (11.7)		Stuss, et al (1987)
PASAT 1.2	Control	10	6/4	23.00 (2.67)	n/a	1 w	33.6 (9.2)	35.0 (7.9)		Stuss, et al (1987)
PASAT 1.2	Control	10	5/5	33.90 (2.88)	n/a	1 w	27.6 (8.1)	32.0 (11.8)		Stuss, et al (1987)
PASAT 1.2	Control	10	6/4	44.20 (3.12)	n/a	1 w	23.0 (15.0)	30.9 (9.7)		Stuss, et al (1987)
PASAT 1.2	Control	10	6/4	55.30 (2.98)	n/a	1 w	8.2 (11.5)	14.5 (12.4)		Stuss, et al (1987)
PASAT 1.2	Control	10	5/5	63.70 (3.13)	n/a	1 w	30.7 (8.7)	37.2 (7.2)		Stuss, et al (1987)
PASAT 1.2	Control	26	20/6	29.70 (12.4)	n/a	1 w	26.3 (10.2)	29.3 (12.0)	*	Stuss, et al (1989)
PASAT 1.2	Control	22	15/7	27.70 (11.6)	n/a	6 d	26.14 (13.13)	30.18 (12.94)	*	Stuss, et al (1989)
PASAT 1.2	Control	10	6/4	31.50	placebo	2 w	33.9 (7.4)	38.0 (8.8)		Thomas, et al (1996)

instrument	group	n	m/f	age	intervention	inter	t #1	t #2	note	citation
PASAT 1.2	Control	10	6/4	31.50	vigabatrin	2 w	33.3 (7.4)	35.0 (7.9)		Thomas, et al (1996)
PASAT 1.2	TBI	26	20/6	30.90 (11.9)	n/a	1 w	17.2 (11.6)	20.9 (13.6)	*	Stuss, et al (1989)
PASAT 1.2	TBI	22	15/7	29.50 (12.6)	n/a	6 d	17.5 (11.39)	25.64 (10.19)	*	Stuss, et al (1989)
PASAT 1.6	Control	30	14/16	61.77 (3.00)	n/a	1 w	30.83 (15.85)	37.1 (15.18)		Stuss, et al (1988)
PASAT 1.6	Control	30	16/14	22.43 (2.67)	n/a	1 w	35.97 (12.97)	43.37 (11.02)		Stuss, et al (1988)
PASAT 1.6	Control	30	14/16	40.63 (2.97)	n/a	1 w	33.1 (12.2)	41.93 (10.56)		Stuss, et al (1988)
PASAT 1.6	Control	10	6/4	23.00 (2.67)	n/a	1 w	41.3 (12.0)	48.8 (6.0)		Stuss, et al (1987)
PASAT 1.6	Control	10	5/5	63.70 (3.13)	n/a	1 w	40.3 (10.7)	45.7 (8.3)		Stuss, et al (1987)
PASAT 1.6	Control	10	6/4	55.30 (2.98)	n/a	1 w	17.6 (15.1)	24.4 (16.6)		Stuss, et al (1987)
PASAT 1.6	Control	10	6/4	44.20 (3.12)	n/a	1 w	30.6 (13.8)	43.0 (9.2)		Stuss, et al (1987)
PASAT 1.6	Control	10	5/5	33.90 (2.88)	n/a	1 w	35.6 (11.7)	43.2 (13.7)		Stuss, et al (1987)
PASAT 1.6	Control	10	5/5	17.30 (0.95)	n/a	1 w	35.3 (14.4)	40.6 (13.2)		Stuss, et al (1987)

instrument	group	n	m/f	age	intervention	inter	t #1	t #2	note	citation
PASAT 1.6	Control	22	15/7	27.70 (11.6)	n/a	6 d	35.1 (15.2)	41.9 (13.8)	*	Stuss, et al (1989)
PASAT 1.6	Control	26	20/6	29.70 (12.4)	n/a	1 w	36.1 (11.8)	40.2 (12.3)	*	Stuss, et al (1989)
PASAT 1.6	Control	10	6/4	31.50	vigabatrin	2 w	37.1 (7.4)	41.0 (8.4)		Thomas, et al (1996)
PASAT 1.6	Control	10	6/4	31.50	placebo	2 w	39.6 (8.8)	40.1 (10.9)		Thomas, et al (1996)
PASAT 1.6	TBI	22	15/7	29.50 (12.6)	n/a	6 d	24.3 (13.6)	36.1 (11.4)	*	Stuss, et al (1989)
PASAT 1.6	TBI	26	20/6	30.90 (11.9)	n/a	1 w	23.4 (15.0)	28.3 (15.4)	*	Stuss, et al (1989)
PASAT 2.0	Control	20	0/20	29.10 (4.70)	n/a	1 m	45.9 (4.7)	49.3 (4.5)	*	Harris, et al (1996)
PASAT 2.0	Control	72	67/5	44.50 (12.4)	n/a	6 m	32.6 (11.7)	35.7 (13.2)		Prevey, et al (1996)
PASAT 2.0	Control	30	14/16	61.77 (3.00)	n/a	1 w	35.6 (14.58)	45.0 (15.3)		Stuss, et al (1988)
PASAT 2.0	Control	30	14/16	40.63 (2.97)	n/a	1 w	41.87 (10.16)	49.23 (8.67)		Stuss, et al (1988)
PASAT 2.0	Control	30	16/14	22.43 (2.67)	n/a	1 w	42.0 (12.5)	50.23 (9.17)		Stuss, et al (1988)
PASAT 2.0	Control	10	5/5	17.30 (0.95)	n/a	1 w	42.8 (15.2)	47.4 (11.6)		Stuss, et al (1987)

instrument	group	n	m/f	age	intervention	inter	t #1	t #2	note	citation
PASAT 2.0	Control	10	6/4	23.00 (2.67)	n/a	1 w	45.7 (8.8)	55.3 (5.0)		Stuss, et al (1987)
PASAT 2.0	Control	10	5/5	33.90 (2.88)	n/a	1 w	42.7 (10.4)	48.7 (10.3)		Stuss, et al (1987)
PASAT 2.0	Control	10	5/5	63.70 (3.13)	n/a	1 w	41.7 (9.6)	51.9 (6.4)		Stuss, et al (1987)
PASAT 2.0	Control	10	6/4	55.30 (2.98)	n/a	1 w	25.5 (16.4)	32.6 (19.8)		Stuss, et al (1987)
PASAT 2.0	Control	10	6/4	44.20 (3.12)	n/a	1 w	45.0 (6.5)	50.6 (7.9)		Stuss, et al (1987)
PASAT 2.0	Control	22	15/7	27.70 (11.6)	n/a	6 d	42.6 (12.4)	50.5 (11.3)	*	Stuss, et al (1989)
PASAT 2.0	Control	26	20/6	29.70 (12.4)	n/a	1 w	41.8 (11.7)	47.2 (11.9)	*	Stuss, et al (1989)
PASAT 2.0	Control	10	6/4	31.50	placebo	2 w	41.5 (8.6)	43.6 (8.4)		Thomas, et al (1996)
PASAT 2.0	Control	10	6/4	31.50	vigabatrin	2 w	40.6 (8.4)	43.1 (7.4)		Thomas, et al (1996)
PASAT 2.0	Epilepsy	26	24/2	43.50 (17.1)	carbamaz	6 m	28.5 (14.1)	30.1 (14.0)		Prevey, et al (1996)
PASAT 2.0	Epilepsy	39	36/3	44.30 (14.2)	valproate	6 m	30.0 (11.5)	27.9 (13.6)		Prevey, et al (1996)
PASAT 2.0	MS	19	6/13	43.37	n/a	8 w	40.0 (4.5)	53.0 (5.2)	*	Bever, et al (1995)

instrument	group	n	m/f	age	intervention	inter	t #1	t #2	note	citation
PASAT 2.0	Pregnant	20	0/20	29.00 (4.60)	normal delivery	1 m	43.7 (5.8)	44.6 (6.9)	*	Harris, et al (1996)
PASAT 2.0	TBI	26	20/6	30.90 (11.9)	n/a	1 w	29.7 (15.1)	33.4 (15.8)	*	Stuss, et al (1989)
PASAT 2.0	TBI	22	15/7	29.50 (12.6)	n/a	6 d	33.6 (12.3)	41.9 (10.4)	*	Stuss, et al (1989)
PASAT 2.4	Control	10	n/a	n/a	n/a	n/a	53.5 (5.8)	54.0		Maddocks, et al (1996)
PASAT 2.4	Control	72	67/5	44.50 (12.4)	n/a	6 m	33.7 (12.4)	38.4 (12.3)		Prevey, et al (1996)
PASAT 2.4	Control	30	14/16	61.77 (3.00)	n/a	1 w	43.47 (13.6)	49.2 (11.4)		Stuss, et al (1988)
PASAT 2.4	Control	30	16/14	22.43 (2.67)	n/a	1 w	47.4 (10.12)	53.73 (7.3)		Stuss, et al (1988)
PASAT 2.4	Control	30	14/16	40.63 (2.97)	n/a	1 w	43.43 (10.16)	52.57 (7.89)		Stuss, et al (1988)
PASAT 2.4	Control	10	5/5	17.30 (0.95)	n/a	1 w	45.7 (12.3)	52.0 (10.2)		Stuss, et al (1987)
PASAT 2.4	Control	10	6/4	23.00 (2.67)	n/a	1 w	51.3 (6.2)	56.8 (4.6)		Stuss, et al (1987)
PASAT 2.4	Control	10	5/5	33.90 (2.88)	n/a	1 w	44.8 (8.1)	51.9 (8.1)		Stuss, et al (1987)
PASAT 2.4	Control	10	6/4	44.20 (3.12)	n/a	1 w	49.1 (7.3)	55.1 (5.2)		Stuss, et al (1987)

instrument	group	n	m/f	age	intervention	inter	t #1	t #2	note	citation
PASAT 2.4	Control	10	6/4	55.30 (2.98)	n/a	1 w	35.3 (15.6)	41.1 (15.8)		Stuss, et al (1987)
PASAT 2.4	Control	10	5/5	63.70 (3.13)	n/a	1 w	47.7 (8.8)	54.0 (5.1)		Stuss, et al (1987)
PASAT 2.4	Control	22	15/7	27.70 (11.6)	n/a	6 d	48.9 (9.7)	53.3 (11.4)	*	Stuss, et al (1989)
PASAT 2.4	Control	26	20/6	29.70 (12.4)	n/a	1 w	47.1 (10.9)	51.3 (11.0)	*	Stuss, et al (1989)
PASAT 2.4	Epilepsy	39	36/3	44.30 (14.2)	valproate	6 m	31.4 (11.4)	29.3 (14.0)		Prevey, et al (1996)
PASAT 2.4	Epilepsy	26	24/2	43.50 (17.1)	carbamaz	6 m	28.3 (15.0)	32.0 (16.0)		Prevey, et al (1996)
PASAT 2.4	TBI	10	n/a	n/a	concussion	n/a	54.2 (5.6)	53.3		Maddocks, et al (1996)
PASAT 2.4	TBI	22	15/7	29.50 (12.6)	n/a	6 d	41.6 (11.3)	48.9 (9.1)	*	Stuss, et al (1989)
PASAT 2.4	TBI	26	20/6	30.90 (11.9)	n/a	1 w	34.1 (12.9)	39.0 (13.1)	*	Stuss, et al (1989)
PASAT 3.0	MS	19	6/13	43.37	n/a	8 w	59.0 (5.7)	63.0 (6.2)	*	Bever, et al (1995)
PASAT 4.0	Control	20	0/20	29.10 (4.70)	n/a	1 m	55.3 (3.4)	57.0 (2.8)	*	Harris, et al (1996)
PASAT 4.0	Pregnant	20	0/20	29.00 (4.60)	normal delivery	1 m	53.6 (3.2)	54.1 (3.3)	*	Harris, et al (1996)

instrument	group	n	m/f	age	intervention	inter	t #1	t #2	note	citation
PASAT 4.0	Renal Failure	9	4/5	65.00	rHuEpo	22.8 w	37.1 (19.1)	47.7 (9.5)		Temple, et al (1995)
PASAT 4.0	Renal Failure	8	3/5	67.50	n/a	19.3 w	29.3 (26.3)	35.5 (23.5)		Temple, et al (1995)
PASAT Delayed Recall (errors)	Control	8	8/0	24.00	metoprolol	3 w	NR	0.0 c		Brooks, et al (1988)
PASAT Delayed Recall (errors)	Control	8	8/0	24.00	atenolol	3 w	NR	0.0 c		Brooks, et al (1988)
PASAT Delayed Recall (errors)	Control	8	8/0	24.00	propranolol	3 w	NR	-0.5 c		Brooks, et al (1988)
PASAT Delayed Recall (errors)	Control	8	8/0	24.00	placebo	3 w	NR	0.0 c		Brooks, et al (1988)
PASAT Delayed Recall (sec)	Control	8	8/0	24.00	placebo	3 w	NR	-7.0 c		Brooks, et al (1988)
PASAT Delayed Recall (sec)	Control	8	8/0	24.00	metoprolol	3 w	NR	0.0 c		Brooks, et al (1988)
PASAT Delayed Recall (sec)	Control	8	8/0	24.00	atenolol	3 w	NR	-4.0 c		Brooks, et al (1988)

instrument	group	n	m/f	age	intervention	inter	t #1	t #2	note	citation
PASAT Delayed Recall (sec)	Control	8	8/0	24.00	propranolol	3 w	NR	-11.0 c		Brooks, et al (1988)
PASAT Serial Addition (errors)	Control	8	8/0	24.00	placebo	3 w	NR	-0.5 c		Brooks, et al (1988)
PASAT Serial Addition (errors)	Control	8	8/0	24.00	propranolol	3 w	NR	-0.5 c		Brooks, et al (1988)
PASAT Serial Addition (errors)	Control	8	8/0	24.00	atenolol	3 w	NR	1.0 c		Brooks, et al (1988)
PASAT Serial Addition (errors)	Control	8	8/0	24.00	metoprolol	3 w	NR	-2.5 c		Brooks, et al (1988)
PASAT Serial Addition (sec)	Control	8	8/0	24.00	placebo	3 w	NR	-10.5 c		Brooks, et al (1988)
PASAT Serial Addition (sec)	Control	8	8/0	24.00	propranolol	3 w	NR	-11.0 c		Brooks, et al (1988)
PASAT Serial Addition (sec)	Control	8	8/0	24.00	metoprolol	3 w	NR	-15.5 c		Brooks, et al (1988)
PASAT Serial Addition (sec)	Control	8	8/0	24.00	atenolol	3 w	NR	2.0 c		Brooks, et al (1988)

Table 46. Paired Associate Tests (PAT)

instrument	group	n	m/f	age	intervention	inter	t #1	t #2	note	citation
PAT (trials)	LD	29	24/5	10.83 (1.40)	methylphenidate	8 w	7.06 (0.52)	3.86 (0.47)		Gittleman-Klein, et al (1976)
PAT (trials)	LD	32	23/9	10.67 (1.30)	placebo	8 w	7.51 (0.47)	5.31 (0.44)		Gittleman-Klein, et al (1976)
paired associates delay [10]	Depression	17	n/a	n/a	trazodone	3 w	4.3 (3.0)	6.1 (2.7)	*	Fudge, et al (1990)
paired associates delay [10]	Depression	21	n/a	n/a	fluoxetine	3 w	3.0 (1.8)	5.4 (2.5)	*	Fudge, et al (1990)
paired associates imm [10]	Depression	17	n/a	n/a	trazodone	3 w	4.7 (2.8)	6.3 (4.7)	*	Fudge, et al (1990)
paired associates imm [10]	Depression	21	n/a	n/a	fluoxetine	3 w	3.4 (2.2)	5.4 (2.0)	*	Fudge, et al (1990)
PALT	Boxers	20	20/0	20.50	n/a	15-18 m	4.6	4.2		Porter, et al (1996)
PALT	Control	24	n/a	58.50	n/a	2.1 y	12.2 (3.4)	12.8 (2.7)		La Rue, et al (1995)
PALT	Control	20	20/0	20.50	n/a	15-18 m	3.9	3.8		Porter, et al (1996)
PALT	early onset DAT relatives	19	n/a	57.10	n/a	4.6 y	13.5 (2.0)	11.9 (4.0)		La Rue, et al (1995)

instrument	group	n	m/f	age	intervention	inter	t #1	t #2	note	citation
PALT	late onset DAT relatives	21	n/a	55.10	n/a	4.4 y	12.7 (3.1)	12.5 (2.7)		La Rue, et al (1995)
PALT (errors)	Orthopedic Injury	25	14/11	10.03 (2.00)	n/a	4 m	8.9 (6.6)	7.1 (6.1)		Chadwick, et al (1981)
PALT (errors)	TBI	25	14/11	10.12 (2.60)	n/a	4 m	14.0 (6.9)	9.2 (5.6)		Chadwick, et al (1981)

Table 47. Peabody Picture Vocabulary Test (PPVT)

instrument	group	n	m/f	age	intervention	inter	t #1	t #2	note	citation
PPVT	CAD	35	23/12	62.30 (8.30)	CE	50.9 d	120.09 (17.15)	118.11 (19.82)		Kelly, et al (1980)
PPVT	Control	14	n/a	76.10	n/a	7d	141.14 (4.61)	142.57 (3.67)		Knotek, et al (1990)
PPVT	Control	81	81/0	4.80	Head Start	~9 m	75.44 (16.2)	82.92 (18.92)		Payne, et al (1972)
PPVT	Control	82	82/0	4.90	Head Start	~9 m	74.3 (17.5)	85.26 (18.4)		Payne, et al (1972)
PPVT	Control	92	0/92	4.70	Head Start	~9 m	76.03 (16.47)	78.46 (15.94)		Payne, et al (1972)
PPVT	Control	77	0/77	4.90	Head Start	~9 m	73.93 (14.41)	83.0 (13.7)		Payne, et al (1972)
PPVT	Control	12	6/6	4.60	play session, different examiner	1-2 w	105.24 (4.68)	113.41 (4.60)		Zigler, et al (1973)

instrument	group	n	m/f	age	intervention	inter	t #1	t #2	note	citation
PPVT	Control	12	6/6	4.60	play session, same examiner	1-2 w	113.83 (4.87)	116.25 (5.08)		Zigler, et al (1973)
PPVT	Control	12	6/6	4.60	same examiner	1-2 w	110.33 (9.50)	115.58 (4.08)		Zigler, et al (1973)
PPVT	Control	12	6/6	4.60	different examiner	1-2 w	114.41 (4.76)	118.08 (3.15)		Zigler, et al (1973)
PPVT	Control (low SES)	12	6/6	4.67	play session, same examiner	1-2 w	81.83 (12.43)	88.58 (8.46)		Zigler, et al (1973)
PPVT	Control (low SES)	12	6/6	4.67	same examiner	1-2 w	78.50 (7.23)	88.99 (6.30)		Zigler, et al (1973)
PPVT	Control (low SES)	12	6/6	4.67	play session, different examiner	1-2 w	91.41 (8.97)	95.83 (10.19)		Zigler, et al (1973)
PPVT	Control (low SES)	12	6/6	4.67	different examiner	1-2 w	75.58 (9.75)	87.25 (9.36)		Zigler, et al (1973)
PPVT	DAT (mild)	10	n/a	79.40	n/a	7 d	109.90 (19.20)	112.60 (18.07)		Knotek, et al (1990)
PPVT	DAT (mod)	13	n/a	80.60	n/a	7d	67.77 (22.06)	71.85 (22.98)		Knotek, et al (1990)
PPVT	HD	40	18/22	40.00 (10.3)	n/a	12 m	115.0 (2.9)	112.4 (3.1)		Bamford, et al (1995)
PPVT	HD	26	12/14	39.00 (10.4)	n/a	12 m	115.0 (3.6)	109.0 (3.6)		Bamford, et al (1995)
PPVT	MR	30	n/a	24.70 (8.80)	n/a	5 min	47.63 (15.15)	52.07 (17.03)	std B /std A	Overton, et al (1972)

instrument	group	n	m/f	age	intervention	inter	t #1	t #2	note	citation
PPVT	MR	30	n/a	24.60 (8.60)	n/a	5 min	51.87 (15.58)	45.53 (15.05)	std A/ auto B	Overton, et al (1972)
PPVT	MR	30	n/a	24.40 (8.70)	n/a	5 min	45.80 (18.14)	51.87 (17.43)	auto B/ std A	Overton, et al (1972)
PPVT	MR	30	n/a	24.40 (8.60)	n/a	5 min	46.60 (16.87)	51.17 (16.09)	std B/ auto A	Overton, et al (1972)
PPVT	MR	30	n/a	24.40 (8.40)	n/a	5 min	43.80 (17.07)	50.83 (17.95)	auto B /auto A	Overton, et al (1972)
PPVT	MR	30	n/a	24.10 (8.60)	n/a	5 min	53.17 (18.34)	48.50 (17.95)	auto A /auto B	Overton, et al (1972)
PPVT	MR	30	n/a	24.00 (8.40)	n/a	5 min	51.30 (16.69)	48.50 (17.70)	std A/ std B	Overton, et al (1972)
PPVT	MR	30	n/a	24.40 (8.90)	n/a	5 min	46.73 (15.16)	45.30 (15.91)	auto A /std B	Overton, et al (1972)
PPVT	PVD	17	14/3	61.40 (7.90)	PVD surgery	51.5 d	125.18 (15.05)	126.29 (14.50)		Kelly, et al (1980)
PPVT (IQ)	Brain Tumor	7	4/3	9.83	radiotherapy	11 m	80.8 (23.3)	81.2 (23.2)		Bordeaux, et al (1988)
PPVT (IQ)	Brain Tumor	7	3/4	10.33	surgery	1 m	111.3 (17.9)	109.8 (19.8)		Bordeaux, et al (1988)
PPVT (IQ)	Control	23	n/a	9.10	n/a	6 m	100.0	104.4		Raskin, et al (1970)
PPVT (IQ)	Control	18	n/a	6.00	n/a	6 m	104.4	102.6		Raskin, et al (1970)
PPVT (IQ)	EMR	26	n/a	9.20	n/a	6 m	74.4	73.5		Raskin, et al (1970)

instrument	group	n	m/f	age	intervention	inter	t #1	t #2	note	citation
PPVT (IQ)	EMR	16	n/a	14.70	n/a	6 m	74.0	73.4		Raskin, et al (1970)
PPVT (IQ)	MR	16	n/a	15.70	n/a	2 w	39.07	42.67	auto/std	Knights, et al (1973)
PPVT (IQ)	MR	16	n/a	15.70	n/a	2 w	43.60	45.20	std/auto	Knights, et al (1973)
PPVT (IQ)	Neuropsych referrals	248	203/45	8.00 (1.70)	n/a	2.65 y	93.1 (17.0)	92.9 (15.2)		Brown, et al (1989)
PPVT (IQ)	Schizophrenia	10	10/0	34.80 (8.69)	clonidine	6 w	93.9 (8.46)	95.3 (8.75)		Fields, et al (1988)
PPVT (raw)	Anemia	27	n/a	4.50	iron supplements	8 w	41.34	47.39		Soewondo (1995)
PPVT (raw)	Anemia	43	n/a	4.50	placebo	8 w	40.56	42.31		Soewondo (1995)
PPVT (raw)	Control	23	n/a	4.80	placebo	8 w	44.85	43.62		Soewondo (1995)
PPVT (raw)	Control	26	n/a	4.80	iron supplements	8 w	37.9	44.6		Soewondo (1995)
PPVT (raw)	Down Syndrome	34	20/14	22.0 - 56.0	n/a	1 y	66.41 (31.79)	65.52 (28.25)	*	Burt, et al (1995)
PPVT (raw)	Language-Poor Children	9	4/5	4.30	tutoring	2.6 m	45.11	48.89		Webster, et al (1989)
PPVT (raw)	Language-Poor Children	10	6/4	4.60	n/a	2.6 m	53.8	59.6		Webster, et al (1989)
PPVT-IIIA	Control	70	n/a	6.00 - 10.90	n/a	42 d	106.6 (11.9)	107.6 (13.3)		Williams, et al (1997)
PPVT-IIIA	Control	67	n/a	2.50 - 5.90	n/a	42 d	106.1 (12.4)	107.9 (14)		Williams, et al (1997)

instrument	group	n	m/f	age	intervention	inter	t #1	t #2	note	citation
PPVT-IIIA	Control	38	n/a	26.0 - 57.9	n/a	42 d	104.8 (10.0)	107.7 (11.3)		Williams, et al (1997)
PPVT-IIIA	Control	51	n/a	12.0 - 17.9	n/a	42 d	101.9 (11.1)	105.1 (15.3)		Williams, et al (1997)
PPVT-IIIB	Control	67	n/a	2.50 - 5.90	n/a	42 d	105.7 (12.4)	107.0 (13.5)		Williams, et al (1997)
PPVT-IIIB	Control	38	n/a	26.0 - 57.9	n/a	42 d	104.9 (11.3)	108.6 (12.1)		Williams, et al (1997)
PPVT-IIIB	Control	51	n/a	12.0 - 17.9	n/a	42 d	102.0 (14.1)	103.2 (14.)		Williams, et al (1997)
PPVT-IIIB	Control	70	n/a	6.00 - 10.90	n/a	42 d	106.3 (11.6)	108.0 (12.5)		Williams, et al (1997)
PPVT-R	Emotionally Disturbed	10	n/a	13.60	n/a	14-18 d	80.50 (18.60)	82.15 (10.96)	Form M/L	Levenson, et al (1988)
PPVT-R	Emotionally Disturbed	10	n/a	13.60	n/a	14-18 d	82.50 (10.85)	80.50 (12.14)	Form L/M	Levenson, et al (1988)
PPVT-R	Psychiatric Inpts	28	15/13	15.50	n/a	15 d	71.6 (15.8)	71.0 (22.1)		Atlas, et al (1990)

Table 48. Pegboard Tests

instrument	group	n	m/f	age	intervention	inter	t #1	t #2	note	citation
Grooved Pegb	Control	21	5/16	34.00	carbamaz/ phenytoin CB	1 m	60.0 (9.0)	57.0 (7.0)	*	Meador, et al (1991)
Grooved Pegb	Control	38	18/20	35.70 (10.5)	n/a	54.7 w	128.3 (17.6)	126.2 (17.2)		Tarter, et al (1990)
Grooved Pegb	Crohn's Disease	22	9/13	37.30 (10.6)	std tx	62.6 w	137.1 (18.9)	131.4 (16.0)		Tarter, et al (1990)
Grooved Pegb	HD (at risk, + genetic marker)	8	1/7	26.20 (2.70)	n/a	2 y	64.1	64.8	*	Giordani, et al (1995)
Grooved Pegb	HD (at risk, - genetic marker)	8	1/7	28.40 (5.20)	n/a	2 y	62.0	59.4	*	Giordani, et al (1995)
Grooved Pegb	Liver Disease	62	23/39	39.20 (10.5)	liver transplant	60.1 w	174.2 (73.6)	148.9 (32.6)		Tarter, et al (1990)
Grooved Pegb DH	Alcoholic (1 yr abstin)	23	23/0	36.80 (6.30)	n/a	1 y	67.2	68.7		Adams, et al (1980)
Grooved Pegb DH	Alcoholic (2.5 yrs abstin)	25	25/0	36.50 (6.30)	n/a	1 y	69.2	69.1		Adams, et al (1980)
Grooved Pegb DH	Brain Tumor	7	4/3	9.83	radiotherapy	11 m	3.3 (10.4)	4.3 (8.7)		Bordeaux, et al (1988)
Grooved Pegb DH	Brain Tumor	7	3/4	10.33	surgery	1 m	6.3 (12.9)	9.6 (1.9)		Bordeaux, et al (1988)
Grooved Pegb DH	Cardiac	22	10/12	47.30 (14.0)	open heart surgery	8.4 d	100.0 (14.7)	102.2 (14.3)	*	Heyer, et al (1995)
Grooved Pegb DH	Cardiac	33	19/14	73.10 (5.50)	open heart surgery	8.4 d	112.2 (14.2)	133.0 (19.4)	*	Heyer, et al (1995)

instrument	group	n	m/f	age	intervention	inter	t #1	t #2	note	citation
Grooved Pegb DH	Control	21	21/0	36.90 (5.90)	n/a	1 y	62.1	63.5		Adams, et al (1980)
Grooved Pegb DH	Control	23	9/14	32.30 (10.3)	n/a	3 w	56.6 (5.9)	58.8 (8.9)		Bornstein, et al (1987)
Grooved Pegb DH	Control	33	15/18	59.10 (9.30)	n/a	10 d	82.3 (15.0)	79.6 (14.7)		McCaffrey, et al (1993)
Grooved Pegb DH	Control	72	67/5	44.50 (12.4)	n/a	6 m	70.7 (12.1)	66.9 (11.9)		Prevey, et al (1996)
Grooved Pegb DH	DAT	10	5/5	74.90	suloctidil 600 mg	12 w	229.6 (161.2)	181.44 (76.33)		McCaffrey, et al (1987)
Grooved Pegb DH	DAT	10	6/4	74.30	suloctidil 450 mg	12 w	428.75 (197.8)	388.75 (244.0)		McCaffrey, et al (1987)
Grooved Pegb DH	DAT	10	8/2	74.10	placebo	12 w	238.14 (169.9)	174.14 (104.9)		McCaffrey, et al (1987)
Grooved Pegb DH	Down Syndrome	34	20/14	22.0 - 56.0	n/a	1 y	147.61 (108.3)	96.90 (54.92)	*	Burt, et al (1995)
Grooved Pegb DH	Epilepsy	32	17/15	33.72 (9.66)	vigabatrin 6 g	18 w	82.42 (16.25)	80.94 (16.09)		Dodrill, et al (1995)
Grooved Pegb DH	Epilepsy	38	21/17	34.26 (9.18)	vigabatrin 3 g	18 w	80.84 (14.27)	79.42 (15.63)		Dodrill, et al (1995)
Grooved Pegb DH	Epilepsy	40	14/26	33.88 (9.77)	placebo	18 w	82.48 (20.43)	76.55 (16.05)		Dodrill, et al (1995)
Grooved Pegb DH	Epilepsy	36	17/19	34.89 (8.38)	vigabatrin 1 g	18 w	81.39 (17.74)	78.44 (18.55)		Dodrill, et al (1995)
Grooved Pegb DH	Epilepsy	26	24/2	43.50 (17.1)	carbamaz	6 m	77.2 (18.7)	77.5 (19.9)		Prevey, et al (1996)

instrument	group	n	m/f	age	intervention	inter	t #1	t #2	note	citation
Grooved Pegb DH	Epilepsy	39	36/3	44.30 (14.2)	valproate	6 m	83.6 (22.2)	84.9 (19.9)		Prevey, et al (1996)
Grooved Pegb DH	HIV+	69	51/18	34.70 (6.30)	n/a	6 m	72.2 (17.1)	69.5 (15.8)	*	Selnes, et al (1992)
Grooved Pegb DH	HIV+	132	132/0	~33.8	n/a	13.3 m	63.5	62.3	*	Selnes, et al (1990)
Grooved Pegb DH	HIV+ (IVDU)	8	5/3	39.00 (8.00)	MSR/placebo	7 d	81.4 (19.9)	69.5 (9.4)	*	Van Dyck, et al (1997)
Grooved Pegb DH	HIV+ (stage 2/3)	14	14/0	31.40 (8.54)	n/a	12.8 m	64.3 (5.8)	62.2 (5.6)		Burgess, et al (1994)
Grooved Pegb DH	HIV+ (stage 4)	6	6/0	36.20 (7.60)	n/a	12.8 m	82.8 (20.2)	78.2 (21.4)		Burgess, et al (1994)
Grooved Pegb DH	HIV-	41	41/0	31.50 (9.32)	n/a	12.8 m	70.0 (9.9)	68.0 (8.6)		Burgess, et al (1994)
Grooved Pegb DH	HIV-	37	27/10	35.60 (7.10)	n/a	6 m	76.7 (29.7)	70.3 (15.1)	*	Selnes, et al (1992)
Grooved Pegb DH	HIV-	132	132/0	~35.6	n/a	13.4 m	63.9	61.4	*	Selnes, et al (1990)
Grooved Pegb DH	Hypertension	25	17/8	50.10 (14.0)	n/a	7-10 d	83.32 (21.31)	78.91 (26.92)		McCaffrey, et al (1992)
Grooved Pegb DH	Left AVM	15	10/5	31.00 (11.0)	surgery	4 m	78.5 (22.4)	77.7 (12.7)	*	Stabell, et al (1994)
Grooved Pegb DH	Right AVM	16	5/11	34.00 (13.0)	surgery	4 m	70.5 (9.2)	75.8 (25.5)	*	Stabell, et al (1994)
Grooved Pegb DH	Substance Abuse	15	8/7	21.10 (4.50)	outpt tx	4 w	68.2 (7.6)	63.0 (7.5)		Cosgrove, et al (1991)

instrument	group	n	m/f	age	intervention	inter	t #1	t #2	note	citation
Grooved Pegb DH	Substance Abuse (PCP)	15	8/7	21.10 (4.50)	outpt tx	4 w	70.3 (9.0)	68.6 (8.3)		Cosgrove, et al (1991)
Grooved Pegb DH	Surgical	13	11/2	74.20 (6.70)	major surgery	6 d	111.3 (16.8)	126.8 (24.9)	*	Heyer, et al (1995)
Grooved Pegb DH + NDH	AIDS	10	10/0	41.70 (5.50)	n/a	6.53 m	127.6 (12.4)	138.1 (19.2)		Hinkin, et al (1995)
Grooved Pegb DH + NDH	Cardiac	158	133/ 25	60.80	CABG w/ ph-stat	7 d	89.1 (21)	103.0 (31.6)	*	Murkin, et al (1995)
Grooved Pegb DH + NDH	Cardiac	158	128/ 30	61.30	CABG w/ nonpulsatile	7 d	89.5 (21.4)	100.0 (27.7)	*	Murkin, et al (1995)
Grooved Pegb DH + NDH	Cardiac	79	66/13	60.90 (8.70)	CABG w/ alpha-stat, pulsatile	7 d	90.5 (21.6)	104.0 (36.6)	*	Murkin, et al (1995)
Grooved Pegb DH + NDH	Cardiac	79	63/16	61.40 (8.40)	CABG w/ ph-stat, nonpulsatile	7 d	90.0 (22.4)	102.0 (29.7)	*	Murkin, et al (1995)
Grooved Pegb DH + NDH	Cardiac	316	264/ 52	60.90 (8.30)	CABG	7 d	89.4 (21.0)	102.0 (31.7)	*	Murkin, et al (1995)
Grooved Pegb DH + NDH	Cardiac	79	70/9	60.20 (8.50)	CABG w/ ph-stat,pulsatile	7 d	88.2 (19.7)	103.0 (33.7)	*	Murkin, et al (1995)
Grooved Pegb DH + NDH	Cardiac	158	136/ 22	60.55	CABG w/ pulsatile	7 d	89.4 (20.6)	103.0 (35.1)	*	Murkin, et al (1995)
Grooved Pegb DH + NDH	Cardiac	158	131/ 27	61.05	CABG w/ alpha-stat	7 d	89.7 (21.0)	101.0 (31.9)	*	Murkin, et al (1995)
Grooved Pegb DH + NDH	Cardiac	79	65/14	61.20 (7.80)	CABG w/ alpha-stat, nonpulsatile	7 d	88.9 (20.5)	98.3 (25.5)	*	Murkin, et al (1995)
Grooved Pegb DH + NDH	Surgical	40	28/12	63.10 (8.40)	non-CABG surgery	7 d	89.4 (22.2)	93.0 (23.8)	*	Murkin, et al (1995)

instrument	group	n	m/f	age	intervention	inter	t #1	t #2	note	citation
Grooved Pegb LH	Cardiac	90	77/13	59.00 (10.6)	CABG/CPB	8 d	87.6 (20.5)	117.7 (29.3)	*	Townes, et al (1989)
Grooved Pegb LH	Control	47	35/12	59.00 (9.81)	n/a	8 d	81.9 (16.2)	81.5 (19.2)	*	Townes, et al (1989)
Grooved Pegb LH (t)	Lung Cancer	11	n/a	~61.0	cranial irradiation	11 m	32.8	35.5		Komaki, et al (1995)
Grooved Pegb NDH	Alcoholic (1 yr abstin)	23	23/0	36.80 (6.30)	n/a	1 y	74.0	74.3		Adams, et al (1980)
Grooved Pegb NDH	Alcoholic (2.5 yrs abstin)	25	25/0	36.50 (6.30)	n/a	1 y	71.8	69.5		Adams, et al (1980)
Grooved Pegb NDH	Brain Tumor	7	3/4	10.33	surgery	1 m	5.5 (9.8)	8.3 (3.8)		Bordeaux, et al (1988)
Grooved Pegb NDH	Brain Tumor	7	4/3	9.83	radiotherapy	11 m	10.0 (2.8)	8.5 (2.1)		Bordeaux, et al (1988)
Grooved Pegb NDH	Cardiac	22	10/12	47.30 (14.0)	open heart surgery	8.4 d	104.4 (14.9)	113.8 (16.6)	*	Heyer, et al (1995)
Grooved Pegb NDH	Cardiac	33	19/14	73.10 (5.50)	open heart surgery	8.4 d	118.3 (15.6)	148.2 (25.3)	*	Heyer, et al (1995)
Grooved Pegb NDH	Control	21	21/0	36.90 (5.90)	n/a	1 y	69.1	69.2		Adams, et al (1980)
Grooved Pegb NDH	Control	23	9/14	32.30 (10.3)	n/a	3 w	59.3 (6.6)	58.8 (6.6)		Bornstein, et al (1987)
Grooved Pegb NDH	Control	33	15/18	59.10 (9.30)	n/a	10 d	88.5 (24.5)	82.9 (15.9)		McCaffrey, et al (1993)
Grooved Pegb NDH	Control	72	67/5	44.50 (12.4)	n/a	6 m	77.5 (15.7)	71.8 (11.9)		Prevey, et al (1996)

instrument	group	n	m/f	age	intervention	inter	t #1	t #2	note	citation
Grooved Pegb NDH	DAT	10	6/4	74.30	suloctidil 450 mg	12 w	436.00 (190.7)	414.25 (215.6)		McCaffrey, et al (1987)
Grooved Pegb NDH	DAT	10	8/2	74.10	placebo	12 w	267.29 (184.0)	206.57 (151.7)		McCaffrey, et al (1987)
Grooved Pegb NDH	DAT	10	5/5	74.90	suloctidil 600 mg	12 w	232.44 (158.4)	199.11 (91.01)		McCaffrey, et al (1987)
Grooved Pegb NDH	Down Syndrome	34	20/14	22.0 - 56.0	n/a	1 y	108.79 (71.29)	81.38 (32.53)	*	Burt, et al (1995)
Grooved Pegb NDH	Epilepsy	40	14/26	33.88 (9.77)	placebo	18 w	85.62 (22.27)	86.28 (18.86)		Dodrill, et al (1995)
Grooved Pegb NDH	Epilepsy	36	17/19	34.89 (8.38)	vigabatrin 1 g	18 w	85.71 (19.27)	83.80 (22.05)		Dodrill, et al (1995)
Grooved Pegb NDH	Epilepsy	38	21/17	34.26 (9.18)	vigabatrin 3 g	18 w	86.00 (15.08)	86.03 (16.41)		Dodrill, et al (1995)
Grooved Pegb NDH	Epilepsy	32	17/15	33.72 (9.66)	vigabatrin 6 g	18 w	80.79 (19.79)	87.03 (15.74)		Dodrill, et al (1995)
Grooved Pegb NDH	Epilepsy	26	24/2	43.50 (17.1)	carbamaz	6 m	86.8 (20.8)	87.6 (22.2)		Prevey, et al (1996)
Grooved Pegb NDH	Epilepsy	39	36/3	44.30 (14.2)	valproate	6 m	87.2 (21.0)	89.6 (19.5)		Prevey, et al (1996)
Grooved Pegb NDH	HIV+	69	51/18	34.70 (6.30)	n/a	6 m	81.4 (25.4)	81.1 (26.1)	*	Selnes, et al (1992)
Grooved Pegb NDH	HIV+	132	132/0	~33.8	n/a	13.3 m	68.3	66.3	*	Selnes, et al (1990)
Grooved Pegb NDH	HIV+ (IVDU)	8	5/3	39.00 (8.00)	MSR/placebo	7 d	88.4 (25.9)	79.6 (16.8)	*	Van Dyck, et al (1997)

instrument	group	n	m/f	age	intervention	inter	t #1	t #2	note	citation
Grooved Pegb NDH	HIV+ (stage 2/3)	14	14/0	31.40 (8.54)	n/a	12.8 m	67.4 (9.3)	65.7 (7.7)		Burgess, et al (1994)
Grooved Pegb NDH	HIV+ (stage 4)	6	6/0	36.20 (7.60)	n/a	12.8 m	82.8 (10.0)	88.2 (28.6)		Burgess, et al (1994)
Grooved Pegb NDH	HIV-	41	41/0	31.50 (9.32)	n/a	12.8 m	73.8 (9.3)	71.5 (9.7)		Burgess, et al (1994)
Grooved Pegb NDH	HIV-	37	27/10	35.60 (7.10)	n/a	6 m	83.0 (26.5)	76.9 (20.2)	*	Selnes, et al (1992)
Grooved Pegb NDH	HIV-	132	132/0	~35.6	n/a	13.4 m	68.8	66.5	*	Selnes, et al (1990)
Grooved Pegb NDH	Hypertension	25	17/8	50.10 (14.0)	n/a	7-10 d	90.00 (20.57)	81.59 (15.79)		McCaffrey, et al (1992)
Grooved Pegb NDH	Left AVM	15	10/5	31.00 (11.0)	surgery	4 m	75.5 (13.5)	73.7 (9.0)	*	Stabell, et al (1994)
Grooved Pegb NDH	Right AVM	16	5/11	34.00 (13.0)	surgery	4 m	79.1 (18.7)	90.4 (32.6)	*	Stabell, et al (1994)
Grooved Pegb NDH	Surgical	13	11/2	74.20 (6.70)	major surgery	6 d	133.1 (43.7)	157.7 (41.9)	*	Heyer, et al (1995)
Grooved Pegb RH	Cardiac	90	77/13	59.00 (10.6)	CABG/CPB	8 d	83.6 (20.5)	110.1 (30.1)	*	Townes, et al (1989)
Grooved Pegb RH	Control	47	35/12	59.00 (9.81)	n/a	8 d	76.9 (18.2)	78.4 (21.8)	*	Townes, et al (1989)
Grooved Pegb RH (t)	Lung Cancer	11	n/a	~61.0	cranial irradiation	11 m	39.0	34.4		Komaki, et al (1995)
Klove Pegb DH Trial 1	Asthma	8	n/a	6.00 - 12.00	placebo	2 w	64.12	63.62		Rappaport, et al (1989)

instrument	group	n	m/f	age	intervention	inter	t #1	t #2	note	citation
Klove Pegb DH Trial 1	Asthma	9	n/a	6.00 - 12.00	theophylline	2 w	75.33	71.88		Rappaport, et al (1989)
Klove Pegb DH Trial 2	Asthma	9	n/a	6.00 - 12.00	theophylline	2 w	70.44	72.0		Rappaport, et al (1989)
Klove Pegb DH Trial 2	Asthma	8	n/a	6.00 - 12.00	placebo	2 w	60.25	60.0		Rappaport, et al (1989)
Klove Pegb NDH Trial 1	Asthma	9	n/a	6.00 - 12.00	theophylline	2 w	90.67	85.44		Rappaport, et al (1989)
Klove Pegb NDH Trial 1	Asthma	8	n/a	6.00 - 12.00	placebo	2 w	79.5	71.12		Rappaport, et al (1989)
Klove Pegb NDH Trial 2	Asthma	9	n/a	6.00 - 12.00	theophylline	2 w	82.11	84.77		Rappaport, et al (1989)
Klove Pegb NDH Trial 2	Asthma	8	n/a	6.00 - 12.00	placebo	2 w	70.25	68.12		Rappaport, et al (1989)
pegb	Control	6	6/0	19.00	75% physical 25% mental	10 d	15.47 (1.94)	31.2 (7.62)		Hird, et al (1991)
pegb	Control	6	0/6	19.00	75% physical 25% mental	10 d	15.12 (1.43)	34.62 (8.0)		Hird, et al (1991)
pegb	Control	6	0/6	19.00	100% mental practice	10 d	15.47 (1.77)	24.42 (4.40)		Hird, et al (1991)
pegb	Control	6	0/6	19.00	100% physical practice	10 d	17.02 (2.35)	45.57 (11.63)		Hird, et al (1991)
pegb	Control	6	0/6	19.00	25% physical 75% mental	10 d	16.57 (2.32)	28.83 (7.37)		Hird, et al (1991)
pegb	Control	6	0/6	19.00	50% physical 50% mental	10 d	14.9 (1.38)	33.57 (13.67)		Hird, et al (1991)

instrument	group	n	m/f	age	intervention	inter	t #1	t #2	note	citation
pegb	Control	6	0/6	19.00	control	10 d	13.87 (1.2)	16.29 (3.0)		Hird, et al (1991)
pegb	Control	6	6/0	19.00	100% mental practice	10 d	16.62 (1.31)	31.17 (7.51)		Hird, et al (1991)
pegb	Control	6	6/0	19.00	100% physical practice	10 d	13.82 (2.21)	30.82 (7.01)		Hird, et al (1991)
pegb	Control	6	6/0	19.00	50% physical 50% mental	10 d	13.85 (1.82)	28.43 (9.43)		Hird, et al (1991)
pegb	Control	6	6/0	19.00	25% physical 75% mental	10 d	13.28 (1.6)	27.0 (5.29)		Hird, et al (1991)
pegb	Control	6	6/0	19.00	control	10 d	15.97 (2.16)	17.15 (3.78)		Hird, et al (1991)
pegb DH	mild Toxic Enceph	13	n/a	36.40 (10.3)	"improved" at retest	18.1 m	69.8 (5.5)	65.0 (7.2)		Morrow, et al (1991)
pegb DH	mild Toxic Enceph	14	n/a	40.10 (6.00)	"unimproved" at retest	15.9 m	85.5 (18.4)	85.9 (20.3)		Morrow, et al (1991)
pegb NDH	mild Toxic Enceph	13	n/a	36.40 (10.3)	"improved" at retest	18.1 m	79.8 (15.5)	70.3 (11.3)		Morrow, et al (1991)
pegb NDH	mild Toxic Enceph	14	n/a	40.10 (6.00)	"unimproved" at retest	15.9 m	88.2 (16.6)	93.2 (28.9)		Morrow, et al (1991)
Purdue Pegb	CVA	9	1/8	74.00	triazolam	3 w	14.9 (1.9)	-0.5 (0.8) c	*	Woo, et al (1991)
Purdue Pegb	CVA	9	2/7	78.00	placebo	3 w	16.1 (1.4)	0.6 (1.2) c	*	Woo, et al (1991)
Purdue Pegb	CVA	8	0/8	77.00	flurazepam	3 w	15.6 (1.8)	-0.5 (0.5) c	*	Woo, et al (1991)

instrument	group	n	m/f	age	intervention	inter	t #1	t #2	note	citation
Purdue Pegb Assemblies	Control	35	11/24	71.70 (7.50)	n/a	8.6 d	28.3 (6.2)	29.3 (6.6)		Desrosiers, et al (1995)
Purdue Pegb Assemblies	Control	14	0/14	27.00 (6.92)	n/a	1 w	11.11 (1.97)	11.52 (2.10)	*	Reddon, et al (1988)
Purdue Pegb Assemblies	Control	12	12/0	31.83 (9.43)	n/a	1 w	10.52 (1.70)	10.94 (1.85)	*	Reddon, et al (1988)
Purdue Pegb Assemblies	Depression	33	14/19	37.40	antidepress	7 w	33.1 (8.3)	33.5 (6.7)		Fromm, et al (1984)
Purdue Pegb Assemblies	MR	16	n/a	29.00 (5.30)	n/a	2 m	17.5 (6.8)	19.9 (6.7)		Guarnaccia, et al (1975)
Purdue Pegb Assemblies (automated)	MR	16	n/a	27.00 (7.10)	n/a	2 m	24.1 (6.8)	22.7 (9.0)		Guarnaccia, et al (1975)
Purdue Pegb BH	Control	35	11/24	71.70 (7.50)	n/a	8.6 d	10.2 (1.8)	10.5 (1.9)		Desrosiers, et al (1995)
Purdue Pegb BH	Control	21	3/18	30.10 (8.20)	n/a	6 m	12.2 (1.0)	12.5 (1.2)		Pulliainen, et al (1994)
Purdue Pegb BH	Control	12	12/0	31.83 (9.43)	n/a	1 w	12.58 (1.44)	12.75 (1.29)	*	Reddon, et al (1988)
Purdue Pegb BH	Control	14	0/14	27.00 (6.92)	n/a	1 w	13.50 (2.38)	13.64 (1.91)	*	Reddon, et al (1988)
Purdue Pegb BH	Depression	33	14/19	37.40	antidepress	7 w	11.8 (2.3)	11.9 (2.3)		Fromm, et al (1984)
Purdue Pegb BH	Epilepsy	23	11/12	26.80 (13.2)	carbamaz	6 m	11.2 (1.4)	11.1 (1.4)		Pulliainen, et al (1994)

instrument	group	n	m/f	age	intervention	inter	t #1	t #2	note	citation
Purdue Pegb BH	Epilepsy	20	9/11	31.50 (11.3)	phenytoin	6 m	10.9 (1.0)	10.5 (0.9)		Pulliainen, et al (1994)
Purdue Pegb BH	IVDU	16	13/3	39.50	n/a	10.4 d	9.93 (0.98)	10.19 (1.78)		Richards, et al (1992)
Purdue Pegb BH	MR	16	n/a	29.00 (5.30)	n/a	2 m	7.7 (2.2)	8.4 (2.5)		Guarnaccia, et al (1975)
Purdue Pegb BH	MS	13	n/a	36.20	placebo	2 y	8.2 (2.5)	7.8 (2.8)		Pliskin, et al (1996)
Purdue Pegb BH	MS	9	n/a	38.90	high dose interferon	2 y	6.7 (3.0)	5.8 (3.4)		Pliskin, et al (1996)
Purdue Pegb BH	MS	8	n/a	38.00	low dose interferon	2 y	6.9 (2.2)	6.5 (2.4)		Pliskin, et al (1996)
Purdue Pegb BH (automated)	MR	16	n/a	27.00 (7.10)	n/a	2 m	8.5 (2.1)	9.0 (2.2)		Guarnaccia, et al (1975)
Purdue Pegb BH (pegs in 30")	Alcoholic (acute)	13	13/0	39.90	inpt tx	8 w	9.9 (1.3)	11.4 (1.5)		Tarter, et al (1971)
Purdue Pegb BH (pegs in 30")	Alcoholic (chronic)	13	13/0	43.80	inpt tx	8 w	9.5 (2.3)	10.2 (2.0)		Tarter, et al (1971)
Purdue Pegb DH	Control	21	3/18	30.10 (8.20)	n/a	6 m	16.2 (1.7)	16.8 (1.6)		Pulliainen, et al (1994)
Purdue Pegb DH	Control	14	0/14	27.00 (6.92)	n/a	1 w	17.00 (2.45)	17.93 (2.06)	*	Reddon, et al (1988)

instrument	group	n	m/f	age	intervention	inter	t #1	t #2	note	citation
Purdue Pegb DH	Control	12	12/0	31.83 (9.43)	n/a	1 w	15.67 (1.50)	16.17 (1.53)	*	Reddon, et al (1988)
Purdue Pegb DH	Depression	33	14/19	37.40	antidepress	7 w	14.9 (2.7)	15.3 (2.2)		Fromm, et al (1984)
Purdue Pegb DH	Epilepsy	23	11/12	26.80 (13.2)	carbamaz	6 m	14.5 (1.7)	15.1 (1.2)		Pulliainen, et al (1994)
Purdue Pegb DH	Epilepsy	20	9/11	31.50 (11.3)	phenytoin	6 m	14.8 (1.2)	14.9 (1.6)		Pulliainen, et al (1994)
Purdue Pegb DH	IVDU	16	13/3	39.50	n/a	10.4 d	13.5 (1.45)	14.28 (1.9)		Richards, et al (1992)
Purdue Pegb DH	MS	9	n/a	38.90	high dose interferon	2 y	8.9 (4.0)	8.1 (4.5)		Pliskin, et al (1996)
Purdue Pegb DH	MS	13	n/a	36.20	placebo	2 y	11.0 (2.2)	9.8 (3.5)		Pliskin, et al (1996)
Purdue Pegb DH	MS	8	n/a	38.00	low dose interferon	2 y	9.9 (3.6)	9.0 (4.0)		Pliskin, et al (1996)
Purdue Pegb LH	Control	35	11/24	71.70 (7.50)	n/a	8.6 d	12.4 (2.1)	12.7 (2.1)		Desrosiers, et al (1995)
Purdue Pegb LH	MR	16	n/a	29.00 (5.30)	n/a	2 m	10.6 (2.2)	11.1 (2.5)		Guarnaccia, et al (1975)
Purdue Pegb LH (auto)	MR	16	n/a	27.00 (7.10)	n/a	2 m	10.6 (2.3)	11.3 (2.8)		Guarnaccia, et al (1975)
Purdue Pegb LH (pegs in 30")	Alcoholic (acute)	13	13/0	39.90	inpt tx	8 w	12.0 (2.2)	13.0 (1.7)		Tarter, et al (1971)

instrument	group	n	m/f	age	intervention	inter	t #1	t #2	note	citation
Purdue Pegb LH (pegs in 30")	Alcoholic (chronic)	13	13/0	43.80	inpt tx	8 w	11.1 (2.5)	12.9 (2.3)		Tarter, et al (1971)
Purdue Pegb NDH	Control	21	3/18	30.10 (8.20)	n/a	6 m	15.0 (1.5)	14.9 (1.3)		Pulliainen, et al (1994)
Purdue Pegb NDH	Control	12	12/0	31.83 (9.43)	n/a	1 w	14.67 (1.67)	15.42 (1.38)	*	Reddon, et al (1988)
Purdue Pegb NDH	Control	14	0/14	27.00 (6.92)	n/a	1 w	16.00 (2.32)	16.71 (1.77)	*	Reddon, et al (1988)
Purdue Pegb NDH	Depression	33	14/19	37.40	antidepress	7 w	14.4 (2.7)	14.5 (2.2)		Fromm, et al (1984)
Purdue Pegb NDH	Epilepsy	20	9/11	31.50 (11.3)	phenytoin	6 m	13.5 (1.2)	13.1 (1.3)		Pulliainen, et al (1994)
Purdue Pegb NDH	Epilepsy	23	11/12	26.80 (13.2)	carbamaz	6 m	13.2 (1.5)	13.7 (1.4)		Pulliainen, et al (1994)
Purdue Pegb NDH	IVDU	16	13/3	39.50	n/a	10.4 d	12.7 (1.25)	13.0 (1.79)		Richards, et al (1992)
Purdue Pegb NDH	MS	9	n/a	38.90	high dose interferon	2 y	8.0 (4.7)	7.1 (3.3)		Pliskin, et al (1996)
Purdue Pegb NDH	MS	8	n/a	38.00	low dose interferon	2 y	8.9 (2.6)	8.5 (2.0)		Pliskin, et al (1996)
Purdue Pegb NDH	MS	13	n/a	36.20	placebo	2 y	9.5 (3.0)	9.5 (2.5)		Pliskin, et al (1996)
Purdue Pegb RH	Control	35	11/24	71.70 (7.50)	n/a	8.6 d	13 (1.9)	13.3 (1.8)		Desrosiers, et al (1995)

instrument	group	n	m/f	age	intervention	inter	t #1	t #2	note	citation
Purdue Pegb RH	MR	16	n/a	29.00 (5.30)	n/a	2 m	10.4 (2.5)	11.2 (2.4)		Guarnaccia, et al (1975)
Purdue Pegb RH (auto)	MR	16	n/a	27.00 (7.10)	n/a	2 m	11.8 (2.1)	12.4 (2.0)		Guarnaccia, et al (1975)
Purdue Pegb RH (pegs in 30")	Alcoholic (acute)	13	13/0	39.90	inpt tx	8 w	13.1 (1.2)	14.2 (1.7)		Tarter, et al (1971)
Purdue Pegb RH (pegs in 30")	Alcoholic (chronic)	13	13/0	43.80	inpt tx	8 w	11.8 (2.2)	13.2 (2.3)		Tarter, et al (1971)
Purdue Pegb RLB	Schizophrenia	11	n/a	21.0 - 61.0	placebo	4 h	44.73	40.64		Serafetinides, et al (1973)
Purdue Pegb RLB	Schizophrenia	13	n/a	21.0 - 61.0	haloperidol	4 h	39.31	39.62		Serafetinides, et al (1973)
Purdue Pegb RLB	Schizophrenia	13	n/a	21.0 - 61.0	drug-free	4 h	40.15	40.31		Serafetinides, et al (1973)
Purdue Pegb RLB	Schizophrenia	11	n/a	21.0 - 61.0	drug-free	4 h	44.82	43.91		Serafetinides, et al (1973)
Purdue Pegb RLB	Schizophrenia	8	n/a	21.0 - 61.0	chlorpromaz	4 h	42.25	41.13		Serafetinides, et al (1973)
Purdue Pegb RLB	Schizophrenia	8	n/a	21.0 - 61.0	drug-free	4 h	36.75	31.13		Serafetinides, et al (1973)
Purdue Pegb RLB	Schizophrenia	9	n/a	21.0 - 61.0	clopenthixol	4 h	32.22	30.44		Serafetinides, et al (1973)
Purdue Pegb RLB	Schizophrenia	9	n/a	21.0 - 61.0	drug-free	4 h	33.56	27.44		Serafetinides, et al (1973)

instrument	group	n	m/f	age	intervention	inter	t #1	t #2	note	citation
Purdue Pegb Total	Schizophrenia	11	n/a	21.0 - 61.0	drug-free	4 h	65.09	65.09		Serafetinides, et al (1973)
Purdue Pegb Total	Schizophrenia	13	n/a	21.0 - 61.0	haloperidol	4 h	56.50	57.50		Serafetinides, et al (1973)
Purdue Pegb Total	Schizophrenia	8	n/a	21.0 - 61.0	chlorpromaz	4 h	61.75	59.75		Serafetinides, et al (1973)
Purdue Pegb Total	Schizophrenia	8	n/a	21.0 - 61.0	drug-free	4 h	52.50	44.25		Serafetinides, et al (1973)
Purdue Pegb Total	Schizophrenia	13	n/a	21.0 - 61.0	drug-free	4 h	60.33	58.17		Serafetinides, et al (1973)
Purdue Pegb Total	Schizophrenia	9	n/a	21.0 - 61.0	clopenthixol	4 h	47.11	46.11		Serafetinides, et al (1973)
Purdue Pegb Total	Schizophrenia	9	n/a	21.0 - 61.0	drug-free	4 h	49.78	39.56		Serafetinides, et al (1973)
Purdue Pegb Total	Schizophrenia	11	n/a	21.0 - 61.0	placebo	4 h	66.27	62.09		Serafetinides, et al (1973)
RCPMB Pegb DH	Alcoholic	10	7/3	25.50	abstin	4 w	73.9	63.1		Goldman, et al (1983)
RCPMB Pegb DH	Alcoholic	10	9/1	35.20	abstin	4 w	72.8	60.9		Goldman, et al (1983)
RCPMB Pegb DH	Alcoholic	11	8/3	50.60	abstin	4 w	95.7	73.5		Goldman, et al (1983)
RCPMB Pegb DH	Control	15	9/6	26.40	n/a	4 w	60.2	53.7		Goldman, et al (1983)
RCPMB Pegb DH	Control	15	15/0	47.50	n/a	4 w	66.3	58.7		Goldman, et al (1983)

instrument	group	n	m/f	age	intervention	inter	t #1	t #2	note	citation
RCPMB Pegb DH	Epilepsy	36	n/a	n/a	carbamaz	3 w	74.53	73.22		Rennick, et al (1974)
RCPMB Pegb DH	Renal Disease	20	n/a	46.50 (11.3)	long-term hemodialysis	1 d	85.6 (20.6)	74.7 (16.7)	*	Ratner, et al (1983)
RCPMB Pegb NDH	Alcoholic	10	9/1	35.20	abstin	4 w	85.0	66.1		Goldman, et al (1983)
RCPMB Pegb NDH	Alcoholic	11	8/3	50.60	abstin	4 w	95.4	74.8		Goldman, et al (1983)
RCPMB Pegb NDH	Alcoholic	10	7/3	25.50	abstin	4 w	82.7	69.9		Goldman, et al (1983)
RCPMB Pegb NDH	Control	15	15/0	47.50	n/a	4 w	71.6	65.5		Goldman, et al (1983)
RCPMB Pegb NDH	Control	15	9/6	26.40	n/a	4 w	61.5	59.2		Goldman, et al (1983)
RCPMB Pegb NDH	Renal Disease	20	n/a	46.50 (11.3)	long-term hemodialysis	1 d	90.2 (21.8)	82.0 (15.5)	*	Ratner, et al (1983)

Table 49. Perceptual Tests

instrument	group	n	m/f	age	intervention	inter	t #1	t #2	note	citation
Gollin Incomplete Figures Test	DAT	32	n/a	70.72	NSAID	1 y	2.97	-0.12 c		Rich, et al (1995)
Gollin Incomplete Figures Test	DAT	117	n/a	69.93	n/a	1 y	3.12	-0.12 c		Rich, et al (1995)

instrument	group	n	m/f	age	intervention	inter	t #1	t #2	note	citation
HVOT	Epilepsy	40	23/17	32.20 (8.20)	n/a	~9 m	25.65 (2.21)	26.20 (2.53)		Hermann, et al (1996)
HVOT	PD	4	3/1	53.50	fetal tissue implanted	12 m	24.9	25.9		Sass, et al (1995)
Mooney Faces Closure (correct)	Schizophrenia	19	13/6	33.70 (6.30)	clozapine	10 w	18.4 (2.5)	20.2 (1.6)		Buchanan, et al (1994)
Mooney Faces Closure (correct)	Schizophrenia	33	n/a	33.7 (6.30)	clozapine	1 y	18.5 (2.2)	19.6 (2.2)		Buchanan, et al (1994)
Mooney Faces Closure (correct)	Schizophrenia	19	15/4	34.00 (6.90)	haloperidol	10 w	19.0 (2.2)	19.4 (2.3)		Buchanan, et al (1994)
Perceptual Speed	DAT	7	n/a	n/a	naloxone	15-60 min	1.52 (2.78)	8.76 (4.10)		Reisberg, et al (1983)
Perceptual Speed	DAT	7	n/a	n/a	placebo	15-60 min	3.62 (5.41)	4.71 (5.34)		Reisberg, et al (1983)
Rapid Visual Discrimination (30")	TBI	15	15/0	18.0 - 56.0	n/a	1-1.5 d	20.07 (3.49)	22.93 (4.83)		desRosiers, et al (1987)
Seguin Form Board (sec)	Control	25	23/2	24.80 (2.08)	diazepam	30 min	14.5 (0.4)	24.0 (1.2)	*	Cooper, et al (1978)
Seguin Form Board (sec)	Control	20	15/5	25.40 (1.76)	n/a	30 min	17.0 (0.5)	14.6 (0.3)	*	Cooper, et al (1978)

instrument	group	n	m/f	age	intervention	inter	t #1	t #2	note	citation
Tactile Form Recog	TBI (sev)	15	13/2	24.80	n/a	11.5 m	1.9	0.7		Drudge, et al (1984)
Tactile Form Recog LH (errors)	Neuropsych referrals	248	203/45	8.00 (1.70)	n/a	2.65 y	1.0 (1.6)	0.61 (1.4)		Brown, et al (1989)
Tactile Form Recog RH (errors)	Neuropsych referrals	248	203/45	8.00 (1.70)	n/a	2.65 y	1.6 (2.0)	0.76 (1.4)		Brown, et al (1989)
Visual Closure	TBI	15	15/0	18.0–56.0	n/a	1-1.5 d	28.00 (9.64)	33.20 (10.65)		desRosiers, et al (1987)

Table 50. Pursuit Rotor Tests

instrument	group	n	m/f	age	intervention	inter	t #1	t #2	note	citation
Lafayette pursuit rotor	Control	6	6/0	19.00	100% physical practice	10 d	4.5 (1.08)	9.78 (0.85)		Hird, et al (1991)
Lafayette pursuit rotor	Control	6	0/6	19.00	100% mental practice	10 d	3.46 (0.46)	6.71 (0.91)		Hird, et al (1991)
Lafayette pursuit rotor	Control	6	0/6	19.00	100% physical practice	10 d	3.58 (1.14)	7.08 (1.5)		Hird, et al (1991)
Lafayette pursuit rotor	Control	6	0/6	19.00	25% physical 75% mental	10 d	3.85 (0.96)	6.61 (0.74)		Hird, et al (1991)
Lafayette pursuit rotor	Control	6	0/6	19.00	50% physical 50% mental	10 d	2.71 (0.78)	6.8 (1.48)		Hird, et al (1991)
Lafayette pursuit rotor	Control	6	0/6	19.00	75% physical 25% mental	10 d	2.47 (0.86)	6.59 (1.88)		Hird, et al (1991)

instrument	group	n	m/f	age	intervention	inter	t #1	t #2	note	citation
Lafayette pursuit rotor	Control	6	6/0	19.00	100% mental practice	10 d	3.8 (0.76)	6.45 (1.26)		Hird, et al (1991)
Lafayette pursuit rotor	Control	6	6/0	19.00	25% physical 75% mental	10 d	4.6 (1.1)	8.17 (1.28)		Hird, et al (1991)
Lafayette pursuit rotor	Control	6	6/0	19.00	50% physical 50% mental	10 d	3.92 (0.71)	8.54 (1.65)		Hird, et al (1991)
Lafayette pursuit rotor	Control	6	6/0	19.00	75% physical 25% mental	10 d	4.4 (1.03)	9.58 (1.34)		Hird, et al (1991)
Lafayette pursuit rotor	Control	6	6/0	19.00	control	10 d	4.34 (1.4)	6.2 (1.21)		Hird, et al (1991)
Lafayette pursuit rotor	Control	6	0/6	19.00	control	10 d	3.64 (1.27)	5.13 (1.18)		Hird, et al (1991)
pursuit rotor (time on target in 20")	Control	38	18/20	35.70 (10.5)	n/a	54.7 w	32.9 (4.7)	35.8 (4.3)		Tarter, et al (1990)
pursuit rotor (time on target in 20")	Crohn's Disease	22	9/13	37.30 (10.6)	std tx	62.6 w	30.3 (4.2)	35.4 (2.6)		Tarter, et al (1990)
pursuit rotor (time on target in 20")	Liver Disease	62	23/39	39.20 (10.5)	liver transplant	60.1 w	28.7 (7.8)	33.4 (5.4)		Tarter, et al (1990)
pursuit rotor - 30rpm (% time on target)	Control	16	n/a	24.50 (7.70)	n/a	1 d	81.71 (6.51)	86.95 (5.95)	*	Ewert, et al (1989)

instrument	group	n	m/f	age	intervention	inter	t #1	t #2	note	citation
pursuit rotor - 30rpm (% time on target)	TBI & PTA	16	n/a	24.50 (7.70)	n/a	1 d	35.25 (24.37)	43.89 (22.45)	*	Ewert, et al (1989)
pursuit rotor - 45 rpm (% time on target)	Control	16	n/a	24.50 (7.70)	n/a	1 d	63.41 (12.67)	78.08 (9.15)	*	Ewert, et al (1989)
pursuit rotor - 45 rpm (% time on target)	TBI & PTA	16	n/a	24.50 (7.70)	n/a	1 d	15.80 (15.43)	22.73 (19.83)	*	Ewert, et al (1989)

Table 51. Randt Memory Test (RMT)

instrument	group	n	m/f	age	intervention	inter	t #1	t #2	note	citation
RMT Acquis & Recall (std)	Substance Abuse	15	8/7	21.10 (4.50)	outpt tx	4 w	85.4 (14.7)	86.3 (16.8)		Cosgrove, et al (1991)
RMT Acquis & Recall (std)	Substance Abuse (PCP)	15	8/7	21.10 (4.50)	outpt tx	4 w	76.7 (15.1)	89.2 (12.6)		Cosgrove, et al (1991)
RMT Acquis (std)	Control	56	18/38	21.36 (1.36)	n/a	1.5 w	96.0 (28.7)	108.0 (32.1)		Franzen, et al (1989)
RMT Acquis [148]	Control	60	26/34	71.24 (5.96)	n/a	12 m	109.91 (10.60)	114.06 (9.97)		Olin, et al (1991)
RMT Acquis/Recall	DAT	10	4/6	68.60 (4.50)	placebo	60 d	62.0 (17.2)	54.0 (16.1)		Agnoli, et al (1992)
RMT Acquis/Recall	DAT	10	4/6	68.60 (4.50)	l-deprenyl	60 d	54.8 (8.6)	64.2 (15.0)		Agnoli, et al (1992)

Practitioner's Guide to Evaluating Change with Neuropsychological Assessment Instruments

instrument	group	n	m/f	age	intervention	inter	t #1	t #2	note	citation
RMT Delayed Recall	DAT	10	4/6	68.60 (4.50)	placebo	60 d	45.8 (7.3)	40.8 (5.4)		Agnoli, et al (1992)
RMT Delayed Recall	DAT	10	4/6	68.60 (4.50)	l-deprenyl	60 d	36.6 (7.2)	47.2 (8.0)		Agnoli, et al (1992)
RMT Delayed Recall (std)	Substance Abuse	15	8/7	21.10 (4.50)	outpt tx	4 w	82.0 (15.6)	74.3 (19.4)		Cosgrove, et al (1991)
RMT Delayed Recall (std)	Substance Abuse (PCP)	15	8/7	21.10 (4.50)	outpt tx	4 w	74.0 (15.3)	81.1 (17.0)		Cosgrove, et al (1991)
RMT Faces	Control	21	3/18	30.10 (8.20)	n/a	6 m	43.4 (5.6)	46.8 (3.3)		Pulliainen, et al (1994)
RMT Faces	Epilepsy	20	9/11	31.50 (11.3)	phenytoin	6 m	43.5 (4.7)	45.5 (3.8)		Pulliainen, et al (1994)
RMT Faces	Epilepsy	23	11/12	26.80 (13.2)	carbamaz	6 m	41.7 (4.4)	44.8 (3.3)		Pulliainen, et al (1994)
RMT Five Items 10' Recall	Control	70	26/44	29.30 (1.15)	n/a	4 y	17.33 (1.4)	17.19 (1.6)		Amato, et al (1995)
RMT Five Items 10' Recall	MS	50	18/32	29.90 (8.48)	n/a	4 y	15.74 (3.4)	16.35 (4.3)		Amato, et al (1995)
RMT Five Items 24 hr Recall	Control	70	26/44	29.30 (1.15)	n/a	4 y	16.21 (2.3)	16.11 (2.4)		Amato, et al (1995)
RMT Five Items 24 hr Recall	MS	50	18/32	29.90 (8.48)	n/a	4 y	14.12 (3.7)	11.80 (3.4)		Amato, et al (1995)

instrument	group	n	m/f	age	intervention	inter	t #1	t #2	note	citation
RMT Five Items Acquis	Control	70	26/44	29.30 (1.15)	n/a	4 y	10.24 (1.6)	10.13 (1.5)		Amato, et al (1995)
RMT Five Items Acquis	MS	50	18/32	29.90 (8.48)	n/a	4 y	9.92 (3.2)	10.14 (3.2)		Amato, et al (1995)
RMT Memory Index	DAT	10	4/6	68.60 (4.50)	l-deprenyl	60 d	37.2 (6.1)	49.0 (12.8)		Agnoli, et al (1992)
RMT Memory Index	DAT	10	4/6	68.60 (4.50)	placebo	60 d	47.0 (13.7)	39.0 (12.7)		Agnoli, et al (1992)
RMT MQ (std)	Control	56	18/38	21.36 (1.36)	n/a	1.5 w	96.0 (18.2)	112.0 (16.4)		Franzen, et al (1989)
RMT Paired Words 10' Recall	Control	70	26/44	29.30 (1.15)	n/a	4 y	21.86 (0.9)	21.91 (0.7)		Amato, et al (1995)
RMT Paired Words 10' Recall	MS	50	18/32	29.90 (8.48)	n/a	4 y	19.88 (3.7)	19.43 (4.8)		Amato, et al (1995)
RMT Paired Words 24 hr Recall	Control	70	26/44	29.30 (1.15)	n/a	4 y	21.26 (1.2)	21.19 (1.2)		Amato, et al (1995)
RMT Paired Words 24 hr Recall	MS	50	18/32	29.90 (8.48)	n/a	4 y	19.16 (4.1)	15.78 (4.8)		Amato, et al (1995)
RMT Paired Words Acquis	Control	70	26/44	29.30 (1.15)	n/a	4 y	14.69 (1.6)	14.79 (1.3)		Amato, et al (1995)
RMT Paired Words Acquis	MS	50	18/32	29.90 (8.48)	n/a	4 y	12.44 (3.0)	12.16 (3.6)		Amato, et al (1995)

instrument	group	n	m/f	age	intervention	inter	t #1	t #2	note	citation
RMT Recall (std)	Control	56	18/38	21.36 (1.36)	n/a	1.5 w	96.0 (30.2)	108.0 (31.3)		Franzen, et al (1989)
RMT Recall [70]	Control	60	26/34	71.24 (5.96)	n/a	12 m	46.39 (6.46)	47.42 (3.20)		Olin, et al (1991)
RMT Short Tale	PD	50	32/18	54.80 (8.70)	n/a	86.7 m	7.2 (3.2)	6.4 (2.9)		Palazzini, et al (1995)
RMT Short Tale	PD w/ Dementia	11	6/5	65.70 (6.10)	n/a	86.7 m	4.5 (2.6)	1.8 (1.6)		Palazzini, et al (1995)
RMT Words	Control	21	3/18	30.10 (8.20)	n/a	6 m	46.2 (3.3)	45.9 (3.4)		Pulliainen, et al (1994)
RMT Words	Epilepsy	24	12/13	28.40 (9.70)	RTL	16.1 m	46.4 (3.8)	46.4 (3.5)		Phillips, et al (1995)
RMT Words	Epilepsy	14	7/7	32.90 (8.30)	LTL	16.1 m	44.8 (3.2)	42.0 (6.0)		Phillips, et al (1995)
RMT Words	Epilepsy	23	11/12	26.80 (13.2)	carbamaz	6 m	44.2 (4.50)	45.0 (4.3)		Pulliainen, et al (1994)
RMT Words	Epilepsy	20	9/11	31.50 (11.3)	phenytoin	6 m	44.7 (3.7)	45.1 (3.2)		Pulliainen, et al (1994)

Table 52. Raven's Progressive Matrices (RPM) Tests

instrument	group	n	m/f	age	intervention	inter	t #1	t #2	note	citation
RCPM	Control	20	6/14	69.40 (4.20)	n/a	1 y	33.5 (2.6)	33.5 (2.6)	*	Fromm, et al (1991)
RCPM	Control	25	n/a	6.50 - 12.50	n/a	3 m	24.9 (5.8)	27.2 (6.3)	*	Raven, et al (1977)

instrument	group	n	m/f	age	intervention	inter	t #1	t #2	note	citation
RCPM	DAT	18	5/13	71.00 (9.40)	n/a	1 y	21.2 (6.3)	20.2 (6.7)	*	Fromm, et al (1991)
RCPM	DAT (mild)	11	10/1	63.00 (8.00)	n/a	26 m	30.0 (4.0)	26.0 (5.0)		Haxby, et al (1990)
RCPM	DAT/MID	30	21/9	67.80 (1.50)	placebo	3 m	13.6 (0.6)	13.5 (0.7)	*	Villardita, et al (1992)
RCPM	DAT/MID	30	15/15	71.70 (1.30)	oxiracetam	3 m	13.2 (0.6)	14.4 (0.6)	*	Villardita, et al (1992)
RCPM	DAT/MID	29	14/15	71.50 (1.30)	oxiracetam	6 m	12.9 (0.6)	13.6 (0.8)	*	Villardita, et al (1992)
RCPM	Disturbed Children	29	n/a	6.50 - 12.50	n/a	3 m	20.5 (6.1)	21.9 (7.2)		Raven, et al (1977)
RCPM	Hypertension	34	n/a	76.10	captopril	24 w	27.4 (5.5)	28.4 (5.5)		Starr, et al (1996)
RCPM	Hypertension	35	n/a	76.10	bendrofluazide	24 w	26.7 (5.1)	28.4 (5.2)		Starr, et al (1996)
RCPM (raw)	MR	16	n/a	15.70	n/a	2 w	10.50	11.25	std/ auto	Knights, et al (1973)
RCPM (raw)	MR	16	n/a	15.70	n/a	2 w	9.38	12.69	auto/ std	Knights, et al (1973)
RPM	Control	70	26/44	29.30 (1.15)	n/a	4 y	48.06 (5.4)	47.94 (5.6)		Amato, et al (1995)
RPM	Control	20	10/10	40.0 - 50.0	n/a	1 w	11.45	12.0		Denney, et al (1990)
RPM	Control	20	10/10	20.0 - 30.0	n/a	1 w	15.95	16.7		Denney, et al (1990)

instrument	group	n	m/f	age	intervention	inter	t #1	t #2	note	citation
RPM	Control	20	10/10	30.0 - 40.0	n/a	1 w	14.9	15.3		Denney, et al (1990)
RPM	Control	20	10/10	30.0 - 40.0	training w/ RPM	1 w	14.4	15.6		Denney, et al (1990)
RPM	Control	20	10/10	40.0 - 50.0	training w/ RPM	1 w	9.55	12.45		Denney, et al (1990)
RPM	Control	20	10/10	20.0 - 30.0	training w/ RPM	1 w	17.55	17.95		Denney, et al (1990)
RPM	Control	77	77/0	50.0+	n/a	n/a	29.0 (10.5)	32.0 (12.0)		Raven, et al (1977)
RPM	Control	44	44/0	20.0 - 30.0	n/a	n/a	48.0 (8.2)	50.0 (8.7)		Raven, et al (1977)
RPM	Control	263	n/a	12.50	n/a	n/a	34.0 (10.8)	40.0 (9.7)		Raven, et al (1977)
RPM	Control	144	144/0	20.0 - 30.0	n/a	n/a	48.0 (8.2)	50.0 (8.7)		Raven, et al (1977)
RPM	Control	106	106/0	40.0 - 50.0	n/a	n/a	35.0 (11.2)	38.0 (11.1)		Raven, et al (1977)
RPM	Control	104	104/0	30.0 - 40.0	n/a	n/a	37.0 (9.5)	41.0 (8.2)		Raven, et al (1977)
RPM	HIV+ (IVDU)	42	31/11	27.0 (5.30)	n/a	12 m	33.7 (5.2)	34.9 (5.5)		Bono, et al (1996)
RPM	HIV- (IVDU)	39	30/9	28.60 (4.90)	n/a	12 m	34.5 (4.6)	35.2 (4.8)		Bono, et al (1996)
RPM	MS	50	18/32	29.90 (8.48)	n/a	4 y	42.78 (9.5)	39.0 (11.0)		Amato, et al (1995)

instrument	group	n	m/f	age	intervention	inter	t #1	t #2	note	citation
RPM (IQ)	Schizophrenia	28	n/a	n/a	n/a	12 m	83.07 (17.44)	92.04 (15.82)		Scottish Schizophrenia Research Group (1988)
RPM (short)	Control	20	12/8	56.40	n/a	10 w	106.0 (11.0)	112.0 (14.0)		Van Den Burg, et al (1985)
RPM (short)	PVD	20	18/2	56.80	major surgery	10 w	105.0 (14.0)	104.0 (14.0)		Van Den Burg, et al (1985)
RPM (short)	TIA	20	13/7	59.60	CE	10 w	101.0 (12.0)	10.0 (13.0)		Van Den Burg, et al (1985)
RPM (std)	CVA (Left)	13	9/4	51.50 (9.50)	early reaction training	3 w	105.2 (10.3)	108.0 (9.0)		Sturm, et al (1991)
RPM (std)	CVA (Left)	14	10/4	49.60 (9.50)	late reaction training	3 w	99.4 (10.8)	102.4 (10.8)	*	Sturm, et al (1991)
RPM (std)	CVA (Right)	8	6/2	51.50 (11.6)	late reaction training	3 w	92.3 (11.1)	94.0 (14.2)	*	Sturm, et al (1991)
RPM (t)	Epilepsy	12	6/6	28.50 (7.00)	phenytoin	3 m	47.25 (6.4)	42.43 (8.5)	*	Gallassi, et al (1988)
RPM (t)	Epilepsy	13	8/5	23.07 (8.90)	carbamaz	3 m	51.24 (8.7)	44.86 (10.2)	*	Gallassi, et al (1988)
RPM [38]	AIDS Dementia Complex	30	29/1	33.80	zdv	6 m	27.1 (10.4)	34.0 (5.9)		Tozzi, et al (1993)
RPM [48]	DAT	34	16/18	62.76 (6.30)	n/a	7.72 m	15.25 (8.54)	10.59 (8.87)		Della Sala, et al (1992)
RPM Advanced	Control	21	3/18	30.10 (8.20)	n/a	6 m	9.9 (1.5)	9.6 (1.5)		Pulliainen, et al (1994)

instrument	group	n	m/f	age	intervention	inter	t #1	t #2	note	citation
RPM Advanced	Epilepsy	20	9/11	31.50 (11.3)	phenytoin	6 m	8.8 (2.6)	9.0 (2.6)		Pulliainen, et al (1994)
RPM Advanced	Epilepsy	23	11/12	26.80 (13.2)	carbamaz	6 m	8.6 (2.0)	9.5 (2.0)		Pulliainen, et al (1994)
mRPM (correct [18])	Control	8	4/4	23.60	sleep deprived	1 d	9.4	-1.9 c		Linde, et al (1992)
mRPM (correct [18])	Control	8	5/3	23.30	n/a	1 d	10.5	0.9 c		Linde, et al (1992)

Table 53. Reaction Time (RT) Tests

instrument	group	n	m/f	age	intervention	inter	t #1	t #2	note	citation
4 choice RT (decision time: msec)	Control	10	n/a	n/a	n/a	n/a	485.4 (32.7)	459.7		Maddocks, et al (1996)
4 choice RT (decision time: msec)	Rugby players	10	n/a	n/a	concussion	n/a	478 (42.9)	499.1		Maddocks, et al (1996)
4 choice RT (movement time: msec)	Control	10	n/a	n/a	n/a	n/a	148.8 (32.1)	127		Maddocks, et al (1996)
4 choice RT (movement time: msec)	Rugby players	10	n/a	n/a	concussion	n/a	131.5 (27.6)	140.9		Maddocks, et al (1996)

instrument	group	n	m/f	age	intervention	inter	t #1	t #2	note	citation
CANTAB Choice RT	Control	16	n/a	46.00 (3.10)	n/a	1 m	625.0 (64.0)	614.0 (73.0)		Jalan, et al (1995)
CANTAB Choice RT	Variceal Hemorrhage	29	19/10	54.30 (5.60)	TIPSS	1 m	836.0 (168.0)	840.0 (223.0)	*	Jalan, et al (1995)
CANTAB Choice RT	Variceal Hemorrhage & Cirrhosis	12	7/5	53.10 (7.10)	variceal band ligation	1 m	865.0 (245.0)	878.0 (221.0)	*	Jalan, et al (1995)
CANTAB Complex RT	Control	10	8/2	31.10 (7.50)	saline	1 w	571.8 (86.7)	567.0 (87.4)		Gooday, et al (1995)
CANTAB Complex RT	Control	10	8/2	31.10 (7.50)	flumazenil	1 w	571.8 (57.1)	582.6 (89.1)		Gooday, et al (1995)
CANTAB Complex RT	Liver Disease	10	8/2	53.90 (7.40)	flumazenil	1 w	762.3 (162.3)	733.5 (139.5)		Gooday, et al (1995)
CANTAB Complex RT	Liver Disease	10	8/2	53.90 (7.40)	saline	1 w	748.5 (106)	842.6 (291.3)		Gooday, et al (1995)
CANTAB Simple RT	Control	10	8/2	31.10 (7.50)	saline	1 w	503.3 (69.7)	521.9 (78.5)		Gooday, et al (1995)
CANTAB Simple RT	Control	10	8/2	31.10 (7.50)	flumazenil	1 w	515.5 (63.5)	526.7 (100.7)		Gooday, et al (1995)
CANTAB Simple RT	Control	16	n/a	46.00 (3.10)	n/a	1 m	586.0 (83.0)	584.0 (83.0)		Jalan, et al (1995)
CANTAB Simple RT	Liver Disease	10	8/2	53.90 (7.40)	saline	1 w	770.0 (232.9)	760.2 (122.4)		Gooday, et al (1995)
CANTAB Simple RT	Liver Disease	10	8/2	53.90 (7.40)	flumazenil	1 w	834.8 (269.9)	700.0 (141.1)		Gooday, et al (1995)

instrument	group	n	m/f	age	intervention	inter	t #1	t #2	note	citation
CANTAB Simple RT	Variceal Hemorrhage	29	19/10	54.30 (5.60)	TIPSS	1 m	885.0 (256.0)	824.0 (282.0)	*	Jalan, et al (1995)
CANTAB Simple RT	Variceal Hemorrhage & Cirrhosis	12	7/5	53.10 (7.10)	variceal band ligation	1 m	861.0 (257.0)	872.0 (229.0)	*	Jalan, et al (1995)
choice RT	Control	10	n/a	27.00	trazadone 100 mg	2 h	25.3	26.5		Curran, et al (1988)
choice RT	Control	10	n/a	27.00	amitriptyline 75 mg	2 h	25.5	26.0		Curran, et al (1988)
choice RT	Control	10	n/a	27.00	amitriptyline 37.5 mg	2 h	24.4	25.0		Curran, et al (1988)
choice RT	Control	10	n/a	27.00	placebo	2 h	25.6	24.7		Curran, et al (1988)
choice RT	Control	10	n/a	27.00	protriptyline 20 mg	2 h	25.0	25.0		Curran, et al (1988)
choice RT	Control	10	n/a	27.00	protriptyline 10 mg	2 h	25.5	24.8		Curran, et al (1988)
choice RT	Control	10	n/a	27.00	trazadone 200 mg	2 h	23.7	25.3		Curran, et al (1988)
choice RT	Control	10	n/a	27.00	viloxazine 100 mg	2 h	22.0	21.1		Curran, et al (1988)
choice RT	Control	10	n/a	27.00	viloxazine 200 mg	2 h	25.0	24.5		Curran, et al (1988)
choice RT (false alarms)	CVA (Left)	13	9/4	51.50 (9.50)	early reaction training	3 w	3.2 (3.0)	3.2 (4.8)	*	Sturm, et al (1991)
choice RT (false alarms)	CVA (Left)	14	10/4	49.60 (9.50)	late reaction training	3 w	5.4 (3.7)	3.9 (3.4)	*	Sturm, et al (1991)

instrument	group	n	m/f	age	intervention	inter	t #1	t #2	note	citation
choice RT (false alarms)	CVA (Right)	8	6/2	51.50 (11.6)	late reaction training	3 w	4.4 (3.5)	3.9 (3.1)	*	Sturm, et al (1991)
choice RT (msec)	Control	21	5/16	34.00	carbamaz/ phenytoin CB	1 m	650.0 (133.0)	668.0 (131.0)	*	Meador, et al (1991)
choice RT (msec)	HD (at risk, + genetic marker)	8	1/7	26.20 (2.70)	n/a	2 y	390.8	401.1	*	Giordani, et al (1995)
choice RT (msec)	HD (at risk, - genetic marker)	8	1/7	28.40 (5.20)	n/a	2 y	396.8	385.2	*	Giordani, et al (1995)
choice RT (msec)	PD	18	11/7	56.90 (8.90)	selegiline	12 w	466.0 (110.0)	458.0 (76.0)		Hietanen (1991)
choice RT (msec)	PD	18	11/7	56.90 (8.90)	placebo	12 w	441.0 (75.0)	450.0 (108.0)		Hietanen (1991)
choice RT (std)	CVA (Left)	14	10/4	49.60 (9.50)	late reaction training	3 w	94.7 (16.5)	97.3 (10.9)	*	Sturm, et al (1991)
choice RT (std)	CVA (Left)	13	9/4	51.50 (9.50)	early reaction training	3 w	91.2 (14.9)	96.3 (14.2)	*	Sturm, et al (1991)
choice RT (std)	CVA (Right)	8	6/2	51.50 (11.6)	late reaction training	3 w	78.8 (14.6)	82.1 (16.6)	*	Sturm, et al (1991)
complex RT	subjective memory impairment	12	6/6	72.00	methylphen	45 min	709.25	768.38		Crook, et al (1977)
complex RT (t)	Epilepsy	13	8/5	23.07 (8.90)	carbamaz	3 m	47.20 (7.4)	49.04 (5.4)	*	Gallassi, et al (1988)
complex RT (t)	Epilepsy	12	6/6	28.50 (7.00)	phenytoin	3 m	44.67 (10.8)	48.54 (8.1)	*	Gallassi, et al (1988)

instrument	group	n	m/f	age	intervention	inter	t #1	t #2	note	citation
CPT-A (mean RT)	Control	216	106/ 110	7.91 (0.47)	n/a	2-3 y	508.66 (70.1)	477.21 (73.93)		Rebok, et al (1997)
CPT-V X (mean RT)	Control	216	106/ 110	7.91 (0.47)	n/a	2-3 y	615.2 (51.3)	527.45 (55.26)		Rebok, et al (1997)
RCPMB RT	Epilepsy	36	n/a	n/a	carbamaz	3 w	442.42	447.97		Rennick, et al (1974)
simple RT (msec)	Control	8	8/0	24.00	propranolol	3 w	NR	8.0 c		Brooks, et al (1988)
simple RT (msec)	Control	8	8/0	24.00	atenolol	3 w	NR	12.5 c		Brooks, et al (1988)
simple RT (msec)	Control	8	8/0	24.00	placebo	3 w	NR	10.5 c		Brooks, et al (1988)
simple RT (msec)	Control	8	8/0	24.00	metoprolol	3 w	NR	5.0 c		Brooks, et al (1988)
simple RT (msec)	HD (at risk, + genetic marker)	8	1/7	26.20 (2.70)	n/a	2 y	295.1	294.1	*	Giordani, et al (1995)
simple RT (msec)	HD (at risk, - genetic marker)	8	1/7	28.40 (5.20)	n/a	2 y	297.1	303.9	*	Giordani, et al (1995)
simple RT (msec)	PD	18	11/7	56.90 (8.90)	selegiline	12 w	415.0 (104.0)	418.0 (116.0)		Hietanen (1991)
simple RT (msec)	PD	18	11/7	56.90 (8.90)	placebo	12 w	392.0 (76.0)	380.0 (70.0)		Hietanen (1991)
simple RT (msec)	subjective memory impairment	12	6/6	72.00	methylphen	45 min	365.00	330.00		Crook, et al (1977)

instrument	group	n	m/f	age	intervention	inter	t #1	t #2	note	citation
simple RT (t)	Epilepsy	12	6/6	28.50 (7.00)	phenytoin	3 m	46.96 (9.9)	51.47 (10.8)	*	Gallassi, et al (1988)
simple RT (t)	Epilepsy	13	8/5	23.07 (8.90)	carbamaz	3 m	51.23 (10.0)	48.62 (6.8)	*	Gallassi, et al (1988)
simple RT auditory	Control	33	15/18	59.10 (9.30)	n/a	10 d	0.37	0.34		McCaffrey, et al (1993)
simple RT auditory (std)	CVA (Left)	13	9/4	51.50 (9.50)	early reaction training	3 w	98.0 (8.0)	101.6 (8.2)	*	Sturm, et al (1991)
simple RT auditory (std)	CVA (Left)	14	10/4	49.60 (9.50)	late reaction training	3 w	96.6 (14.2)	97.3 (9.0)	*	Sturm, et al (1991)
simple RT auditory (std)	CVA (Right)	8	6/2	51.50 (11.6)	late reaction training	3 w	73.3 (37.5)	72.5 (34.3)	*	Sturm, et al (1991)
simple RT left	Control	16	6/10	27.90	placebo	1 d	492.1 (142.9)	479.6 (167.4)	*	Gigli, et al (1993)
simple RT left	Control	16	6/10	27.90	brotizolam	1 d	491.8 (191.3)	495.4 (203.8)	*	Gigli, et al (1993)
simple RT right	Control	16	6/10	27.90	brotizolam	1 d	481.5 (193.3)	507.8 (213.9)	*	Gigli, et al (1993)
simple RT right	Control	16	6/10	27.90	placebo	1 d	485.9 (132.9)	470.4 (121.3)	*	Gigli, et al (1993)
simple RT visual (std)	CVA (Left)	13	9/4	51.50 (9.50)	early reaction training	3 w	95.4 (13.2)	100.9 (8.7)	*	Sturm, et al (1991)
simple RT visual (std)	CVA (Left)	14	10/4	49.60 (9.50)	late reaction training	3 w	98.7 (10.2)	94.6 (11.9)	*	Sturm, et al (1991)

instrument	group	n	m/f	age	intervention	inter	t #1	t #2	note	citation
simple RT visual (std)	CVA (Right)	8	6/2	51.50 (11.6)	late reaction training	3 w	62.4 (41.5)	64.3 (32.5)	*	Sturm, et al (1991)
symbol digit substitution test (avg RT)	Control	12	12/0	26.00	placebo	~1 h	1.58 (0.43)	1.68 (0.47)		Cook, et al (1991)
symbol digit substitution test (avg RT)	Control	12	12/0	26.00	methanol	~1 h	1.67 (0.57)	1.69 (0.53)		Cook, et al (1991)

Table 54. Repeatable Cognitive Perceptual Motor Battery (RCPMB)

instrument	group	n	m/f	age	intervention	inter	t #1	t #2	note	citation
RCPMB CFF (errors)	Epilepsy	36	n/a	n/a	carbamaz	3 w	20.361	19.722		Rennick, et al (1974)
RCPMB Color Naming	Alcoholic	10	9/1	35.20	abstin	4 w	130.9	116.6		Goldman, et al (1983)
RCPMB Color Naming	Alcoholic	10	7/3	25.50	abstin	4 w	125.4	113.8		Goldman, et al (1983)
RCPMB Color Naming	Alcoholic	11	8/3	50.60	abstin	4 w	139.5	125.9		Goldman, et al (1983)
RCPMB Color Naming	Control	15	9/6	26.40	n/a	4 w	121.0	106.9		Goldman, et al (1983)
RCPMB Color Naming	Control	15	15/0	47.50	n/a	4 w	116.5	105.1		Goldman, et al (1983)

instrument	group	n	m/f	age	intervention	inter	t #1	t #2	note	citation
RCPMB Color Naming	Epilepsy	71	n/a	n/a	anticonvulsant	n/a	175.0	168.0		Clifford, et al (1976)
RCPMB Color Naming	Epilepsy	36	n/a	n/a	carbamaz	3 w	149.08	155.72		Rennick, et al (1974)
RCPMB Color Naming (errors)	Renal Disease	20	n/a	46.50 (11.3)	long-term hemodialysis	1 d	1.2 (1.4)	0.8 (1.5)	*	Ratner, et al (1983)
RCPMB Color Naming (time)	Renal Disease	20	n/a	46.50 (11.3)	long-term hemodialysis	1 d	129.7 (23.9)	122.0 (19.5)	*	Ratner, et al (1983)
RCPMB D Span	Epilepsy	36	n/a	n/a	carbamaz	3 w	10.44	10.33		Rennick, et al (1974)
RCPMB D Sym	Alcoholic	11	8/3	50.60	abstin	4 w	38.4	46.3		Goldman, et al (1983)
RCPMB D Sym	Alcoholic	10	9/1	35.20	abstin	4 w	49.2	59.0		Goldman, et al (1983)
RCPMB D Sym	Alcoholic	10	7/3	25.50	abstin	4 w	49.2	53.1		Goldman, et al (1983)
RCPMB D Sym	Boxers	20	20/0	20.50	n/a	15-18 m	73.6	74.0		Porter, et al (1996)
RCPMB D Sym	Control	15	15/0	47.50	n/a	4 w	55.7	59.6		Goldman, et al (1983)
RCPMB D Sym	Control	15	9/6	26.40	n/a	4 w	60.7	69.5		Goldman, et al (1983)
RCPMB D Sym	Control	20	20/0	20.50	n/a	15-18 m	71.1	72.1		Porter, et al (1996)

instrument	group	n	m/f	age	intervention	inter	t #1	t #2	note	citation
RCPMB D Sym	Epilepsy	71	n/a	n/a	anticonvulsant	n/a	7.5	7.97		Clifford, et al (1976)
RCPMB D Sym	Epilepsy	36	n/a	n/a	carbamaz	3 w	8.50	8.53		Rennick, et al (1974)
RCPMB Digit Vigilance	Cardiac	90	77/13	59.00 (10.6)	CABG/CPB	8 d	124.4 (37.1)	170.2 (66.4)	*	Townes, et al (1989)
RCPMB Digit Vigilance	Control	47	35/12	59.00 (9.81)	n/a	8 d	111.2 (26.7)	109.3 (25.1)	*	Townes, et al (1989)
RCPMB FTT DH	Alcoholic	10	7/3	25.50	abstin	4 w	44.2	51.6		Goldman, et al (1983)
RCPMB FTT DH	Alcoholic	11	8/3	50.60	abstin	4 w	39.9	50.5		Goldman, et al (1983)
RCPMB FTT DH	Alcoholic	10	9/1	35.20	abstin	4 w	46.7	52.1		Goldman, et al (1983)
RCPMB FTT DH	Boxers	20	20/0	20.50	n/a	15-18 m	49.0	46.3		Porter, et al (1996)
RCPMB FTT DH	Control	15	15/0	47.50	n/a	4 w	52.3	56.2		Goldman, et al (1983)
RCPMB FTT DH	Control	15	9/6	26.40	n/a	4 w	49.3	50.5		Goldman, et al (1983)
RCPMB FTT DH	Control	20	20/0	20.50	n/a	15-18 m	50.9	51.1		Porter, et al (1996)
RCPMB FTT DH	Epilepsy	36	n/a	n/a	carbamaz	3 w	45.14	45.61		Rennick, et al (1974)
RCPMB FTT NDH	Alcoholic	10	9/1	35.20	abstin	4 w	41.3	46.6		Goldman, et al (1983)

instrument	group	n	m/f	age	intervention	inter	t #1	t #2	note	citation
RCPMB FTT NDH	Alcoholic	11	8/3	50.60	abstin	4 w	35.4	44.0		Goldman, et al (1983)
RCPMB FTT NDH	Alcoholic	10	7/3	25.50	abstin	4 w	43.1	48.8		Goldman, et al (1983)
RCPMB FTT NDH	Boxers	20	20/0	20.50	n/a	15-18 m	44.7	43.6		Porter, et al (1996)
RCPMB FTT NDH	Control	15	15/0	47.50	n/a	4 w	48.7	50.8		Goldman, et al (1983)
RCPMB FTT NDH	Control	15	9/6	26.40	n/a	4 w	46.5	46.8		Goldman, et al (1983)
RCPMB FTT NDH	Control	20	20/0	20.50	n/a	15-18 m	49.5	49.7		Porter, et al (1996)
RCPMB Grip Strength DH	Epilepsy	36	n/a	n/a	carbamaz	3 w	36.24	35.36		Rennick, et al (1974)
RCPMB Pegb DH	Alcoholic	10	9/1	35.20	abstin	4 w	72.8	60.9		Goldman, et al (1983)
RCPMB Pegb DH	Alcoholic	10	7/3	25.50	abstin	4 w	73.9	63.1		Goldman, et al (1983)
RCPMB Pegb DH	Alcoholic	11	8/3	50.60	abstin	4 w	95.7	73.5		Goldman, et al (1983)
RCPMB Pegb DH	Control	15	15/0	47.50	n/a	4 w	66.3	58.7		Goldman, et al (1983)
RCPMB Pegb DH	Control	15	9/6	26.40	n/a	4 w	60.2	53.7		Goldman, et al (1983)
RCPMB Pegb DH	Epilepsy	36	n/a	n/a	carbamaz	3 w	74.53	73.22		Rennick, et al (1974)

instrument	group	n	m/f	age	intervention	inter	t #1	t #2	note	citation
RCPMB Pegb DH	Renal Disease	20	n/a	46.50 (11.3)	long-term hemodialysis	1 d	85.6 (20.6)	74.7 (16.7)	*	Ratner, et al (1983)
RCPMB Pegb NDH	Alcoholic	10	9/1	35.20	abstin	4 w	85.0	66.1		Goldman, et al (1983)
RCPMB Pegb NDH	Alcoholic	10	7/3	25.50	abstin	4 w	82.7	69.9		Goldman, et al (1983)
RCPMB Pegb NDH	Alcoholic	11	8/3	50.60	abstin	4 w	95.4	74.8		Goldman, et al (1983)
RCPMB Pegb NDH	Control	15	9/6	26.40	n/a	4 w	61.5	59.2		Goldman, et al (1983)
RCPMB Pegb NDH	Control	15	15/0	47.50	n/a	4 w	71.6	65.5		Goldman, et al (1983)
RCPMB Pegb NDH	Renal Disease	20	n/a	46.50 (11.3)	long-term hemodialysis	1 d	90.2 (21.8)	82.0 (15.5)	*	Ratner, et al (1983)
RCPMB RT	Epilepsy	36	n/a	n/a	carbamaz	3 w	442.42	447.97		Rennick, et al (1974)
RCPMB TMT-A	Boxers	20	20/0	20.50	n/a	15-18 m	26.2	26.1		Porter, et al (1996)
RCPMB TMT-A	Control	20	20/0	20.50	n/a	15-18 m	31.6	31.6		Porter, et al (1996)
RCPMB TMT-B	Alcoholic	11	8/3	50.60	abstin	4 w	159.2	110.2		Goldman, et al (1983)
RCPMB TMT-B	Alcoholic	10	7/3	25.50	abstin	4 w	105.8	60.8		Goldman, et al (1983)
RCPMB TMT-B	Alcoholic	10	9/1	35.20	abstin	4 w	100.1	67.8		Goldman, et al (1983)

instrument	group	n	m/f	age	intervention	inter	t #1	t #2	note	citation
RCPMB TMT-B	Boxers	20	20/0	20.50	n/a	15-18 m	53.8	53.4		Porter, et al (1996)
RCPMB TMT-B	Control	15	15/0	47.50	n/a	4 w	79.5	67.1		Goldman, et al (1983)
RCPMB TMT-B	Control	15	9/6	26.40	n/a	4 w	62.7	45.7		Goldman, et al (1983)
RCPMB TMT-B	Control	20	20/0	20.50	n/a	15-18 m	70.9	70.1		Porter, et al (1996)
RCPMB TMT-B	Epilepsy	71	n/a	n/a	anticonvulsant	n/a	140.0	116.05		Clifford, et al (1976)
RCPMB TMT-B	Epilepsy	36	n/a	n/a	carbamaz	3 w	79.61	87.03		Rennick, et al (1974)
RCPMB Visual Search	Alcoholic	10	7/3	25.50	abstin	4 w	170.8	133.7		Goldman, et al (1983)
RCPMB Visual Search	Alcoholic	11	8/3	50.60	abstin	4 w	280.8	177.3		Goldman, et al (1983)
RCPMB Visual Search	Alcoholic	10	9/1	35.20	abstin	4 w	176.9	119.5		Goldman, et al (1983)
RCPMB Visual Search	Cardiac	90	77/13	59.00 (10.6)	CABG/CPB	8 d	186.3 (102.1)	350.3 (206.7)	*	Townes, et al (1989)
RCPMB Visual Search	Control	15	15/0	47.50	n/a	4 w	152.0	107.2		Goldman, et al (1983)
RCPMB Visual Search	Control	15	9/6	26.40	n/a	4 w	135.7	110.1		Goldman, et al (1983)

instrument	group	n	m/f	age	intervention	inter	t #1	t #2	note	citation
RCPMB Visual Search	Control	47	35/12	59.00 (9.81)	n/a	8 d	143.1 (52.0)	134.6 (46.1)	*	Townes, et al (1989)
RCPMB Visual Search	Epilepsy	71	n/a	n/a	anticonvulsant	n/a	11.3	9.8		Clifford, et al (1976)
RCPMB Visual Search	Epilepsy	36	n/a	n/a	carbamaz	3 w	7.83	8.88		Rennick, et al (1974)
RCPMB Writing Time DH	Epilepsy	36	n/a	n/a	carbamaz	3 w	5.69	6.22		Rennick, et al (1974)

Table 55. Rey Auditory Verbal Learning Test (RAVLT)

instrument	group	n	m/f	age	intervention	inter	t #1	t #2	note	citation
RAVLT	Control	16	n/a	60.0+	placebo	1 d	11.0	10.0		Richardson, et al (1985)
RAVLT	Control	14	n/a	60.0+	scopolamine	1 d	8.0	6.0		Richardson, et al (1985)
RAVLT	DAT (mild – mod)	46	19/27	70.31 (7.15)	idebenone	45 d	17.31 (1.41)	20.14 (1.64)	*	Bergamasco, et al (1994)
RAVLT	DAT (mild – mod)	46	24/22	69.85 (5.81)	placebo	45 d	14.07 (0.91)	14.95 (0.87)	*	Bergamasco, et al (1994)
RAVLT	HIV+ (IVDU)	8	5/3	39.00 (8.00)	MSR/placebo	7 d	7.5 (2.2)	7.5 (2.6)	*	Van Dyck, et al (1997)
RAVLT Intrus	Cardiac	104	84/20	59.10 (8.30)	CPB	8-9 d	1.1 (1.4)	2.0 (2.3)		Vingerhoets, et al (1996)

instrument	group	n	m/f	age	intervention	inter	t #1	t #2	note	citation
RAVLT Intrus	Cardiac	88	75/13	58.90 (8.20)	CPB	6 m	1.1 (1.5)	1.2 (1.6)		Vingerhoets, et al (1996)
RAVLT Intrus	Control	30	26/4	29.90 (6.20)	CVLT admin first	2-4 h	NR	1.8 (3.3)		Crossen, et al (1994)
RAVLT Intrus	Vascular/ Thoracic	16	14/2	58.60 (9.20)	surgery	6 m	1.4 (2.3)	1.6 (1.9)		Vingerhoets, et al (1996)
RAVLT Intrus	Vascular/ Thoracic	18	16/2	61.40 (9.70)	surgery	8-9 d	1.8 (3.1)	1.6 (1.7)		Vingerhoets, et al (1996)
RAVLT Persev	Control	30	26/4	29.90 (6.20)	CVLT admin first	2-4 h	NR	5.5 (4.5)		Crossen, et al (1994)
RAVLT Recog	Control	30	15/15	n/a	n/a	27.0 d	25.20 (3.15)	24.57 (3.67)	AF	Crawford, et al (1989b)
RAVLT Recog	Control	30	15/15	n/a	n/a	27.0 d	25.30 (2.47)	26.67 (2.47)		Crawford, et al (1989b)
RAVLT Recog	Control	30	26/4	29.90 (6.20)	CVLT admin first	2-4 h	NR	13.8 (1.1)		Crossen, et al (1994)
RAVLT Recog	Control	42	n/a	45.80	n/a	1 m	13.6 (1.8)	14.0 (1.2)	AF	Delaney, et al (1992)
RAVLT Recog	Control	51	25/26	31.30 (12.7)	n/a	6 – 14 d	13.84 (1.50)	13.51 (1.57)	AF	Geffen, et al (1994)
RAVLT Recog	Control	16	6/10	27.90	brotizolam	1 d	10.77 (3.79)	10.62 (2.33)	*	Gigli, et al (1993)
RAVLT Recog	Control	16	6/10	27.90	placebo	1 d	10.62 (1.83)	10.39 (2.29)	*	Gigli, et al (1993)
RAVLT Recog	Epilepsy	38	21/17	34.26 (9.18)	vigabatrin 3 g	18 w	13.90 (4.42)	13.08 (3.97)		Dodrill, et al (1995)

instrument	group	n	m/f	age	intervention	inter	t #1	t #2	note	citation
RAVLT Recog	Epilepsy	36	17/19	34.89 (8.38)	vigabatrin 1 g	18 w	14.58 (4.74)	14.47 (4.69)		Dodrill, et al (1995)
RAVLT Recog	Epilepsy	40	14/26	33.88 (9.77)	placebo	18 w	14.33 (3.41)	14.50 (3.26)		Dodrill, et al (1995)
RAVLT Recog	Epilepsy	32	17/15	33.72 (9.66)	vigabatrin 6 g	18 w	14.10 (4.45)	14.61 (3.64)		Dodrill, et al (1995)
RAVLT Recog	Epilepsy	28	17/11	27.00 (5.90)	LTL	9.4 m	12.3	10.6		Ivnik, et al (1987)
RAVLT Recog	Epilepsy	35	17/18	28.40 (9.60)	RTL	9.4 m	13.0	13.8		Ivnik, et al (1987)
RAVLT Recog	Lung Cancer	14	12/2	63.00	chemotherapy	~5 d	27.0 (2.1)	26.1 (2.8)	*	Van Oosterhout, et al (1995)
RAVLT Recog	Spinal Cord Injury	67	54/13	32.00 (14.7)	n/a	38 w	12.96 (2.76)	13.17 (2.18)		Richards, et al (1988)
RAVLT Recog	VA Inpts	44	n/a	45.86 (14.0)	n/a	140.0 min	10.59 (2.75)	8.95 (3.58)	alt/ std	Ryan, et al (1986)
RAVLT Recog	VA Inpts	41	n/a	45.86 (14.0)	n/a	140.0 min	10.78 (3.51)	10.18 (3.10)	std /alt	Ryan, et al (1986)
RAVLT Recog (10', errors)	Control	8	4/4	21.80 (4.20)	placebo	60 min	1.88 (1.73)	1.50 (1.31)	AF	Kirkby, et al (1995)
RAVLT Recog (10', errors)	Control	5	1/4	68.40 (6.10)	lorazepam	60 min	2.40 (1.68)	7.60 (7.44)	AF	Kirkby, et al (1995)
RAVLT Recog (10', errors)	Control	9	4/5	26.40 (7.70)	lorazepam	60 min	1.78 (1.72)	2.11 (3.02)	AF	Kirkby, et al (1995)
RAVLT Recog (10', errors)	Control	4	0/4	67.30 (0.50)	placebo	60 min	2.25 (0.96)	1.75 (1.26)	AF	Kirkby, et al (1995)

instrument	group	n	m/f	age	intervention	inter	t #1	t #2	note	citation
RAVLT Recog (10', hits)	Control	9	4/5	26.40 (7.70)	lorazepam	60 min	11.0 (2.00)	8.00 (3.81)	AF	Kirkby, et al (1995)
RAVLT Recog (10', hits)	Control	8	4/4	21.80 (4.20)	placebo	60 min	9.25 (3.28)	7.75 (1.98)	AF	Kirkby, et al (1995)
RAVLT Recog (10', hits)	Control	5	1/4	68.40 (6.10)	lorazepam	60 min	10.0 (1.41)	8.40 (2.41)	AF	Kirkby, et al (1995)
RAVLT Recog (10', hits)	Control	4	0/4	67.30 (0.50)	placebo	60 min	8.25 (1.89)	5.50 (3.11)	AF	Kirkby, et al (1995)
RAVLT Recog B	Control	51	25/26	31.30 (12.7)	n/a	6 – 14 d	7.57 (2.93)	6.96 (2.76)	AF	Geffen, et al (1994)
RAVLT Total	AIDS	10	10/0	41.70 (5.50)	n/a	6.53 m	48.5 (9.2)	48.0 (10.1)		Hinkin, et al (1995)
RAVLT Total	AIDS Dementia Complex	30	29/1	33.80	zdv	6 m	44.2 (11.0)	49.2 (8.1)		Tozzi, et al (1993)
RAVLT Total	Alcoholic	16	16/0	37.50 (11.1)	inpt tx	3-4 w	46.7 (8.9)	47.6 (9.2)		Unkenstein, et al (1991)
RAVLT Total	BMT	25	14/11	~12.0	BMT	8.2 m	40.5 (14.3)	49.9 (12.5)		Phipps, et al (1995)
RAVLT Total	Cardiac	88	75/13	58.90 (8.20)	CPB	6 m	42.9 (7.9)	46.1 (9.5)		Vingerhoets, et al (1996)
RAVLT Total	Cardiac	104	84/20	59.10 (8.30)	CPB	8-9 d	41.7 (8.1)	38.5 (9.3)		Vingerhoets, et al (1996)
RAVLT Total	Control	30	26/4	29.90 (6.20)	CVLT admin first	2-4 h	NR	52.3 (8.0)		Crossen, et al (1994)

instrument	group	n	m/f	age	intervention	inter	t #1	t #2	note	citation
RAVLT Total	Control	51	25/26	31.30 (12.7)	n/a	6 – 14 d	50.25 (7.08)	50.88 (8.02)	AF	Geffen, et al (1994)
RAVLT Total	Control	10	8/2	31.10 (7.50)	saline	1 w	62.0 (6.1)	61.4 (6.6)		Gooday, et al (1995)
RAVLT Total	Control	10	8/2	31.10 (7.50)	flumazenil	1 w	61.9 (5.8)	57.6 (7.9)		Gooday, et al (1995)
RAVLT Total	Control	37	n/a	~6.00	n/a	~6 m	NR	7.15 c	*	Neyens, et al (1996)
RAVLT Total	Control	20	12/8	56.40	n/a	10 w	40.0 (9.0)	44.0 (11.0)		Van Den Burg, et al (1985)
RAVLT Total	DAT/MID	30	15/15	71.70 (1.30)	oxiracetam	3 m	18.5 (1.1)	20.6 (1.1)	*	Villardita, et al (1992)
RAVLT Total	DAT/MID	29	14/15	71.50 (1.30)	oxiracetam	6 m	18.3 (1.2)	20.1 (1.1)	*	Villardita, et al (1992)
RAVLT Total	DAT/MID	30	21/9	67.80 (1.50)	placebo	3 m	18.8 (1.1)	18.4 (1.1)	*	Villardita, et al (1992)
RAVLT Total	Epilepsy	32	17/15	33.72 (9.66)	vigabatrin 6 g	18 w	44.28 (11.15)	43.28 (9.79)		Dodrill, et al (1995)
RAVLT Total	Epilepsy	38	21/17	34.26 (9.18)	vigabatrin 3 g	18 w	41.87 (9.24)	40.05 (10.27)		Dodrill, et al (1995)
RAVLT Total	Epilepsy	36	17/19	34.89 (8.38)	vigabatrin 1 g	18 w	40.89 (11.54)	40.69 (9.84)		Dodrill, et al (1995)
RAVLT Total	Epilepsy	40	14/26	33.88 (9.77)	placebo	18 w	45.92 (10.88)	45.58 (9.18)		Dodrill, et al (1995)
RAVLT Total	Epilepsy	20	8/12	34.60 (9.80)	LTL	4.1 m	45.5	39.1		Ivnik, et al (1993)

instrument	group	n	m/f	age	intervention	inter	t #1	t #2	note	citation
RAVLT Total	Epilepsy	20	12/8	29.90 (10.1)	RTL	3.8 m	48.7	51.7		Ivnik, et al (1993)
RAVLT Total	HIV+	132	132/0	~33.8	n/a	13.3 m	52.9	51.2		Selnes, et al (1990)
RAVLT Total	HIV-	132	132/0	~35.6	n/a	13.4 m	51.9	51.0		Selnes, et al (1990)
RAVLT Total	Liver Disease	10	8/2	53.90 (7.40)	flumazenil	1 w	40.6 (5.7)	37.0 (9.3)		Gooday, et al (1995)
RAVLT Total	Liver Disease	10	8/2	53.90 (7.40)	saline	1 w	38.3 (8.8)	35.7 (7.5)		Gooday, et al (1995)
RAVLT Total	Lung Cancer	14	12/2	63.00	chemotherapy	~5 d	32.5 (9.3)	35.6 (11.6)	*	Van Oosterhout, et al (1995)
RAVLT Total	PVD	20	18/2	56.80	major surgery	10 w	31.0 (7.0)	34.0 (9.0)		Van Den Burg, et al (1985)
RAVLT Total	Schizophrenia (acute)	39	24/15	28.60 (8.60)	n/a	1 y	45.8 (11.4)	48.6 (10.0)		Sweeney, et al (1991)
RAVLT Total	Schizophrenia Inpts	35	29/6	23.71 (4.50)	neuroleptics	1-2 y	45.8 (15.6)	47.4 (13.9)		Nopoulos, et al (1994)
RAVLT Total	TIA	20	13/7	59.60	CE	10 w	35.0 (11.0)	37.0 (12.0)		Van Den Burg, et al (1985)
RAVLT Total	VA Inpts	44	n/a	45.86 (14.0)	n/a	140.0 min	31.91 (10.36)	33.30 (11.44)	alt/ std	Ryan, et al (1986)
RAVLT Total	VA Inpts	41	n/a	45.86 (14.0)	n/a	140.0 min	37.98 (10.27)	33.78 (12.05)	std/ alt	Ryan, et al (1986)
RAVLT Total	Vascular/ Thoracic	16	14/2	58.60 (9.20)	surgery	6 m	44.6 (7.9)	43.4 (8.3)		Vingerhoets, et al (1996)

instrument	group	n	m/f	age	intervention	inter	t #1	t #2	note	citation
RAVLT Total	Vascular/ Thoracic	18	16/2	61.40 (9.70)	surgery	8-9 d	40.6 (8.7)	37.3 (10.0)		Vingerhoets, et al (1996)
RAVLT Total Persev	Cardiac	104	84/20	59.10 (8.30)	CPB	8-9 d	2.5 (2.8)	2.8 (3.4)		Vingerhoets, et al (1996)
RAVLT Total Persev	Cardiac	88	75/13	58.90 (8.20)	CPB	6 m	2.4 (2.8)	3.0 (2.9)		Vingerhoets, et al (1996)
RAVLT Total Persev	Vascular/ Thoracic	16	14/2	58.60 (9.20)	surgery	6 m	2.8 (3.6)	2.8 (2.3)		Vingerhoets, et al (1996)
RAVLT Total Persev	Vascular/ Thoracic	18	16/2	61.40 (9.70)	surgery	8-9 d	3.3 (3.3)	2.0 (2.3)		Vingerhoets, et al (1996)
RAVLT Trial 1	BMT	25	14/11	~12.0	BMT	8.2 m	4.5 (2.2)	5.8 (2.1)		Phipps, et al (1995)
RAVLT Trial 1	Cardiac	88	75/13	58.90 (8.20)	CPB	6 m	5.4 (1.6)	6.2 (1.8)		Vingerhoets, et al (1996)
RAVLT Trial 1	Cardiac	104	84/20	59.10 (8.30)	CPB	8-9 d	5.2 (1.6)	4.9 (1.9)		Vingerhoets, et al (1996)
RAVLT Trial 1	Control	63	8/55	56.22 (11.0)	n/a	~6 m	NR	-0.40 (1.96) c		Bruggemans, et al (1997)
RAVLT Trial 1	Control	30	15/15	n/a	n/a	27.0 d	7.53 (1.76)	7.50 (2.13)	AF	Crawford, et al (1989b)
RAVLT Trial 1	Control	30	15/15	n/a	n/a	27.0 d	7.87 (1.76)	10.53 (2.39)		Crawford, et al (1989b)
RAVLT Trial 1	Control	30	26/4	29.90 (6.20)	CVLT admin first	2-4 h	NR	6.8 (1.5)		Crossen, et al (1994)
RAVLT Trial 1	Control	42	n/a	45.80	n/a	1m	6.0 (2.1)	6.1 (2.2)	AF	Delaney, et al (1992)

instrument	group	n	m/f	age	intervention	inter	t #1	t #2	note	citation
RAVLT Trial 1	Control	51	25/26	31.30 (12.7)	n/a	6 – 14 d	6.67 (1.29)	6.98 (1.71)	AF	Geffen, et al (1994)
RAVLT Trial 1	Control	8	4/4	21.80 (4.20)	placebo	60 min	7.75 (1.28)	8.00 (1.31)	AF	Kirkby, et al (1995)
RAVLT Trial 1	Control	9	4/5	26.40 (7.70)	lorazepam	60 min	8.00 (2.00)	7.33 (2.18)	AF	Kirkby, et al (1995)
RAVLT Trial 1	Control	4	0/4	67.30 (0.50)	placebo	60 min	6.50 (1.29)	6.50 (0.58)	AF	Kirkby, et al (1995)
RAVLT Trial 1	Control	5	1/4	68.40 (6.10)	lorazepam	60 min	7.60 (1.52)	4.80 (1.79)	AF	Kirkby, et al (1995)
RAVLT Trial 1	Control	47	14/33	72.90 (1.40)	n/a	1 y	5.1 (2.0)	5.4 (1.7)	*	Mitrushina, et al (1991b)
RAVLT Trial 1	Control	40	6/34	68.20 (1.20)	n/a	1 y	6.0 (1.6)	6.2 (1.8)	*	Mitrushina, et al (1991b)
RAVLT Trial 1	Control	16	4/12	78.30 (2.50)	n/a	1 y	5.1 (1.5)	5.8 (1.2)	*	Mitrushina, et al (1991b)
RAVLT Trial 1	Control	19	2/17	62.20 (2.50)	n/a	1 y	6.7 (1.6)	6.4 (1.3)	*	Mitrushina, et al (1991b)
RAVLT Trial 1	Control	72	67/5	44.50 (12.4)	n/a	6 m	6.4 (2.4)	6.3 (2.1)		Prevey, et al (1996)
RAVLT Trial 1	Control	47	47/0	37.70 (6.00)	n/a	1 y	6.89 (2.11)	7.79 (2.26)	*	Uchiyama, et al (1995)
RAVLT Trial 1	Epilepsy	35	17/18	28.40 (9.60)	RTL	9.4 m	6.4	7.4		Ivnik, et al (1987)
RAVLT Trial 1	Epilepsy	28	17/11	27.00 (5.90)	LTL	9.4 m	6.1	5.9		Ivnik, et al (1987)

instrument	group	n	m/f	age	intervention	inter	t #1	t #2	note	citation
RAVLT Trial 1	Epilepsy	39	36/3	44.30 (14.2)	valproate	6 m	5.6 (1.7)	5.9 (1.6)		Prevey, et al (1996)
RAVLT Trial 1	Epilepsy	26	24/2	43.50 (17.1)	carbamaz	6 m	5.8 (2.1)	5.2 (1.6)		Prevey, et al (1996)
RAVLT Trial 1	Myasthenia Gravis	11	7/4	49.00	prednisolone	3-11 m	6.2 (2.0)	5.5 (2.5)		Glennerster, et al (1996)
RAVLT Trial 1	Ocular Disease	50	27/23	42.00 (17.0)	steroid tx	~8 d	5.2 (1.8)	5.0 (1.6)		Naber, et al (1996)
RAVLT Trial 1	Renal Failure	9	4/5	65.00	rHuEpo	22.8 w	6.0 (1.9)	6.7 (3.0)		Temple, et al (1995)
RAVLT Trial 1	Renal Failure	8	3/5	67.50	n/a	19.3 w	5.0 (1.3)	5.9 (1.9)		Temple, et al (1995)
RAVLT Trial 1	VA Inpts	44	n/a	45.86 (14.0)	n/a	140.0 min	4.27 (1.61)	4.59 (1.69)	alt/ std	Ryan, et al (1986)
RAVLT Trial 1	VA Inpts	41	n/a	45.86 (14.0)	n/a	140.0 min	4.80 (1.72)	4.66 (1.94)	std/ alt	Ryan, et al (1986)
RAVLT Trial 1	Vascular/ Thoracic	18	16/2	61.40 (9.70)	surgery	8-9 d	5.2 (1.8)	4.9 (1.7)		Vingerhoets, et al (1996)
RAVLT Trial 1	Vascular/ Thoracic	16	14/2	58.60 (9.20)	surgery	6 m	6.0 (1.2)	5.6 (1.1)		Vingerhoets, et al (1996)
RAVLT Trial 2	Cardiac	88	75/13	58.90 (8.20)	CPB	6 m	7.7 (2.0)	8.6 (2.2)		Vingerhoets, et al (1996)
RAVLT Trial 2	Cardiac	104	84/20	59.10 (8.30)	CPB	8-9 d	7.4 (2.0)	7.0 (2.0)		Vingerhoets, et al (1996)
RAVLT Trial 2	Control	30	15/15	n/a	n/a	27.0 d	11.10 (2.19)	12.87 (1.81)		Crawford, et al (1989b)

instrument	group	n	m/f	age	intervention	inter	t #1	t #2	note	citation
RAVLT Trial 2	Control	30	15/15	n/a	n/a	27.0 d	10.40 (2.43)	10.27 (2.16)	AF	Crawford, et al (1989b)
RAVLT Trial 2	Control	30	26/4	29.90 (6.20)	CVLT admin first	2-4 h	NR	9.9 (2.3)		Crossen, et al (1994)
RAVLT Trial 2	Control	51	25/26	31.30 (12.7)	n/a	6 – 14 d	9.08 (1.96)	9.18 (2.03)	AF	Geffen, et al (1994)
RAVLT Trial 2	Control	72	67/5	44.50 (12.4)	n/a	6 m	8.9 (2.1)	8.5 (2.6)		Prevey, et al (1996)
RAVLT Trial 2	Control	47	47/0	37.70 (6.00)	n/a	1 y	9.98 (2.44)	10.26 (2.43)	*	Uchiyama, et al (1995)
RAVLT Trial 2	Epilepsy	28	17/11	27.00 (5.90)	LTL	9.4 m	8.1	7.8		Ivnik, et al (1987)
RAVLT Trial 2	Epilepsy	35	17/18	28.40 (9.60)	RTL	9.4 m	8.5	9.7		Ivnik, et al (1987)
RAVLT Trial 2	Epilepsy	39	36/3	44.30 (14.2)	valproate	6 m	8.5 (1.9)	7.9 (2.1)		Prevey, et al (1996)
RAVLT Trial 2	Epilepsy	26	24/2	43.50 (17.1)	carbamaz	6 m	7.5 (3.3)	7.6 (2.0)		Prevey, et al (1996)
RAVLT Trial 2	Ocular Disease	50	27/23	42.00 (17.0)	steroid tx	~8 d	7.7 (2.4)	6.5 (2.1)		Naber, et al (1996)
RAVLT Trial 2	VA Inpts	41	n/a	45.86 (14.0)	n/a	140.0 min	6.63 (2.05)	6.32 (2.65)	std/ alt	Ryan, et al (1986)
RAVLT Trial 2	VA Inpts	44	n/a	45.86 (14.0)	n/a	140.0 min	5.80 (2.12)	6.07 (2.10)	alt/ std	Ryan, et al (1986)
RAVLT Trial 2	Vascular/ Thoracic	16	14/2	58.60 (9.20)	surgery	6 m	7.9 (2.0)	7.4 (1.9)		Vingerhoets, et al (1996)

instrument	group	n	m/f	age	intervention	inter	t #1	t #2	note	citation
RAVLT Trial 2	Vascular/ Thoracic	18	16/2	61.40 (9.70)	surgery	8-9 d	7.0 (2.3)	7.7 (1.5)		Vingerhoets, et al (1996)
RAVLT Trial 3	Cardiac	88	75/13	58.90 (8.20)	CPB	6 m	9.0 (2.0)	9.7 (2.2)		Vingerhoets, et al (1996)
RAVLT Trial 3	Cardiac	104	84/20	59.10 (8.30)	CPB	8-9 d	8.7 (2.1)	8.1 (2.4)		Vingerhoets, et al (1996)
RAVLT Trial 3	Control	30	15/15	n/a	n/a	27.0 d	11.57 (2.56)	11.87 (2.00)	AF	Crawford, et al (1989b)
RAVLT Trial 3	Control	30	15/15	n/a	n/a	27.0 d	11.93 (2.00)	13.67 (1.40)		Crawford, et al (1989b)
RAVLT Trial 3	Control	30	26/4	29.90 (6.20)	CVLT admin first	2-4 h	NR	11.2 (2.1)		Crossen, et al (1994)
RAVLT Trial 3	Control	42	n/a	45.80	n/a	1m	10.1 (2.4)	10.0 (2.4)	AF	Delaney, et al (1992)
RAVLT Trial 3	Control	51	25/26	31.30 (12.7)	n/a	6 – 14 d	10.82 (2.09)	10.86 (1.85)	AF	Geffen, et al (1994)
RAVLT Trial 3	Control	72	67/5	44.50 (12.4)	n/a	6 m	10.4 (2.4)	10.1 (2.4)		Prevey, et al (1996)
RAVLT Trial 3	Control	47	47/0	37.70 (6.00)	n/a	1 y	11.32 (2.46)	11.89 (2.26)	*	Uchiyama, et al (1995)
RAVLT Trial 3	Epilepsy	35	17/18	28.40 (9.60)	RTL	9.4 m	10.3	11.1		Ivnik, et al (1987)
RAVLT Trial 3	Epilepsy	28	17/11	27.00 (5.90)	LTL	9.4 m	9.8	8.2		Ivnik, et al (1987)
RAVLT Trial 3	Epilepsy	26	24/2	43.50 (17.1)	carbamaz	6 m	9.1 (2.8)	9.3 (2.2)		Prevey, et al (1996)

instrument	group	n	m/f	age	intervention	inter	t #1	t #2	note	citation
RAVLT Trial 3	Epilepsy	39	36/3	44.30 (14.2)	valproate	6 m	9.4 (2.3)	8.6 (2.6)		Prevey, et al (1996)
RAVLT Trial 3	Ocular Disease	50	27/23	42.00 (17.0)	steroid tx	~8 d	9.5 (2.4)	7.9 (2.4)		Naber, et al (1996)
RAVLT Trial 3	VA Inpts	44	n/a	45.86 (14.0)	n/a	140.0 min	6.82 (2.36)	6.98 (2.65)	alt/ std	Ryan, et al (1986)
RAVLT Trial 3	VA Inpts	41	n/a	45.86 (14.0)	n/a	140.0 min	7.63 (2.43)	7.05 (2.85)	std/ alt	Ryan, et al (1986)
RAVLT Trial 3	Vascular/ Thoracic	18	16/2	61.40 (9.70)	surgery	8-9 d	8.6 (1.9)	7.7 (2.2)		Vingerhoets, et al (1996)
RAVLT Trial 3	Vascular/ Thoracic	16	14/2	58.60 (9.20)	surgery	6 m	9.4 (1.9)	9.1 (2.0)		Vingerhoets, et al (1996)
RAVLT Trial 4	Cardiac	88	75/13	58.90 (8.20)	CPB	6 m	9.9 (2.0)	10.4 (2.2)		Vingerhoets, et al (1996)
RAVLT Trial 4	Cardiac	104	84/20	59.10 (8.30)	CPB	8-9 d	9.7 (2.1)	8.9 (2.4)		Vingerhoets, et al (1996)
RAVLT Trial 4	Control	30	15/15	n/a	n/a	27.0 d	12.33 (1.88)	12.70 (1.82)	AF	Crawford, et al (1989b)
RAVLT Trial 4	Control	30	15/15	n/a	n/a	27.0 d	13.03 (1.59)	13.90 (1.35)		Crawford, et al (1989b)
RAVLT Trial 4	Control	30	26/4	29.90 (6.20)	CVLT admin first	2-4 h	NR	12.2 (2.1)		Crossen, et al (1994)
RAVLT Trial 4	Control	51	25/26	31.30 (12.7)	n/a	6 – 14 d	11.59 (1.99)	11.49 (2.18)	AF	Geffen, et al (1994)
RAVLT Trial 4	Control	72	67/5	44.50 (12.4)	n/a	6 m	11.2 (2.4)	10.9 (2.6)		Prevey, et al (1996)

instrument	group	n	m/f	age	intervention	inter	t #1	t #2	note	citation
RAVLT Trial 4	Control	47	47/0	37.70 (6.00)	n/a	1 y	12.15 (2.29)	12.64 (2.17)	*	Uchiyama, et al (1995)
RAVLT Trial 4	Epilepsy	28	17/11	27.00 (5.90)	LTL	9.4 m	10.8	9.2		Ivnik, et al (1987)
RAVLT Trial 4	Epilepsy	35	17/18	28.40 (9.60)	RTL	9.4 m	10.9	11.7		Ivnik, et al (1987)
RAVLT Trial 4	Epilepsy	39	36/3	44.30 (14.2)	valproate	6 m	10.6 (2.3)	9.6 (2.6)		Prevey, et al (1996)
RAVLT Trial 4	Epilepsy	26	24/2	43.50 (17.1)	carbamaz	6 m	9.8 (3.2)	10.1 (2.4)		Prevey, et al (1996)
RAVLT Trial 4	VA Inpts	44	n/a	45.86 (14.0)	n/a	140.0 min	7.39 (2.66)	7.50 (3.10)	alt/ std	Ryan, et al (1986)
RAVLT Trial 4	VA Inpts	41	n/a	45.86 (14.0)	n/a	140.0 min	9.27 (2.73)	7.39 (3.11)	std/ alt	Ryan, et al (1986)
RAVLT Trial 4	Vascular/ Thoracic	18	16/2	61.40 (9.70)	surgery	8-9 d	9.2 (2.7)	8.6 (2.8)		Vingerhoets, et al (1996)
RAVLT Trial 4	Vascular/ Thoracic	16	14/2	58.60 (9.20)	surgery	6 m	10.1 (2.3)	10.6 (2.5)		Vingerhoets, et al (1996)
RAVLT Trial 5	AIDS	10	10/0	41.70 (5.50)	n/a	6.53 m	12.2 (2.3)	11.7 (2.0)		Hinkin, et al (1995)
RAVLT Trial 5	Anorexia	18	0/18	n/a	refeeding tx	69.8 d	13.6 (1.6)	14.1 (1.3)		Szmukler, et al (1992)
RAVLT Trial 5	Cardiac	104	84/20	59.10 (8.30)	CPB	8-9 d	10.8 (2.1)	9.6 (2.4)		Vingerhoets, et al (1996)
RAVLT Trial 5	Cardiac	88	75/13	58.90 (8.20)	CPB	6 m	11.0 (2.1)	11.2 (2.4)		Vingerhoets, et al (1996)

instrument	group	n	m/f	age	intervention	inter	t #1	t #2	note	citation
RAVLT Trial 5	Control	63	8/55	56.22 (11.0)	n/a	~6 m	NR	0.17 (1.74) c		Bruggemans, et al (1997)
RAVLT Trial 5	Control	30	15/15	n/a	n/a	27.0 d	13.33 (1.56)	14.13 (1.14)		Crawford, et al (1989b)
RAVLT Trial 5	Control	30	15/15	n/a	n/a	27.0 d	12.87 (1.80)	12.90 (2.11)	AF	Crawford, et al (1989b)
RAVLT Trial 5	Control	30	26/4	29.90 (6.20)	CVLT admin first	2-4 h	NR	12.3 (2.1)		Crossen, et al (1994)
RAVLT Trial 5	Control	42	n/a	45.80	n/a	1m	11.6 (2.5)	11.8 (2.8)	AF	Delaney, et al (1992)
RAVLT Trial 5	Control	51	25/26	31.30 (12.7)	n/a	6 – 14 d	12.1 (1.85)	12.37 (2.07)	AF	Geffen, et al (1994)
RAVLT Trial 5	Control	16	4/12	78.30 (2.50)	n/a	1 y	10.3 (2.4)	10.6 (3.2)	*	Mitrushina, et al (1991b)
RAVLT Trial 5	Control	47	14/33	72.90 (1.40)	n/a	1 y	10.4 (2.7)	10.1 (3.3)	*	Mitrushina, et al (1991b)
RAVLT Trial 5	Control	40	6/34	68.20 (1.20)	n/a	1 y	11.8 (2.5)	11.7 (2.5)	*	Mitrushina, et al (1991b)
RAVLT Trial 5	Control	19	2/17	62.20 (2.50)	n/a	1 y	12.4 (2.6)	12.3 (2.5)	*	Mitrushina, et al (1991b)
RAVLT Trial 5	Control	72	67/5	44.50 (12.4)	n/a	6 m	11.7 (2.3)	11.6 (2.5)		Prevey, et al (1996)
RAVLT Trial 5	Control	18	0/18	n/a	n/a	108.4 d	14.0 (1.0)	13.4 (1.6)		Szmukler, et al (1992)
RAVLT Trial 5	Control	47	47/0	37.70 (6.00)	n/a	1 y	12.64 (1.91)	12.89 (2.0)	*	Uchiyama, et al (1995)

instrument	group	n	m/f	age	intervention	inter	t #1	t #2	note	citation
RAVLT Trial 5	Epilepsy	35	17/18	28.40 (9.60)	RTL	9.4 m	11.5	12.6		Ivnik, et al (1987)
RAVLT Trial 5	Epilepsy	28	17/11	27.00 (5.90)	LTL	9.4 m	10.3	9.4		Ivnik, et al (1987)
RAVLT Trial 5	Epilepsy	39	36/3	44.30 (14.2)	valproate	6 m	10.7 (2.6)	10.2 (2.8)		Prevey, et al (1996)
RAVLT Trial 5	Epilepsy	26	24/2	43.50 (17.1)	carbamaz	6 m	10.4 (3.0)	10.7 (2.7)		Prevey, et al (1996)
RAVLT Trial 5	HIV+	132	132/0	~33.8	n/a	13.3 m	12.7	12.4		Selnes, et al (1990)
RAVLT Trial 5	HIV-	132	132/0	~35.6	n/a	13.4 m	12.7	12.1		Selnes, et al (1990)
RAVLT Trial 5	VA Inpts	41	n/a	45.86 (14.0)	n/a	140.0 min	9.63 (2.91)	8.37 (2.91)	std/ alt	Ryan, et al (1986)
RAVLT Trial 5	VA Inpts	44	n/a	45.86 (14.0)	n/a	140.0 min	7.64 (2.69)	8.16 (3.32)	alt/ std	Ryan, et al (1986)
RAVLT Trial 5	Vascular/ Thoracic	18	16/2	61.40 (9.70)	surgery	8-9 d	10.6 (2.0)	9.4 (3.1)		Vingerhoets, et al (1996)
RAVLT Trial 5	Vascular/ Thoracic	16	14/2	58.60 (9.20)	surgery	6 m	11.1 (2.3)	10.9 (2.5)		Vingerhoets, et al (1996)
RAVLT Trial 6	Cardiac	88	75/13	58.90 (8.20)	CPB	6 m	4.5 (1.8)	4.7 (1.8)		Vingerhoets, et al (1996)
RAVLT Trial 6	Cardiac	104	84/20	59.10 (8.30)	CPB	8-9 d	8.3 (2.6)	6.9 (2.9)		Vingerhoets, et al (1996)
RAVLT Trial 6	Cardiac	88	75/13	58.90 (8.20)	CPB	6 m	8.3 (2.6)	9.1 (2.8)		Vingerhoets, et al (1996)

instrument	group	n	m/f	age	intervention	inter	t #1	t #2	note	citation
RAVLT Trial 6	Cardiac	104	84/20	59.10 (8.30)	CPB	8-9 d	4.3 (1.8)	4.2 (1.7)		Vingerhoets, et al (1996)
RAVLT Trial 6	Control	30	15/15	n/a	n/a	27.0 d	11.40 (2.58)	11.93 (2.77)	AF	Crawford, et al (1989b)
RAVLT Trial 6	Control	30	15/15	n/a	n/a	27.0 d	11.93 (1.95)	13.43 (1.68)		Crawford, et al (1989b)
RAVLT Trial 6	Control	30	15/15	n/a	n/a	27.0 d	6.70 (2.40)	7.70 (2.29)		Crawford, et al (1989b)
RAVLT Trial 6	Control	30	15/15	n/a	n/a	27.0 d	6.63 (1.70)	6.23 (1.91)	AF	Crawford, et al (1989b)
RAVLT Trial 6	Control	30	26/4	29.90 (6.20)	CVLT admin first	2-4 h	NR	7.2 (2.2)		Crossen, et al (1994)
RAVLT Trial 6	Control	42	n/a	45.80	n/a	1m	9.9 (3.2)	9.9 (3.3)	AF	Delaney, et al (1992)
RAVLT Trial 6	Control	51	25/26	31.30 (12.7)	n/a	6 – 14 d	5.86 (1.6)	5.84 (1.82)	AF	Geffen, et al (1994)
RAVLT Trial 6	Epilepsy	38	21/17	34.26 (9.18)	vigabatrin 3 g	18 w	5.24 (1.85)	5.08 (2.29)		Dodrill, et al (1995)
RAVLT Trial 6	Epilepsy	32	17/15	33.72 (9.66)	vigabatrin 6 g	18 w	5.66 (2.01)	5.16 (1.67)		Dodrill, et al (1995)
RAVLT Trial 6	Epilepsy	40	14/26	33.88 (9.77)	placebo	18 w	5.75 (2.05)	5.03 (1.73)		Dodrill, et al (1995)
RAVLT Trial 6	Epilepsy	36	17/19	34.89 (8.38)	vigabatrin 1 g	18 w	5.00 (2.10)	4.69 (1.88)		Dodrill, et al (1995)
RAVLT Trial 6	Epilepsy	28	17/11	27.00 (5.90)	LTL	9.4 m	5.5	4.3		Ivnik, et al (1987)

instrument	group	n	m/f	age	intervention	inter	t #1	t #2	note	citation
RAVLT Trial 6	Epilepsy	28	17/11	27.00 (5.90)	LTL	9.4 m	7.9	6.4		Ivnik, et al (1987)
RAVLT Trial 6	Epilepsy	35	17/18	28.40 (9.60)	RTL	9.4 m	9.7	10.5		Ivnik, et al (1987)
RAVLT Trial 6	Epilepsy	35	17/18	28.40 (9.60)	RTL	9.4 m	4.9	5.6		Ivnik, et al (1987)
RAVLT Trial 6	Renal Failure	9	4/5	65.00	rHuEpo	22.8 w	8.4 (2.3)	9.4 (3.2)		Temple, et al (1995)
RAVLT Trial 6	Renal Failure	8	3/5	67.50	n/a	19.3 w	6.4 (2.0)	7.5 (3.4)		Temple, et al (1995)
RAVLT Trial 6	VA Inpts	41	n/a	45.86 (14.0)	n/a	140.0 min	7.05 (3.69)	5.27 (3.53)	std/ alt	Ryan, et al (1986)
RAVLT Trial 6	VA Inpts	44	n/a	45.86 (14.0)	n/a	140.0 min	5.59 (3.05)	5.36 (3.65)	alt/ std	Ryan, et al (1986)
RAVLT Trial 6	Vascular/ Thoracic	16	14/2	58.60 (9.20)	surgery	6 m	4.8 (1.1)	4.8 (1.4)		Vingerhoets, et al (1996)
RAVLT Trial 6	Vascular/ Thoracic	18	16/2	61.40 (9.70)	surgery	8-9 d	7.2 (2.5)	6.3 (4.2)		Vingerhoets, et al (1996)
RAVLT Trial 6	Vascular/ Thoracic	16	14/2	58.60 (9.20)	surgery	6 m	7.6 (3.0)	8.8 (3.1)		Vingerhoets, et al (1996)
RAVLT Trial 6	Vascular/ Thoracic	18	16/2	61.40 (9.70)	surgery	8-9 d	4.5 (1.2)	4.6 (1.6)		Vingerhoets, et al (1996)
RAVLT Trial 7	Cardiac	88	75/13	58.90 (8.20)	CPB	6 m	8.3 (2.7)	9.2 (2.9)		Vingerhoets, et al (1996)
RAVLT Trial 7	Cardiac	104	84/20	59.10 (8.30)	CPB	8-9 d	8.3 (2.7)	6.6 (3.1)		Vingerhoets, et al (1996)

instrument	group	n	m/f	age	intervention	inter	t #1	t #2	note	citation
RAVLT Trial 7	Control	30	26/4	29.90 (6.20)	CVLT admin first	2-4 h	NR	11.0 (3.4)		Crossen, et al (1994)
RAVLT Trial 7	Control	51	25/26	31.30 (12.7)	n/a	6 – 14 d	10.65 (2.67)	10.88 (2.94)	AF	Geffen, et al (1994)
RAVLT Trial 7	Control	16	6/10	27.90	placebo	1 d	41.22 (8.15)	36.14 (13.47)	*	Gigli, et al (1993)
RAVLT Trial 7	Control	16	6/10	27.90	brotizolam	1 d	38.71 (9.2)	37.43 (7.81)	*	Gigli, et al (1993)
RAVLT Trial 7	Control	40	6/34	68.20 (1.20)	n/a	1 y	9.5 (3.0)	9.9 (3.2)	*	Mitrushina, et al (1991b)
RAVLT Trial 7	Control	47	14/33	72.90 (1.40)	n/a	1 y	8.7 (3.5)	8.4 (3.6)	*	Mitrushina, et al (1991b)
RAVLT Trial 7	Control	19	2/17	62.20 (2.50)	n/a	1 y	10.7 (3.2)	10.8 (3.2)	*	Mitrushina, et al (1991b)
RAVLT Trial 7	Control	16	4/12	78.30 (2.50)	n/a	1 y	8.4 (3.5)	8.5 (3.8)	*	Mitrushina, et al (1991b)
RAVLT Trial 7	Control	72	67/5	44.50 (12.4)	n/a	6 m	10.0 (2.9)	9.7 (2.9)		Prevey, et al (1996)
RAVLT Trial 7	Epilepsy	38	21/17	34.26 (9.18)	vigabatrin 3 g	18 w	7.63 (3.30)	7.55 (3.45)		Dodrill, et al (1995)
RAVLT Trial 7	Epilepsy	36	17/19	34.89 (8.38)	vigabatrin 1 g	18 w	7.53 (3.55)	7.58 (3.86)		Dodrill, et al (1995)
RAVLT Trial 7	Epilepsy	32	17/15	33.72 (9.66)	vigabatrin 6 g	18 w	7.72 (3.92)	8.06 (3.57)		Dodrill, et al (1995)
RAVLT Trial 7	Epilepsy	40	14/26	33.88 (9.77)	placebo	18 w	8.58 (3.38)	8.20 (3.25)		Dodrill, et al (1995)

instrument	group	n	m/f	age	intervention	inter	t #1	t #2	note	citation
RAVLT Trial 7	Epilepsy	26	24/2	43.50 (17.1)	carbamaz	6 m	8.7 (3.3)	8.5 (3.0)		Prevey, et al (1996)
RAVLT Trial 7	Epilepsy	39	36/3	44.30 (14.2)	valproate	6 m	8.3 (3.6)	7.8 (3.2)		Prevey, et al (1996)
RAVLT Trial 7	Myasthenia Gravis	11	7/4	49.00	prednisolone	3-11 m	10.0 (3.1)	9.5 (3.9)		Glennerster, et al (1996)
RAVLT Trial 7	Renal Failure	9	4/5	65.00	rHuEpo	22.8 w	8.6 (2.4)	10.9 (3.2)		Temple, et al (1995)
RAVLT Trial 7	Renal Failure	8	3/5	67.50	n/a	19.3 w	6.1 (2.2)	7.8 (3.6)		Temple, et al (1995)
RAVLT Trial 7	Vascular/ Thoracic	16	14/2	58.60 (9.20)	surgery	6 m	7.5 (2.7)	8.4 (2.9)		Vingerhoets, et al (1996)
RAVLT Trial 7	Vascular/ Thoracic	18	16/2	61.40 (9.70)	surgery	8-9 d	7.1 (2.1)	6.0 (3.9)		Vingerhoets, et al (1996)
RAVLT Trial 8	AIDS	10	10/0	41.70 (5.50)	n/a	6.53 m	10.7 (2.9)	10.3 (2.7)		Hinkin, et al (1995)
RAVLT Trial 8	Cardiac	104	84/20	59.10 (8.30)	CPB	8-9 d	13.1 (1.8)	12.1 (2.3)		Vingerhoets, et al (1996)
RAVLT Trial 8	Cardiac	88	75/13	58.90 (8.20)	CPB	6 m	13.1 (1.8)	13.8 (1.3)		Vingerhoets, et al (1996)
RAVLT Trial 8	Control	63	8/55	56.22 (11.0)	n/a	~6 m	NR	-0.38 (2.31) c		Bruggemans, et al (1997)
RAVLT Trial 8	Control	42	n/a	45.80	n/a	1m	9.9 (3.1)	9.2 (3.5)	AF	Delaney, et al (1992)
RAVLT Trial 8	Control	51	25/26	31.30 (12.7)	n/a	6 – 14 d	10.76 (2.81)	10.39 (3.02)	AF	Geffen, et al (1994)

instrument	group	n	m/f	age	intervention	inter	t #1	t #2	note	citation
RAVLT Trial 8	Control	10	8/2	31.10 (7.50)	saline	1 w	12.4 (1.4)	11.9 (1.8)		Gooday, et al (1995)
RAVLT Trial 8	Control	10	8/2	31.10 (7.50)	flumazenil	1 w	12.8 (1.9)	11.8 (2.2)		Gooday, et al (1995)
RAVLT Trial 8	Control	37	n/a	~6.00	n/a	~6 m	NR	1.26 c	*	Neyens, et al (1996)
RAVLT Trial 8	Control	72	67/5	44.50 (12.4)	n/a	6 m	9.7 (3.0)	8.9 (3.1)		Prevey, et al (1996)
RAVLT Trial 8	Control	20	12/8	56.40	n/a	10 w	8.0 (2.8)	8.9 (3.5)		Van Den Burg, et al (1985)
RAVLT Trial 8	DAT/MID	30	15/15	71.70 (1.30)	oxiracetam	3 m	2.3 (0.3)	2.8 (0.2)	*	Villardita, et al (1992)
RAVLT Trial 8	DAT/MID	30	21/9	67.80 (1.50)	placebo	3 m	2.4 (0.3)	2.5 (0.2)	*	Villardita, et al (1992)
RAVLT Trial 8	DAT/MID	29	14/15	71.50 (1.30)	oxiracetam	6 m	2.2 (0.3)	2.8 (0.3)	*	Villardita, et al (1992)
RAVLT Trial 8	Epilepsy	40	14/26	33.88 (9.77)	placebo	18 w	8.33 (3.62)	7.70 (3.44)		Dodrill, et al (1995)
RAVLT Trial 8	Epilepsy	38	21/17	34.26 (9.18)	vigabatrin 3 g	18 w	7.16 (3.23)	7.21 (3.32)		Dodrill, et al (1995)
RAVLT Trial 8	Epilepsy	36	17/19	34.89 (8.38)	vigabatrin 1 g	18 w	7.28 (3.45)	6.78 (3.62)		Dodrill, et al (1995)
RAVLT Trial 8	Epilepsy	32	17/15	33.72 (9.66)	vigabatrin 6 g	18 w	7.58 (4.09)	7.84 (4.30)		Dodrill, et al (1995)
RAVLT Trial 8	Epilepsy	28	17/11	27.00 (5.90)	LTL	9.4 m	7.1	5.0		Ivnik, et al (1987)

instrument	group	n	m/f	age	intervention	inter	t #1	t #2	note	citation
RAVLT Trial 8	Epilepsy	35	17/18	28.40 (9.60)	RTL	9.4 m	8.6	9.6		Ivnik, et al (1987)
RAVLT Trial 8	Epilepsy	39	36/3	44.30 (14.2)	valproate	6 m	8.0 (3.5)	7.8 (3.7)		Prevey, et al (1996)
RAVLT Trial 8	Epilepsy	26	24/2	43.50 (17.1)	carbamaz	6 m	8.3 (3.7)	8.4 (3.3)		Prevey, et al (1996)
RAVLT Trial 8	Liver Disease	10	8/2	53.90 (7.40)	saline	1 w	5.8 (2.9)	4.8 (1.8)		Gooday, et al (1995)
RAVLT Trial 8	Liver Disease	10	8/2	53.90 (7.40)	flumazenil	1 w	7.0 (3.4)	6.1 (3.2)		Gooday, et al (1995)
RAVLT Trial 8	Lung Cancer	14	12/2	63.00	chemotherapy	~5 d	6.4 (2.6)	6.6 (2.6)	*	Van Oosterhout, et al (1995)
RAVLT Trial 8	PVD	20	18/2	56.80	major surgery	10 w	5.5 (2.5)	6.9 (2.5)		Van Den Burg, et al (1985)
RAVLT Trial 8	Schizophrenia Inpts	35	29/6	23.71 (4.50)	neuroleptics	1-2 y	6.6 (3.7)	5.4 (3.5)		Nopoulos, et al (1994)
RAVLT Trial 8	Spinal Cord Injury	67	54/13	32.00 (14.7)	n/a	38 w	10.15 (4.78)	10.02 (3.43)		Richards, et al (1988)
RAVLT Trial 8	TIA	20	13/7	59.60	CE	10 w	7.0 (3.2)	7.3 (3.4)		Van Den Burg, et al (1985)
RAVLT Trial 8	Vascular/ Thoracic	18	16/2	61.40 (9.70)	surgery	8-9 d	12.9 (2.0)	11.9 (3.3)		Vingerhoets, et al (1996)
RAVLT Trial 8	Vascular/ Thoracic	16	14/2	58.60 (9.20)	surgery	6 m	13.6 (1.6)	13.9 (1.2)		Vingerhoets, et al (1996)

instrument	group	n	m/f	age	intervention	inter	t #1	t #2	note	citation
RAVLT Trial 8 (% forg)	Epilepsy	35	17/18	28.40 (9.60)	RTL	9.4 m	25.7	25.7		Ivnik, et al (1987)
RAVLT Trial 8 (% forg)	Epilepsy	28	17/11	27.00 (5.90)	LTL	9.4 m	37.6	48.5		Ivnik, et al (1987)
RAVLT Trial 8 (% ret)	Epilepsy	20	12/8	29.90 (10.1)	RTL	3.8 m	70.1	81.9		Ivnik, et al (1993)
RAVLT Trial 8 (% ret)	Epilepsy	20	8/12	34.60 (9.80)	LTL	4.1 m	62.7	43.9		Ivnik, et al (1993)
RAVLT Trial 8 (10')	Control	4	0/4	67.30 (0.50)	placebo	60 min	3.25 (1.28)	1.50 (0.58)	AF	Kirkby, et al (1995)
RAVLT Trial 8 (10')	Control	5	1/4	68.40 (6.10)	lorazepam	60 min	4.00 (1.23)	0.80 (1.10)	AF	Kirkby, et al (1995)
RAVLT Trial 8 (10')	Control	9	4/5	26.40 (7.70)	lorazepam	60 min	7.00 (2.92)	2.22 (2.54)	AF	Kirkby, et al (1995)
RAVLT Trial 8 (10')	Control	8	4/4	21.80 (4.20)	placebo	60 min	4.38 (1.92)	3.25 (1.28)	AF	Kirkby, et al (1995)
RAVLT Trial 8 (15')	Control	16	6/10	27.90	brotizolam	1 d	6.95 (2.19)	6.04 (2.17)	*	Gigli, et al (1993)
RAVLT Trial 8 (15')	Control	16	6/10	27.90	placebo	1 d	7.04 (3.22)	5.22 (4.05)	*	Gigli, et al (1993)
RAVLT Trials 2-5	Myasthenia Gravis	11	7/4	49.00	prednisolone	3-11 m	40.9 (9.9)	40.8 (10.6)		Glennerster, et al (1996)
RAVLT-2 Recog	Control	37	37/0	37.50 (6.90)	n/a	1 y	13.95 (1.73)	13.97 (1.30)	*	Uchiyama, et al (1995)

instrument	group	n	m/f	age	intervention	inter	t #1	t #2	note	citation
RAVLT-2 Recog	Control	47	47/0	37.70 (6.00)	n/a	1 y	13.64 (1.54)	13.87 (1.62)	*	Uchiyama, et al (1995)
RAVLT-2 Total Intrus	Control	47	47/0	37.70 (6.00)	n/a	1 y	2.4 (1.73)	3.32 (3.14)	*	Uchiyama, et al (1995)
RAVLT-2 Total Intrus	Control	37	37/0	37.50 (6.90)	n/a	1 y	4.51 (3.08)	3.6 (4.19)	*	Uchiyama, et al (1995)
RAVLT-2 Trial 1	Control	37	37/0	37.50 (6.90)	n/a	1 y	6.78 (1.65)	7.19 (1.79)	*	Uchiyama, et al (1995)
RAVLT-2 Trial 2	Control	37	37/0	37.50 (6.90)	n/a	1 y	9.22 (1.93)	10.19 (2.05)	*	Uchiyama, et al (1995)
RAVLT-2 Trial 3	Control	37	37/0	37.50 (6.90)	n/a	1 y	10.84 (1.83)	11.84 (1.94)	*	Uchiyama, et al (1995)
RAVLT-2 Trial 4	Control	37	37/0	37.50 (6.90)	n/a	1 y	11.65 (1.62)	12.35 (2.21)	*	Uchiyama, et al (1995)
RAVLT-2 Trial 5	Control	37	37/0	37.50 (6.90)	n/a	1 y	12.05 (1.96)	12.46 (1.84)	*	Uchiyama, et al (1995)
RAVLT-2 Trial 6	Control	37	37/0	37.50 (6.90)	n/a	1 y	6.60 (1.69)	6.6 (1.77)	*	Uchiyama, et al (1995)
RAVLT-2 Trial 6	Control	47	47/0	37.70 (6.00)	n/a	1 y	6.74 (2.18)	6.56 (2.17)	*	Uchiyama, et al (1995)
RAVLT-2 Trial 7	Control	47	47/0	37.70 (6.00)	n/a	1 y	11.26 (2.82)	11.72 (2.58)	*	Uchiyama, et al (1995)
RAVLT-2 Trial 7	Control	37	37/0	37.50 (6.90)	n/a	1 y	10.32 (2.59)	10.89 (2.84)	*	Uchiyama, et al (1995)

instrument	group	n	m/f	age	intervention	inter	t #1	t #2	note	citation
RAVLT-2 Trial 8	Control	47	47/0	37.70 (6.00)	n/a	1 y	10.98 (3.1)	11.49 (2.79)	*	Uchiyama, et al (1995)
RAVLT-2 Trial 8	Control	37	37/0	37.50 (6.90)	n/a	1 y	10.24 (2.33)	10.6 (3.24)	*	Uchiyama, et al (1995)

Table 56. Rivermead Behavioural Memory Test (RBMT)

instrument	group	n	m/f	age	intervention	inter	t #1	t #2	note	citation
RBMT	Control	16	n/a	46.00 (3.10)	n/a	1 m	21.4 (0.5)	22.1 (0.6)		Jalan, et al (1995)
RBMT	Variceal Hemorrhage	29	19/10	54.30 (5.60)	TIPSS	1 m	16.6 (0.7)	17.7 (0.6)	*	Jalan, et al (1995)
RBMT	Variceal Hemorrhage & Cirrhosis	12	7/5	53.10 (7.10)	variceal band ligation	1 m	15.3 (1.3)	14.9 (0.9)	*	Jalan, et al (1995)
RBMT Delay	HIV+ (stage 2/3)	14	14/0	31.40 (8.54)	n/a	12.8 m	9.0 (3.7)	10.3 (3.8)		Burgess, et al (1994)
RBMT Delay	HIV+ (stage 4)	6	6/0	36.20 (7.60)	n/a	12.8 m	7.4 (1.9)	7.5 (4.9)		Burgess, et al (1994)
RBMT Delay	HIV-	41	41/0	31.50 (9.32)	n/a	12.8 m	8.5 (2.9)	9.7 (3.3)		Burgess, et al (1994)
RBMT Imm	HIV+ (stage 2/3)	14	14/0	31.40 (8.54)	n/a	12.8 m	11.0 (4.3)	11.5 (4.6)		Burgess, et al (1994)
RBMT Imm	HIV+ (stage 4)	6	6/0	36.20 (7.60)	n/a	12.8 m	8.7 (1.2)	8.4 (4.2)		Burgess, et al (1994)

instrument	group	n	m/f	age	intervention	inter	t #1	t #2	note	citation
RBMT Imm	HIV-	41	41/0	31.50 (9.32)	n/a	12.8 m	9.8 (3.1)	10.7 (3.6)		Burgess, et al (1994)
RBMT Prospective [6]	Control	60	26/34	71.24 (5.96)	n/a	12 m	4.33 (1.24)	5.20 (1.44)		Olin, et al (1991)

Table 57. Rod and Frame Tests

instrument	group	n	m/f	age	intervention	inter	t #1	t #2	note	citation
Portable Rod and Frame Test	Control	31	0/31	20.00	n/a	~9 m	2.15 (1.93)	2.50 (2.12)		Applebaum (1978)
Rod and Frame (Left Tilt)	Alcoholic Inpts	91	91/0	42.20 (10.0)	n/a	12-22 d	-1.80 (1.40)	-1.4 (0.90)		Eckardt, et al (1979)
Rod and Frame (Left Tilt)	Medical Inpts	20	20/0	45.60 (11.1)	n/a	12-22 d	-2.80 (1.80)	-2.0 (1.60)		Eckardt, et al (1979)
Rod and Frame (Right Tilt)	Alcoholic Inpts	91	91/0	42.20 (10.0)	n/a	12-22 d	-1.20 (1.0)	-1.0 (1.0)		Eckardt, et al (1979)
Rod and Frame (Right Tilt)	Medical Inpts	20	20/0	45.60 (11.1)	n/a	12-22 d	-1.90 (1.40)	-1.80 (1.30)		Eckardt, et al (1979)
Rod and Frame Test (avg error)	Control	26	13/13	28.80 (8.20)	n/a	4 w	7.1 (7.7)	5.9 (6.6)		Killian, et al (1984)
Rod and Frame Test (avg error)	Depression	6	4/2	26.30 (6.30)	std meds	4 w	5.3 (3.4)	4.0 (3.5)		Killian, et al (1984)
Rod and Frame Test (avg error)	Depression	26	12/4	37.10 (12.7)	no meds	4 w	8.3 (8.4)	7.6 (8.2)		Killian, et al (1984)
Rod and Frame Test (avg error)	Schizophrenia	34	17/17	24.30 (6.40)	d/c meds	4 w	10.3 (9.0)	9.1 (9.6)		Killian, et al (1984)

instrument	group	n	m/f	age	intervention	inter	t #1	t #2	note	citation
Rod and Frame Test (avg error)	Schizophrenia	13	8/5	24.10 (3.10)	std meds	4 w	5.7 (7.2)	4.6 (7.0)		Killian, et al (1984)

Table 58. Seashore Rhythm Test (SeaRT)

instrument	group	n	m/f	age	intervention	inter	t #1	t #2	note	citation
SeaRT	Alcoholic	4	4/0	48.75	minimal alcohol	18.75 m	22.5	23.7		Johnson-Greene, et al (1997)
SeaRT	Alcoholic	2	2/0	48.50	excessive alcohol	18.5 m	29.0	27.5		Johnson-Greene, et al (1997)
SeaRT	Alcoholic Inpts	91	91/0	42.20 (10.0)	n/a	16.8 d	24.1 (3.1)	25.3 (2.7)		Eckardt, et al (1981)
SeaRT	Alcoholic Inpts	91	91/0	42.20 (10.0)	n/a	12-22 d	24.0 (3.1)	25.3 (2.7)		Eckardt, et al (1979)
SeaRT	CVD	17	15/2	62.00	CE	20w	23.67 (5.15)	22.47 (4.31)		Matarazzo, et al (1979)
SeaRT	CVD	16	n/a	60.00	n/a	12w	23.48 (2.12)	25.86 (2.66)		Matarazzo, et al (1979)
SeaRT	Control	23	9/14	32.30 (10.3)	n/a	3 w	27.7 (2.1)	27.6 (2.1)		Bornstein, et al (1987)
SeaRT	Control	102	65/37	24.52	n/a	12 m	28.0	28.0	*	Dikmen, et al (1990)
SeaRT	Control	29	29/0	24.00	n/a	20w	27.24 (1.94)	27.76 (1.48)		Matarazzo, et al (1979)
SeaRT	Control	33	15/18	59.10 (9.30)	n/a	10 d	26.4 (3.1)	26.2 (3.2)		McCaffrey, et al (1993)

instrument	group	n	m/f	age	intervention	inter	t #1	t #2	note	citation
SeaRT	Control	10	5/5	70.0 - 79.0	n/a	1 d	NR	2.4 c		Peak (1970)
SeaRT	Control	10	5/5	60.0 - 69.0	n/a	1 d	NR	0.3 c		Peak (1970)
SeaRT	Control	10	5/5	50.0 - 59.0	n/a	1 d	NR	-0.4 c		Peak (1970)
SeaRT	Control	10	5/5	40.0 - 49.0	n/a	1 d	NR	0.7 c		Peak (1970)
SeaRT	Control	174	174/0	24.0 - 85.0	n/a	2 y	3.67	3.64	*	Schludermann, et al (1983)
SeaRT	Control	86	86/0	24.0 - 85.0	n/a	2 y	3.71	3.72	*	Schludermann, et al (1983)
SeaRT	Epilepsy	14	8/6	41.20 (10.5)	sabeluzole	12 w	25.3 (3.6)	24.7 (2.9)		Aldenkamp, et al (1995)
SeaRT	Epilepsy	19	11/8	40.00 (8.00)	placebo	12 w	24.3 (3.2)	23.7 (3.8)		Aldenkamp, et al (1995)
SeaRT	Epilepsy	17	7/10	27.44 (6.04)	meds	6-12 m	23.53 (4.02)	21.41 (5.20)	*	Dodrill, et al (1975)
SeaRT	Epilepsy	21	n/a	22.30 (7.60)	improved WAIS re-test	20.5 m	21.5 (4.0)	22.0 (4.7)		Seidenberg, et al (1981)
SeaRT	Epilepsy	19	n/a	20.30 (4.30)	slightly improved WAIS re-test	20.1 m	23.7 (10.6)	25.0 (3.2)		Seidenberg, et al (1981)
SeaRT	Epilepsy	18	n/a	20.30 (5.40)	stable WAIS on re-test	21.6 m	21.3 (5.3)	21.9 (4.2)		Seidenberg, et al (1981)

instrument	group	n	m/f	age	intervention	inter	t #1	t #2	note	citation
SeaRT	Epilepsy (sz continued)	26	n/a	~21.0	n/a	20.7 m	21.35 (4.36)	21.85 (4.29)		Seidenberg, et al (1981)
SeaRT	Epilepsy (sz remitted)	24	n/a	~21.0	n/a	20.7 m	22.00 (4.39)	23.17 (3.94)		Seidenberg, et al (1981)
SeaRT	Medical Inpts	20	20/0	45.60 (11.1)	n/a	22.9 d	24.0 (4.2)	24.9 (3.7)		Eckardt, et al (1981)
SeaRT	Medical Inpts	20	20/0	45.60 (11.1)	n/a	12-22 d	24.0 (4.2)	24.9 (3.7)		Eckardt, et al (1979)
SeaRT	Psychiatric Inpts	231	83/148	30.70	ECT	4 - 5 w	23.3 (5.3)	23.0 (4.6)		Malloy, et al (1982)
SeaRT	Psychiatric Inpts	231	83/148	30.70	ECT	4 - 5 w	6.9 (4.4)	7.0 (3.4)		Malloy, et al (1982)
SeaRT	Schizophrenia (chronic)	35	n/a	47.00	n/a	52w	24.09 (4.26)	24.29 (3.9)		Matarazzo, et al (1979)
SeaRT	TBI	31	20/11	24.16	n/a	12 m	22.0	26.0	*	Dikmen, et al (1990)
SeaRT	TBI (severe)	15	13/2	24.80	n/a	11.5 m	22.4	25.7		Drudge, et al (1984)
SeaRT (errors)	Alcoholic (1 yr abstin)	23	23/0	36.80 (6.30)	n/a	1 y	3.7	4.5		Adams, et al (1980)
SeaRT (errors)	Alcoholic (2.5 yrs abstin)	25	25/0	36.50 (6.30)	n/a	1 y	3.2	2.2		Adams, et al (1980)
SeaRT (errors)	Alcoholic Inpts	25	25/0	44.84	n/a	4 w	5.20 (4.26)	5.16 (3.80)		Claiborn, et al (1981)
SeaRT (errors)	Cardiac	135	120/15	55.40	CABG	3 m	3.9	3.7	*	Klonoff, et al (1989)

instrument	group	n	m/f	age	intervention	inter	t #1	t #2	note	citation
SeaRT (errors)	CAD	20	n/a	57.20 (7.20)	CE	6 m	7.9	6.2		Parker, et al (1983)
SeaRT (errors)	CAD	17	n/a	57.20 (7.20)	n/a	6 m	7.9	6.1		Parker, et al (1983)
SeaRT (errors)	CAD	36	n./a	61.10 (8.30)	CE	6 m	7.7	6.9	*	Parker, et al (1986)
SeaRT (errors)	CAD	17	n/a	57.90 (8.40)	n/a	6 m	7.4	6.7	*	Parker, et al (1986)
SeaRT (errors)	Control	21	21/0	36.90 (5.90)	n/a	1 y	4.3	4.5		Adams, et al (1980)
SeaRT (errors)	Control	25	25/0	28.68	n/a	4 w	3.04 (2.98)	2.48 (2.12)		Claiborn, et al (1981)
SeaRT (errors)	Depression	33	14/19	37.40	antidepress	7 w	5.6 (4.6)	5.0 (4.4)		Fromm, et al (1984)
SeaRT (errors)	Psychiatric Inpts	12	12/0	40.17	n/a	4 w	5.25 (4.83)	3.75 (3.31)		Claiborn, et al (1981)
SeaRT (errors)	Substance Abuse	15	8/7	21.10 (4.50)	outpt tx	4 w	3.6 (2.2)	4.3 (2.5)		Cosgrove, et al (1991)
SeaRT (errors)	Substance Abuse (PCP)	15	8/7	21.10 (4.50)	outpt tx	4 w	4.9 (3.2)	5.1 (4.4)		Cosgrove, et al (1991)
SeaRT (errors)	Surgical	17	n/a	57.20 (7.20)	surgery	6 m	5.6	4.8		Parker, et al (1983)
SeaRT (errors)	Surgical	26	n/a	55.30 (6.80)	surgery (non-CE)	6 m	5.5	5.0	*	Parker, et al (1986)
SeaRT (errors)	TBI	27	23/4	24.62	n/a	12 m	25.25	25.52		Dikmen, et al (1983)

instrument	group	n	m/f	age	intervention	inter	t #1	t #2	note	citation
SeaRT (t)	ALL	31	16/15	8.38 (3.19)	n/a	2.0 y	50.7 (9.1)	51.3 (9.7)		Berg, et al (1983)
SeaRT (t)	ALL w/ Somnolence	48	27/21	8.63 (3.15)	n/a	2.25 y	53.7 (139.0)	54.3 (14.6)		Berg, et al (1983)

Table 59. Selective Reminding Tests (SRT)

instrument	group	n	m/f	age	intervention	inter	t #1	t #2	note	citation
BSRT CLTR	Brain Tumor	7	4/3	9.83	radiotherapy	11 m	8.7 (4.2)	7.5 (5.1)		Bordeaux, et al (1988)
BSRT CLTR	Brain Tumor	7	3/4	10.33	surgery	1 m	12.7 (7.9)	14.5 (10.2)		Bordeaux, et al (1988)
BSRT CLTR	Cardiac	22	10/12	47.30 (14.0)	open heart surgery	8.4 d	80.0 (25.8)	51.0 (18.1)	*	Heyer, et al (1995)
BSRT CLTR	Cardiac	33	19/14	73.10 (5.50)	open heart surgery	8.4 d	47.1 (20.0)	25.0 (13.3)	*	Heyer, et al (1995)
BSRT CLTR	Control	102	65/37	24.52	n/a	12 m	83.0	83.0	*	Dikmen, et al (1990)
BSRT CLTR	Control	10	5/5	20.50 (2.60)	n/a	1 w	99.55 (29.45)	108.13 (29.01)	AF, *	Hannay, et al (1985)
BSRT CLTR	Control	110	110/0	19.30 (1.30)	n/a	~3 m	93.7 (33.9)	113.0 (30.0)		Macciocchi (1990)
BSRT CLTR	Control	21	5/16	34.00	carbamaz/ phenytoin CB	1 m	48.0 (10.0)	50.0 (13.0)	*	Meador, et al (1991)
BSRT CLTR	Control (overweight)	24	24/0	40.70 (8.30)	placebo	8 w	58.2 (27.1)	58.3 (27.6)		Hatsukami, et al (1986)

instrument	group	n	m/f	age	intervention	inter	t #1	t #2	note	citation
BSRT CLTR	Control (overweight)	26	26/0	37.20 (4.80)	naltrexone	8 w	52.4 (19.1)	60.8 (26.8)		Hatsukami, et al (1986)
BSRT CLTR	DAT	14	n/a	53.0 - 81.0	lithium carbonate	7 d	4.0 (2.0)	4.4 (1.7)	*	Brinkman, et al (1984)
BSRT CLTR	HD (at risk, + genetic marker)	8	1/7	26.20 (2.70)	n/a	2 y	54.8	57.0	*	Giordani, et al (1995)
BSRT CLTR	HD (at risk, - genetic marker)	8	1/7	28.40 (5.20)	n/a	2 y	54.9	52.8	*	Giordani, et al (1995)
BSRT CLTR	Spinal Cord Injury	67	54/13	32.00 (14.7)	n/a	38 w	57.84 (32.49)	54.38 (34.55)		Richards, et al (1988)
BSRT CLTR	Surgical	13	11/2	74.20 (6.70)	major surgery	6 d	60.1 (32.4)	58.6 (34.4)	*	Heyer, et al (1995)
BSRT CLTR	TBI	31	20/11	24.16	n/a	12 m	2.0	50.0	*	Dikmen, et al (1990)
BSRT CLTR	TIA/CVA	34	34/0	60.30	CE	8-16 d	19.00	17.77		Cushman, et al (1984)
BSRT Cued Recall	Control	10	5/5	20.50 (2.60)	n/a	1 w	10.2 (1.29)	10.55 (1.04)	AF	Hannay, et al (1985)
BSRT DR	Cardiac	90	77/13	59.00 (10.6)	CABG/CPB	8 d	15.9 (2.8)	3.2 (2.8)	*	Townes, et al (1989)
BSRT DR	Control	10	5/5	20.50 (2.60)	n/a	1 w	11.1 (1.45)	11.1 (1.85)	AF, *	Hannay, et al (1985)
BSRT DR	Control	47	35/12	59.00 (9.81)	n/a	8 d	6.8 (2.4)	6.3 (2.5)	*	Townes, et al (1989)
BSRT DR	Control (overweight)	24	24/0	40.70 (8.30)	placebo	8 w	7.1 (2.2)	7.2 (2.1)		Hatsukami, et al (1986)

instrument	group	n	m/f	age	intervention	inter	t #1	t #2	note	citation
BSRT DR	Control (overweight)	26	26/0	37.20 (4.80)	naltrexone	8 w	8.0 (1.4)	7.3 (2.1)		Hatsukami, et al (1986)
BSRT DR	DAT	14	n/a	60.0 - 80.0	placebo	6 m	0.5 (1.0)	0.1 (0.3)		Sano, et al (1992)
BSRT DR	DAT	13	n/a	60.0 - 80.0	acetyl levocarnitine	6 m	0.8 (0.8)	0.6 (1.6)		Sano, et al (1992)
BSRT DR	MS & Fatigue	16	4/12	40.00 (6.40)	amantadine hydrochloride	6 w	8.1 (2.8)	8.9 (3.6)		Geisler, et al (1996)
BSRT DR	MS & Fatigue	16	2/14	40.00 (5.60)	placebo	6 w	8.3 (2.9)	8.9 (3.1)		Geisler, et al (1996)
BSRT DR	MS & Fatigue	13	4/9	41.00 (6.20)	pemoline	6 w	6.3 (2.7)	7.5 (2.6)		Geisler, et al (1996)
BSRT DR [10]	Mountain climbers	35	34/1	24.0 - 45.0	Climb of 5,000-8,000 meters	~1 m	7.41 (2.15)	7.35 (2.50)		Hornbein, et al (1989)
BSRT DR [10]	Mountain climbers	6	6/0	21.0 - 31.0	progressive decompression	~43 d	8.14 (1.86)	6.83 (1.47)		Hornbein, et al (1989)
BSRT Intrus	Control	10	5/5	20.50 (2.60)	n/a	1 w	2.48 (4.48)	2.18 (3.76)	AF, *	Hannay, et al (1985)
BSRT Intrus	DAT	14	n/a	53.0 - 81.0	lithium carbonate	7 d	5.6 (1.5)	11.9 (3.4)	*	Brinkman, et al (1984)
BSRT Last Trial	Cardiac	90	77/13	59.00 (10.6)	CABG/CPB	8 d	8.5 (1.7)	6.4 (2.6)	*	Townes, et al (1989)
BSRT Last Trial	Control	47	35/12	59.00 (9.81)	n/a	8 d	8.9 (1.3)	9.0 (1.2)	*	Townes, et al (1989)
BSRT LTR	Cardiac	33	19/14	73.10 (5.50)	open heart surgery	8.4 d	85.6 (31.0)	57.4 (25.2)	*	Heyer, et al (1995)

instrument	group	n	m/f	age	intervention	inter	t #1	t #2	note	citation
BSRT LTR	Cardiac	22	10/12	47.30 (14.0)	open heart surgery	8.4 d	104.4 (32.3)	90.6 (15.3)	*	Heyer, et al (1995)
BSRT LTR	Control	10	5/5	20.50 (2.60)	n/a	1 w	116.3 (19.02)	121.03 (17.04)	AF, *	Hannay, et al (1985)
BSRT LTR	Control (overweight)	26	26/0	37.20 (4.80)	naltrexone	8 w	69.2 (14.4)	75.9 (17.2)		Hatsukami, et al (1986)
BSRT LTR	Control (overweight)	24	24/0	40.70 (8.30)	placebo	8 w	74.2 (19.3)	74.4 (19.6)		Hatsukami, et al (1986)
BSRT LTR	DAT	14	n/a	53.0 - 81.0	lithium carbonate	7 d	22.3 (9.3)	18.9 (5.5)	*	Brinkman, et al (1984)
BSRT LTR	MS & Fatigue	16	4/12	40.00 (6.40)	amantadine hydrochloride	6 w	37.9 (17.8)	42.2 (17.5)		Geisler, et al (1996)
BSRT LTR	MS & Fatigue	16	2/14	40.00 (5.60)	placebo	6 w	50.2 (11.6)	45.2 (11.4)		Geisler, et al (1996)
BSRT LTR	MS & Fatigue	13	4/9	41.00 (6.20)	pemoline	6 w	30.7 (12.4)	36.1 (16.7)		Geisler, et al (1996)
BSRT LTR	Surgical	13	11/2	74.20 (6.70)	major surgery	6 d	95.2 (27.1)	90.2 (31.2)	*	Heyer, et al (1995)
BSRT LTR	TIA/CVA	34	34/0	60.30	CE	8-16 d	45.36	43.35		Cushman, et al (1984)
BSRT LTS	Brain Tumor	7	4/3	9.83	radiotherapy	11 m	8.3 (2.7)	8.2 (5.0)		Bordeaux, et al (1988)
BSRT LTS	Brain Tumor	7	3/4	10.33	surgery	1 m	11.6 (9.7)	11.8 (5.1)		Bordeaux, et al (1988)
BSRT LTS	Control	10	5/5	20.50 (2.60)	n/a	1 w	121.4 (16.52)	125.25 (13.84)	AF, *	Hannay, et al (1985)

instrument	group	n	m/f	age	intervention	inter	t #1	t #2	note	citation
BSRT LTS	Control (overweight)	24	24/0	40.70 (8.30)	placebo	8 w	79.3 (17.9)	80.1 (16.8)		Hatsukami, et al (1986)
BSRT LTS	Control (overweight)	26	26/0	37.20 (4.80)	naltrexone	8 w	74.2 (14.2)	80.3 (16.1)		Hatsukami, et al (1986)
BSRT LTS	DAT	14	n/a	53.0 - 81.0	lithium carbonate	7 d	28.0 (10.0)	25.7 (7.2)	*	Brinkman, et al (1984)
BSRT LTS	DAT	13	n/a	71.70 (6.40)	placebo	1 m	7.5 (6.8)	6.4 (5.3)	AF	Green, et al (1992)
BSRT LTS	DAT	11	n/a	71.70 (6.40)	oxiracetam	1 m	6.5 (7.7)	6.5 (4.0)	AF	Green, et al (1992)
BSRT LTS	Spinal Cord Injury	67	54/13	32.00 (14.7)	n/a	38 w	86.90 (31.34)	84.20 (32.10)		Richards, et al (1988)
BSRT LTS	TIA/CVA	34	34/0	60.30	CE	8-16 d	48.58	45.17		Cushman, et al (1984)
BSRT Multiple Choice	Control	10	5/5	20.50 (2.60)	n/a	1 w	11.95 (0.22)	11.9 (0.38)	AF, *	Hannay, et al (1985)
BSRT Recog	DAT	14	n/a	60.0 - 80.0	placebo	6 m	6.4 (2.0)	5.2 (2.6)		Sano, et al (1992)
BSRT Recog	DAT	13	n/a	60.0 - 80.0	acetyl levocarnitine	6 m	7.1 (3.2)	6.5 (3.1)		Sano, et al (1992)
BSRT Reminders	Control	10	5/5	20.50 (2.60)	n/a	1 w	30.98 (11.13)	27.85 (10.68)	AF, *	Hannay, et al (1985)
BSRT RLTR	Control	10	5/5	20.50 (2.60)	n/a	1 w	16.8 (14.24)	12.95 (14.64)	AF, *	Hannay, et al (1985)
BSRT STR	Control	10	5/5	20.50 (2.60)	n/a	1 w	8.4 (8.01)	6.8 (6.25)	AF, *	Hannay, et al (1985)

instrument	group	n	m/f	age	intervention	inter	t #1	t #2	note	citation
BSRT Sum Recall	Cardiac	90	77/13	59.00 (10.6)	CABG/CPB	8 d	72.8 (16.3)	56.7 (21.4)	*	Townes, et al (1989)
BSRT Sum Recall	Control	102	65/37	24.52	n/a	12 m	90.0	90.0	*	Dikmen, et al (1990)
BSRT Sum Recall	Control	10	5/5	20.50 (2.60)	n/a	1 w	124.58 (11.99)	127. 78 (11.16)	AF, *	Hannay, et al (1985)
BSRT Sum Recall	Control	47	35/12	59.00 (9.81)	n/a	8 d	79.4 (11.2)	77.9 (11.1)	*	Townes, et al (1989)
BSRT Sum Recall	MS & Fatigue	13	4/9	41.00 (6.20)	pemoline	6 w	45.9 (7.4)	49.2 (10.1)		Geisler, et al (1996)
BSRT Sum Recall	MS & Fatigue	16	4/12	40.00 (6.40)	amantadine hydrochloride	6 w	48.9 (10.1)	52.3 (10.1)		Geisler, et al (1996)
BSRT Sum Recall	MS & Fatigue	16	2/14	40.00 (5.60)	placebo	6 w	50.9 (6.9)	53.5 (6.7)		Geisler, et al (1996)
BSRT Sum Recall	TBI	31	20/11	24.16	n/a	12 m	45.0	80.0	*	Dikmen, et al (1990)
BSRT Total	CVD	15	n/a	60.00 (4.57)	LCE	2-3 m	68.77 (18.53)	69.38 (21.02)		Greiffenstein, et al (1988)
BSRT Total	CVD	15	n/a	60.32 (4.02)	RCE	2-3 m	70.53 (16.72)	77.53 (16.72)		Greiffenstein, et al (1988)
BSRT Total	CVD	15	n/a	59.76 (3.74)	n/a	2 w	73.44 (24.82)	75.44 (22.47)		Greiffenstein, et al (1988)
BSRT Total	Control (overweight)	24	24/0	40.70 (8.30)	placebo	8 w	82.1 (11.6)	82.3 (12.8)		Hatsukami, et al (1986)
BSRT Total	Control (overweight)	26	26/0	37.20 (4.80)	naltrexone	8 w	79.1 (8.4)	83.8 (9.9)		Hatsukami, et al (1986)

instrument	group	n	m/f	age	intervention	inter	t #1	t #2	note	citation
BSRT Total	DAT	14	n/a	53.0 - 81.0	lithium carbonate	7 d	46.9 (8.8)	47.4 (9.0)	*	Brinkman, et al (1984)
BSRT Total	DAT	13	n/a	60.0 - 80.0	acetyl levocarnitine	6 m	22.1 (7.3)	21.2 (8.8)		Sano, et al (1992)
BSRT Total	DAT	14	n/a	60.0 - 80.0	placebo	6 m	21.4 (7.6)	16.0 (10.0)		Sano, et al (1992)
BSRT Total	Down Syndrome	34	20/14	22.0 - 56.0	n/a	1 y	23.69 (9.89)	24.28 (8.42)	*	Burt, et al (1995)
BSRT Total	TIA/CVA	34	34/0	60.30	CE	8-16 d	65.96	68.70		Cushman, et al (1984)
BSRT Total [72]	DAT	11	n/a	71.70 (6.40)	oxiracetam	1 m	22.2 (10.3)	23.9 (7.8)	AF	Green, et al (1992)
BSRT Total [72]	DAT	13	n/a	71.70 (6.40)	placebo	1 m	23.2 (7.6)	23.1 (8.7)	AF	Green, et al (1992)
BSRT Trials to Learn List	Cardiac	90	77/13	59.00 (10.6)	CABG/CPB	8 d	9.6 (2.2)	10.8 (0.7)	*	Townes, et al (1989)
BSRT Trials to Learn List	Control	47	35/12	59.00 (9.81)	n/a	8 d	9.6 (2.2)	9.7 (2.1)	*	Townes, et al (1989)
SRT	TBI (mild - mod)	7	7/0	25.00	CDP-choline	1 m	76.0	111.0		Levin (1991)
SRT	TBI (mild - mod)	7	7/0	20.00	placebo	1 m	117.0	106.0		Levin (1991)
SRT (% consistency)	HD	26	12/14	39.00 (10.4)	n/a	12 m	54.1 (4.1)	49.0 (4.5)		Bamford, et al (1995)
SRT (mean words)	HD	40	18/22	40.00 (10.3)	n/a	12 m	6.5 (0.2)	5.9 (0.3)		Bamford, et al (1995)

instrument	group	n	m/f	age	intervention	inter	t #1	t #2	note	citation
SRT (mean words)	HD	26	12/14	39.00 (10.4)	n/a	12 m	6.5 (0.3)	6.0 (0.4)		Bamford, et al (1995)
SRT CLTR	Control	30	n/a	~6.80	n/a	4-5 h	27.4 (11.2)	26.7 (10.7)		Morgan (1982)
SRT CLTR	IVDU	16	13/3	39.50	n/a	10.4 d	33.19 (13.95)	41.44 (16.83)		Richards, et al (1992)
SRT CLTR (non-verbal)	Brain Tumor	7	3/4	10.33	surgery	1 m	8.8 (4.2)	8.7 (4.4)		Bordeaux, et al (1988)
SRT CLTR (non-verbal)	Brain Tumor	7	4/3	9.83	radiotherapy	11 m	8.5 (4.2)	9.0 (5.4)		Bordeaux, et al (1988)
SRT Delayed Recog	CVA/Control	71	n/a	70.70	"declined"	9-12 m	NR	-1.2 (1.9) c		Desmond, et al (1995)
SRT Delayed Recog	CVA/Control	300	n/a	70.70	"improved/ stable"	9-12 m	NR	-0.2 (1.6) c		Desmond, et al (1995)
SRT Delayed Recog	IVDU	16	13/3	39.50	n/a	10.4 d	11.81 (0.4)	12.0 (0.0)		Richards, et al (1992)
SRT DR	Control	16	10/6	64.00 (1.70)	n/a	1 w	11.3 (0.7)	10.9 (1.0)	*	Claus, et al (1991)
SRT DR	CVA/Control	300	n/a	70.70	"improved/ stable"	9-12 m	NR	0.3 (1.9) c		Desmond, et al (1995)
SRT DR	CVA/Control	71	n/a	70.70	"declined"	9-12 m	NR	-1.8 (1.9) c		Desmond, et al (1995)
SRT DR	DAT	17	7/1	64.00 (1.70)	n/a	1 w	1.3 (0.4)	1.4 (0.4)	*	Claus, et al (1991)
SRT DR	IVDU	16	13/3	39.50	n/a	10.4 d	7.56 (2.78)	8.81 (2.34)		Richards, et al (1992)

instrument	group	n	m/f	age	intervention	inter	t #1	t #2	note	citation
SRT DR	Schizophrenia	36	28/8	35.50 (9.80)	clozapine	6 w	6.6 (2.9)	6.7 (2.9)	*	Hagger, et al (1993)
SRT Imm Recall	Schizophrenia	36	28/8	35.50 (9.80)	clozapine	6 w	7.4 (2.5)	7.4 (2.2)	*	Hagger, et al (1993)
SRT Intrus	IVDU	16	13/3	39.50	n/a	10.4 d	1.25 (1.06)	0.81 (1.22)		Richards, et al (1992)
SRT Locations	TBI (mild - mod)	7	7/0	25.00	CDP-choline	1 m	67.0	94.0		Levin (1991)
SRT Locations	TBI (mild - mod)	7	7/0	20.00	placebo	1 m	95.0	95.0		Levin (1991)
SRT LTR	Control	30	n/a	~6.80	n/a	4-5 h	32.5 (8.7)	31.3 (8.9)		Morgan (1982)
SRT LTR	CVA/Control	71	n/a	70.70	"declined"	9-12 m	NR	-6.6 (8.7) c		Desmond, et al (1995)
SRT LTR	CVA/Control	300	n/a	70.70	"improved/ stable"	9-12 m	NR	5.1 (9.6) c		Desmond, et al (1995)
SRT LTR	IVDU	16	13/3	39.50	n/a	10.4 d	40.62 (12.75)	48.81 (12.91)		Richards, et al (1992)
SRT LTS	Control	30	n/a	~6.80	n/a	4-5 h	34.5 (7.8)	33.2 (8.7)		Morgan (1982)
SRT LTS	IVDU	16	13/3	39.50	n/a	10.4 d	43.62 (12.47)	51.38 (11.94)		Richards, et al (1992)
SRT LTS	MS	19	6/13	43.37	n/a	8 w	37.0 (3.2)	39.0 (3.0)	*	Bever, et al (1995)
SRT LTS (non-verbal)	Brain Tumor	7	3/4	10.33	surgery	1 m	9.1 (5.6)	9.9 (2.9)		Bordeaux, et al (1988)

instrument	group	n	m/f	age	intervention	inter	t #1	t #2	note	citation
SRT LTS (non-verbal)	Brain Tumor	7	4/3	9.83	radiotherapy	11 m	8.2 (4.9)	7.7 (6.8)		Bordeaux, et al (1988)
SRT Objects (total of 7 objects across 10 trials)	DAT	14	8/6	66.50	tacrine	3 m	30.7 (13.3)	30.4 (20.2)	*	Maltby, et al (1994)
SRT Objects (total of 7 objects across 10 trials)	DAT	18	9/9	71.10	placebo	3 m	36.8 (21.2)	32.6 (20.3)	*	Maltby, et al (1994)
SRT Recall/Trial	Control	30	n/a	~6.80	n/a	4-5 h	6.1 (0.8)	6.2 (0.8)		Morgan (1982)
SRT Total Recall	Control	16	10/6	64.00 (1.70)	n/a	1 w	49.1 (3.4)	48.9 (3.4)	*	Claus, et al (1991)
SRT Total Recall	CVA/Control	300	n/a	70.70	"improved/ stable"	9-12 m	NR	2.9 (6.5) c		Desmond, et al (1995)
SRT Total Recall	CVA/Control	71	n/a	70.70	"declined"	9-12 m	NR	-6.2 (5.9) c		Desmond, et al (1995)
SRT Total Recall	DAT	17	7/1	64.00 (1.70)	n/a	1 w	11.4 (1.9)	12.4 (1.8)	*	Claus, et al (1991)
SRT Total Recall	IVDU	16	13/3	39.50	n/a	10.4 d	49.81 (8.64)	56.44 (8.24)		Richards, et al (1992)
SRT Words (total of 10 words across 10 trials)	DAT	14	8/6	66.50	tacrine	3 m	34.9 (15.1)	37.8 (17.8)	*	Maltby, et al (1994)

instrument	group	n	m/f	age	intervention	inter	t #1	t #2	note	citation
SRT Words (total of 10 words across 10 trials)	DAT	18	9/9	71.10	placebo	3 m	35.5 (15.9)	37.0 (15.8)	*	Maltby, et al (1994)

Table 60. Shipley Hartford Institute of Living Scale (SHILS)

instrument	group	n	m/f	age	intervention	inter	t #1	t #2	note	citation
SHILS Abstract	Alcoholic Inpts	91	91/0	42.20 (10.0)	n/a	12-22 d	9.3 (4.7)	11.6 (4.7)		Eckardt, et al (1979)
SHILS Abstract	Control	38	18/20	35.70 (10.5)	n/a	54.7 w	17.2 (1.8)	17.1 (1.7)		Tarter, et al (1990)
SHILS Abstract	Crohn's Disease	22	9/13	37.30 (10.6)	std tx	62.6 w	16.1 (2.9)	16.9 (2.3)		Tarter, et al (1990)
SHILS Abstract	Liver Disease	62	23/39	39.20 (10.5)	liver transplant	60.1 w	14.9 (2.9)	15.8 (3.1)		Tarter, et al (1990)
SHILS Abstract	Medical Inpts	20	20/0	45.60 (11.1)	n/a	12-22 d	10.8 (5.1)	11.8 (4.7)		Eckardt, et al (1979)
SHILS Abstract (IQ)	Cardiac	90	77/13	59.00 (10.6)	CABG/CPB	7 m	92.8 (20.7)	97.6 (21.4)		Townes, et al (1989)
SHILS Abstract (IQ)	Control	47	35/12	59.00 (9.81)	n/a	7 m	102.3 (19.6)	103.0 (19.8)		Townes, et al (1989)
SHILS CQ	Alcoholic Inpts	91	91/0	42.20 (10.0)	n/a	12-22 d	79.5 (13.9)	87.8 (15.4)		Eckardt, et al (1979)
SHILS CQ	Cardiac	90	77/13	59.00 (10.6)	CABG/CPB	7 m	81.0 (16.3)	84.1 (17.2)		Townes, et al (1989)

instrument	group	n	m/f	age	intervention	inter	t #1	t #2	note	citation
SHILS CQ	Control	47	35/12	59.00 (9.81)	n/a	7 m	88.4	88.4 (15.8)		Townes, et al (1989)
SHILS CQ	Medical Inpts	20	20/0	45.60 (11.1)	n/a	12-22 d	82.4 (16.8)	85.6 (16.0)		Eckardt et al (1979)
SHILS Verbal	Alcoholic Inpts	91	91/0	42.20 (10.0)	n/a	12-22 d	28.5 (5.1)	29.0 (5.5)		Eckardt, et al (1979)
SHILS Verbal	Medical Inpts	20	20/0	45.60 (11.1)	n/a	12-22 d	30.9 (4.6)	31.5 (5.3)		Eckardt, et al (1979)
SHILS Vocabulary	Control	38	18/20	35.70 (10.5)	n/a	54.7 w	18.1 (1.2)	18.4 (1.3)		Tarter, et al (1990)
SHILS Vocabulary	Crohn's Disease	22	9/13	37.30 (10.6)	std tx	62.6 w	17.9 (1.5)	18.5 (0.9)		Tarter, et al (1990)
SHILS Vocabulary	Liver Disease	62	23/39	39.20 (10.5)	liver transplant	60.1 w	17.1 (2.3)	17.5 (2.1)		Tarter, et al (1990)
SHILS Vocabulary (IQ)	Cardiac	90	77/13	59.00 (10.6)	CABG/CPB	7 m	119.0 (15.9)	122.2 (14.0)		Townes, et al (1989)
SHILS Vocabulary (IQ)	Control	47	35/12	59.00 (9.81)	n/a	7 m	124.8 (12.9)	126.6 (11.8)		Townes, et al (1989)

Table 61. Speech Sounds Perception Test (SSPT)

instrument	group	n	m/f	age	intervention	inter	t #1	t #2	note	citation
mSSPT (correct)	Renal Disease	20	n/a	46.50 (11.3)	long-term hemodialysis	1 d	16.0 (2.7)	17.7 (1.7)	*	Ratner, et al (1983)
SSPT	Alcoholic	2	2/0	48.50	excessive alcohol	18.5 m	7.5	12.5		Johnson-Greene, et al (1997)
SSPT	Alcoholic	4	4/0	48.75	minimal alcohol	18.75 m	11.0	15.0		Johnson-Greene, et al (1997)
SSPT	Alcoholic Inpts	91	91/0	42.20 (10.0)	n/a	12-22 d	50.0 (6.8)	51.3 (4.7)		Eckardt, et al (1979)
SSPT	CVD	17	15/2	62.00	CE	20w	12.87 (6.29)	11.8 (4.57)		Matarazzo, et al (1979)
SSPT	CVD	16	n/a	60.00	n/a	12w	6.44 (1.94)	6.82 (2.06)		Matarazzo, et al (1979)
SSPT	Control	23	9/14	32.30 (10.3)	n/a	3 w	55.0 (3.5)	56.0 (2.3)		Bornstein, et al (1987)
SSPT	Control	102	65/37	24.52	n/a	12 m	4.0	3.0	*	Dikmen, et al (1990)
SSPT	Control	29	29/0	24.00	n/a	20w	3.79 (1.74)	3.31 (1.93)		Matarazzo, et al (1979)
SSPT	Control	33	15/18	59.10 (9.30)	n/a	10 d	54.8 (3.0)	55.1 (2.8)		McCaffrey, et al (1993)
SSPT	Control	86	86/0	24.0 - 85.0	n/a	2 y	4.55	4.28	*	Schludermann, et al (1983)
SSPT	Control	174	174/0	24.0 - 85.0	n/a	2 y	4.64	4.62	*	Schludermann, et al (1983)

instrument	group	n	m/f	age	intervention	inter	t #1	t #2	note	citation
SSPT	Epilepsy	17	7/10	27.44 (6.04)	meds	6-12 m	8.71 (4.55)	9.65 (7.38)	*	Dodrill, et al (1975)
SSPT	Epilepsy	21	n/a	22.30 (7.60)	improved WAIS re-test	20.5 m	10.4 (6.4)	9.6 (6.0)		Seidenberg, et al (1981)
SSPT	Epilepsy	18	n/a	20.30 (5.40)	stable WAIS on re-test	21.6 m	11.1 (15.1)	12.7 (8.6)		Seidenberg, et al (1981)
SSPT	Epilepsy	19	n/a	20.30 (4.30)	slightly improved WAIS re-test	20.1 m	10.6 (7.5)	8.9 (2.8)		Seidenberg, et al (1981)
SSPT	Epilepsy (sz continued)	26	n/a	~21.0	n/a	20.7 m	12.12 (7.89)	11.96 (7.51)		Seidenberg, et al (1981)
SSPT	Epilepsy (sz remitted)	24	n/a	~21.0	n/a	20.7 m	9.75 (5.29)	9.17 (5.36)		Seidenberg, et al (1981)
SSPT	Medical Inpts	20	20/0	45.60 (11.1)	n/a	12-22 d	50.2 (5.5)	52.2 (4.5)		Eckardt, et al (1979)
SSPT	Psychiatric Inpts	231	83/148	30.70	ECT	4 - 5 w	12.0 (7.0)	10.5 (5.9)		Malloy, et al (1982)
SSPT	Schizophrenia (chronic)	35	n/a	47.00	n/a	52w	7.34 (5.24)	6.94 (6.26)		Matarazzo, et al (1979)
SSPT	TBI	31	20/11	24.16	n/a	12 m	11.0	6.0	*	Dikmen, et al (1990)
SSPT	TBI (severe)	15	13/2	24.80	n/a	11.5 m	10.1	7.4		Drudge, et al (1984)
SSPT (correct)	Alcoholic Inpts	91	91/0	42.20 (10.0)	n/a	16.8 d	50.0 (6.8)	51.3 (4.7)		Eckardt, et al (1981)

instrument	group	n	m/f	age	intervention	inter	t #1	t #2	note	citation
SSPT (correct)	Medical Inpts	20	20/0	45.60 (11.1)	n/a	22.9 d	50.2 (5.5)	52.2 (4.7)		Eckardt, et al (1981)
SSPT (correct)	Neuropsych referrals	248	203/ 45	8.00 (1.70)	n/a	2.65 y	14.9 (6.9)	19.2 (6.5)		Brown, et al (1989)
SSPT (errors)	Alcoholic (1 yr abstin)	23	23/0	36.80 (6.30)	n/a	1 y	6.1	5.6		Adams, et al (1980)
SSPT (errors)	Alcoholic (2.5 yrs abstin)	25	25/0	36.50 (6.30)	n/a	1 y	4.3	4.0		Adams, et al (1980)
SSPT (errors)	Alcoholic Inpts	25	25/0	44.84	n/a	4 w	11.04 (6.36)	10.52 (6.67)		Claiborn, et al (1981)
SSPT (errors)	CAD	17	n/a	57.20 (7.20)	n/a	6 m	12.7	12.0		Parker, et al (1983)
SSPT (errors)	CAD	20	n/a	57.20 (7.20)	CE	6 m	12.0	10.2		Parker, et al (1983)
SSPT (errors)	CAD	17	n/a	57.90 (8.40)	n/a	6 m	12.4	11.9	*	Parker, et al (1986)
SSPT (errors)	CAD	36	n./a	61.10 (8.30)	CE	6 m	11.5	10.3	*	Parker, et al (1986)
SSPT (errors)	Control	21	21/0	36.90 (5.90)	n/a	1 y	5.3	4.6		Adams, et al (1980)
SSPT (errors)	Control	25	25/0	28.68	n/a	4 w	6.32 (3.58)	5.56 (4.04)		Claiborn, et al (1981)
SSPT (errors)	Depression	33	14/19	37.40	antidepress	7 w	7.0 (6.0)	5.7 (3.1)		Fromm, et al (1984)

instrument	group	n	m/f	age	intervention	inter	t #1	t #2	note	citation
SSPT (errors)	Psychiatric Inpts	12	12/0	40.17	n/a	4 w	10.33 (6.61)	8.42 (5.27)		Claiborn, et al (1981)
SSPT (errors)	Surgical	17	n/a	57.20 (7.20)	surgery	6 m	9.7	9.2		Parker, et al (1983)
SSPT (errors)	Surgical	26	n/a	55.30 (6.80)	surgery (non-CE)	6 m	8.7	8.1	*	Parker, et al (1986)
SSPT (errors)	TBI	27	23/4	24.62	n/a	12 m	10.62	7.85		Dikmen, et al (1983)
SSPT (short form)	Cardiac	135	120/15	55.40	CABG	3 m	6.1	5.1	*	Klonoff, et al (1989)
SSPT (t)	ALL	31	16/15	8.38 (3.19)	n/a	2.0 y	49.8 (9.9)	49.1 (8.4)		Berg, et al (1983)
SSPT (t)	ALL w/ Somnolence	48	27/21	8.63 (3.15)	n/a	2.25 y	50.0 (12.3)	47.6 (8.9)		Berg, et al (1983)

Table 62. Stroop Tests

instrument	group	n	m/f	age	intervention	inter	t #1	t #2	note	citation
mStroop CW	Control	22	5/17	~21.00	DHA	3 m	50.8 (11.4)	57.4 (15.2)		Hamazaki, et al (1996)
mStroop CW	Control	19	7/12	~21.00	placebo	3 m	51.1 (12.7)	59.3 (14.6)		Hamazaki, et al (1996)
mStroop CW (errors)	Cardiac	23	16/7	42.78	cardiac valvular replacement (complicated)	8 m	6.95 (3.04)	7.78 (3.19)		Sotaniemi, et al (1981)

instrument	group	n	m/f	age	intervention	inter	t #1	t #2	note	citation
mStroop CW (errors)	Cardiac	26	17/9	40.16	cardiac valvular replacement (uncomplicated)	8 m	9.08 (1.44)	9.35 (1.35)		Sotaniemi, et al (1981)
mStroop CW (time)	Cardiac	26	17/9	40.16	cardiac valvular replacement (uncomplicated)	3 m	7.46 (2.56)	7.81 (2.50)		Sotaniemi, et al (1981)
mStroop CW (time)	Cardiac	23	16/7	42.78	cardiac valvular replacement (complicated)	3 m	5.48 (3.75)	5.96 (3.42)		Sotaniemi, et al (1981)
mStroop W time - C time	Control	12	12/0	22.40 (5.00)	n/a	50 min	86.7 (18.6)	60.9 (15.0)	*	Sacks, et al (1991)
Stroop (derived)	Schizophrenia	33	n/a	~33.70 (6.30)	clozapine	1 y	-9.0 (8.9)	-5.8 (9.3)		Buchanan, et al (1994)
Stroop (derived)	Schizophrenia	19	15/4	34.00 (6.90)	haloperidol	10 w	-8.9 (9.8)	-6.7 (7.3)		Buchanan, et al (1994)
Stroop (derived)	Schizophrenia	19	13/6	33.70 (6.30)	clozapine	10 w	-7.25 (7.8)	-5.7 (10.5)		Buchanan, et al (1994)
Stroop C	Control	40	17/23	18.00 - 25.00	practice	< 5 d	81.22 (9.38)	93.80 (16.85)	*	Connor, et al (1988)
Stroop C	Control	12	12/0	26.00	methanol	~1 h	80.3	82.3		Cook, et al (1991)
Stroop C	Control	12	12/0	26.00	placebo	~1 h	81.4	80.4		Cook, et al (1991)
Stroop C	Control	60	15/45	20.15 (1.79)	n/a	1-2 w	82.19 (14.94)	87.52 (14.68)		Franzen, et al (1987)
Stroop C	Control	21	5/16	34.00	carbamaz/ phenytoin CB	1 m	71.0 (14.0)	71.0 (13.0)	*	Meador, et al (1991)

instrument	group	n	m/f	age	intervention	inter	t #1	t #2	note	citation
Stroop C	Control	21	21/0	31.45 (5.53)	n/a	18 m	83.50 (8.26)	84.05 (8.24)		Saykin, et al (1991)
Stroop C	Control	38	18/20	35.70 (10.50)	n/a	54.7 w	13.0 (2.5)	12.6 (2.3)		Tarter, et al (1990)
Stroop C	Control	18	12/6	37.20 (9.70)	n/a	76.5 d	220.33 (51.73)	198.64 (51.02)		Verdoux, et al (1995)
Stroop C	Control (Clinic/ Volunteer)	15	5/10	33.90 (8.40)	n/a	20.7 d	84.2 (8.5)	87.4 (8.0)		Goulet Fisher, et al (1986)
Stroop C	Crohn's Disease	22	9/13	37.30 (10.60)	std tx	62.6 w	13.5 (3.2)	12.1 (3.5)		Tarter, et al (1990)
Stroop C	Depression	15	6/9	28.50 (10.60)	inpt tx	19.5 d	64.1 (9.2)	68.8 (13.6)		Goulet Fisher, et al (1986)
Stroop C	HD (at risk, + genetic marker)	8	1/7	26.20 (2.70)	n/a	2 y	76.4	79.6	*	Giordani, et al (1995)
Stroop C	HD (at risk, - genetic marker)	8	1/7	28.40 (5.20)	n/a	2 y	81.0	79.5	*	Giordani, et al (1995)
Stroop C	HIV+/ARC	8	8/0	33.57 (6.35)	n/a	18 m	59.40 (9.81)	67.00 (17.38)		Saykin, et al (1991)
Stroop C	HIV+/PGL	13	13/0	31.15 (4.91)	n/a	18 m	69.00 (13.37)	75.91 (13.00)		Saykin, et al (1991)
Stroop C	Liver Disease	62	23/39	39.20 (10.50)	liver transplant	60.1 w	16.5 (6.3)	13.2 (2.8)		Tarter, et al (1990)
Stroop C	Lung Cancer	14	12/2	63.00	chemotherapy	~5 d	63.0 (9.5)	57.1 (9.2)	*	Van Oosterhout et al (1995)

instrument	group	n	m/f	age	intervention	inter	t #1	t #2	note	citation
Stroop C	PD	19	13/6	54.30	pergolide	~6 w	76.4 (27.7)	77.5 (19.11)		Stern, et al (1984)
Stroop C	Schizophrenia	18	12/6	37.90 (10.80)	n/a	84.3 d	365.8 (108.2)	271.0 (62.80)		Verdoux, et al (1995)
Stroop C (correct per 100")	Schizophrenia Inpts	35	29/6	23.71 (4.50)	neuroleptics	1-2 y	120.0 (30.0)	130.0 (30.0)		Nopoulos, et al (1994)
Stroop C (sec)	Control	26	n/a	~9.00	n/a	~6 m	NR	-9.15 c		Neyens, et al (1996)
Stroop C (sec)	HD	26	12/14	39.00 (10.40)	n/a	12 m	100.0 (6.0)	124.0 (10.0)		Bamford, et al (1995)
Stroop C (sec)	HD	40	18/22	40.00 (10.30)	n/a	12 m	108.0 (8.0)	120.0 (10.0)		Bamford, et al (1995)
Stroop C (sec)	Orthopedic Injury	25	14/11	10.03 (2.00)	n/a	4 m	20.6 (5.5)	21.4 (6.5)		Chadwick, et al (1981)
Stroop C (sec)	PD	18	11/7	56.90 (8.90)	selegiline	12 w	56.0 (18.0)	61.0 (22.0)		Hietanen (1991)
Stroop C (sec)	PD	18	11/7	56.90 (8.90)	placebo	12 w	57.0 (14.0)	57.0 (13.0)		Hietanen (1991)
Stroop C (sec)	Spinal Cord Injury	67	54/13	32.00 (14.70)	n/a	38 w	82.59 (36.04)	72.46 (22.21)		Richards, et al (1988)
Stroop C (sec)	TBI	25	14/11	10.12 (2.60)	n/a	4 m	36.8 (20.9)	23.4 (7.3)		Chadwick, et al (1981)
Stroop C (t)	Control	72	67/5	44.50 (12.40)	n/a	6 m	45.0 (9.2)	45.7 (10.3)		Prevey, et al (1996)

instrument	group	n	m/f	age	intervention	inter	t #1	t #2	note	citation
Stroop C (t)	Epilepsy	26	24/2	43.50 (17.10)	carbamaz	6 m	41.9 (11.9)	40.9 (8.9)		Prevey, et al (1996)
Stroop C (t)	Epilepsy	39	36/3	44.30 (14.20)	valproate	6 m	41.6 (11.3)	40.0 (10.4)		Prevey, et al (1996)
Stroop C (t)	MS	9	n/a	38.90	high dose interferon	2 y	42.0 (10.3)	43.4 (9.9)		Pliskin, et al (1996)
Stroop C (t)	MS	8	n/a	38.00	low dose interferon	2 y	40.5 (7.1)	43.3 (7.6)		Pliskin, et al (1996)
Stroop C (t)	MS	13	n/a	36.20	placebo	2 y	42.2 (6.6)	42.8 (7.6)		Pliskin, et al (1996)
Stroop CW	AIDS Dementia Complex	30	29/1	33.80	zdv	6 m	94.8 (79.3)	66.6 (21.5)		Tozzi, et al (1993)
Stroop CW	Control	40	17/23	18.00 - 25.00	practice	< 5 d	49.75 (7.53)	70.62 (15.74)	*	Connor, et al (1988)
Stroop CW	Control	12	12/0	26.00	placebo	~1 h	63.2	68.1		Cook, et al (1991)
Stroop CW	Control	12	12/0	26.00	methanol	~1 h	65.6	65.9		Cook, et al (1991)
Stroop CW	Control	60	15/45	20.15 (1.79)	n/a	1-2 w	48.9 (11.57)	52.73 (10.96)		Franzen, et al (1987)
Stroop CW	Control	26	13/13	28.80 (8.20)	n/a	4 w	2.8 (4.4)	2.0 (2.4)		Killian, et al (1984)
Stroop CW	Control	20	10/10	34.00 (12.40)	n/a	4 w	46.5 (11.2)	47.6 (13.7)		McGrath, et al (1997)
Stroop CW	Control	21	5/16	34.00	carbamaz/ phenytoin CB	1 m	38.0 (7.0)	39.0 (6.0)	*	Meador, et al (1991)

instrument	group	n	m/f	age	intervention	inter	t #1	t #2	note	citation
Stroop CW	Control	21	21/0	31.45 (5.53)	n/a	18 m	48.90 (7.17)	48.35 (7.39)		Saykin, et al (1991)
Stroop CW	Control	38	18/20	35.70 (10.50)	n/a	54.7 w	22.6 (6.1)	21.7 (4.6)		Tarter, et al (1990)
Stroop CW	Control (Clinic/ Volunteer)	15	5/10	33.90 (8.40)	n/a	20.7 d	48.4 (8.9)	52.2 (8.2)		Goulet Fisher, et al (1986)
Stroop CW	Crohn's Disease	22	9/13	37.30 (10.60)	std tx	62.6 w	25.4 (10.8)	22.4 (9.0)		Tarter, et al (1990)
Stroop CW	DAT (mild)	11	10/1	63.00 (8.00)	n/a	26 m	24.0 (8.0)	18.0 (11.0)		Haxby, et al (1990)
Stroop CW	Depression	15	6/9	28.50 (10.60)	inpt tx	19.5 d	35.5 (9.8)	40.9 (10.3)		Goulet Fisher, et al (1986)
Stroop CW	Depression	26	12/4	37.10 (12.70)	no meds	4 w	3.1 (4.2)	2.7 (2.3)		Killian, et al (1984)
Stroop CW	Depression	6	4/2	26.30 (6.30)	std meds	4 w	3.3 (2.3)	1.8 (1.7)		Killian, et al (1984)
Stroop CW	Epilepsy	32	17/15	33.72 (9.66)	vigabatrin 6 g	18 w	133.16 (52.64)	138.47 (44.46)		Dodrill, et al (1995)
Stroop CW	Epilepsy	36	17/19	34.89 (8.38)	vigabatrin 1 g	18 w	135.56 (45.80)	129.19 (46.70)		Dodrill, et al (1995)
Stroop CW	Epilepsy	38	21/17	34.26 (9.18)	vigabatrin 3 g	18 w	134.60 (46.53)	145.37 (61.09)		Dodrill, et al (1995)
Stroop CW	Epilepsy	40	14/26	33.88 (9.77)	placebo	18 w	128.08 (56.02)	125.76 (49.47)		Dodrill, et al (1995)

instrument	group	n	m/f	age	intervention	inter	t #1	t #2	note	citation
Stroop CW	Epilepsy	3	n/a	9.00	barbituate anticonvulsants	7.7 w	49.0	45.7		Willis, et al (1997)
Stroop CW	Epilepsy	8	n/a	9.20	barbituate anticonvulsants	7.7 w	46.4	56.5		Willis, et al (1997)
Stroop CW	HD (at risk, + genetic marker)	8	1/7	26.20 (2.70)	n/a	2 y	46.1	46.4	*	Giordani, et al (1995)
Stroop CW	HD (at risk, - genetic marker)	8	1/7	28.40 (5.20)	n/a	2 y	45.4	45.6	*	Giordani, et al (1995)
Stroop CW	HIV+/ARC	8	8/0	33.57 (6.35)	n/a	18 m	31.00 (4.00)	39.00 (7.39)		Saykin, et al (1991)
Stroop CW	HIV+/PGL	13	13/0	31.15 (4.91)	n/a	18 m	40.25 (11.41)	45.55 (10.81)		Saykin, et al (1991)
Stroop CW	Liver Disease	62	23/39	39.20 (10.50)	liver transplant	60.1 w	32.2 (11.8)	24.7 (8.8)		Tarter, et al (1990)
Stroop CW	Lung Cancer	14	12/2	63.00	chemotherapy	~5 d	134.1 (36.2)	110.9 (27.0)	*	Van Oosterhout et al (1995)
Stroop CW	Mania	16	1/15	40.60 (12.80)	std tx	4 w	26.1 (8.6)	29.5 (12.3)		McGrath, et al (1997)
Stroop CW	PD	19	13/6	54.30	pergolide	~6 w	153.1 (57.99)	160.8 (68.14)		Stern, et al (1984)
Stroop CW	Schizophrenia	34	17/17	24.30 (6.40)	d/c meds	4 w	11.5 (9.4)	8.2 (9.4)		Killian, et al (1984)
Stroop CW	Schizophrenia	13	8/5	24.10 (3.10)	std meds	4 w	7.8 (6.5)	7.5 (7.9)		Killian, et al (1984)

instrument	group	n	m/f	age	intervention	inter	t #1	t #2	note	citation
Stroop CW	Schizophrenia	31	21/10	31.50 (8.90)	std tx	4 w	26.0 (9.5)	30.0 (10.5)		McGrath, et al (1997)
Stroop CW (correct in 100")	Schizophrenia Inpts	35	29/6	23.71 (4.50)	neuroleptics	1-2 y	60.0 (20.0)	80.0 (20.0)		Nopoulos, et al (1994)
Stroop CW (errors in 100")	Control	16	16/0	20.80	n/a	2 w	5.25 (3.9)	1.81 (1.8)		Merill, et al (1994)
Stroop CW (errors in 100")	Control (Sonar Operator)	16	16/0	21.80	n/a	2 w	2.81 (3.4)	2.19 (1.9)		Merill, et al (1994)
Stroop CW (errors)	Epilepsy	40	14/26	33.88 (9.77)	placebo	18 w	4.81 (3.89)	3.97 (3.83)		Dodrill, et al (1995)
Stroop CW (errors)	Epilepsy	36	17/19	34.89 (8.38)	vigabatrin 1 g	18 w	5.11 (4.69)	4.81 (3.93)		Dodrill, et al (1995)
Stroop CW (errors)	Epilepsy	38	21/17	34.26 (9.18)	vigabatrin 3 g	18 w	5.26 (4.43)	5.50 (4.86)		Dodrill, et al (1995)
Stroop CW (errors)	Epilepsy	32	17/15	33.72 (9.66)	vigabatrin 6 g	18 w	4.53 (4.20)	5.09 (4.12)		Dodrill, et al (1995)
Stroop CW (sec to complete 100)	Control	16	16/0	20.80	n/a	2 w	92.38 (13.2)	78.25 (13.1)		Merill, et al (1994)
Stroop CW (sec to complete 100)	Control (Sonar Operator)	16	16/0	21.80	n/a	2 w	85.69 (22.4)	78.75 (15.6)		Merill, et al (1994)
Stroop CW (sec)	ALS	12	n/a	49.40 (11.80)	high dose interferon	5 d	129.5 (42.5)	127.7 (60.1)	*	Poutiainen, et al (1994)

instrument	group	n	m/f	age	intervention	inter	t #1	t #2	note	citation
Stroop CW (sec)	ALS	3	n/a	52.30 (8.10)	placebo	5 d	131.3 (56.1)	106.7 (42.1)	*	Poutiainen, et al (1994)
Stroop CW (sec)	Control	26	n/a	~9.00	n/a	~6 m	NR	-21.78 c	*	Neyens, et al (1996)
Stroop CW (sec)	HD	40	18/22	40.00 (10.30)	n/a	12 m	200.0 (17.0)	199.0 (16.0)		Bamford, et al (1995)
Stroop CW (sec)	HD	26	12/14	39.00 (10.40)	n/a	12 m	189.0 (19.0)	215.0 (25.0)		Bamford, et al (1995)
Stroop CW (sec)	PD	18	11/7	56.90 (8.90)	selegiline	12 w	123.0 (39.0)	159.0 (132.0)		Hietanen (1991)
Stroop CW (sec)	PD	18	11/7	56.90 (8.90)	placebo	12 w	116.0 (37.0)	111.0 (40.0)		Hietanen (1991)
Stroop CW (sec)	Spinal Cord Injury	67	54/13	32.00 (14.70)	n/a	38 w	146.5 (68.31)	142.9 (46.04)		Richards, et al (1988)
Stroop CW (t)	Control	72	67/5	44.50 (12.40)	n/a	6 m	44.8 (9.9)	45.7 (11.6)		Prevey, et al (1996)
Stroop CW (t)	Dyspepsia	6	3/3	53.00	ranitidine	8 w	30.0	32.0	*	Nwokolo, et al (1994)
Stroop CW (t)	Dyspepsia	8	4/4	50.00	TDB	8 w	25.0	27.0	*	Nwokolo, et al (1994)
Stroop CW (t)	Epilepsy	4	2/2	23.00	lamotrigine/ placebo	12 w	39.0	37.0	*	Banks, et al (1991)
Stroop CW (t)	Epilepsy	6	2/4	33.30	placebo/ lamotrigine	12 w	33.3	33.3	*	Banks, et al (1991)
Stroop CW (t)	Epilepsy	26	24/2	43.50 (17.10)	carbamaz	6 m	42.2 (10.9)	43.7 (8.9)		Prevey, et al (1996)
Stroop CW (t)	Epilepsy	39	36/3	44.30 (14.20)	valproate	6 m	42.3 (11.1)	43.1 (10.4)		Prevey, et al (1996)

instrument	group	n	m/f	age	intervention	inter	t #1	t #2	note	citation
Stroop CW (t)	MS	13	n/a	36.20	placebo	2 y	40.3 (10.0)	42.9 (9.8)		Pliskin, et al (1996)
Stroop CW (t)	MS	8	n/a	38.00	low dose interferon	2 y	40.4 (9.3)	45.5 (5.8)		Pliskin, et al (1996)
Stroop CW (t)	MS	9	n/a	38.90	high dose interferon	2 y	42.9 (11.5)	44.4 (8.9)		Pliskin, et al (1996)
Stroop CW (z)	PD	20	9/11	57.90	posteroventral pallidotomy	3 m	-0.55	-0.87		Scott, et al (1998)
Stroop CW - W	Control	26	n/a	~9.00	n/a	~6 m	NR	-12.63 c	*	Neyens, et al (1996)
Stroop CW time - C time	Control	15	8/7	41.00 (12.00)	n/a	29.0 d	57.0 (14.0)	48.0 (14.0)		Trichard, et al (1995)
Stroop CW time - C time	Major Depression	23	12/11	47.00 (14.00)	n/a	29.0 d	92.0 (45.0)	75.0 (36)		Trichard, et al (1995)
Stroop Interference	Control	63	8/55	56.22 (11.00)	n/a	~6 m	NR	-8.13 (14.3)c		Bruggemans, et al (1997)
Stroop Interference	Control	21	3/18	30.10 (8.20)	n/a	6 m	29.0 (10.9)	24.8 (7.2)		Pulliainen, et al (1994)
Stroop Interference	Epilepsy	20	9/11	31.50 (11.30)	phenytoin	6 m	30.3 (12.3)	26.4 (9.1)		Pulliainen, et al (1994)
Stroop Interference	Epilepsy	23	11/12	26.80 (13.20)	carbamaz	6 m	29.3 (9.1)	28.4 (9.8)		Pulliainen, et al (1994)
Stroop Interference	Lung Cancer	14	12/2	63.00	chemotherapy	~5 d	71.1 (32.2)	53.8 (23.3)	*	Van Oosterhout et al (1995)

instrument	group	n	m/f	age	intervention	inter	t #1	t #2	note	citation
Stroop Interference (sec)	Orthopedic Injury	25	14/11	10.03 (2.00)	n/a	4 m	38.3 (13.8)	37.5 (13.8)		Chadwick, et al (1981)
Stroop Interference (sec)	TBI	25	14/11	10.12 (2.60)	n/a	4 m	49.0 (21.4)	45.5 (15.8)		Chadwick, et al (1981)
Stroop Interference (t)	MS	9	n/a	38.90	high dose interferon	2 y	51.4 (9.3)	49.9 (6.1)		Pliskin, et al (1996)
Stroop Interference (t)	MS	8	n/a	38.00	low dose interferon	2 y	51.1 (3.4)	49.4 (7.7)		Pliskin, et al (1996)
Stroop Interference (t)	MS	13	n/a	36.20	placebo	2 y	46.5 (8.1)	49.2 (7.9)		Pliskin, et al (1996)
Stroop Naming (sec)	ALS	3	n/a	52.30 (8.10)	placebo	5 d	76.3 (30.0)	69.7 (17.8)	*	Poutiainen, et al (1994)
Stroop Naming (sec)	ALS	12	n/a	49.40 (11.80)	high dose interferon	5 d	61.4 (9.2)	62.4 (12.8)	*	Poutiainen, et al (1994)
Stroop Part 1	Control	102	65/37	24.52	n/a	12 m	39.0	39.0	*	Dikmen, et al (1990)
Stroop Part 1	TBI	31	20/11	24.16	n/a	12 m	76.0	50.0	*	Dikmen, et al (1990)
Stroop Part 2	Control	102	65/37	24.52	n/a	12 m	91.0	85.0	*	Dikmen, et al (1990)
Stroop Part 2	TBI	31	20/11	24.16	n/a	12 m	254.0	119.0	*	Dikmen, et al (1990)
Stroop Reading & Naming-Correct	Control	10	6/4	31.50	vigabatrin	2 w	105.5 (9.7)	109.2 (4.5)		Thomas, et al (1996)

instrument	group	n	m/f	age	intervention	inter	t #1	t #2	note	citation
Stroop Reading & Naming-Correct	Control	10	6/4	31.50	placebo	2 w	107.3 (8.3)	110.5 (2.8)		Thomas, et al (1996)
Stroop Reading & Naming-Latency	Control	10	6/4	31.50	vigabatrin	2 w	104.8 (16.9)	101.6 (16.3)		Thomas, et al (1996)
Stroop Reading & Naming-Latency	Control	10	6/4	31.50	placebo	2 w	101.4 (13.9)	105.9 (18.8)		Thomas, et al (1996)
Stroop Speed	Control	21	3/18	30.10 (8.20)	n/a	6 m	23.3 (3.1)	23.4 (3.2)		Pulliainen, et al (1994)
Stroop Speed	Epilepsy	23	11/12	26.80 (13.20)	carbamaz	6 m	25.4 (4.9)	26.3 (5.8)		Pulliainen, et al (1994)
Stroop Speed	Epilepsy	20	9/11	31.50 (11.30)	phenytoin	6 m	26.4 (7.0)	26.9 (5.6)		Pulliainen, et al (1994)
Stroop W	Control	40	17/23	18.00 - 25.00	practice	< 5 d	113.52 (14.72)	123.22 (19.28)	*	Connor, et al (1988)
Stroop W	Control	60	15/45	20.15 (1.79)	n/a	1-2 w	112.15 (18.63)	117.64 (17.56)		Franzen, et al (1987)
Stroop W	Control	21	5/16	34.00	carbamaz/ phenytoin CB	1 m	96.0 (12.0)	97.0 (14.0)	*	Meador, et al (1991)
Stroop W	Control	21	21/0	31.45 (5.53)	n/a	18 m	110.90 (11.26)	114.30 (11.93)		Saykin, et al (1991)
Stroop W	Control	38	18/20	35.70 (10.50)	n/a	54.7 w	8.6 (1.6)	9.0 (1.6)		Tarter, et al (1990)

instrument	group	n	m/f	age	intervention	inter	t #1	t #2	note	citation
Stroop W	Control	18	12/6	37.20 (9.70)	n/a	76.5 d	94.87 (21.3)	94.29 (20.84)		Verdoux, et al (1995)
Stroop W	Control (Clinic/ Volunteer)	15	5/10	33.90 (8.40)	n/a	20.7 d	116.7 (14.7)	117.8 (18.6)		Goulet Fisher, et al (1986)
Stroop W	Crohn's Disease	22	9/13	37.30 (10.60)	std tx	62.6 w	9.4 (1.9)	8.6 (2.2)		Tarter, et al (1990)
Stroop W	Depression	15	6/9	28.50 (10.60)	inpt tx	19.5 d	93.6 (20.4)	97.9 (22.6)		Goulet Fisher, et al (1986)
Stroop W	Epilepsy	32	17/15	33.72 (9.66)	vigabatrin 6 g	18 w	54.62 (17.47)	56.50 (15.59)		Dodrill, et al (1995)
Stroop W	Epilepsy	36	17/19	34.89 (8.38)	vigabatrin 1 g	18 w	53.03 (21.71)	53.31 (19.01)		Dodrill, et al (1995)
Stroop W	Epilepsy	40	14/26	33.88 (9.77)	placebo	18 w	53.81 (19.88)	54.24 (19.08)		Dodrill, et al (1995)
Stroop W	Epilepsy	38	21/17	34.26 (9.18)	vigabatrin 3 g	18 w	56.03 (15.14)	64.60 (25.53)		Dodrill, et al (1995)
Stroop W	HD (at risk, + genetic marker)	8	1/7	26.20 (2.70)	n/a	2 y	104.0	98.8	*	Giordani, et al (1995)
Stroop W	HD (at risk, - genetic marker)	8	1/7	28.40 (5.20)	n/a	2 y	109.1	103.1	*	Giordani, et al (1995)
Stroop W	HIV+/ARC	8	8/0	33.57 (6.35)	n/a	18 m	74.20 (15.16)	85.86 (15.45)		Saykin, et al (1991)
Stroop W	HIV+/PGL	13	13/0	31.15 (4.91)	n/a	18 m	97.00 (27.85)	105.45 (19.08)		Saykin, et al (1991)

instrument	group	n	m/f	age	intervention	inter	t #1	t #2	note	citation
Stroop W	Liver Disease	62	23/39	39.20 (10.50)	liver transplant	60.1 w	10.8 (3.0)	9.4 (2.1)		Tarter, et al (1990)
Stroop W	Lung Cancer	14	12/2	63.00	chemotherapy	~5 d	50.4 (6.3)	47.9 (8.4)	*	Van Oosterhout et al (1995)
Stroop W	PD	19	13/6	54.30	pergolide	~6 w	49.4 (13.10)	54.5 (13.96)		Stern, et al (1984)
Stroop W	Schizophrenia	18	12/6	37.90 (10.80)	n/a	84.3 d	113.07 (38.07)	107.64 (24.21)		Verdoux, et al (1995)
Stroop W (correct in 100")	Schizophrenia Inpts	35	29/6	23.71 (4.50)	neuroleptics	1-2 y	190.0 (50.0)	190.0 (60.0)		Nopoulos, et al (1994)
Stroop W (errors)	Epilepsy	38	21/17	34.26 (9.18)	vigabatrin 3 g	18 w	1.08 (1.30)	1.24 (1.57)		Dodrill, et al (1995)
Stroop W (errors)	Epilepsy	40	14/26	33.88 (9.77)	placebo	18 w	0.78 (1.16)	0.81 (1.15)		Dodrill, et al (1995)
Stroop W (errors)	Epilepsy	32	17/15	33.72 (9.66)	vigabatrin 6 g	18 w	1.03 (1.56)	1.19 (1.31)		Dodrill, et al (1995)
Stroop W (errors)	Epilepsy	36	17/19	34.89 (8.38)	vigabatrin 1 g	18 w	0.97 (1.23)	0.92 (1.32)		Dodrill, et al (1995)
Stroop W (sec)	Control	26	n/a	~9.00	n/a	~6 m	NR	-0.52 c	*	Neyens, et al (1996)
Stroop W (sec)	Control	15	8/7	41.00 (12.00)	n/a	29.0 d	38.0 (6.5)	36.5 (5.0)		Trichard, et al (1995)
Stroop W (sec)	Major Depression	23	12/11	47.00 (14.00)	n/a	29.0 d	50.0 (11.5)	47.5 (9.5)		Trichard, et al (1995)

instrument	group	n	m/f	age	intervention	inter	t #1	t #2	note	citation
Stroop W (sec)	Orthopedic Injury	25	14/11	10.03 (2.00)	n/a	4 m	13.0 (3.0)	12.5 (3.2)		Chadwick, et al (1981)
Stroop W (sec)	Spinal Cord Injury	67	54/13	32.00 (14.70)	n/a	38 w	62.69 (30.06)	52.0 (14.19)		Richards, et al (1988)
Stroop W (sec)	TBI	25	14/11	10.12 (2.60)	n/a	4 m	23.1 (16.2)	17.3 (7.8)		Chadwick, et al (1981)
Stroop W (t)	Control	72	67/5	44.50 (12.40)	n/a	6 m	46.3 (8.8)	46.7 (10.8)		Prevey, et al (1996)
Stroop W (t)	Epilepsy	26	24/2	43.50 (17.10)	carbamaz	6 m	42.3 (9.3)	43.8 (8.5)		Prevey, et al (1996)
Stroop W (t)	Epilepsy	39	36/3	44.30 (14.20)	valproate	6 m	42.5 (9.7)	42.6 (9.9)		Prevey, et al (1996)
Stroop W (t)	MS	13	n/a	36.20	placebo	2 y	41.9 (6.1)	44.2 (7.8)		Pliskin, et al (1996)
Stroop W (t)	MS	9	n/a	38.90	high dose interferon	2 y	40.2 (10.4)	43.0 (6.5)		Pliskin, et al (1996)
Stroop W (t)	MS	8	n/a	38.00	low dose interferon	2 y	44.6 (11.6)	47.1 (9.7)		Pliskin, et al (1996)
Stroop W - C	Control	26	13/13	28.80 (8.20)	n/a	4 w	86.2 (24.7)	76.6 (19.2)		Killian, et al (1984)
Stroop W - C	Depression	6	4/2	26.30 (6.30)	std meds	4 w	100.5 (74.8)	75.1 (18.1)		Killian, et al (1984)
Stroop W - C	Depression	26	12/4	37.10 (12.70)	no meds	4 w	118.3 (45.4)	95.5 (46.2)		Killian, et al (1984)

instrument	group	n	m/f	age	intervention	inter	t #1	t #2	note	citation
Stroop W - C	Schizophrenia	13	8/5	24.10 (3.10)	std meds	4 w	155.7 (80.9)	136.6 (58.2)		Killian, et al (1984)
Stroop W - C	Schizophrenia	34	17/17	24.30 (6.40)	d/c meds	4 w	134.6 (51.8)	120.4 (54.2)		Killian, et al (1984)

Table 63. Symbol Digit Modalities Test (SDMT)

instrument	group	n	m/f	age	intervention	inter	t #1	t #2	note	citation
SDMT	Control	8	8/0	24.00	placebo	3 w	NR	3.0 c		Brooks, et al (1988)
SDMT	Control	8	8/0	24.00	metoprolol	3 w	NR	7.5 c		Brooks, et al (1988)
SDMT	Control	8	8/0	24.00	propranolol	3 w	NR	4.0 c		Brooks, et al (1988)
SDMT	Control	8	8/0	24.00	atenolol	3 w	NR	0.5 c		Brooks, et al (1988)
SDMT	Control	63	8/55	56.22 (11.0)	n/a	~6 m	NR	3.79 (4.56)c		Bruggemans, et al (1997)
SDMT	Control	33	15/18	59.10 (9.30)	n/a	10 d	46.9 (9.4)	47.9 (11.0)		McCaffrey, et al (1993)
SDMT	Control	21	5/16	34.00	carbamaz/ phenytoin CB	1 m	53.0 (8.0)	52.0 (8.0)	*	Meador, et al (1991)
SDMT	Control	16	n/a	60.0+	placebo	1 d	33.0	36.0		Richardson, et al (1985)
SDMT	Control	14	n/a	60.0+	scopolamine	1 d	24.0	28.0		Richardson, et al (1985)
SDMT	Control	39	39/0	37.60 (7.20)	n/a	1y	56.21 (8.69)	56.95 (7.27)	*	Uchiyama, et al (1994)

instrument	group	n	m/f	age	intervention	inter	t #1	t #2	note	citation
SDMT	Epilepsy	32	17/15	33.72 (9.66)	vigabatrin 6 g	18 w	41.72 (11.76)	41.31 (11.38)		Dodrill, et al (1995)
SDMT	Epilepsy	38	21/17	34.26 (9.18)	vigabatrin 3 g	18 w	39.76 (10.73)	40.18 (10.96)		Dodrill, et al (1995)
SDMT	Epilepsy	36	17/19	34.89 (8.38)	vigabatrin 1 g	18 w	40.69 (13.52)	41.14 (12.52)		Dodrill, et al (1995)
SDMT	Epilepsy	40	14/26	33.88 (9.77)	placebo	18 w	42.56 (11.03)	43.51 (12.23)		Dodrill, et al (1995)
SDMT	Epilepsy	20	9/11	31.50 (11.3)	phenytoin	6 m	49.6 (13.1)	49.0 (9.1)		Pulliainen, et al (1994)
SDMT	Epilepsy	23	11/12	26.80 (13.2)	carbamaz	6 m	50.6 (11.0)	56.1 (6.2)		Pulliainen, et al (1994)
SDMT	HIV+	69	51/18	34.70 (6.30)	n/a	6 m	40.5 (10.0)	42.3 (8.9)	*	Selnes, et al (1992)
SDMT	HIV+	132	132/0	~33.8	n/a	13.3 m	56.9	59.2		Selnes, et al (1990)
SDMT	HIV-	37	27/10	35.60 (7.10)	n/a	6 m	38.5 (9.0)	42.9 (9.5)	*	Selnes, et al (1992)
SDMT	HIV-	132	132/0	~35.6	n/a	13.4 m	57.5	59.7		Selnes, et al (1990)
SDMT	MS	19	6/13	43.37	n/a	8 w	32.0 (4.2)	37.0 (4.1)	*	Bever, et al (1995)
SDMT Oral	Aphasia	15	n/a	n/a	n/a	22.6 m	13.0	13.7		Smith (1982)

instrument	group	n	m/f	age	intervention	inter	t #1	t #2	note	citation
SDMT Oral	Aphasia	24	n/a	n/a	tx	20.6 m	21.7	24.5		Smith (1982)
SDMT Oral	BMT	25	14/11	~12.0	BMT	8.2 m	46.8 (21.4)	51.4 (21.6)		Phipps, et al (1995)
SDMT Oral	Control	80	32/48	34.80 (11.2)	n/a	29.4 d	64.99 (11.91)	69.15 (11.97)		Smith (1982)
SDMT Oral	MS & Fatigue	16	2/14	40.00 (5.60)	placebo	6 w	53.4 (13.4)	58.3 (16.8)		Geisler, et al (1996)
SDMT Oral	MS & Fatigue	13	4/9	41.00 (6.20)	pemoline	6 w	49.2 (14.5)	49 (16.6)		Geisler, et al (1996)
SDMT Oral	MS & Fatigue	16	4/12	40.00 (6.40)	amantadine hydrochloride	6 w	50.8 (17.5)	57.8 (19.7)		Geisler, et al (1996)
SDMT Recall	Control	39	39/0	37.60 (7.20)	n/a	1y	6.05 (2.31)	7.49 (2.3)	*	Uchiyama, et al (1994)
SDMT Recall	HIV+	69	51/18	34.70 (6.30)	n/a	6 m	5.0 (2.6)	5.1 (2.5)	*	Selnes, et al (1992)
SDMT Recall	HIV-	37	27/10	35.60 (7.10)	n/a	6 m	4.2 (2.7)	4.8 (2.2)	*	Selnes, et al (1992)
SDMT Written	Aphasia	24	n/a	n/a	tx	20.6 m	23.7	24.9		Smith (1982)
SDMT Written	Aphasia	15	n/a	n/a	n/a	22.6 m	13.4	13.9		Smith (1982)
SDMT Written	BMT	25	14/11	~12.0	BMT	8.2 m	41.6 (19.4)	41.7 (18.0)		Phipps, et al (1995)

instrument	group	n	m/f	age	intervention	inter	t #1	t #2	note	citation
SDMT Written	Control	80	32/48	34.80 (11.2)	n/a	29.4 d	56.79 (9.84)	60.46 (11.16)		Smith (1982)
SDMT Written	MS & Fatigue	16	2/14	40.00 (5.60)	placebo	6 w	45.1 (10.9)	46.6 (14.2)		Geisler, et al (1996)
SDMT Written	MS & Fatigue	13	4/9	41.00 (6.20)	pemoline	6 w	39.6 (11.9)	40.4 (12.9)		Geisler, et al (1996)
SDMT Written	MS & Fatigue	16	4/12	40.00 (6.40)	amantadine hydrochloride	6 w	40.4 (17.9)	48.6 (15.7)		Geisler, et al (1996)
SDMT-2	Control	20	20/0	40.04 (7.05)	n/a	1y	55.65 (10.71)	58.05 (12.78)	*	Uchiyama, et al (1994)
SDMT-2 Recall	Control	20	20/0	40.04 (7.05)	n/a	1y	7.1 (2.1)	7.25 (2.12)	*	Uchiyama, et al (1994)

Table 64. Tactual Performance Test (TPT)

instrument	group	n	m/f	age	intervention	inter	t #1	t #2	note	citation
TPT BH	Alcoholic (1 yr abstin)	23	23/0	36.80 (6.30)	n/a	1 y	2.3	2.7		Adams, et al (1980)
TPT BH	Alcoholic (2.5 yrs abstin)	25	25/0	36.50 (6.30)	n/a	1 y	2.4	2.5		Adams, et al (1980)
TPT BH	Alcoholic (detoxed)	17	n/a	44.47	abstin	1 y	2.39 (8.98)	2.56 (2.97)		Long, et al (1974)
TPT BH	Alcoholic Inpts	25	25/0	44.84	n/a	4 w	4.80 (3.38)	3.23 (1.35)		Claiborn, et al (1981)

instrumenct	group	n	m/f	age	intervention	inter	t #1	t #2	note	citation
TPT BH	Alcoholic Inpts	91	91/0	42.20 (10.0)	n/a	12-22 d	4.6 (3.2)	2.9 (1.6)		Eckardt, et al (1979)
TPT BH	Control	21	21/0	36.90 (5.90)	n/a	1 y	2.5	2.2		Adams, et al (1980)
TPT BH	Control	25	25/0	28.68	n/a	4 w	2.12 (0.72)	1.61 (0.65)		Claiborn, et al (1981)
TPT BH	Depression	33	14/19	37.40	antidepress	7 w	4.35 (2.78)	3.35 (2.29)		Fromm, et al (1984)
TPT BH	Medical Inpts	20	20/0	45.60 (11.1)	n/a	12-22 d	6.7 (4.2)	5.8 (4.3)		Eckardt, et al (1979)
TPT BH	Neuropsych referrals	248	203/45	8.00 (1.70)	n/a	2.65 y	3.1 (2.6)	1.9 (1.7)		Brown, et al (1989)
TPT BH	Psychiatric Inpts	12	12/0	40.17	n/a	4 w	3.88 (2.32)	3.30 (2.38)		Claiborn, et al (1981)
TPT BH	Psychiatric Inpts	231	83/148	30.70	ECT	4 – 5 w	7.24 (14.73)	6.61 (14.1)		Malloy, et al (1982)
TPT BH (min/block)	TBI	27	23/4	24.62	n/a	12 m	0.46	0.29		Dikmen, et al (1983)
TPT DH	Alcoholic (1 yr abstin)	23	23/0	36.80 (6.30)	n/a	1 y	6.0	5.6		Adams, et al (1980)
TPT DH	Alcoholic (2.5 yrs abstin)	25	25/0	36.50 (6.30)	n/a	1 y	6.7	4.9		Adams, et al (1980)
TPT DH	Alcoholic Inpts	25	25/0	44.84	n/a	4 w	9.57 (7.02)	5.98 (3.55)		Claiborn, et al (1981)

instrumenct	group	n	m/f	age	intervention	inter	t #1	t #2	note	citation
TPT DH	Alcoholic Inpts	91	91/0	42.20 (10.0)	n/a	12-22 d	8.2 (3.7)	5.7 (2.8)		Eckardt, et al (1979)
TPT DH	Control	21	21/0	36.90 (5.90)	n/a	1 y	5.6	5.0		Adams, et al (1980)
TPT DH	Control	25	25/0	28.68	n/a	4 w	4.89 (1.82)	3.25 (1.20)		Claiborn, et al (1981)
TPT DH	Depression	33	14/19	37.40	antidepress	7 w	7.17 (2.61)	5.75 (2.47)		Fromm, et al (1984)
TPT DH	HIV+ (IVDU)	18	10/8	29.80 (5.40)	drug tx	17.7 m	5.5 (1.9)	6.0 (2.7)		Hestad, et al (1996)
TPT DH	HIV- (IVDU)	30	16/14	27.90 (4.90)	drug tx	14.9 m	5.9 (2.2)	4.7 (1.5)		Hestad, et al (1996)
TPT DH	Medical Inpts	20	20/0	45.60 (11.1)	n/a	12-22 d	8.2 (3.9)	8.6 (4.5)		Eckardt, et al (1979)
TPT DH	Neuropsych referrals	248	203/45	8.00 (1.70)	n/a	2.65 y	6.7 (3.6)	4.9 (3.0)		Brown, et al (1989)
TPT DH	Psychiatric Inpts	12	12/0	40.17	n/a	4 w	7.93 (4.08)	5.21 (2.52)		Claiborn, et al (1981)
TPT DH	TBI	17	15/2	23.50 (5.10)	n/a	12.6 m	6.84	6.725		Prigatano, et al (1984)
TPT DH	TBI	18	15/3	26.10 (8.30)	rehab	7.5 m	7.71	8.08		Prigatano, et al (1984)
TPT DH (min./block)	TBI	27	23/4	24.62	n/a	12 m	0.86	0.56		Dikmen, et al (1983)

instrumenct	group	n	m/f	age	intervention	inter	t #1	t #2	note	citation
TPT LH	Alcoholic (detoxed)	17	n/a	44.47	abstin	1 y	5.62 (0.24)	4.04 (6.39)		Long, et al (1974)
TPT LH	Psychiatric Inpts	231	83/ 148	30.70	ECT	4 - 5 w	11.67 (19.05)	11.35 (18.1)		Malloy, et al (1982)
TPT Localization	Alcoholic	4	4/0	48.75	minimal alcohol	18.75 m	2.0	4.3		Johnson-Greene, et al (1997)
TPT Localization	Alcoholic	2	2/0	48.50	excessive alcohol	18.5 m	5.0	5.5		Johnson-Greene, et al (1997)
TPT Localization	Alcoholic (1 yr abstin)	23	23/0	36.80 (6.30)	n/a	1 y	4.6	5.0		Adams, et al (1980)
TPT Localization	Alcoholic (2.5 yrs abstin)	25	25/0	36.50 (6.30)	n/a	1 y	4.7	4.6		Adams, et al (1980)
TPT Localization	Alcoholic (detoxed)	17	n/a	44.47	abstin	1 y	4.41 (2.21)	4.41 (2.6)		Long, et al (1974)
TPT Localization	Alcoholic Inpts	25	25/0	44.84	n/a	4 w	1.80 (1.58)	3.44 (2.69)		Claiborn, et al (1981)
TPT Localization	Alcoholic Inpts	91	91/0	42.20 (10.0)	n/a	16.8 d	2.9 (2.3)	4.2 (2.6)		Eckardt, et al (1981)
TPT Localization	Alcoholic Inpts	91	91/0	42.20 (10.0)	n/a	12- 22 d	2.9 (2.3)	4.2 (2.5)		Eckardt, et al (1979)
TPT Localization	Alcoholic Inpts	27	27/0	50.40 (6.22)	n/a	14 m	3.5 (2.73)	0.4 (1.72)c		Schau, et al (1980)
TPT Localization	CAD	20	n/a	57.20 (7.20)	CE	6 m	1.5	1.1		Parker, et al (1983)

instrumenct	group	n	m/f	age	intervention	inter	t #1	t #2	note	citation
TPT Localization	CAD	17	n/a	57.20 (7.20)	n/a	6 m	1.9	2.8		Parker, et al (1983)
TPT Localization	CAD	36	n./a	61.10 (8.30)	CE	6 m	1.7	1.2	*	Parker, et al (1986)
TPT Localization	CAD	17	n/a	57.90 (8.40)	n/a	6 m	1.8	2.7	*	Parker, et al (1986)
TPT Localization	CVD	16	n/a	60.00	n/a	12 w	1.06 (1.13)	1.1 (1.08)		Matarazzo, et al (1979)
TPT Localization	CVD	17	15/2	62.00	CE	20 w	2.2 (1.93)	1.53 (1.77)		Matarazzo, et al (1979)
TPT Localization	Control	21	21/0	36.90 (5.90)	n/a	1 y	3.7	5.0		Adams, et al (1980)
TPT Localization	Control	23	9/14	32.30 (10.3)	n/a	3 w	5.1 (2.3)	6.3 (2.9)		Bornstein, et al (1987)
TPT Localization	Control	25	25/0	28.68	n/a	4 w	4.56 (1.71)	6.12 (2.07)		Claiborn, et al (1981)
TPT Localization	Control	102	65/37	24.52	n/a	12 m	5.0	6.0	*	Dikmen, et al (1990)
TPT Localization	Control	9	4/5	53.10 (7.30)	n/a	5.8 y	5.8 (1.2)	6.0 (1.9)		Elias, et al (1989)
TPT Localization	Control	18	8/10	48.50 (10.1)	n/a	5.6 y	5.0 (1.7)	5.2 (2.1)		Elias, et al (1989)
TPT Localization	Control	102	~69/ 33	~26.0	n/a	12 m	5.0	6.0		Fraser, et al (1988)

instrumenct	group	n	m/f	age	intervention	inter	t #1	t #2	note	citation
TPT Localization	Control	29	29/0	24.00	n/a	20 w	5.34 (2.41)	7.1 (1.82)		Matarazzo, et al (1979)
TPT Localization	Control	27	27/0	49.50	n/a	14 m	4.2 (2.26)	0.88 (0.3) c		Schau, et al (1980)
TPT Localization	Control	86	86/0	24.0 - 85.0	n/a	2 y	3.47	3.97	*	Schludermann, et al (1983)
TPT Localization	Control	174	174/0	24.0 - 85.0	n/a	2 y	3.77	4.12	*	Schludermann, et al (1983)
TPT Localization	Depression	33	14/19	37.40	antidepress	7 w	3.7 (2.5)	4.1 (2.7)		Fromm, et al (1984)
TPT Localization	Epilepsy	17	7/10	27.44 (6.04)	meds	6-12 m	2.76 (2.25)	2.88 (2.29)	*	Dodrill, et al (1975)
TPT Localization	Epilepsy	18	n/a	20.30 (5.40)	stable WAIS on re-test	21.6 m	2.9 (2.5)	2.9 (2.2)		Seidenberg, et al (1981)
TPT Localization	Epilepsy	19	n/a	20.30 (4.30)	slightly improved WAIS re-test	20.1 m	3.1 (1.8)	4.1 (2.1)		Seidenberg, et al (1981)
TPT Localization	Epilepsy	21	n/a	22.30 (7.60)	improved WAIS re-test	20.5 m	3.1 (2.8)	4.05 (2.8)		Seidenberg, et al (1981)
TPT Localization	Epilepsy (sz continued)	26	n/a	~21.0	n/a	20.7 m	3.19 (2.12)	3.31 (2.40)		Seidenberg, et al (1981)
TPT Localization	Epilepsy (sz remitted)	24	n/a	~21.0	n/a	20.7 m	2.63 (2.36)	4.04 (2.39)		Seidenberg, et al (1981)
TPT Localization	HD (at risk, + genetic marker)	8	1/7	26.20 (2.70)	n/a	2 y	6.0	5.5	*	Giordani, et al (1995)

instrumenct	group	n	m/f	age	intervention	inter	t #1	t #2	note	citation
TPT Localization	HD (at risk, - genetic marker)	8	1/7	28.40 (5.20)	n/a	2 y	4.1	5.0	*	Giordani, et al (1995)
TPT Localization	Hypertension	19	8/11	46.80 (9.60)	n/a	5.6 y	4.3 (2.2)	3.8 (1.8)		Elias, et al (1989)
TPT Localization	Hypertension	10	6/4	52.20 (3.10)	n/a	5.7 y	4.0 (1.9)	3.6 (1.9)		Elias, et al (1989)
TPT Localization	Medical Inpts	20	20/0	45.60 (11.1)	n/a	22.9 d	2.2 (2.6)	4.0 (2.6)		Eckardt, et al (1981)
TPT Localization	Medical Inpts	20	20/0	45.60 (11.1)	n/a	12-22 d	2.2 (2.6)	4.0 (2.6)		Eckardt, et al (1979)
TPT Localization	Neuropsych referrals	248	203/ 45	8.00 (1.70)	n/a	2.65 y	1.4 (1.6)	2.2 (1.8)		Brown, et al (1989)
TPT Localization	Psychiatric Inpts	12	12/0	40.17	n/a	4 w	2.83 (2.66)	3.33 (2.67)		Claiborn, et al (1981)
TPT Localization	Psychiatric Inpts	231	83/ 148	30.70	ECT	4 – 5 w	2.6 (2.0)	3.1 (2.3)		Malloy, et al (1982)
TPT Localization	Schizophrenia (chronic)	35	n/a	47.00	n/a	52 w	1.26 (1.46)	2.2 (1.91)		Matarazzo, et al (1979)
TPT Localization	Surgical	17	n/a	57.20 (7.20)	surgery	6 m	1.7	1.6	*	Parker, et al (1986)
TPT Localization	Surgical	26	n/a	55.30 (6.80)	surgery (non-CE)	6 m	2.7	2.9	*	Parker, et al (1986)
TPT Localization	TBI	31	20/11	24.16	n/a	12 m	1.0	3.0	*	Dikmen, et al (1990)
TPT Localization	TBI	27	23/4	24.62	n/a	12 m	3.51	4.18		Dikmen, et al (1983)

instrumenct	group	n	m/f	age	intervention	inter	t #1	t #2	note	citation
TPT Localization	TBI (did not return to work)	13	3/10	24.00	n/a	12 m	0.0	3.0		Fraser, et al (1988)
TPT Localization	TBI (did return to work)	35	26/9	29.00	n/a	12 m	5.0	5.0		Fraser, et al (1988)
TPT Localization	TBI (in litigation)	20	14/6	41.85 (10.2)	n/a	14.45 m	2.60 (1.90)	1.75 (1.25)		Reitan, et al (1996)
TPT Localization	TBI (not in litigation)	20	17/3	29.65 (14.9)	n/a	12.00 m	3.25 (1.65)	4.35 (2.52)		Reitan, et al (1996)
TPT Localization	TBI (sev)	15	13/2	24.80	n/a	11.5 m	1.3	3.0		Drudge, et al (1984)
TPT Memory	Alcoholic	4	4/0	48.75	minimal alcohol	18.75 m	6.5	7.5		Johnson-Greene, et al (1997)
TPT Memory	Alcoholic	2	2/0	48.50	excessive alcohol	18.5 m	8.5	7.0		Johnson-Greene, et al (1997)
TPT Memory	Alcoholic (1 yr abstin)	23	23/0	36.80 (6.30)	n/a	1 y	8.4	8.2		Adams, et al (1980)
TPT Memory	Alcoholic (2.5 yrs abstin)	25	25/0	36.50 (6.30)	n/a	1 y	8.2	8.4		Adams, et al (1980)
TPT Memory	Alcoholic (detoxed)	17	n/a	44.47	abstin	1 y	7.53 (1.84)	7.12 (1.54)		Long, et al (1974)
TPT Memory	Alcoholic Inpts	25	25/0	44.84	n/a	4 w	8.44 (1.36)	8.60 (1.26)		Claiborn, et al (1981)
TPT Memory	Alcoholic Inpts	91	91/0	42.20 (10.0)	n/a	16.8 d	7.1 (1.6)	7.9 (1.4)		Eckardt, et al (1981)
TPT Memory	Alcoholic Inpts	91	91/0	42.20 (10.0)	n/a	12-22 d	7.1 (1.6)	7.9 (1.3)		Eckardt, et al (1979)

instrumenct	group	n	m/f	age	intervention	inter	t #1	t #2	note	citation
TPT Memory	CAD	20	n/a	57.20 (7.20)	CE	6 m	5.8	5.2		Parker, et al (1983)
TPT Memory	CAD	17	n/a	57.20 (7.20)	n/a	6 m	5.5	5.9		Parker, et al (1983)
TPT Memory	CAD	36	n./a	61.10 (8.30)	CE	6 m	5.3	4.9	*	Parker, et al (1986)
TPT Memory	CAD	17	n/a	57.90 (8.40)	n/a	6 m	5.5	5.7	*	Parker, et al (1986)
TPT Memory	CVD	17	15/2	62.00	CE	20 w	5.8 (1.52)	4.93 (2.58)		Matarazzo, et al (1979)
TPT Memory	CVD	16	n/a	60.00	n/a	12 w	5.44 (1.08)	5.03 (1.25)		Matarazzo, et al (1979)
TPT Memory	Control	21	21/0	36.90 (5.90)	n/a	1 y	7.9	8.3		Adams, et al (1980)
TPT Memory	Control	23	9/14	32.30 (10.3)	n/a	3 w	8.4 (0.9)	8.9 (1.0)		Bornstein, et al (1987)
TPT Memory	Control	25	25/0	28.68	n/a	4 w	8.76 (1.27)	9.24 (1.01)		Claiborn, et al (1981)
TPT Memory	Control	102	65/37	24.52	n/a	12 m	8.0	9.0	*	Dikmen, et al (1990)
TPT Memory	Control	18	8/10	48.50 (10.1)	n/a	5.6 y	7.7 (1.0)	7.6 (1.3)		Elias, et al (1989)
TPT Memory	Control	9	4/5	53.10 (7.30)	n/a	5.8 y	8.1 (0.9)	8.3 (1.1)		Elias, et al (1989)
TPT Memory	Control	29	29/0	24.00	n/a	20 w	8.38 (0.82)	8.72 (0.88)		Matarazzo, et al (1979)

instrumenct	group	n	m/f	age	intervention	inter	t #1	t #2	note	citation
TPT Memory	Control	174	174/0	24.0 - 85.0	n/a	2 y	7.11	7.38	*	Schludermann, et al (1983)
TPT Memory	Control	86	86/0	24.0 - 85.0	n/a	2 y	6.86	7.20	*	Schludermann, et al (1983)
TPT Memory	Depression	33	14/19	37.40	antidepress	7 w	7.1 (2.1)	7.8 (1.4)		Fromm, et al (1984)
TPT Memory	Epilepsy	17	7/10	27.44 (6.04)	meds	6-12 m	7.59 (1.33)	7.59 (1.77)	*	Dodrill, et al (1975)
TPT Memory	Epilepsy	21	n/a	22.30 (7.60)	improved WAIS re-test	20.5 m	6.5 (2.1)	7.3 (1.5)		Seidenberg, et al (1981)
TPT Memory	Epilepsy	19	n/a	20.30 (4.30)	slightly improved WAIS re-test	20.1 m	6.3 (1.2)	6.9 (1.6)		Seidenberg, et al (1981)
TPT Memory	Epilepsy	18	n/a	20.30 (5.40)	stable WAIS on re-test	21.6 m	5.6 (2.3)	5.9 (2.1)		Seidenberg, et al (1981)
TPT Memory	Epilepsy (sz continued)	26	n/a	~21.0	n/a	20.7 m	5.92 (1.83)	6.42 (1.75)		Seidenberg, et al (1981)
TPT Memory	Epilepsy (sz remitted)	24	n/a	~21.0	n/a	20.7 m	6.21 (1.96)	6.96 (1.94)		Seidenberg, et al (1981)
TPT Memory	HD (at risk, + genetic marker)	8	1/7	26.20 (2.70)	n/a	2 y	8.2	8.1	*	Giordani, et al (1995)
TPT Memory	HD (at risk, - genetic marker)	8	1/7	28.40 (5.20)	n/a	2 y	7.1	7.1	*	Giordani, et al (1995)
TPT Memory	Hypertension	10	6/4	52.20 (3.10)	n/a	5.7 y	6.8 (1.4)	6.7 (1.0)		Elias, et al (1989)

instrumenct	group	n	m/f	age	intervention	inter	t #1	t #2	note	citation
TPT Memory	Hypertension	19	8/11	46.80 (9.60)	n/a	5.6 y	7.1 (1.4)	6.9 (1.7)		Elias, et al (1989)
TPT Memory	Medical Inpts	20	20/0	45.60 (11.1)	n/a	22.9 d	6.5 (1.6)	7.3 (1.3)		Eckardt, et al (1981)
TPT Memory	Medical Inpts	20	20/0	45.60 (11.1)	n/a	12-22 d	6.5 (1.6)	7.3 (1.3)		Eckardt, et al (1979)
TPT Memory	Neuropsych referrals	248	203/45	8.00 (1.70)	n/a	2.65 y	3.0 (1.7)	4.1 (1.5)		Brown, et al (1989)
TPT Memory	Psychiatric Inpts	12	12/0	40.17	n/a	4 w	8.50 (1.17)	8.58 (1.17)		Claiborn, et al (1981)
TPT Memory	Psychiatric Inpts	231	83/148	30.70	ECT	4 – 5 w	6.0 (2.1)	6.6 (2.1)		Malloy, et al (1982)
TPT Memory	Schizophrenia (chronic)	35	n/a	47.00	n/a	52 w	4.6 (2.13)	5.49 (2.3)		Matarazzo, et al (1979)
TPT Memory	Surgical	17	n/a	57.20 (7.20)	surgery	6 m	6.4	6.4		Parker, et al (1983)
TPT Memory	Surgical	26	n/a	55.30 (6.80)	surgery (non-CE)	6 m	6.7	6.6	*	Parker, et al (1986)
TPT Memory	TBI	31	20/11	24.16	n/a	12 m	4.0	7.0	*	Dikmen, et al (1990)
TPT Memory	TBI	27	23/4	24.62	n/a	12 m	6.66	7.26		Dikmen, et al (1983)
TPT Memory	TBI (sev)	15	13/2	24.80	n/a	11.5 m	4.9	7.3		Drudgc, ct al (1984)
TPT Memory (Imp Rating)	Control	10	n/a	48.60 (8.20)	n/a	5.6 y	0.80	0.80 (0.42)	*	Elias, et al (1986)
TPT Memory (Imp Rating)	Hypertension	11	n/a	51.20 (4.50)	n/a	5.7 y	1.09 (0.54)	1.27 (0.65)	*	Elias, et al (1986)

instrumenct	group	n	m/f	age	intervention	inter	t #1	t #2	note	citation
TPT NDH	Alcoholic (1 yr abstin)	23	23/0	36.80 (6.30)	n/a	1 y	4.5	4.5		Adams, et al (1980)
TPT NDH	Alcoholic (2.5 yrs abstin)	25	25/0	36.50 (6.30)	n/a	1 y	4.2	3.5		Adams, et al (1980)
TPT NDH	Alcoholic Inpts	25	25/0	44.84	n/a	4 w	7.80 (5.92)	5.71 (3.39)		Claiborn, et al (1981)
TPT NDH	Alcoholic Inpts	91	91/0	42.20 (10.0)	n/a	12-22 d	7.0 (3.9)	4.6 (2.6)		Eckardt, et al (1979)
TPT NDH	Control	21	21/0	36.90 (5.90)	n/a	1 y	4.2	3.7		Adams, et al (1980)
TPT NDH	Control	25	25/0	28.68	n/a	4 w	3.50 (1.34)	2.58 (0.85)		Claiborn, et al (1981)
TPT NDH	Depression	33	14/19	37.40	antidepress	7 w	6.17 (2.86)	4.83 (2.92)		Fromm, et al (1984)
TPT NDH	Medical Inpts	20	20/0	45.60 (11.1)	n/a	12-22 d	7.7 (4.0)	7.2 (4.5)		Eckardt, et al (1979)
TPT NDH	Neuropsych referrals	248	203/45	8.00 (1.70)	n/a	2.65 y	5.3 (3.7)	3.4 (2.6)		Brown, et al (1989)
TPT NDH	Psychiatric Inpts	12	12/0	40.17	n/a	4 w	5.53 (2.99)	4.57 (2.96)		Claiborn, et al (1981)
TPT NDH	TBI	18	15/3	26.10 (8.30)	rehab	7.5 m	7.46	6.43		Prigatano, et al (1984)
TPT NDH	TBI	17	15/2	23.50 (5.10)	n/a	12.6 m	6.44	6.43		Prigatano, et al (1984)
TPT NDH (min/block)	TBI	27	23/4	24.62	n/a	12 m	0.70	0.43		Dikmen, et al (1983)

instrumenct	group	n	m/f	age	intervention	inter	t #1	t #2	note	citation
TPT RH	Alcoholic (detoxed)	17	n/a	44.47	abstin	1 y	6.41 (6.13)	5.51 (4.43)		Long, et al (1974)
TPT RH	Psychiatric Inpts	231	83/148	30.70	ECT	4 - 5 w	12.24 (14.6)	10.60 (12.43)		Malloy, et al (1982)
TPT Total	Alcoholic	4	4/0	48.75	minimal alcohol	18.75 m	24.6	20.0		Johnson-Greene, et al (1997)
TPT Total	Alcoholic	2	2/0	48.50	excessive alcohol	18.5 m	10.7	12.3		Johnson-Greene, et al (1997)
TPT Total	Alcoholic (1 yr abstin)	23	23/0	36.80 (6.30)	n/a	1 y	12.6	13.0		Adams, et al (1980)
TPT Total	Alcoholic (2.5 yrs abstin)	25	25/0	36.50 (6.30)	n/a	1 y	13.0	10.7		Adams et al (1980)
TPT Total	Alcoholic (detoxed)	17	n/a	44.47	abstin	1 y	14.41 (5.18)	12.10 (4.36)		Long, et al (1974)
TPT Total	Alcoholic Inpts	91	91/0	42.20 (10.0)	n/a	16.8 d	19.7 (9.8)	13.2 (6.1)		Eckardt, et al (1981)
TPT Total	Alcoholic Inpts	91	91/0	42.20 (10.0)	n/a	12-22 d	19.7 (9.8)	13.2 (6.1)		Eckardt, et al (1979)
TPT Total	Alcoholic Inpts	27	27/0	50.40 (6.22)	n/a	14 m	1260.0 (842.9)	-19.6 (532.7) c		Schau, et al (1980)
TPT Total	CAD	20	n/a	57.20 (7.20)	CE	6 m	25.9	24.0		Parker, et al (1983)
TPT Total	CAD	17	n/a	57.20 (7.20)	n/a	6 m	25.0	23.3		Parker, et al (1983)

instrumenct	group	n	m/f	age	intervention	inter	t #1	t #2	note	citation
TPT Total	CAD	17	n/a	57.90 (8.40)	n/a	6 m	24.5	23.1	*	Parker, et al (1986)
TPT Total	CAD	36	n/a	61.10 (8.30)	CE	6 m	26.4	24.3	*	Parker, et al (1986)
TPT Total	CVD	17	15/2	62.00	CE	20 w	22.79 (6.08)	22.72 (7.64)		Matarazzo, et al (1979)
TPT Total	CVD	16	n/a	60.00	n/a	12 w	32.48 (5.88)	30.67 (5.13)		Matarazzo, et al (1979)
TPT Total	Control	21	21/0	36.90 (5.90)	n/a	1 y	12.3	10.9		Adams, et al (1980)
TPT Total	Control	23	9/14	32.30 (10.3)	n/a	3 w	10.7 (4.2)	7.4 (2.6)		Bornstein, et al (1987)
TPT Total	Control	102	65/37	24.52	n/a	12 m	0.35	0.29	*	Dikmen, et al (1990)
TPT Total	Control	29	29/0	24.00	n/a	20 w	9.36 (2.73)	8.19 (2.7)		Matarazzo, et al (1979)
TPT Total	Control	27	27/0	49.50	n/a	14 m	764.0 (316.5)	-86.5 (206.2) c		Schau, et al (1980)
TPT Total	Control	86	86/0	24.0 - 85.0	n/a	2 y	13.87	12.88	*	Schludermann, et al (1983)
TPT Total	Control	174	174/0	24.0 - 85.0	n/a	2 y	13.75	12.42	*	Schludermann, et al (1983)
TPT Total	Epilepsy	17	7/10	27.44 (6.04)	meds	6-12 m	0.71 (0.42)	1.81 (3.13)	*	Dodrill, et al (1975)

instrumenct	group	n	m/f	age	intervention	inter	t #1	t #2	note	citation
TPT Total	Medical Inpts	20	20/0	45.60 (11.1)	n/a	22.9 d	22.6 (10.8)	21.6 (12.4)		Eckardt, et al (1981)
TPT Total	Medical Inpts	20	20/0	45.60 (11.1)	n/a	12-22 d	22.6 (10.8)	21.6 (12.4)		Eckardt, et al (1979)
TPT Total	Psychiatric Inpts	231	83/ 148	30.70	ECT	4 – 5 w	27.31 (28.42)	25.06 (29.14)		Malloy, et al (1982)
TPT Total	Schizophrenia (chronic)	35	n/a	47.00	n/a	52 w	27.8 (11.78)	24.2 (11.75)		Matarazzo, et al (1979)
TPT Total	Surgical	17	n/a	57.20 (7.20)	surgery	6 m	21.5	20.4		Parker, et al (1983)
TPT Total	Surgical	26	n/a	55.30 (6.80)	surgery (non-CE)	6 m	20.5	18.6	*	Parker, et al (1986)
TPT Total	TBI	31	20/11	24.16	n/a	12 m	1.24	0.48	*	Dikmen, et al (1990)
TPT Total	TBI (sev)	15	13/2	24.80	n/a	11.5 m	23.5	17.7		Drudge, et al (1984)
TPT Total (min/block)	Epilepsy	21	n/a	22.30 (7.60)	improved WAIS re-test	20.5 m	1.18 (1.2)	0.65 (0.35)		Seidenberg, et al (1981)
TPT Total (min/block)	Epilepsy	19	n/a	20.30 (4.30)	slightly improved WAIS re-test	20.1 m	0.90 (0.69)	0.75 (0.76)		Seidenberg, et al (1981)
TPT Total (min/block)	Epilepsy	18	n/a	20.30 (5.40)	stable WAIS on re-test	21.6 m	1.2 (1.2)	1.1 (0.7)		Seidenberg, et al (1981)
TPT Total (min/block)	Epilepsy (sz continued)	26	n/a	~21.0	n/a	20.7 m	1.00 (0.67)	0.92 (0.75)		Seidenberg, et al (1981)

instrumenct	group	n	m/f	age	intervention	inter	t #1	t #2	note	citation
TPT Total (min/block)	Epilepsy (sz remitted)	24	n/a	~21.0	n/a	20.7 m	1.33 (1.44)	0.82 (0.57)		Seidenberg, et al (1981)
TPT Total (min/block)	HD (at risk, + genetic marker)	8	1/7	26.20 (2.70)	n/a	2 y	0.4	0.4	*	Giordani, et al (1995)
TPT Total (min/block)	HD (at risk, - genetic marker)	8	1/7	28.40 (5.20)	n/a	2 y	0.4	0.4	*	Giordani, et al (1995)
TPT Total (min/block)	TBI	27	23/4	24.62	n/a	12 m	0.69	0.45		Dikmen, et al (1983)
TPT-6 BH	Cardiac	79	79/0	55.5 (8.01)	CABG	3 m	1.05 (0.59)	0.97 (0.49)	*	Clark, et al (1988)
TPT-6 BH (t)	ALL	31	16/15	8.38 (3.19)	n/a	2.0 y	50.7 (9.9)	50.3 (25.6)		Berg, et al (1983)
TPT-6 BH (t)	ALL w/ Somnolence	48	27/21	8.63 (3.15)	n/a	2.25 y	48.8 (9.2)	50.7 (17.8)		Berg, et al (1983)
TPT-6 DH	Cardiac	79	79/0	55.5 (8.01)	CABG	3 m	2.37 (1.16)	2.07 (0.86)	*	Clark, et al (1988)
TPT-6 DH (t)	ALL	31	16/15	8.38 (3.19)	n/a	2.0 y	51.4 (8.3)	52.5 (26.1)		Berg, et al (1983)
TPT-6 DH (t)	ALL w/ Somnolence	48	27/21	8.63 (3.15)	n/a	2.25 y	50.6 (9.9)	47.3 (13.9)		Berg, et al (1983)
TPT-6 Localization	Cardiac	79	79/0	55.5 (8.01)	CABG	3 m	3.33 (1.59)	3.47 (1.67)	*	Clark, et al (1988)
TPT-6 Localization	Cardiac	135	120/15	55.40	CABG	3 m	3.2	3.4	*	Klonoff, et al (1989)

instrumenct	group	n	m/f	age	intervention	inter	t #1	t #2	note	citation
TPT-6 Localization (t)	ALL	31	16/15	8.38 (3.19)	n/a	2.0 y	46.7 (12.1)	50.0 (16.7)		Berg, et al (1983)
TPT-6 Localization (t)	ALL w/ Somnolence	48	27/21	8.63 (3.15)	n/a	2.25 y	52.3 (8.6)	48.9 (9.5)		Berg, et al (1983)
TPT-6 Memory	Cardiac	79	79/0	55.5 (8.01)	CABG	3 m	4.46 (1.11)	4.64 (1.09)	*	Clark, et al (1988)
TPT-6 Memory	Cardiac	135	120/ 15	55.40	CABG	3 m	4.4	4.6	*	Klonoff, et al (1989)
TPT-6 Memory (t)	ALL	31	16/15	8.38 (3.19)	n/a	2.0 y	53.1 (11.7)	49.6 (19.1)		Berg, et al (1983)
TPT-6 Memory (t)	ALL w/ Somnolence	48	27/21	8.63 (3.15)	n/a	2.25 y	50.2 (9.7)	51.3 (8.8)		Berg, et al (1983)
TPT-6 NDH	Cardiac	79	79/0	55.5 (8.01)	CABG	3 m	1.74 (0.86)	1.83 (1.10)	*	Clark, et al (1988)
TPT-6 NDH (t)	ALL	31	16/15	8.38 (3.19)	n/a	2.0 y	48.6 (10.1)	52.8 (29.8)		Berg, et al (1983)
TPT-6 NDH (t)	ALL w/ Somnolence	48	27/21	8.63 (3.15)	n/a	2.25 y	48.3 (8.5)	49.3 (10.9)		Berg, et al (1983)
TPT-6 Total	Cardiac	79	79/0	55.5 (8.01)	CABG	3 m	5.16 (2.29)	4.87 (2.16)	*	Clark, et al (1988)
TPT-6 Total	Cardiac	135	120/ 15	55.40	CABG	3 m	5.2	4.9	*	Klonoff, et al (1989)

Table 65. Token Tests

instrument	group	n	m/f	age	intervention	inter	t #1	t #2	note	citation
AAT Token Test	CVA	36	n/a	~68.0	placebo	12 w	NR	4.67 (8.9)%c	*	Enderby, et al (1994)
AAT Token Test	CVA	30	n/a	~64.0	piracetam	12 w	NR	8.6 (10.5) %c	*	Enderby, et al (1994)
MAE Token Test	Depression	9	6/3	50.20 (18.5)	right ECT	2 d	40.2	40.7	*	Kronfol, et al (1978)
MAE Token Test	Depression	9	6/3	48.30 (17.8)	left ECT	2 d	41.0	40.3	*	Kronfol, et al (1978)
MAE Token Test	Epilepsy	40	23/17	32.20 (8.20)	n/a	~9 m	41.85 (2.48)	41.62 (3.59)		Hermann, et al (1996)
MAE Token Test (t)	Lung Cancer	11	n/a	~61.0	cranial irradiation	11 m	44.3	46.7		Komaki, et al (1995)
mToken Test II (sec)	PD/Tremor	12	7/5	56.00	left thalamotomy	~6 d	13.0	18.0		Vilkki, et al (1974)
mToken Test II (sec)	PD/Tremor	13	8/5	56.00	right thalamotomy	~6 d	10.8	9.9		Vilkki, et al (1974)
mToken Test IV (sec)	PD/Tremor	12	7/5	56.00	left thalamotomy	~6 d	22.0	49.0		Vilkki, et al (1974)
mToken Test IV (sec)	PD/Tremor	13	8/5	56.00	right thalamotomy	~6 d	14.3	13.2		Vilkki, et al (1974)
mToken Test Naming (sec)	PD/Tremor	12	7/5	56.00	left thalamotomy	~6 d	55.8	94.8		Vilkki, et al (1974)

instrument	group	n	m/f	age	intervention	inter	t #1	t #2	note	citation
mToken Test Naming (sec)	PD/Tremor	13	8/5	56.00	right thalamotomy	~6 d	49.8	47.3		Vilkki, et al (1974)
Token Test	Control	22	12/10	65.82 (5.20)	n/a	2 y	156.3 (0.77)	156.33 (1.19)		Rebok, et al (1990)
Token Test	DAT	51	16/35	67.29 (7.94)	n/a	2 y	148.6 (9.33)	136.06 (22.90)		Rebok, et al (1990)
Token Test	DAT	32	n/a	70.72	NSAID	1 y	136.6	16.94 c		Rich, et al (1995)
Token Test	DAT	117	n/a	69.93	n/a	1 y	129.1	10.28 c		Rich, et al (1995)
Token Test	DAT (declining)	12	3/9	56.20 (6.40)	n/a	1 y	NR	-7.9 (5.0) c		Piccini, et al (1995)
Token Test	DAT (mild - mod)	46	24/22	69.85 (5.81)	placebo	45 d	22.84 (0.82)	22.79 (0.83)	*	Bergamasco, et al (1994)
Token Test	DAT (mild - mod)	46	19/27	70.31 (7.15)	idebenone	45 d	23.8 (0.89)	24.48 (0.92)	*	Bergamasco, et al (1994)
Token Test	DAT (stable)	19	3/16	61.00 (6.40)	n/a	1 y	NR	-3.2 (2.3) c		Piccini, et al (1995)
Token Test (raw)	PD	20	9/11	57.90	posteroventral pallidotomy	3 m	161.0	160.0		Scott, et al (1998)
Token Test (shortened)	Control	70	26/44	29.30 (1.15)	n/a	4 y	34.54 (0.5)	34.63 (0.6)		Amato, et al (1995)
Token Test (shortened)	Left AVM	15	10/5	31.00 (11.0)	surgery	4 m	35.4 (1.0)	32.2 (10.6)	*	Stabell, et al (1994)
Token Test (shortened)	MS	50	18/32	29.90 (8.48)	n/a	4 y	34.26 (1.4)	33.57 (2.7)		Amato, et al (1995)

instrument	group	n	m/f	age	intervention	inter	t #1	t #2	note	citation
Token Test (shortened)	Right AVM	16	5/11	34.00 (13.0)	surgery	4 m	35.5 (0.6)	35.8 (0.2)	*	Stabell, et al (1994)
Token Test [13]	Control	38	18/20	35.70 (10.5)	n/a	54.7 w	12.6 (0.6)	12.8 (0.6)		Tarter, et al (1990)
Token Test [13]	Crohn's Disease	22	9/13	37.30 (10.6)	std tx	62.6 w	12.0 (1.4)	12.6 (0.6)		Tarter, et al (1990)
Token Test [13]	Liver Disease	62	23/39	39.20 (10.5)	liver transplant	60.1 w	11.7 (1.6)	12.2 (1.1)		Tarter, et al (1990)
Token Test [22]	DAT	13	n/a	71.70 (6.40)	placebo	1 m	19.0 (2.3)	18.3 (2.6)	AF	Green, et al (1992)
Token Test [22]	DAT	11	n/a	71.70 (6.40)	oxiracetam	1 m	19.6 (2.5)	19.6 (2.2)	AF	Green, et al (1992)
Token Test [36]	DAT	34	16/18	62.76 (6.30)	n/a	7.72 m	26.81 (5.89)	20.77 (8.23)		Della Sala, et al (1992)

Table 66. Tower of London Tests

instrument	group	n	m/f	age	intervention	inter	t #1	t #2	note	citation
mTower of London (% Correct Trial 1)	TBI	57	33/24	10.01	n/a	33.01 m	55.15	70.06		Levin, et al (1997)
mTower of London (% Correct	TBI	57	33/24	10.01	n/a	33.01 m	90.05	98.02		Levin, et al (1997)

instrument	group	n	m/f	age	intervention	inter	t #1	t #2	note	citation
Trial 3)										
mTower of London (Broken Rules)	TBI	57	33/24	10.01	n/a	33.01 m	0.34	6.05		Levin, et al (1997)
mTower of London (Planning Time)	TBI	57	33/24	10.01	n/a	33.01 m	5.39	5.49		Levin, et al (1997)

Table 67. Trail Making Tests (TMT)

instrument	group	n	m/f	age	intervention	inter	t #1	t #2	note	citation
RCPMB TMT-A	Boxers	20	20/0	20.50	n/a	15-18 m	26.2	26.1		Porter, et al (1996)
RCPMB TMT-A	Control	20	20/0	20.50	n/a	15-18 m	31.6	31.6		Porter, et al (1996)
RCPMB TMT-B	Alcoholic	10	9/1	35.20	abstin	4 w	100.1	67.8		Goldman, et al (1983)
RCPMB TMT-B	Alcoholic	10	7/3	25.50	abstin	4 w	105.8	60.8		Goldman, et al (1983)
RCPMB TMT-B	Alcoholic	11	8/3	50.60	abstin	4 w	159.2	110.2		Goldman, et al (1983)
RCPMB TMT-B	Boxers	20	20/0	20.50	n/a	15-18 m	53.8	53.4		Porter, et al (1996)
RCPMB TMT-B	Control	15	15/0	47.50	n/a	4 w	79.5	67.1		Goldman, et al (1983)

instrument	group	n	m/f	age	intervention	inter	t #1	t #2	note	citation
RCPMB TMT-B	Control	15	9/6	26.40	n/a	4 w	62.7	45.7		Goldman, et al (1983)
RCPMB TMT-B	Control	20	20/0	20.50	n/a	15-18 m	70.9	70.1		Porter, et al (1996)
RCPMB TMT-B	Epilepsy	71	n/a	n/a	anticonvul	n/a	140.0	116.05		Clifford, et al (1976)
RCPMB TMT-B	Epilepsy	36	n/a	n/a	carbamaz	3 w	79.61	87.03		Rennick, et al (1974)
TMT-A	AIDS	10	10/0	41.70 (5.50)	n/a	6.53 m	37.1 (12.3)	30.0 (7.2)		Hinkin, et al (1995)
TMT-A	Alcohol Dependent	16	16/0	42.38 (10.6)	placebo program	3 w	37.13 (16.75)	36.06 (13.34)		Roehrich, et al (1993)
TMT-A	Alcohol Dependent	15	15/0	43.13 (11.5)	n/a	3 w	42.93 (13.4)	40.07 (12.41)		Roehrich, et al (1993)
TMT-A	Alcohol Dependent	15	15/0	42.07 (9.80)	neuropsych remediation	3 w	34.07 (10.45)	26.27 (7.81)		Roehrich, et al (1993)
TMT-A	Alcohol Dependent	15	15/0	42.07 (10.9)	ecological remediation	3 w	37.93 (14.58)	30.07 (11.03)		Roehrich, et al (1993)
TMT-A	Alcoholic	24	24/0	51.00 (6.38)	inpt tx	12-16 m	47.2 (23.80)	39.4 (20.30)		O'Leary, et al (1977)
TMT-A	Alcoholic (1 yr abstin)	23	23/0	36.80 (6.30)	n/a	1 y	26.6	28.2		Adams, et al (1980)
TMT-A	Alcoholic (2.5 yrs abstin)	25	25/0	36.50 (6.30)	n/a	1 y	22.7	28.8		Adams, et al (1980)
TMT-A	Alcoholic (detoxed)	17	n/a	44.47	abstin	1 y	9.53 (6.87)	9.65 (6.85)		Long, et al (1974)

instrument	group	n	m/f	age	intervention	inter	t #1	t #2	note	citation
TMT-A	Alcoholic Inpts	25	25/0	44.84	n/a	4 w	55.56 (31.43)	38.40 (14.56)		Claiborn, et al (1981)
TMT-A	Alcoholic Inpts	91	91/0	42.20 (10.0)	n/a	16.8 d	39.9 (13.8)	32.3 (12.2)		Eckardt, et al (1981)
TMT-A	Alcoholic Inpts	91	91/0	42.20 (10.0)	n/a	12-22 d	39.9 (13.8)	32.2 (12.1)		Eckardt, et al (1979)
TMT-A	Anorexia	18	0/18	n/a	refeeding tx	69.8 d	25.1 (7.5)	22.6 (8.1)		Szmukler, et al (1992)
TMT-A	Brain Tumor	7	3/4	10.33	surgery	1 m	-0.2 (9.9)	4.1 (6.9)		Bordeaux, et al (1988)
TMT-A	Brain Tumor	7	4/3	9.83	radiotherapy	11 m	5.0 (6.9)	5.6 (5.2)		Bordeaux, et al (1988)
TMT-A	Cardiac	33	19/14	73.10 (5.50)	open heart surgery	8.4 d	42.4 (12.6)	56.8 (21.0)	*	Heyer, et al (1995)
TMT-A	Cardiac	22	10/12	47.30 (14.0)	open heart surgery	8.4 d	25.8 (6.0)	21.0 (4.8)	*	Heyer, et al (1995)
TMT-A	Cardiac	135	120/15	55.40	CABG	3 m	37.3	35.3	*	Klonoff, et al (1989)
TMT-A	Cardiac	17	12/5	50.00 (10.5)	heart transplant	36.0 m	46.0 (12.39)	49.0 (19.94)		Roman, et al (1997)
TMT-A	Cardiac	245	198/47	54.70	CABG/cardiac operation	6 m	40.79 (19.0)	37.06 (15.79)		Savageau, et al (1982a)
TMT-A	Cardiac	227	184/43	54.50	cardiac operation	10-12 d	42.66 (22.81)	45.74 (24.80)		Savageau, et al (1982b)
TMT-A	Cardiac	90	77/13	59.00 (10.6)	CABG/CPB	8 d	35.2 (14.7)	46.3 (22.2)	*	Townes, et al (1989)

instrument	group	n	m/f	age	intervention	inter	t #1	t #2	note	citation
TMT-A	Carotid Artery Occlusion	11	3/8	65.27	CE	6 w	125.0	73.8		King, et al (1977)
TMT-A	CVD	15	n/a	60.00 (4.57)	LCE	2-3 m	71.23 (23.96)	63.61 (23.70)		Greiffenstein, et al (1988)
TMT-A	CVD	15	n/a	60.32 (4.02)	RCE	2-3 m	69.46 (42.95)	50.92 (24.35)		Greiffenstein, et al (1988)
TMT-A	CVD	15	n/a	59.76 (3.74)	n/a	2 w	65.15 (20.26)	52.53 (18.17)		Greiffenstein, et al (1988)
TMT-A	CVD	17	15/2	62.00	CE	20 w	57.8 (19.8)	51.0 (16.89)		Matarazzo, et al (1979)
TMT-A	CVD	16	n/a	60.00	n/a	12 w	36.4 (8.26)	34.22 (7.14)		Matarazzo, et al (1979)
TMT-A	Control	21	21/0	36.90 (5.90)	n/a	1 y	25.8	22.7		Adams, et al (1980)
TMT-A	Control	23	9/14	32.30 (10.3)	n/a	3 w	25.6 (6.8)	21.5 (5.6)		Bornstein, et al (1987)
TMT-A	Control	63	8/55	56.22 (11.0)	n/a	~6 m	NR	-4.91 (9.10)c		Bruggemans, et al (1997)
TMT-A	Control	25	25/0	28.68	n/a	4 w	33.0 (11.44)	26.64 (8.67)		Claiborn, et al (1981)
TMT-A	Control	11	9/2	31.60 (5.00)	n/a	6 m	24.5 (6.6)	18.5 (2.7)		Di Stefano, et al (1996)
TMT-A	Control	102	65/37	24.52	n/a	12 m	19.0	19.0	*	Dikmen, et al (1990)
TMT-A	Control	1017	436/ 581	74.30 (5.40)	n/a	2 y	50.7 (25.9)	53.8 (30.9)		Ganguli, et al (1996)

instrument	group	n	m/f	age	intervention	inter	t #1	t #2	note	citation
TMT-A	Control	8	4/4	21.80 (4.20)	placebo	60 min	27.9 (15.9)	27.6 (16.8)	A/C	Kirkby, et al (1995)
TMT-A	Control	9	4/5	26.40 (7.70)	lorazepam	60 min	26.7 (8.93)	27.4 (8.68)	A/C	Kirkby, et al (1995)
TMT-A	Control	4	0/4	67.30 (0.50)	placebo	60 min	33.3 (2.61)	33.4 (8.56)	A/C	Kirkby, et al (1995)
TMT-A	Control	5	1/4	68.40 (6.10)	lorazepam	60 min	37.0 (4.55)	45.8 (17.5)	A/C	Kirkby, et al (1995)
TMT-A	Control	29	29/0	24.00	n/a	20 w	21.76 (5.65)	21.72 (5.86)		Matarazzo, et al (1979)
TMT-A	Control	40	6/34	68.20 (1.20)	n/a	1 y	44.1 (13.9)	41.6 (14.1)	*	Mitrushina, et al (1991b)
TMT-A	Control	47	14/33	72.90 (1.40)	n/a	1 y	47.2 (13.7)	45.0 (13.2)	*	Mitrushina, et al (1991b)
TMT-A	Control	19	2/17	62.20 (2.50)	n/a	1 y	41.0 (9.5)	38.0 (11.7)	*	Mitrushina, et al (1991b)
TMT-A	Control	16	4/12	78.30 (2.50)	n/a	1 y	56.0 (20.7)	51.9 (18.1)	*	Mitrushina, et al (1991b)
TMT-A	Control	26	n/a	~9.00	n/a	~6 m	NR	-6.04 c	*	Neyens, et al (1996)
TMT-A	Control	12	12/0	31.50	hypoxia	15 min	27.1	52.6		Noble, et al (1993)
TMT-A	Control	12	12/0	31.60	n/a	15 min	23.3	20.0		Noble, et al (1993)
TMT-A	Control	20	20/0	49.90 (7.34)	n/a	12-16 m	31.2 (7.44)	26.6 (9.64)		O'Leary, et al (1977)

instrument	group	n	m/f	age	intervention	inter	t #1	t #2	note	citation
TMT-A	Control	16	10/6	12.60	n/a	1 m	28.0 (10.0)	20.0 (7.0)		Pieters, et al (1992)
TMT-A	Control	21	3/18	30.10 (8.20)	n/a	6 m	30.9 (10.0)	27.3 (6.2)		Pulliainen, et al (1994)
TMT-A	Control	14	6/8	11.20	n/a	4-6 h	55.8 (6.3)	59.9 (7.2)		Reich, et al (1990)
TMT-A	Control	21	21/0	31.45 (5.53)	n/a	18 m	23.75 (6.82)	22.05 (7.56)		Saykin, et al (1991)
TMT-A	Control	30	16/14	22.43 (2.67)	n/a	1 w	21.48 (6.44)	19.68 (7.32)		Stuss, et al (1988)
TMT-A	Control	30	14/16	61.77 (3.00)	n/a	1 w	36.73 (13.68	29.3 (14.73)		Stuss, et al (1988)
TMT-A	Control	30	14/16	40.63 (2.97)	n/a	1 w	27.58 (9.43)	22.95 (6.23)		Stuss, et al (1988)
TMT-A	Control	10	6/4	23.00 (2.67)	n/a	1 w	18.5 (5.1)	16.2 (5.0)		Stuss, et al (1987)
TMT-A	Control	10	5/5	33.90 (2.88)	n/a	1 w	21.9 (6.3)	18.4 (2.9)		Stuss, et al (1987)
TMT-A	Control	10	5/5	63.70 (3.13)	n/a	1 w	37.3 (14.7)	29.9 (8.9)		Stuss, et al (1987)
TMT-A	Control	10	6/4	55.30 (2.98)	n/a	1 w	38.5 (18.2)	32.7 (23.8)		Stuss, et al (1987)
TMT-A	Control	10	5/5	17.30 (0.95)	n/a	1 w	21.8 (5.3)	22.2 (8.7)		Stuss, et al (1987)
TMT-A	Control	10	6/4	44.20 (3.12)	n/a	1 w	29.2 (9.0)	26.5 (7.5)		Stuss, et al (1987)

instrument	group	n	m/f	age	intervention	inter	t #1	t #2	note	citation
TMT-A	Control	22	15/7	27.70 (11.6)	n/a	6 d	20.9 (6.9)	17.4 (4.1)	*	Stuss, et al (1989)
TMT-A	Control	26	20/6	29.70 (12.4)	n/a	1 w	22.4 (7.9)	21.4 (6.8)	*	Stuss, et al (1989)
TMT-A	Control	18	0/18	n/a	n/a	108.4 d	20.0 (4.7)	17.8 (4.2)		Szmukler, et al (1992)
TMT-A	Control	38	18/20	35.70 (10.5)	n/a	54.7 w	24.6 (7.0)	21.8 (5.8)		Tarter, et al (1990)
TMT-A	Control	47	35/12	59.00 (9.81)	n/a	8 d	30.3 (8.6)	28.7 (9.2)	*	Townes, et al (1989)
TMT-A	Control (CDR-0)	30	15/15	70.9 (4.6)	n/a	1 y	27.6 (7.8)	25.4 (5.2)	*	Botwinick, et al (1986)
TMT-A	Control (overweight)	24	24/0	40.70 (8.30)	placebo	8 w	23.9 (8.2)	20.3 (4.7)		Hatsukami, et al (1986)
TMT-A	Control (overweight)	26	26/0	37.20 (4.80)	naltrexone	8 w	25.1 (9.4)	22.4 (7.1)		Hatsukami, et al (1986)
TMT-A	Control (Clinic/ Volunteer)	15	5/10	33.90 (8.40)	n/a	20.7 d	22.7 (9.2)	21.3 (6.2)		Goulet Fisher, et al (1986)
TMT-A	Crohn's Disease	22	9/13	37.30 (10.6)	std tx	62.6 w	30.1 (1.0)	26.5 (9.8)		Tarter, et al (1990)
TMT-A	DAT	10	6/4	74.30	suloctidil 450 mg	12 w	334.60 (243.0)	327.80 (255.2)		McCaffrey, et al (1987)
TMT-A	DAT	10	5/5	74.90	suloctidil 600 mg	12 w	88.67 (46.05)	100.89 (62.93)		McCaffrey, et al (1987)

instrument	group	n	m/f	age	intervention	inter	t #1	t #2	note	citation
TMT-A	DAT	10	8/2	74.10	placebo	12 w	132.29 (97.58)	140.86 (95.47)		McCaffrey, et al (1987)
TMT-A	DAT (CDR-1)	18	7/11	71.40 (4.40)	n/a	1 y	14.0 (7.7)	12.0 (34.1)	*	Botwinick, et al (1986)
TMT-A	Depression	33	14/19	37.40	antidepress	7 w	37.9 (21.0)	32.8 (14.4)		Fromm, et al (1984)
TMT-A	Depression	15	6/9	28.50 (10.6)	inpt tx	19.5 d	36.9 (8.9)	28.9 (8.2)		Goulet Fisher, et al (1986)
TMT-A	Depression w/ Melancholia	7	5/2	9.50	tricyclic antidepress	3 - 6 m	17.6 (5.8)	15.8 (1.5)		Stanton, et al (1981)
TMT-A	Depression	4	4/2	11.00	tricyclic antidepress	3 - 6 m	24.8 (21.0)	21.8 (11.3)		Stanton, et al (1981)
TMT-A	Diabetes	14	6/8	10.50	mild hypoglycemia	4-6 h	48.2 (17.6)	56.1 (7.2)		Reich, et al (1990)
TMT-A	Diabetes	10	5/5	12.20	hypoglycemia	4-6 h	49.6 (15.3)	42.3 (35.9)		Reich, et al (1990)
TMT-A	Dyspepsia	8	4/4	50.00	TDB	8 w	34.0	29.0	*	Nwokolo, et al (1994)
TMT-A	Dyspepsia	6	3/3	53.00	ranitidine	8 w	62.0	47.0	*	Nwokolo, et al (1994)
TMT-A	Epilepsy	17	7/10	27.44 (6.04)	meds	6-12 m	37.29 (18.21)	48.00 (26.83)	*	Dodrill, et al (1975)
TMT-A	Epilepsy	40	23/17	32.20 (8.20)	n/a	~9 m	33.35 (11.43)	31.10 (12.52)		Hermann, et al (1996)
TMT-A	Epilepsy	16	10/6	12.60	n/a	1 m	35.0 (12.0)	25.0 (9.0)		Pieters, et al (1992)

instrument	group	n	m/f	age	intervention	inter	t #1	t #2	note	citation
TMT-A	Epilepsy	23	11/12	26.80 (13.2)	carbamaz	6 m	34.9 (11.3)	33.3 (12.8)		Pulliainen, et al (1994)
TMT-A	Epilepsy	20	9/11	31.50 (11.3)	phenytoin	6 m	36.3 (10.7)	33.8 (11.4)		Pulliainen, et al (1994)
TMT-A	Epilepsy	18	n/a	20.30 (5.40)	stable WAIS on re-test	21.6 m	45.6 (16.9)	47.2 (17.9)		Seidenberg, et al (1981)
TMT-A	Epilepsy	21	n/a	22.30 (7.60)	improved WAIS re-test	20.5 m	39.4 (17.2)	32.6 (15.0)		Seidenberg, et al (1981)
TMT-A	Epilepsy	19	n/a	20.30 (4.30)	slightly improved WAIS re-test	20.1 m	40.3 (12.2)	34.0 (15.9)		Seidenberg, et al (1981)
TMT-A	Epilepsy (sz continued)	26	n/a	~21.0	n/a	20.7 m	42.54 (16.40)	42.85 (19.57)		Seidenberg, et al (1981)
TMT-A	Epilepsy (sz remitted)	24	n/a	~21.0	n/a	20.7 m	42.29 (17.10)	34.50 (15.46)		Seidenberg, et al (1981)
TMT-A	HD (at risk, + genetic marker)	8	1/7	26.20 (2.70)	n/a	2 y	28.0	28.0	*	Giordani, et al (1995)
TMT-A	HD (at risk, - genetic marker)	8	1/7	28.40 (5.20)	n/a	2 y	26.8	24.4	*	Giordani, et al (1995)
TMT-A	HIV+	46	n/a	~33.0	n/a	7.4 m	42.0 (19.0)	38.0 (17.0)		McKegney, et al (1990)
TMT-A	HIV+	69	51/18	34.70 (6.30)	n/a	6 m	35.7 (12.6)	32.1 (11.3)	*	Selnes, et al (1992)

instrument	group	n	m/f	age	intervention	inter	t #1	t #2	note	citation
TMT-A	HIV+ (asx)	19	10/19	30.30	n/a	4 y	37.6 (15.2)	39.2 (11.9)		Silberstein, et al (1993)
TMT-A	HIV+ (IVDU)	42	31/11	27.00 (5.30)	n/a	12 m	40.4 (12.0)	37.4 (11.0)		Bono, et al (1996)
TMT-A	HIV+ (IVDU)	18	10/8	29.80 (5.40)	drug tx	17.7 m	28.6 (9.3)	38.6 (11.2)		Hestad, et al (1996)
TMT-A	HIV+ (IVDU)	8	5/3	39.00 (8.00)	MSR/placebo	7 d	32.1 (8.7)	25.4 (6.0)	*	Van Dyck, et al (1997)
TMT-A	HIV+ (stage 2/3)	14	14/0	31.40 (8.54)	n/a	12.8 m	27.6 (7.3)	27.4 (7.1)		Burgess, et al (1994)
TMT-A	HIV+ (stage 4)	6	6/0	36.20 (7.60)	n/a	12.8 m	39.1 (23.2)	42.3 (9.1)		Burgess, et al (1994)
TMT-A	HIV+ (sx)	21	9/12	28.50	n/a	4y	42.1 (31.6)	46.9 (28.3)		Silberstein, et al (1993)
TMT-A	HIV+/ARC	8	8/0	33.57 (6.35)	n/a	18 m	28.71 (9.36)	26.86 (6.39)		Saykin, et al (1991)
TMT-A	HIV+/PGL	13	13/0	31.15 (4.91)	n/a	18 m	24.75 (6.15)	22.08 (5.09)		Saykin, et al (1991)
TMT-A	HIV-	41	41/0	31.50 (9.32)	n/a	12.8 m	28.6 (8.3)	26.4 (7.1)		Burgess, et al (1994)
TMT-A	HIV-	45	n/a	~33.0	n/a	7.4 m	38.0 (15.0)	37.0 (16.0)		McKegney, et al (1990)
TMT-A	HIV-	37	27/10	35.60 (7.10)	n/a	6 m	33.6 (11.7)	29.7 (10.1)	*	Selnes, et al (1992)
TMT-A	HIV-	81	45/36	29.70	n/a	4 y	37.3 (15.2)	36.9 (17.1)		Silberstein, et al (1993)

instrument	group	n	m/f	age	intervention	inter	t #1	t #2	note	citation
TMT-A	HIV- (IVDU)	39	30/9	28.60 (4.90)	n/a	12 m	39.4 (12.0)	37.1 (13.0)		Bono, et al (1996)
TMT-A	HIV- (IVDU)	30	16/14	27.90 (4.90)	drug tx	14.9 m	35.4 (11.7)	35.8 (11.4)		Hestad, et al (1996)
TMT-A	Hydroceph	14	9/5	66.00 (14.2)	extracranial shunting	27.37 w	151.67 (69.91)	135.33 (80.03)		Stambrook, et al (1988)
TMT-A	Hypertension	25	17/8	50.10 (14.0)	n/a	7-10 d	35.75 (12.81)	33.86 (14.98)		McCaffrey, et al (1992)
TMT-A	Hypertension	34	n/a	76.10	captopril	24 w	47.0 (22.0)	39.0 (17.0)		Starr, et al (1996)
TMT-A	Hypertension	35	n/a	76.10	bendrofluaz	24 w	47.0 (19.0)	42.0 (19.0)		Starr, et al (1996)
TMT-A	IVDU	16	13/3	39.50	n/a	10.4 d	42.06 (14.27)	39.75 (14.21)		Richards, et al (1992)
TMT-A	Korsakoff's Syndrome	10	9/1	63.00 (10.0)	fluvoxamine	3 w	46.0 (13.0)	43.0 (11.0)	*	Martin, et al (1995)
TMT-A	Left AVM	15	10/5	31.00 (11.0)	surgery	4 m	41.7 (17.5)	46.8 (19.8)	*	Stabell, et al (1994)
TMT-A	Liver Disease	62	23/39	39.20 (10.5)	liver transplant	60.1 w	35.4 (16.0)	32.5 (28.4)		Tarter, et al (1990)
TMT-A	Lung Cancer	14	12/2	63.00	chemotherapy	~5 d	50.5 (23.3)	45.2 (16.6)	*	Van Oosterhout, et al (1995)
TMT-A	Medical Inpts	20	20/0	45.60 (11.1)	n/a	22.9 d	49.1 (27.3)	41.1 (19.8)		Eckardt, et al (1981)
TMT-A	Medical Inpts	20	20/0	45.60 (11.1)	n/a	12-22 d	49.1 (27.3)	41.0 (19.8)		Eckardt, et al (1979)

instrument	group	n	m/f	age	intervention	inter	t #1	t #2	note	citation
TMT-A	MS & Fatigue	16	4/12	40.00 (6.40)	amantadine hydrochloride	6 w	37.6 (10.9)	30.9 (9.4)		Geisler, et al (1996)
TMT-A	MS & Fatigue	16	2/14	40.00 (5.60)	placebo	6 w	36.8 (15.2)	36.2 (14.2)		Geisler, et al (1996)
TMT-A	MS & Fatigue	13	4/9	41.00 (6.20)	pemoline	6 w	44.9 (17.6)	41.0 (18.5)		Geisler, et al (1996)
TMT-A	Naphtha Exposure	185	n/a	36.00	n/a	1 y	30.9 (10.4)	28.5 (9.2)		White, et al (1994)
TMT-A	Neurological	64	n/a	40.70 (16.7)	n/a	imm	51.1 (15)	49.0 (15.3)	A/C	Franzen, et al (1996)
TMT-A	Neuro-psychiatric	192	n/a	42.80 (16.6)	n/a	imm	47.3 (13.6)	41.4 (15.9)	A/C	Franzen, et al (1996)
TMT-A	Ocular Disease	50	27/23	42.00 (17.0)	steroid tx	~8 d	43.4 (24.3)	39.5 (21.1)		Naber, et al (1996)
TMT-A	Orthopedic	134	39/95	69.00	epidural anesthesia	1 w	53.3 (38.3)	-2.3 (23.0)c	*	Williams-Russo, et al (1995)
TMT-A	Orthopedic	128	38/90	69.00	general anesthesia	1 w	50.9 (33.9)	0.1 (15.2)c	*	Williams-Russo, et al (1995)
TMT-A	PD	4	3/1	53.50	fetal tissue implanted	12 m	81.1	67.5		Sass, et al (1995)
TMT-A	Psychiatric	64	n/a	43.60 (17.9)	n/a	imm	49.9 (14.7)	44.3 (14.9)	A/C	Franzen, et al (1996)
TMT-A	Psychiatric Inpts	12	12/0	40.17	n/a	4 w	36.50 (13.62)	30.08 (12.77)		Claiborn, et al (1981)
TMT-A	Psychiatric Inpts	231	83/148	30.70	ECT	4 - 5 w	40.6 (22.3)	37.8 (20.0)		Malloy, et al (1982)

instrument	group	n	m/f	age	intervention	inter	t #1	t #2	note	citation
TMT-A	Renal Disease	20	n/a	46.50 (11.3)	long-term hemodialysis	1 d	53.4 (18.5)	44.0 (11.7)	*	Ratner, et al (1983)
TMT-A	Renal Failure	9	4/5	65.00	rHuEpo	22.8 w	30.0	35.0		Temple, et al (1995)
TMT-A	Renal Failure	8	3/5	67.50	n/a	19.3 w	60.5	56.5		Temple, et al (1995)
TMT-A	Right AVM	16	5/11	34.00 (13.0)	surgery	4 m	33.9 (12.9)	38.8 (15.3)	*	Stabell, et al (1994)
TMT-A	Schizophrenia	10	8/2	71.00	risperidone	4 w	179.2 (93.0)	134.4 (86.8)		Berman, et al (1996)
TMT-A	Schizophrenia	10	10/0	34.80 (8.69)	clonidine	6 w	43.7 (24.54)	40.8 (27.71)		Fields, et al (1988)
TMT-A	Schizophrenia (acute)	39	24/15	28.60 (8.60)	n/a	1 y	38.9 (19.2)	32.6 (18.3)		Sweeney, et al (1991)
TMT-A	Schizophrenia (chronic)	35	n/a	47.00	n/a	52 w	56.17 (17.42)	45.97 (20.28)		Matarazzo, et al (1979)
TMT-A	Substance Abuse	64	n/a	44.30 (15.0)	n/a	imm	34.8 (13.3)	30.9 (13.7)	A/C	Franzen, et al (1996)
TMT-A	Substance Abuse Inpts (Black)	43	43/0	~29.0	n/a	7-10 d	33.65 (9.22)	31.71 (5.12)		McCaffrey, et al (1989)
TMT-A	Substance Abuse Inpts (Caucasian)	66	66/0	~29.0	n/a	7-10 d	28.58 (8.56)	28.79 (7.21)		McCaffrey, et al (1989)

instrument	group	n	m/f	age	intervention	inter	t #1	t #2	note	citation
TMT-A	Substance Abuse Inpts (Caucasian)	4	0/4	~29.0	n/a	7-10 d	35.36 (11.27)	28.0 (0.0)		McCaffrey, et al (1989)
TMT-A	Substance Abuse Inpts (Hispanic)	6	6/0	~29.0	n/a	7-10 d	24.50 (5.86)	23.33 (1.53)		McCaffrey, et al (1989)
TMT-A	Surgical	13	11/2	74.20 (6.70)	major surgery	6 d	45.9 (24.5)	41.8 (17.1)	*	Heyer, et al (1995)
TMT-A	Surgical	8	3/5	66.87	major surgery	6 w	49.8	54.0		King, et al (1977)
TMT-A	TBI	15	15/0	18.0 - 56.0	n/a	1-1.5 d	39.60 (15.07)	42.13 (16.91)	A/C	desRosiers, et al (1987)
TMT-A	TBI	31	20/11	24.16	n/a	12 m	64.0	30.0	*	Dikmen, et al (1990)
TMT-A	TBI	27	23/4	24.62	n/a	12 m	40.03	29.85		Dikmen, et al (1983)
TMT-A	TBI	18	15/3	26.10 (8.30)	rehab	7.5 m	60.8	45.3		Prigatano, et al (1984)
TMT-A	TBI	17	15/2	23.50 (5.10)	n/a	12.6 m	49.3	44.3		Prigatano, et al (1984)
TMT-A	TBI	26	20/6	30.90 (11.9)	n/a	1 w	34.1 (17.9)	30.8 (14.9)	*	Stuss, et al (1989)
TMT-A	TBI	22	15/7	29.50 (12.6)	n/a	6 d	25.9 (9.1)	21.3 (9.8)	*	Stuss, et al (1989)
TMT-A	TBI (sev)	15	13/2	24.80	n/a	11.5 m	95.6	35.6		Drudge, et al (1984)
TMT-A	TIA/CVA	34	34/0	60.30	CE	8-16 d	104.1	80.0		Cushman, et al (1984)

instrument	group	n	m/f	age	intervention	inter	t #1	t #2	note	citation
TMT-A	mild Toxic Enceph	14	n/a	40.10 (6.00)	"unimproved" at retest	15.9 m	36.0 (10.8)	37.3 (6.2)		Morrow, et al (1991)
TMT-A	mild Toxic Enceph	13	n/a	36.40 (10.3)	"improved" at retest	18.1 m	36.5 (12.7)	30.7 (9.9)		Morrow, et al (1991)
TMT-A	Whiplash	21	8/13	35.50 (10.5)	n/a	6 m	24.2 (9.8)	22.0 (13.3)	*	Di Stefano, et al (1995)
TMT-A	Whiplash	58	26/32	29.60 (8.90)	n/a	6 m	23.6 (8.7)	20.7 (7.3)		Di Stefano, et al (1996)
TMT-A	Whiplash (asx at 6 mos)	67	28/36	29.00 (8.50)	n/a	6 m	22.7 (7.8)	20.4 (7.2)		Radanov, et al (1993)
TMT-A	Whiplash (sx at 6 mos)	31	9/19	36.50 (10.2)	n/a	6 m	26.3 (9.7)	23.3 (8.7)		Radanov, et al (1993)
TMT-A	Whiplash w/ continuing sx	21	8/13	35.40 (11.0)	n/a	6 m	27.0 (9.6)	26.2 (9.9)	*	Di Stefano, et al (1995)
TMT-A	Whiplash w/ continuing sx	28	9/19	34.10 (10.2)	n/a	6 m	25.6 (8.5)	22.8 (9.3)		Di Stefano, et al (1996)
TMT-A (errors)	Cardiac	245	198/47	54.70	CABG/cardiac operation	6 m	0.16 (0.51)	0.140 (0.413)		Savageau, et al (1982a)
TMT-A (errors)	Cardiac	227	184/43	54.50	cardiac operation	10-12 d	0.17 (0.53)	0.23 (0.54)		Savageau, et al (1982b)
TMT-A (errors)	Control	16	10/6	12.60	n/a	1 m	0.21 (0.23)	0.12 (0.16)		Pieters, et al (1992)
TMT-A (errors)	Epilepsy	16	10/6	12.60	n/a	1 m	0.11 (0.17)	0.10 (0.12)		Pieters, et al (1992)
TMT-A (errors)	IVDU	16	13/3	39.50	n/a	10.4 d	0.0 (0.0)	0.12 (0.34)		Richards, et al (1992)

instrument	group	n	m/f	age	intervention	inter	t #1	t #2	note	citation
TMT-A (errors)	Naphtha Exposure	185	n/a	36.00	n/a	1 y	0.20 (0.51)	0.11 (0.38)		White, et al (1994)
TMT-A (t)	ALL	31	16/15	8.38 (3.19)	n/a	2.0 y	50.2 (11.3)	50.3 (14.5)		Berg, et al (1983)
TMT-A (t)	ALL w/ Somnolence	48	27/21	8.63 (3.15)	n/a	2.25 y	49.7 (23.1)	46.7 (11.8)		Berg, et al (1983)
TMT-A (t)	Lung Cancer	11	n/a	~61.0	cranial irradiation	11 m	30.0	28.3		Komaki, et al (1995)
TMT-B	AIDS	10	10/0	41.70 (5.50)	n/a	6.53 m	105.6 (46.7)	89.9 (22.5)		Hinkin, et al (1995)
TMT-B	AIDS Dementia Complex	30	29/1	33.80	zdv	6 m	192.2 (129.8)	161.1 (108.5)		Tozzi, et al (1993)
TMT-B	Alcohol Dependent	15	15/0	43.13 (11.5)	n/a	3 w	80.33 (20.09)	79.73 (20.23)		Roehrich, et al (1993)
TMT-B	Alcohol Dependent	16	16/0	42.38 (10.6)	placebo	3 w	72.75 (21.75)	69.37 (18.44)		Roehrich, et al (1993)
TMT-B	Alcohol Dependent	15	15/0	42.07 (10.9)	ecological remediation	3 w	99.8 (35.25)	71.46 (37.94)		Roehrich, et al (1993)
TMT-B	Alcohol Dependent	15	15/0	42.07 (9.80)	neuropsych remediation	3 w	85.73 (46.14)	53.0 (15.9)		Roehrich, et al (1993)
TMT-B	Alcoholic	24	24/0	51.00 (6.38)	inpt tx	12-16 m	112.8 (61.56)	96.9 (47.09)		O'Leary, et al (1977)
TMT-B	Alcoholic (1 yr abstin)	23	23/0	36.80 (6.30)	n/a	1 y	63.3	67.9		Adams, et al (1980)

instrument	group	n	m/f	age	intervention	inter	t #1	t #2	note	citation
TMT-B	Alcoholic (2.5 yrs abstin)	25	25/0	36.50 (6.30)	n/a	1 y	57.2	67.3		Adams, et al (1980)
TMT-B	Alcoholic (detoxed)	17	n/a	44.47	abstin	1 y	5.06 (6.13)	5.71 (4.43)		Long, et al (1974)
TMT-B	Alcoholic Inpts	25	25/0	44.84	n/a	4 w	130.96 (61.91)	132.64 (79.48)		Claiborn, et al (1981)
TMT-B	Alcoholic Inpts	91	91/0	42.20 (10.0)	n/a	16.8 d	97.3 (35.5)	81.6 (35.4)		Eckardt, et al (1981)
TMT-B	Alcoholic Inpts	91	91/0	42.20 (10.0)	n/a	12-22 d	97.3 (45.5)	80.7 (34.6)		Eckardt, et al (1979)
TMT-B	Alcoholic Inpts	27	27/0	50.40 (6.22)	n/a	14 m	90.0 (39.2)	-18.8 (30.6)c		Schau, et al (1980)
TMT-B	Anorexia	18	0/18	n/a	refeeding tx	69.8 d	56.9 (12.8)	46.8 (15.4)		Szmukler, et al (1992)
TMT-B	Brain Tumor	7	4/3	9.83	radiotherapy	11 m	3.0 (7.6)	6.8 (4.2)		Bordeaux, et al (1988)
TMT-B	Brain Tumor	7	3/4	10.33	surgery	1 m	0.8 (7.2)	3.2 (7.0)		Bordeaux, et al (1988)
TMT-B	Breast Cancer	20	3/17	39.28 (9.38)	ABMT	~12 d	79.7 (28.6)	103.4 (38.6)		Ahles, et al (1996)
TMT-B	Cardiac	22	10/12	47.30 (14.0)	open heart surgery	8.4 d	65.4 (14.8)	65.2 (14.2)	*	Heyer, et al (1995)
TMT-B	Cardiac	33	19/14	73.10 (5.50)	open heart surgery	8.4 d	101.4 (23.5)	144.3 (47.3)	*	Heyer, et al (1995)

instrument	group	n	m/f	age	intervention	inter	t #1	t #2	note	citation
TMT-B	Cardiac	135	120/15	55.40	CABG	3 m	86.4	84.6	*	Klonoff, et al (1989)
TMT-B	Cardiac	17	12/5	50.00 (10.5)	heart transplant	36.0 m	79.0 (26.68)	79.0 (27.61)		Roman, et al (1997)
TMT-B	Cardiac	245	198/47	54.70	CABG/cardiac operation	6 m	98.53 (40.71)	87.52 (44.58)		Savageau, et al (1982)
TMT-B	Cardiac	227	184/43	54.50	cardiac operation	10-12 d	99.86 (41.67)	119.68 (75.27)		Savageau, et al (1982)
TMT-B	Cardiac	90	77/13	59.00 (10.6)	CABG/CPB	8 d	97.0 (43.2)	140.3 (80.8)	*	Townes, et al (1989)
TMT-B	CAD	20	n/a	57.20 (7.20)	CE	6 m	161.2	146.9		Parker, et al (1983)
TMT-B	CAD	17	n/a	57.20 (7.20)	n/a	6 m	190.6	154.3		Parker, et al (1983)
TMT-B	CAD	36	n./a	61.10 (8.30)	CE	6 m	160.2	140.7	*	Parker, et al (1986)
TMT-B	CAD	17	n/a	57.90 (8.40)	n/a	6 m	175.3	128.9	*	Parker, et al (1986)
TMT-B	Carotid Artery Occlusion	11	3/8	65.27	CE	6 w	242.0	193.4		King, et al (1977)
TMT-B	CVD	15	n/a	60.32 (4.02)	RCE	2-3 m	224.23 (156.9)	158.92 (134.4)		Greiffenstein, et al (1988)
TMT-B	CVD	15	n/a	59.76 (3.74)	n/a	2 w	167.62 (83.29)	189.38 (144.1)		Greiffenstein, et al (1988)

instrument	group	n	m/f	age	intervention	inter	t #1	t #2	note	citation
TMT-B	CVD	15	n/a	60.00 (4.57)	LCE	2-3 m	205.62 (84.98)	185.00 (78.54)		Greiffenstein, et al (1988)
TMT-B	CVD	17	15/2	62.00	CE	20w	174.33 (67.23)	178.53 (91.25)		Matarazzo, et al (1979)
TMT-B	CVD	16	n/a	60.00	n/a	12w	146.36 (10.46)	158.66 (11.12)		Matarazzo, et al (1979)
TMT-B	Control	21	21/0	36.90 (5.90)	n/a	1 y	65.6	57.0		Adams, et al (1980)
TMT-B	Control	23	9/14	32.30 (10.3)	n/a	3 w	52.1 (15.1)	47.4 (16.5)		Bornstein, et al (1987)
TMT-B	Control	63	8/55	56.22 (11.0)	n/a	~6 m	NR	-10.06 (20.13) c		Bruggemans, et al (1997)
TMT-B	Control	25	25/0	28.68	n/a	4 w	65.72 (18.27)	60.96 (22.32)		Claiborn, et al (1981)
TMT-B	Control	11	9/2	31.60 (5.00)	n/a	6 m	57.3 (15.2)	49.8 (17.1)		Di Stefano, et al (1996)
TMT-B	Control	102	65/37	24.52	n/a	12 m	48.0	45.0	*	Dikmen, et al (1990)
TMT-B	Control	101	101/0	78.50 (7.20)	n/a	2.6 y	125.0	114.5		Frank, et al (1996)
TMT-B	Control	141	0/141	78.50 (6.60)	n/a	2.7 y	135.1	120.4		Frank, et al (1996)
TMT-B	Control	102	~69/ 33	~26.0	n/a	12 m	48.0	45.0		Fraser, et al (1988)

instrument	group	n	m/f	age	intervention	inter	t #1	t #2	note	citation
TMT-B	Control	1017	436/581	74.30 (5.40)	n/a	2 y	132.3 (64.7)	147.6 (72.2)		Ganguli, et al (1996)
TMT-B	Control	20	0/20	29.10 (4.70)	n/a	1 m	38.0 (11.6)	33.3 (10.7)	*	Harris, et al (1996)
TMT-B	Control	4	0/4	67.30 (0.50)	placebo	60 min	71.5 (20.0)	92.2 (25.4)	B/D	Kirkby, et al (1995)
TMT-B	Control	5	1/4	68.40 (6.10)	lorazepam	60 min	93.9 (34.2)	135.8 (26.2)	B/D	Kirkby, et al (1995)
TMT-B	Control	9	4/5	26.40 (7.70)	lorazepam	60 min	56.8 (19.8)	64.6 (20.6)	B/D	Kirkby, et al (1995)
TMT-B	Control	8	4/4	21.80 (4.20)	placebo	60 min	67.0 (30.5)	59.4 (22.8)	B/D	Kirkby, et al (1995)
TMT-B	Control	110	110/0	19.30 (1.30)	n/a	~3 m	51.4 (15.3)	41.1 (13.7)		Macciocchi (1990)
TMT-B	Control	29	29/0	24.00	n/a	20w	54.17 (12.54)	51.28 (12.29)		Matarazzo, et al (1979)
TMT-B	Control	33	15/18	59.10 (9.30)	n/a	10 d	88.0 (25.9)	75.5 (24.0)		McCaffrey, et al (1993)
TMT-B	Control	20	18/2	26.00	hypoglycemia	2 w	26.70 (8.61)	29.85 (10.26)		McCrimmon, et al (1996)
TMT-B	Control	20	18/2	26.00	euglycemia	2 w	28.20 (12.58)	25.80 (11.60)		McCrimmon, et al (1996)
TMT-B	Control	19	2/17	62.20 (2.50)	n/a	1 y	85.3 (28.9)	87.5 (38.5)	*	Mitrushina, et al (1991b)

instrument	group	n	m/f	age	intervention	inter	t #1	t #2	note	citation
TMT-B	Control	40	6/34	68.20 (1.20)	n/a	1 y	94.6 (37.4)	85.0 (31.6)	*	Mitrushina, et al (1991b)
TMT-B	Control	47	14/33	72.90 (1.40)	n/a	1 y	102.3 (41.0)	99.6 (35.3)	*	Mitrushina, et al (1991b)
TMT-B	Control	16	4/12	78.30 (2.50)	n/a	1 y	133.7 (58.0)	122.6 (52.0)	*	Mitrushina, et al (1991b)
TMT-B	Control	26	n/a	~9.00	n/a	~6 m	NR	-8.78 c	*	Neyens, et al (1996)
TMT-B	Control	12	12/0	31.50	hypoxia	15 min	35.7	52.7		Noble, et al (1993)
TMT-B	Control	12	12/0	31.60	n/a	15 min	47.4	34.5		Noble, et al (1993)
TMT-B	Control	20	20/0	49.90 (7.34)	n/a	12-16 m	65.4 (18.59)	64.6 (16.36)		O'Leary, et al (1977)
TMT-B	Control	16	10/6	12.60	n/a	1 m	76.0 (47.0)	42.0 (21.0)		Pieters, et al (1992)
TMT-B	Control	21	3/18	30.10 (8.20)	n/a	6 m	69.7 (18.1)	61.9 (14.0)		Pulliainen, et al (1994)
TMT-B	Control	14	6/8	11.20	n/a	4-6 h	56.6 (7.7)	62.3 (4.3)		Reich, et al (1990)
TMT-B	Control	21	21/0	31.45 (5.53)	n/a	18 m	49.25 (13.76)	46.70 (16.21)		Saykin, et al (1991)
TMT-B	Control	27	27/0	49.50	n/a	14 m	69.0 (38.67)	2.1 (32.7)c		Schau, et al (1980)
TMT-B	Control	30	16/14	22.43 (2.67)	n/a	1 w	48.77 (18.66)	42.18 (15.54)		Stuss, et al (1988)

instrument	group	n	m/f	age	intervention	inter	t #1	t #2	note	citation
TMT-B	Control	30	14/16	61.77 (3.00)	n/a	1 w	76.97 (30.52)	67.10 (28.37)		Stuss, et al (1988)
TMT-B	Control	30	14/16	40.63 (2.97)	n/a	1 w	61.30 (17.88)	61.52 (22.79)		Stuss, et al (1988)
TMT-B	Control	10	5/5	63.70 (3.13)	n/a	1 w	73.3 (20.3)	67.3 (23.2)		Stuss, et al (1987)
TMT-B	Control	10	5/5	17.30 (0.95)	n/a	1 w	49.0 (21.1)	41.8 (13.1)		Stuss, et al (1987)
TMT-B	Control	10	6/4	23.00 (2.67)	n/a	1 w	41.6 (11.4)	34.0 (12.7)		Stuss, et al (1987)
TMT-B	Control	10	5/5	33.90 (2.88)	n/a	1 w	46.3 (13.7)	46.8 (11.4)		Stuss, et al (1987)
TMT-B	Control	10	6/4	55.30 (2.98)	n/a	1 w	83.1 (44.3)	71.4 (41.3)		Stuss, et al (1987)
TMT-B	Control	10	6/4	44.20 (3.12)	n/a	1 w	64.1 (16.3)	64.4 (23.0)		Stuss, et al (1987)
TMT-B	Control	22	15/7	27.70 (11.6)	n/a	6 d	47.4 (16.5)	38.5 (11.0)	*	Stuss, et al (1989)
TMT-B	Control	26	20/6	29.70 (12.4)	n/a	1 w	53.4 (20.6)	44.6 (17.7)	*	Stuss, et al (1989)
TMT-B	Control	18	0/18	n/a	n/a	108.4 d	48.3 (10.7)	42.5 (9.1)		Szmukler, et al (1992)
TMT-B	Control	38	18/20	35.70 (10.5)	n/a	54.7 w	50.8 (12.7)	50.0 (12.7)		Tarter, et al (1990)
TMT-B	Control	47	35/12	59.00 (9.81)	n/a	8 d	79.9 (33.9)	75.5 (46.1)	*	Townes, et al (1989)

instrument	group	n	m/f	age	intervention	inter	t #1	t #2	note	citation
TMT-B	Control (overweight)	24	24/0	40.70 (8.30)	placebo	8 w	25.0 (12.6)	22.6 (9.1)		Hatsukami, et al (1986)
TMT-B	Control (overweight)	26	26/0	37.20 (4.80)	naltrexone	8 w	29.5 (12.3)	24.0 (8.8)		Hatsukami, et al (1986)
TMT-B	Control (Clinic/ Volunteer)	15	5/10	33.90 (8.40)	n/a	20.7 d	55.3 (26.4)	56.6 (25.4)		Goulet Fisher, et al (1986)
TMT-B	Coronary Artery Disease	298	264/ 34	53.40 (7.40)	CABG	9.4 d	116.7 (46.0)	140.0 (86.9)		Shaw, et al (1986)
TMT-B	Crohn's Disease	22	9/13	37.30 (10.6)	std tx	62.6 w	67.4 (26.4)	69.2 (30.8)		Tarter, et al (1990)
TMT-B	DAT	34	34/0	83.90 (4.30)	n/a	2.1 y	216.0	248.6		Frank, et al (1996)
TMT-B	DAT	34	34/0	83.90 (4.30)	n/a	2.1 y	216.2	233.2		Frank, et al (1996)
TMT-B	DAT	10	6/4	74.30	suloctidil 450 mg	12 w	510.0 (180.0)	405.5 (236.1)		McCaffrey, et al (1987)
TMT-B	DAT	10	8/2	74.10	placebo	12 w	175.9 (59.8)	285.3 (220.7)		McCaffrey, et al (1987)
TMT-B	DAT	10	5/5	74.90	suloctidil 600 mg	12 w	238.3 (129.8)	246.2 (147.7)		McCaffrey, et al (1987)
TMT-B	DAT (at risk)	50	0/50	84.10 (5.10)	n/a	2.3 y	215.3	203.9		Frank, et al (1996)
TMT-B	DAT (at risk)	32	32/0	83.30 (6.70)	n/a	2.0 y	175.8	155.9		Frank, et al (1996)

instrument	group	n	m/f	age	intervention	inter	t #1	t #2	note	citation
TMT-B	DAT (mild)	11	10/1	63.00 (8.00)	n/a	26 m	192.0 (155.0)	281.0 (182.0)		Haxby, et al (1990)
TMT-B	Depression	33	14/19	37.40	antidepress	7 w	89.9 (52.1)	75.9 (37.2)		Fromm, et al (1984)
TMT-B	Depression	15	6/9	28.50 (10.6)	inpt tx	19.5 d	90.2 (46.9)	66.9 (25.9)		Goulet Fisher, et al (1986)
TMT-B	Depression w/ Melancholia	7	5/2	9.50	tricyclic antidepress	3 - 6 m	45.0 (10.4)	39.8 (12.0)		Stanton, et al (1981)
TMT-B	Depression w/o Melancholia	4	4/2	11.00	tricyclic antidepress	3 - 6 m	63.0 (41.6)	56.0 (43.2)		Stanton, et al (1981)
TMT-B	Diabetes	10	5/5	12.20	hypoglycemia	4-6 h	48.5 (12.9)	45.5 (19.9)		Reich, et al (1990)
TMT-B	Diabetes	14	6/8	10.50	mild hypoglycemia	4-6 h	47.5 (13.5)	57.0 (6.7)		Reich, et al (1990)
TMT-B	Dyspepsia	6	3/3	53.00	ranitidine	8 w	116.0	102.0	*	Nwokolo, et al (1994)
TMT-B	Dyspepsia	8	4/4	50.00	TDB	8 w	57.0	59.0	*	Nwokolo, et al (1994)
TMT-B	Epilepsy	17	7/10	27.44 (6.04)	meds	6-12 m	111.6 (88.3)	192.1 (149.2)	*	Dodrill, et al (1975)
TMT-B	Epilepsy	40	23/17	32.20 (8.20)	n/a	~9 m	77.95 (35.10)	81.26 (50.07)		Hermann, et al (1996)
TMT-B	Epilepsy	16	10/6	12.60	n/a	1 m	82.0 (35.0)	65.0 (31.0)		Pieters, et al (1992)
TMT-B	Epilepsy	20	9/11	31.50 (11.3)	phenytoin	6 m	85.5 (41.8)	83.1 (41.3)		Pulliainen, et al (1994)

instrument	group	n	m/f	age	intervention	inter	t #1	t #2	note	citation
TMT-B	Epilepsy	23	11/12	26.80 (13.2)	carbamaz	6 m	78.6 (28.6)	76.1 (26)		Pulliainen, et al (1994)
TMT-B	Epilepsy	19	n/a	20.30 (4.30)	slightly improved WAIS re-test	20.1 m	95.8 (42.9)	80.4 (48.8)		Seidenberg, et al (1981)
TMT-B	Epilepsy	18	n/a	20.30 (5.40)	stable WAIS on re-test	21.6 m	121.4 (65.1)	142.5 (79.1)		Seidenberg, et al (1981)
TMT-B	Epilepsy	21	n/a	22.30 (7.60)	improved WAIS re-test	20.5 m	123.2 (89.4)	97.9 (80.5)		Seidenberg, et al (1981)
TMT-B	Epilepsy (sz continued)	26	n/a	~21.0	n/a	20.7 m	116.58 (79.24)	123.54 (80.76)		Seidenberg, et al (1981)
TMT-B	Epilepsy (sz remitted)	24	n/a	~21.0	n/a	20.7 m	122.63 (66.33)	102.79 (73.73)		Seidenberg, et al (1981)
TMT-B	HD	40	18/22	40.00 (10.3)	n/a	12 m	205.0 (22.0)	258.0 (27.0)		Bamford, et al (1995)
TMT-B	HD	26	12/14	39.00 (10.4)	n/a	12 m	187.0 (24.0)	255.0 (34.0)		Bamford, et al (1995)
TMT-B	HD (at risk, + genetic marker)	8	1/7	26.20 (2.70)	n/a	2 y	45.1	47.9	*	Giordani, et al (1995)
TMT-B	HD (at risk, - genetic marker)	8	1/7	28.40 (5.20)	n/a	2 y	55.5	52.1	*	Giordani, et al (1995)
TMT-B	Hematologic D/O	14	2/12	39.28 (9.38)	ABMT	~12 d	73.3 (20.3)	79.7 (25.8)		Ahles, et al (1996)

instrument	group	n	m/f	age	intervention	inter	t #1	t #2	note	citation
TMT-B	HIV+	46	n/a	~33.0	n/a	7.4 m	110.0 (58.0)	110.0 (76.0)		McKegney, et al (1990)
TMT-B	HIV+	69	51/18	34.70 (6.30)	n/a	6 m	104.3 (49.4)	85.4 (33.6)	*	Selnes, et al (1992)
TMT-B	HIV+ (asx)	19	10/19	30.30	n/a	4y	117.8 (52.7)	124.4 (50.8)		Silberstein, et al (1993)
TMT-B	HIV+ (IVDU)	42	31/11	27.00 (5.30)	n/a	12 m	112.5 (40.0)	99.1 (39.0)		Bono, et al (1996)
TMT-B	HIV+ (IVDU)	8	5/3	39.00 (8.00)	MSR/placebo	7 d	100.9 (48.4)	85.1 (37.3)	*	Van Dyck, et al (1997)
TMT-B	HIV+ (stage 2/3)	14	14/0	31.40 (8.54)	n/a	12.8 m	60.8 (16.8)	67.2 (22.3)		Burgess, et al (1994)
TMT-B	HIV+ (stage 4)	6	6/0	36.20 (7.60)	n/a	12.8 m	101.0 (44.3)	89.2 (36.8)		Burgess, et al (1994)
TMT-B	HIV+ (sx)	21	9/12	28.50	n/a	4y	101.4 (33.4)	118.0 (42.9)		Silberstein, et al (1993)
TMT-B	HIV+/ARC	8	8/0	33.57 (6.35)	n/a	18 m	69.43 (23.39)	78.71 (16.94)		Saykin, et al (1991)
TMT-B	HIV+/PGL	13	13/0	31.15 (4.91)	n/a	18 m	63.92 (26.42)	63.31 (29.92)		Saykin, et al (1991)
TMT-B	HIV-	41	41/0	31.50 (9.32)	n/a	12.8 m	63.5 (25.2)	60.9 (19.6)		Burgess, et al (1994)
TMT-B	HIV-	45	n/a	~33.0	n/a	7.4 m	110.0 (46.0)	93.0 (46.0)		McKegney, et al (1990)
TMT-B	HIV-	37	27/10	35.60 (7.10)	n/a	6 m	96.8 (49.3)	85.5 (39.9)	*	Selnes, et al (1992)

instrument	group	n	m/f	age	intervention	inter	t #1	t #2	note	citation
TMT-B	HIV-	81	45/36	29.70	n/a	4 y	107.9 (46.3)	96.6 (36.7)		Silberstein, et al (1993)
TMT-B	HIV- (IVDU)	39	30/9	28.60 (4.90)	n/a	12 m	104.1 (35.0)	95.6 (31.0)		Bono, et al (1996)
TMT-B	Hydroceph	14	9/5	66.00 (14.2)	extracranial shunting	27.37 w	402.0 (89.31)	419.25 (30.7)		Stambrook, et al (1988)
TMT-B	Hypertension	25	17/8	50.10 (14.0)	n/a	7-10 d	91.6 (49.8)	87.1 (53.0)		McCaffrey, et al (1992)
TMT-B	IVDU	16	13/3	39.50	n/a	10.4 d	105.79 (42.98)	98.73 (40.44)		Richards, et al (1992)
TMT-B	Left AVM	15	10/5	31.00 (11.0)	surgery	4 m	104.6 (55.5)	120.8 (74.2)	*	Stabell, et al (1994)
TMT-B	Liver Disease	62	23/39	39.20 (10.5)	liver transplant	60.1 w	84.3 (40.4)	73.5 (43.2)		Tarter, et al (1990)
TMT-B	Lung Cancer	14	12/2	63.00	chemotherapy	~5 d	77.0 (26.4)	75.4 (30.4)	*	Van Oosterhout, et al (1995)
TMT-B	Medical Inpts	20	20/0	45.60 (11.1)	n/a	22.9 d	130.4 (89.2)	116.8 (69.1)		Eckardt, et al (1981)
TMT-B	Medical Inpts	20	20/0	45.60 (11.1)	n/a	12-22 d	130.4 (89.2)	116.8 (69.1)		Eckardt, et al (1979)
TMT-B	MS & Fatigue	13	4/9	41.00 (6.20)	pemoline	6 w	103.5 (33.6)	94.4 (60.0)		Geisler, et al (1996)
TMT-B	MS & Fatigue	16	2/14	40.00 (5.60)	placebo	6 w	92.1 (30.1)	83.1 (29.2)		Geisler, et al (1996)
TMT-B	MS & Fatigue	16	4/12	40.00 (6.40)	amantadine hydrochloride	6 w	73.3 (32.0)	68.9 (31.2)		Geisler, et al (1996)

instrument	group	n	m/f	age	intervention	inter	t #1	t #2	note	citation
TMT-B	Naphtha Exposure	185	n/a	36.00	n/a	1 y	75.7 (39.5)	74.8 (45.8)		White, et al (1994)
TMT-B	Neurological	64	n/a	40.70 (16.7)	n/a	imm	161.3 (60.3)	124.4 (53.4)	B/D	Franzen, et al (1996)
TMT-B	Neuro-psychiatric	192	n/a	42.80 (16.6)	n/a	imm	147.5 (48.3)	140.4 (51.2)	B/D	Franzen, et al (1996)
TMT-B	Ocular Disease	50	27/23	42.00 (17.0)	steroid tx	~8 d	90.4 (40.0)	87.0 (32.3)		Naber, et al (1996)
TMT-B	Orthopedic	134	39/95	69.00	epidural anesthesia	1 w	124.4 (77.2)	1.2 (44.4)c	*	Williams-Russo, et al (1995)
TMT-B	Orthopedic	128	38/90	69.00	general anesthesia	1 w	131.5 (79.0)	7.2 (50.0)c	*	Williams-Russo, et al (1995)
TMT-B	PD	18	11/7	56.90 (8.90)	selegiline	12 w	159.0 (71.0)	132.0 (34.0)		Hietanen (1991)
TMT-B	PD	18	11/7	56.90 (8.90)	placebo	12 w	135.0 (50.0)	180.0 (126.0)		Hietanen (1991)
TMT-B	PD	4	3/1	53.50	fetal tissue implanted	12 m	152.3	200.3		Sass, et al (1995)
TMT-B	PVD	50	36/14	57.40 (6.40)	major surgery	7.5 d	112.8 (37.0)	108.1 (35.0)		Shaw, et al (1987)
TMT-B	Pregnant	20	0/20	29.00 (4.60)	normal delivery	1 m	41.2 (12.7)	38.6 (10.7)	*	Harris, et al (1996)
TMT-B	Psychiatric	64	n/a	43.60 (17.9)	n/a	imm	151.4 (59.6)	137.8 (75.8)	B/D	Franzen, et al (1996)
TMT-B	Psychiatric Inpts	12	12/0	40.17	n/a	4 w	102.58 (59.86)	76.83 (37.44)		Claiborn, et al (1981)

instrument	group	n	m/f	age	intervention	inter	t #1	t #2	note	citation
TMT-B	Psychiatric Inpts	231	83/ 148	30.70	ECT	4 - 5 w	136.2 (125.0)	104.9 (83.5)		Malloy, et al (1982)
TMT-B	Right AVM	16	5/11	34.00 (13.0)	surgery	4 m	73.7 (24.6)	81.3 (25.5)	*	Stabell, et al (1994)
TMT-B	Schizophrenia	10	10/0	34.80 (8.69)	clonidine	6 w	122.8 (69.26)	82.1 (39.15)		Fields, et al (1988)
TMT-B	Schizophrenia	15	10/5	35.00	std neuroleptics	~15 m	123.0 (51.1)	124.9 (46.2)		Goldberg, et al (1993)
TMT-B	Schizophrenia (acute)	39	24/15	28.60 (8.60)	n/a	1 y	90.1 (53.7)	71.3 (36.2)		Sweeney, et al (1991)
TMT-B	Schizophrenia (chronic)	35	n/a	47.00	n/a	52w	152.57 (93.76)	150.83 (87.28)		Matarazzo, et al (1979)
TMT-B	Schizophrenia Inpts	35	29/6	23.71 (4.50)	neuroleptics	1-2 y	119.6 (46.5)	97.8 (39.2)		Nopoulos, et al (1994)
TMT-B	Substance Abuse	15	8/7	21.10 (4.50)	outpt tx	4 w	81.0 (20.5)	70.2 (23.4)		Cosgrove, et al (1991)
TMT-B	Substance Abuse	64	n/a	44.30 (15.0)	n/a	imm	129.8 (61.4)	124.4 (58.6)	B/D	Franzen, et al (1996)
TMT-B	Substance Abuse (PCP)	15	8/7	21.10 (4.50)	outpt tx	4 w	99.2 (35.2)	79.7 (23.4)		Cosgrove, et al (1991)
TMT-B	Substance Abuse Inpts (Black)	43	43/0	~29.0	n/a	7-10 d	91.91 (30.88)	85.18 (25.23)		McCaffrey, et al (1989)
TMT-B	Substance Abuse Inpts (Black)	3	0/3	~29.0	n/a	7-10 d	92.00 (8.72)	83.33 (21.55)		McCaffrey, et al (1989)

instrument	group	n	m/f	age	intervention	inter	t #1	t #2	note	citation
TMT-B	Substance Abuse Inpts (Caucasian)	66	66/0	~29.0	n/a	7-10 d	72.85 (28.06)	66.26 (24.88)		McCaffrey, et al (1989)
TMT-B	Substance Abuse Inpts (Caucasian)	4	0/4	~29.0	n/a	7-10 d	88.18 (26.14)	63.27 (17.58)		McCaffrey, et al (1989)
TMT-B	Substance Abuse Inpts (Hispanic)	6	6/0	~29.0	n/a	7-10 d	73.83 (11.43)	62.50 (18.52)		McCaffrey, et al (1989)
TMT-B	Surgical	13	11/2	74.20 (6.70)	major surgery	6 d	94.6 (39.5)	93.7 (64.0)	*	Heyer, et al (1995)
TMT-B	Surgical	8	3/5	66.87	major surgery	6 w	182.0	202.3		King, et al (1977)
TMT-B	Surgical	17	n/a	57.20 (7.20)	surgery	6 m	110.0	93.0		Parker, et al (1983)
TMT-B	Surgical	26	n/a	55.30 (6.80)	surgery (non-CE)	6 m	97.7	91.4	*	Parker, et al (1986)
TMT-B	TBI	15	15/0	18.0 - 56.0	n/a	1-1.5 d	120.47 (53.69)	102.93 (52.52)	B/D	desRosiers, et al (1987)
TMT-B	TBI	31	20/11	24.16	n/a	12 m	140.0	66.0	*	Dikmen, et al (1990)
TMT-B	TBI	27	23/4	24.62	n/a	12 m	87.66	71.37		Dikmen, et al (1983)
TMT-B	TBI	18	15/3	26.10 (8.30)	rehab	7.5 m	163.2	133.2		Prigatano, et al (1984)
TMT-B	TBI	17	15/2	23.50 (5.10)	n/a	12.6 m	125.8	110.4		Prigatano, et al (1984)
TMT-B	TBI	26	20/6	30.90 (11.9)	n/a	1 w	79.8 (29.0)	77.4 (38.5)	*	Stuss, et al (1989)

instrument	group	n	m/f	age	intervention	inter	t #1	t #2	note	citation
TMT-B	TBI	22	15/7	29.50 (12.6)	n/a	6 d	64.3 (42.2)	49.5 (25.3)	*	Stuss, et al (1989)
TMT-B	TBI (did not return to work)	13	3/10	24.00	n/a	12 m	101.0	67.0		Fraser, et al (1988)
TMT-B	TBI (returned to work)	35	26/9	29.00	n/a	12 m	66.0	56.0		Fraser, et al (1988)
TMT-B	TBI (in litigation)	20	14/6	41.85 (10.2)	n/a	14.45 m	118.25 (64.55)	153.50 (79.96)		Reitan, et al (1996)
TMT-B	TBI (not in litigation)	20	17/3	29.65 (14.9)	n/a	12.00 m	109.00 (63.91)	89.40 (53.76)		Reitan, et al (1996)
TMT-B	TBI (sev)	15	13/2	24.80	n/a	11.5 m	192.3	77.2		Drudge, et al (1984)
TMT-B	TIA/CVA	34	34/0	60.30	CE	8-16 d	232.3	222.2		Cushman, et al (1984)
TMT-B	mild Toxic Enceph	13	n/a	36.40 (10.3)	"improved" at retest	18.1 m	106.8 (45.9)	72.3 (21.6)		Morrow, et al (1991)
TMT-B	mild Toxic Enceph	14	n/a	40.10 (6.00)	"unimproved" at retest	15.9 m	91.0 (33.7)	108.0 (38.8)		Morrow, et al (1991)
TMT-B	Whiplash	21	8/13	35.50 (10.5)	n/a	6 m	67.1 (27.6)	61.0 (21.3)	*	Di Stefano, et al (1995)
TMT-B	Whiplash	58	26/32	29.60 (8.90)	n/a	6 m	71.1 (30.8)	62.0 (23.7)		Di Stefano, et al (1996)
TMT-B	Whiplash (asx at 6 mos)	67	28/36	29.00 (8.50)	n/a	6 m	69.8 (31.2)	59.9 (23.4)		Radanov, et al (1993)

instrument	group	n	m/f	age	intervention	inter	t #1	t #2	note	citation
TMT-B	Whiplash (sx at 6 mos)	31	9/19	36.50 (10.2)	n/a	6 m	74.0 (23.5)	69.3 (24.4)		Radanov, et al (1993)
TMT-B	Whiplash w/ continuing sx	21	8/13	35.40 (11.0)	n/a	6 m	76.4 (20.6)	77.9 (23.8)	*	Di Stefano, et al (1995)
TMT-B	Whiplash w/ continuing sx	28	9/19	34.10 (10.2)	n/a	6 m	71.0 (25.0)	66.1 (24.6)		Di Stefano, et al (1996)
TMT-B (%ile)	Epilepsy	4	2/2	23.00	lamotrigine/ placebo	12 w	26.5	26.5	*	Banks, et al (1991)
TMT-B (%ile)	Epilepsy	6	2/4	33.30	placebo/ lamotrigine	12 w	32.5	28.3	*	Banks, et al (1991)
TMT-B (derived)	Schizophrenia	19	13/6	33.70 (6.30)	clozapine	10 w	0.08 (0.14)	0.17 (0.18)		Buchanan, et al (1994)
TMT-B (derived)	Schizophrenia	19	15/4	34.00 (6.90)	haloperidol	10 w	0.06 (0.16)	0.17 (0.27)		Buchanan, et al (1994)
TMT-B (derived)	Schizophrenia	33	n/a	~33.7 (6.30)	clozapine	1 y	0.10 (0.17)	0.18 (0.19)		Buchanan, et al (1994)
TMT-B (errors)	Cardiac	245	198/47	54.70	CABG/cardiac operation	6 m	0.91 (1.6)	0.82 (1.5)		Savageau, et al (1982a)
TMT-B (errors)	Cardiac	227	184/43	54.50	cardiac operation	10-12 d	0.91 (1.3)	1.43 (2.2)		Savageau, et al (1982b)
TMT-B (errors)	Control	16	10/6	12.60	n/a	1 m	0.43 (0.53)	0.38 (0.51)		Pieters, et al (1992)
TMT-B (errors)	Epilepsy	16	10/6	12.60	n/a	1 m	0.32 (0.38)	0.37 (0.59)		Pieters, et al (1992)

instrument	group	n	m/f	age	intervention	inter	t #1	t #2	note	citation
TMT-B (errors)	IVDU	16	13/3	39.50	n/a	10.4 d	1.07 (1.49)	0.47 (0.74)		Richards, et al (1992)
TMT-B (errors)	Naphtha Exposure	185	n/a	36.00	n/a	1 y	0.78 (1.68)	1.05 (2.80)		White, et al (1994)
TMT-B (Imp Rating)	Control	10	n/a	48.60 (8.20)	n/a	5.6 y	0.50 (0.71)	0.20 (0.42)	*	Elias, et al (1986)
TMT-B (Imp Rating)	Hypertension	11	n/a	51.20 (4.50)	n/a	5.7 y	0.91 (0.83)	0.73 (0.47)	*	Elias, et al (1986)
TMT-B (t)	ALL	31	16/15	8.38 (3.19)	n/a	2.0 y	50.9 (8.9)	51.9 (12.2)		Berg, et al (1983)
TMT-B (t)	ALL w/ Somnolence	48	27/21	8.63 (3.15)	n/a	2.25 y	48.6 (13.4)	52.4 (11.0)		Berg, et al (1983)
TMT-B (t)	Epilepsy	13	8/5	23.07 (8.90)	carbamaz	3 m	48.79 (9.5)	50.21 (8.7)	*	Gallassi, et al (1988)
TMT-B (t)	Epilepsy	12	6/6	28.50 (7.00)	phenytoin	3 m	43.93 (7.2)	47.19 (10.1)	*	Gallassi, et al (1988)
TMT-B (t)	Lung Cancer	11	n/a	~61.0	cranial irradiation	11 m	35.4	32.1		Komaki, et al (1995)
TMT-B (t)	MS	13	n/a	36.20	placebo	2 y	41.1 (8.2)	41.2 (10.8)		Pliskin, et al (1996)
TMT-B (t)	MS	8	n/a	38.00	low dose interferon	2 y	40.9 (15.7)	39.9 (13)		Pliskin, et al (1996)
TMT-B (t)	MS	9	n/a	38.90	high dose interferon	2 y	32.8 (8.0)	38.0 (3.4)		Pliskin, et al (1996)

instrument	group	n	m/f	age	intervention	inter	t #1	t #2	note	citation
TMT-B - A	Control	20	10/10	34.00 (12.4)	n/a	4 w	32.6 (20.2)	36.9 (24.1)		McGrath, et al (1997)
TMT-B - A	Mania	16	1/15	40.60 (12.8)	std tx	4 w	65.1 (50.8)	62.9 (34.6)		McGrath, et al (1997)
TMT-B - A	Schizophrenia	31	21/10	31.50 (8.90)	std tx	4 w	81.3 (56.5)	60.8 (44.1)		McGrath, et al (1997)
TMT-C	Neurological	64	n/a	40.70 (16.7)	n/a	imm	42.5 (14.3)	43.7 (14.7)	C/A	Franzen, et al (1996)
TMT-C	Neuro-psychiatric	192	n/a	42.80 (16.6)	n/a	imm	41.3 (13.9)	39.8 (14.1)	C/A	Franzen, et al (1996)
TMT-C	Psychiatric	64	n/a	43.60 (17.9)	n/a	imm	43.0 (14.2)	38.0 (14.2)	C/A	Franzen, et al (1996)
TMT-C	Substance Abuse	64	n/a	44.30 (15.0)	n/a	imm	38.5 (14.6)	37.5 (15.1)	C/A	Franzen, et al (1996)
TMT-C	TBI	15	15/0	18.0 - 56.0	n/a	1-1.5 d	39.00 (10.16)	41.87 (15.23)	C/A	desRosiers, et al (1987)
TMT-D	Neurological	64	n/a	40.70 (16.7)	n/a	imm	166.5 (61.3)	140.9 (58.7)	D/B	Franzen, et al (1996)
TMT-D	Neuro-psychiatric	192	n/a	42.80 (16.6)	n/a	imm	143.1 (48.3)	132.3 (50.7)	D/B	Franzen, et al (1996)
TMT-D	Psychiatric	64	n/a	43.60 (17.9)	n/a	imm	128.2 (68.7)	117.6 (58.6)	D/B	Franzen, et al (1996)
TMT-D	Substance Abuse	64	n/a	44.30 (15.0)	n/a	imm	134.5 (64.1)	138.5 (69.3)	D/B	Franzen, et al (1996)

instrument	group	n	m/f	age	intervention	inter	t #1	t #2	note	citation
TMT-D	TBI	15	15/0	18.0 - 56.0	n/a	1-1.5 d	121.27 (61.78)	109.20 (54.29)	D/B	desRosiers, et al (1987)
TMT-Total	Alcoholic (detoxed)	17	n/a	44.47	abstin	1 y	14.59 (2.91)	15.35 (2.74)		Long, et al (1974)

Table 68. Verbal Fluency Tests

instrument	group	n	m/f	age	intervention	inter	t #1	t #2	note	citation
COWAT	Breast Cancer	20	3/17	39.28 (9.38)	ABMT	~12 d	39.9 (12.9)	35.2 (8.3)		Ahles, et al (1996)
COWAT	CAD	35	23/12	62.30 (8.30)	CE	50.9 d	40.51 (11.87)	44.60 (12.66)		Kelly, et al (1980)
COWAT	Control	63	8/55	56.22 (11.0)	n/a	~6 m	NR	4.38 (6.09)c	NKA	Bruggemans, et al (1997)
COWAT	Control	110	110/0	19.30 (1.30)	n/a	~3 m	44.8 (9.0)	49.3 (9.5)		Macciocchi (1990)
COWAT	Control	20	10/10	34.00 (12.4)	n/a	4 w	39.1 (8.4)	42.4 (8.0)	CFL/ PRW	McGrath, et al (1997)
COWAT	Control	60	26/34	71.24 (5.96)	n/a	12 m	40.33 (9.79)	40.00 (11.24)	FAS	Olin, et al (1991)
COWAT	Control	120	60/60	40.50	n/a	6 m	39.7 (10.48)	42.5 (9.9)	CFL/ PRW	Ruff, et al (1996)
COWAT	DAT	13	n/a	71.70 (6.40)	placebo	1 m	13.2 (7.5)	13.9 (8.7)	2 lett, AF	Green, et al (1992)

instrument	group	n	m/f	age	intervention	inter	t #1	t #2	note	citation
COWAT	DAT	11	n/a	71.70 (6.40)	oxiracetam	1 m	18.7 (8.9)	15.5 (5.7)	2 lett, AF	Green, et al (1992)
COWAT	Dementia	<35	n/a	66.00 (9.60)	n/a	19.0 m	28.6 (12.3)	24.5 (10.2)		Jones, et al (1992)
COWAT	Epilepsy	11	n/a	25.90 (7.00)	RTL	1 w	28.8 (8.7)	17.3 (10.5)		Loring, et al (1994)
COWAT	Epilepsy	18	n/a	28.10 (6.70)	LTL	1 y	24.1 (4.6)	28.5 (7.6)		Loring, et al (1994)
COWAT	Epilepsy	12	n/a	29.00 (6.40)	LTL	1 w	23.2 (7.8)	10.9 (9.4)		Loring, et al (1994)
COWAT	Epilepsy	16	n/a	25.70 (6.40)	RTL	1 y	32.2 (6.2)	33.4 (6.5)		Loring, et al (1994)
COWAT	HD	26	12/14	39.00 (10.4)	n/a	12 m	24.4 (2.1)	24.2 (2.2)	FAS	Bamford, et al (1995)
COWAT	HD	40	18/22	40.00 (10.3)	n/a	12 m	23.0 (1.6)	23.9 (2.1)	FAS	Bamford, et al (1995)
COWAT	Hematologic D/O	14	2/12	39.28 (9.38)	ABMT	~12 d	37.1 (5.2)	34.3 (5.5)		Ahles, et al (1996)
COWAT	HIV+ (IVDU)	8	5/3	39.00 (8.00)	MSR/placebo	7 d	11.5 (6.3)	12.7 (6.1)	*	Van Dyck, et al (1997)
COWAT	IVDU	16	13/3	39.50	n/a	10.4 d	33.4 (9.15)	37.0 (9.72)	CFL	Richards, et al (1992)
COWAT	Mania	16	1/15	40.60 (12.8)	std tx	4 w	34.6 (10.8)	34.4 (12.6)	CFL/ PRW	McGrath, et al (1997)

instrument	group	n	m/f	age	intervention	inter	t #1	t #2	note	citation
COWAT	Orthopedic	128	38/90	69.00	general anesthesia	1 w	33.9 (12.7)	0.5 (6.6) c	*	Williams-Russo, et al (1995)
COWAT	Orthopedic	134	39/95	69.00	epidural anesthesia	1 w	36.6 (12.8)	-0.8 (7.2) c	*	Williams-Russo, et al (1995)
COWAT	PVD	17	14/3	61.40 (7.90)	PVD surgery	51.5 d	41.06 (11.64)	40.53 (11.52)		Kelly, et al (1980)
COWAT	Pseudo-dementia	<35	n/a	66.00 (9.60)	n/a	19.0 m	30.7 (11.7)	32.3 (7.2)		Jones, et al (1992)
COWAT	Schizophrenia	33	n/a	~33.7 (6.30)	clozapine	1 y	33.6 (11.8)	38.8 (13.8)		Buchanan, et al (1994)
COWAT	Schizophrenia	19	15/4	34.00 (6.90)	haloperidol	10 w	34.0 (10.3)	34.7 (11.4)		Buchanan, et al (1994)
COWAT	Schizophrenia	19	13/6	33.70 (6.30)	clozapine	10 w	35.7 (13.6)	36.2 (14.6)		Buchanan, et al (1994)
COWAT	Schizophrenia	36	28/8	35.50 (9.80)	clozapine	6 w	30.4 (14.1)	34.9 (16.2)	FAS, *	Hagger, et al (1993)
COWAT	Schizophrenia	31	21/10	31.50 (8.90)	std tx	4 w	33.7 (12.5)	36.8 (11.9)	CFL/ PRW	McGrath, et al (1997)
COWAT	Schizophrenia Inpts	35	29/6	23.71 (4.50)	neuroleptics	1-2 y	35.7 (13.6)	38.3 (12.1)		Nopoulos, et al (1994)
DRS Verbal Fluency	DAT/MID	29	14/15	71.50 (1.30)	oxiracetam	6 m	6.4 (0.4)	7.9 (0.6)	*	Villardita, et al (1992)
DRS Verbal Fluency	DAT/MID	30	15/15	71.70 (1.30)	oxiracetam	3 m	6.5 (0.4)	8.8 (0.5)	*	Villardita, et al (1992)

instrument	group	n	m/f	age	intervention	inter	t #1	t #2	note	citation
DRS Verbal Fluency	DAT/MID	30	21/9	67.80 (1.50)	placebo	3 m	6.3 (0.5)	6.4 (0.4)	*	Villardita, et al (1992)
MAE COWAT	Dementia (2° to steroid)	6	6/0	49.67	steriods d/c or reduced	10.9 m	6.0	12.5		Varney, et al (1984)
MAE COWAT	Depression	9	6/3	50.20 (18.5)	right ECT	2 d	32.8	28.7	*	Kronfol, et al (1978)
MAE COWAT	Depression	9	6/3	48.30 (17.8)	left ECT	2 d	37.9	37.0	*	Kronfol, et al (1978)
MAE COWAT	Epilepsy	40	23/17	32.20 (8.20)	n/a	~9 m	33.00 (11.10)	32.00 (7.51)		Hermann, et al (1996)
MAE COWAT (t)	Lung Cancer	11	n/a	~61.0	cranial irradiation	11 m	38.6	38.4		Komaki, et al (1995)
Thurstone Verbal Fluency	DAT	10	8/2	74.10	placebo	12 w	11.50 (11.50)	9.50 (10.75)		McCaffrey, et al (1987)
Thurstone Verbal Fluency	DAT	10	6/4	74.30	suloctidil 450 mg	12 w	13.80 (9.47)	12.60 (10.60)		McCaffrey, et al (1987)
Thurstone Verbal Fluency	DAT	10	5/5	74.90	suloctidil 600 mg	12 w	18.50 (11.94)	14.25 (12.07)		McCaffrey, et al (1987)
Verbal Fluency	AIDS	10	10/0	41.70 (5.50)	n/a	6.53 m	40.3 (12.6)	40.7 (12.8)	FAS	Hinkin, et al (1995)
Verbal Fluency	Alcoholic	10	10/0	33.05 (7.09)	placebo	1 h	40.0	42.6	CFL/ PRW CB	Mallick, et al (1993)

instrument	group	n	m/f	age	intervention	inter	t #1	t #2	note	citation
Verbal Fluency	Alcoholic	10	10/0	33.05 (7.09)	lorazepam	1 h	37.3	44.1	CFL/ PRW CB	Mallick, et al (1993)
Verbal Fluency	Aphasia (acute)	17	10/7	61.40 (14.9)	n/a	6-8 w	16.9 (13.7)	20.9 (17.9)	anim, food, cloth	Roberts, et al (1994)
Verbal Fluency	Aphasia (chronic)	16	10/6	53.30 (11.3)	n/a	6-8 w	27.4 (11.5)	31.6 (11.7)	anim, food, cloth	Roberts, et al (1994)
Verbal Fluency	Brain Tumor	7	4/3	9.83	radiotherapy	11 m	8.8 (1.7)	7.5 (2.1)		Bordeaux, et al (1988)
Verbal Fluency	Brain Tumor	7	3/4	10.33	surgery	1 m	9.6 (3.0)	9.8 (1.6)		Bordeaux, et al (1988)
Verbal Fluency	Brain Tumor (post-surgery)	12	5/7	31.80 (8.60)	radiation tx	3 m	33.1 (11.0)	36.5 (15)	FAS, *	Armstrong, et al (1995)
Verbal Fluency	Brain Tumor (post-surgery)	12	5/7	31.80 (8.60)	radiation tx	3 m	20.0 (5.3)	18.7 (5.8)	anim, *	Armstrong, et al (1995)
Verbal Fluency	Cardiac	135	120/ 15	55.40	CABG	3 m	39.1	40.9	*	Klonoff, et al (1989)
Verbal Fluency	Cardiac	17	12/5	50.00 (10.5)	heart transplant	36.0 m	36.0 (10.62)	35.0 (10.52)	FAS	Roman, et al (1997)
Verbal Fluency	Continuing Care Inpts	10	0/10	79.00	n/a	1 d	36.0	39.0	categ, AF	Gregory, et al (1983)

instrument	group	n	m/f	age	intervention	inter	t #1	t #2	note	citation
Verbal Fluency	Continuing Care Inpts	10	0/10	79.00	n/a	1 d	32.0	40.0	categ	Gregory, et al (1983)
Verbal Fluency	Control	50	n/a	71.90 (0.90)	n/a	2 y	14.9 (0.6)	17.0 (1.0)	categ	Flicker, et al (1993)
Verbal Fluency	Control	101	101/0	78.50 (7.20)	n/a	2.6 y	19.1	16.3	anim	Frank, et al (1996)
Verbal Fluency	Control	141	0/141	78.50 (6.60)	n/a	2.7 y	17.4	16.2	anim	Frank, et al (1996)
Verbal Fluency	Control	20	6/14	69.40 (4.20)	n/a	1 y	20.6 (5.3)	22.9 (6.4)	categ, *	Fromm, et al (1991)
Verbal Fluency	Control	1017	436/ 581	74.30 (5.40)	n/a	2 y	26.8 (5.8)	26.0 (6.3)	fruit, anim	Ganguli, et al (1996)
Verbal Fluency	Control	1017	436/ 581	74.30 (5.40)	n/a	2 y	22.2 (7.5)	21.9 (7.6)	PS	Ganguli, et al (1996)
Verbal Fluency	Control	4	0/4	67.30 (0.50)	placebo	60 min	42.5 (6.19)	42.8 (6.19)	CFL/ PRW	Kirkby, et al (1995)
Verbal Fluency	Control	8	4/4	21.80 (4.20)	placebo	60 min	36.5 (4.24)	39.3 (11.3)	CFL/ PRW	Kirkby, et al (1995)
Verbal Fluency	Control	9	4/5	26.40 (7.70)	lorazepam	60 min	46.7 (9.68)	49.4 (13.2)	CFL/ PRW	Kirkby, et al (1995)
Verbal Fluency	Control	5	1/4	68.40 (6.10)	lorazepam	60 min	53.2 (2.39)	42.6 (3.36)	CFL/ PRW	Kirkby, et al (1995)
Verbal Fluency	Control	10	10/0	31.30 (6.14)	placebo	1 h	50.9	55.0	CFL/ PRW CB	Mallick, et al (1993)

instrument	group	n	m/f	age	intervention	inter	t #1	t #2	note	citation
Verbal Fluency	Control	10	10/0	31.30 (6.14)	lorazepam	1 h	61.1	63.6	CFL/ PRW CB	Mallick, et al (1993)
Verbal Fluency	Control	47	n/a	~68.0	n/a	1 y	18.4 (5.4)	19.7 (4.8)	anim	Morris, et al (1989)
Verbal Fluency	Control	72	67/5	44.50 (12.4)	n/a	6 m	18.2 (6.1)	20.8 (6.1)	H	Prevey, et al (1996)
Verbal Fluency	Control	22	12/10	65.82 (5.20)	n/a	2 y	60.00 (13.13)	73.09 (16.82)	anim, food, city	Rebok, et al (1990)
Verbal Fluency	Control	21	21/0	31.45 (5.53)	n/a	18 m	45.20 (8.37)	48.45 (8.49)	CFL	Saykin, et al (1991)
Verbal Fluency	Control	15	8/7	41.00 (12.0)	n/a	29.0 d	39.0 (5.5)	37.0 (10.5)	MPD/ FAS	Trichard, et al (1995)
Verbal Fluency	Control	15	8/7	41.00 (12.0)	n/a	29.0 d	23.0 (7.5)	23.0 (6.0)	anim	Trichard, et al (1995)
Verbal Fluency	Control	20	12/8	56.40	n/a	10 w	17.0 (4.6)	18.1 (4.7)	prof	Van Den Burg, et al (1985)
Verbal Fluency	Control	20	12/8	56.40	n/a	10 w	23.1 (7.0)	22.4 (5.5)	anim	Van Den Burg, et al (1985)
Verbal Fluency	Control	18	12/6	37.20 (9.70)	n/a	76.5 d	11.51 (3.37)	12.87 (3.22)	lett	Verdoux, et al (1995)
Verbal Fluency	Control (CDR-0)	30	15/15	70.9 (4.6)	n/a	1 y	26.8 (6.6)	30.8 (9.1)	SP, *	Botwinick, et al (1986)
Verbal Fluency	Control w/ APOE-E4	20	5/15	80.35 (4.75)	n/a	3.32 y	18.80 (8.27)	19.75 (7.51)	food	Small, et al (1998)

instrument	group	n	m/f	age	intervention	inter	t #1	t #2	note	citation
Verbal Fluency	Control w/ APOE-E4	20	5/15	80.35 (4.75)	n/a	3.32 y	12.36 (5.44)	12.95 (5.3)	NS	Small, et al (1998)
Verbal Fluency	Control w/o APOE-E4	54	16/38	82.04 (5.26)	n/a	3.21 y	12.51 (5.19)	12.45 (5.14)	NS	Small, et al (1998)
Verbal Fluency	Control w/o APOE-E4	54	16/38	82.04 (5.26)	n/a	3.21 y	19.89 (7.17)	18.85 (6.19)	food	Small, et al (1998)
Verbal Fluency	CVA	19	n/a	~65.0	n/a	104.0 d	35.6	40.1		Bowler, et al (1994)
Verbal Fluency	CVA/Control	300	n/a	70.70	"improved/ stable"	9-12 m	NR	0.4 (2.3) c	CFL	Desmond, et al (1995)
Verbal Fluency	CVA/Control	71	n/a	70.70	"declined"	9-12 m	NR	-1.5 (3.4) c	categ	Desmond, et al (1995)
Verbal Fluency	CVA/Control	300	n/a	70.70	"improved/ stable"	9-12 m	NR	0.2 (2.9) c	categ	Desmond, et al (1995)
Verbal Fluency	CVA/Control	71	n/a	70.70	"declined"	9-12 m	NR	-0.8 (2.4) c	CFL	Desmond, et al (1995)
Verbal Fluency	DAT	14	n/a	53.0 - 81.0	lithium carbonate	7 d	10.8 (2.2)	16.4 (2.7)	categ, *	Brinkman, et al (1984)
Verbal Fluency	DAT	14	n/a	53.0 - 81.0	lithium carbonate	7 d	12.1 (2.3)	10.9 (2.4)	lett, *	Brinkman, et al (1984)
Verbal Fluency	DAT	34	34/0	83.90 (4.30)	n/a	2.1 y	11.2	8.7	anim	Frank, et al (1996)
Verbal Fluency	DAT	34	34/0	83.90 (4.30)	n/a	2.1 y	12.0	8.4	anim	Frank, et al (1996)
Verbal Fluency	DAT	18	5/13	71.00 (9.40)	n/a	1 y	10.5 (4.7)	9.1 (4.0)	categ, *	Fromm, et al (1991)

instrument	group	n	m/f	age	intervention	inter	t #1	t #2	note	citation
Verbal Fluency	DAT	18	9/9	71.10	placebo	3 m	22.4 (13.2)	20.5 (13.1)	*	Maltby, et al (1994)
Verbal Fluency	DAT	14	8/6	66.50	tacrine	3 m	23.1 (15)	22.6 (14.9)	*	Maltby, et al (1994)
Verbal Fluency	DAT	430	198/ 232	70.90 (8.00)	n/a	1 y	8.1 (4.1)	-1.8 (3.0) c	anim, *	Morris, et al (1993)
Verbal Fluency	DAT	52	n/a	~71.0	n/a	1 y	8.9 (4.6)	7.6 (5.0)	anim, *	Morris, et al (1989)
Verbal Fluency	DAT	51	16/35	67.29 (7.94)	n/a	2 y	17.44 (10.23)	6.38 (7.43)	anim, food, city	Rebok, et al (1990)
Verbal Fluency	DAT	32	n/a	70.72	NSAID	1 y	19.59	3.67 c	categ	Rich, et al (1995)
Verbal Fluency	DAT	117	n/a	69.93	n/a	1 y	14.74	6.31 c	categ	Rich, et al (1995)
Verbal Fluency	DAT	14	n/a	60.0 - 80.0	placebo	6 m	23.4 (13.0)	23.4 (13.0)	categ	Sano, et al (1992)
Verbal Fluency	DAT	14	n/a	60.0 - 80.0	placebo	6 m	34.5 (30.7)	26.3 (25.9)	lett	Sano, et al (1992)
Verbal Fluency	DAT	13	n/a	60.0 - 80.0	acetyl levocarnitine	6 m	24.8 (33.1)	26.8 (32.7)	lett	Sano, et al (1992)
Verbal Fluency	DAT	13	n/a	60.0 - 80.0	acetyl levocarnitine	6 m	23.8 (6.5)	23.8 (6.5)	categ	Sano, et al (1992)
Verbal Fluency	DAT (advanced)	39	n/a	72.20 (1.20)	n/a	2 y	2.9 (1.5)	1.5 (1.1)	categ	Flicker, et al (1993)
Verbal Fluency	DAT (at risk)	50	0/50	84.10 (5.10)	n/a	2.3 y	13.6	11.5	anim	Frank, et al (1996)

instrument	group	n	m/f	age	intervention	inter	t #1	t #2	note	citation
Verbal Fluency	DAT (at risk)	32	32/0	83.30 (6.70)	n/a	2.0 y	14.9	12.2	anim	Frank, et al (1996)
Verbal Fluency	DAT (CDR-1)	18	7/11	71.40 (4.40)	n/a	1 y	16.1 (10.3)	14.7 (11.1)	SP, *	Botwinick, et al (1986)
Verbal Fluency	DAT (declining)	12	3/9	56.20 (6.40)	n/a	1 y	NR	-10.6 (7.4) c	categ	Piccini, et al (1995)
Verbal Fluency	DAT (early)	47	n/a	69.80 (1.20)	n/a	2 y	9.4 (0.7)	8.7 (0.8)	categ	Flicker, et al (1993)
Verbal Fluency	DAT (early)	47	n/a	69.80 (1.20)	n/a	2 y	9.4 (0.7)	8.7 (0.8)	categ	Flicker, et al (1993)
Verbal Fluency	DAT (mild)	11	10/1	63.00 (8.00)	n/a	26 m	34.0 (13.0)	29.0 (11.0)	FAS	Haxby, et al (1990)
Verbal Fluency	DAT (stable)	19	3/16	61.00 (6.40)	n/a	1 y	NR	-4.4 (2.9) c	categ	Piccini, et al (1995)
Verbal Fluency	Epilepsy	14	8/6	41.20 (10.5)	sabeluzole	12 w	24.8 (10.5)	27.8 (8.9)	categ	Aldenkamp, et al (1995)
Verbal Fluency	Epilepsy	19	11/8	40.00 (8.00)	placebo	12 w	26.5	27.8	categ	Aldenkamp, et al (1995)
Verbal Fluency	Epilepsy	36	17/19	34.89 (8.38)	vigabatrin 1 g	18 w	26.19 (13.52)	29.19 (15.56)	CFL/ PRW	Dodrill, et al (1995)
Verbal Fluency	Epilepsy	38	21/17	34.26 (9.18)	vigabatrin 3 g	18 w	25.63 (10.11)	26.11 (12.08)	CFL/ PRW	Dodrill, et al (1995)
Verbal Fluency	Epilepsy	32	17/15	33.72 (9.66)	vigabatrin 6 g	18 w	26.38 (10.11)	26.31 (10.14)	CFL/ PRW	Dodrill, et al (1995)
Verbal Fluency	Epilepsy	40	14/26	33.88 (9.77)	placebo	18 w	26.18 (9.68)	26.23 (8.29)	CFL/ PRW	Dodrill, et al (1995)

instrument	group	n	m/f	age	intervention	inter	t #1	t #2	note	citation
Verbal Fluency	Epilepsy	11	n/a	25.90 (7.00)	RTL	1 w	16.9 (5.1)	14.4 (9.1)	anim	Loring, et al (1994)
Verbal Fluency	Epilepsy	12	n/a	29.00 (6.40)	LTL	1 w	13.0 (2.8)	5.9 (4.2)	anim	Loring, et al (1994)
Verbal Fluency	Epilepsy	18	n/a	28.10 (6.70)	LTL	1 y	17.0 (3.9)	17.1 (4.4)	anim	Loring, et al (1994)
Verbal Fluency	Epilepsy	16	n/a	25.70 (6.40)	RTL	1 y	16.8 (4.6)	16.6 (5.2)	anim	Loring, et al (1994)
Verbal Fluency	Epilepsy	26	24/2	43.50 (17.1)	carbamaz	6 m	14.8 (6.4)	15.7 (6.0)	H	Prevey, et al (1996)
Verbal Fluency	Epilepsy	39	36/3	44.30 (14.2)	valproate	6 m	15.4 (5.2)	15.6 (5.0)	H	Prevey, et al (1996)
Verbal Fluency	HIV+	132	132/0	~33.8	n/a	13.3 m	45.0	46.7	FAS/ PRW	Selnes, et al (1990)
Verbal Fluency	HIV+ (IVDU)	42	31/11	27.00 (5.30)	n/a	12 m	18.9 (4.3)	19.3 (3.7)	fruit, color, anim, town	Bono, et al (1996)
Verbal Fluency	HIV+ (stage 2/3)	14	14/0	31.40 (8.54)	n/a	12.8 m	67.2 (14.7)	65.6 (17.4)	anim, object, fruit	Burgess, et al (1994)
Verbal Fluency	HIV+ (stage 2/3)	14	14/0	31.40 (8.54)	n/a	12.8 m	46.1 (10.4)	47.6 (8.7)	FAS	Burgess, et al (1994)
Verbal Fluency	HIV+ (stage 4)	6	6/0	36.20 (7.60)	n/a	12.8 m	60.8 (3.5)	52.5 (10.5)	anim, object, fruit	Burgess, et al (1994)

instrument	group	n	m/f	age	intervention	inter	t #1	t #2	note	citation
Verbal Fluency	HIV+ (stage 4)	6	6/0	36.20 (7.60)	n/a	12.8 m	36.7 (12.5)	44.0 (13.6)	FAS	Burgess, et al (1994)
Verbal Fluency	HIV+/ARC	8	8/0	33.57 (6.35)	n/a	18 m	38.43 (7.18)	33.86 (12.52)	CFL	Saykin, et al (1991)
Verbal Fluency	HIV+/PGL	13	13/0	31.15 (4.91)	n/a	18 m	41.85 (8.14)	48.54 (12.72)	CFL	Saykin, et al (1991)
Verbal Fluency	HIV-	41	41/0	31.50 (9.32)	n/a	12.8 m	42.5 (13)	44.0 (12.8)	FAS	Burgess, et al (1994)
Verbal Fluency	HIV-	41	41/0	31.50 (9.32)	n/a	12.8 m	66.9 (16.7)	64.7 (17.4)	anim, object, fruit	Burgess, et al (1994)
Verbal Fluency	HIV-	132	132/0	~35.6	n/a	13.4 m	44.4	48.6	FAS/ PRW	Selnes, et al (1990)
Verbal Fluency	HIV- (IVDU)	39	30/9	28.60 (4.90)	n/a	12 m	19.6 (4.1)	20.2 (3.9)	fruit, color, anim, town	Bono, et al (1996)
Verbal Fluency	IVDU	16	13/3	39.50	n/a	10.4 d	19.6 (6.21)	19.31 (5.8)	anim	Richards, et al (1992)
Verbal Fluency	Left AVM	15	10/5	31.00 (11.0)	surgery	4m	17.8 (3.7)	17.5 (8.6)	*	Stabell, et al (1994)
Verbal Fluency	Major Depression	23	12/11	47.00 (14.0)	n/a	29.0 d	15.5 (4.5)	18.5 (5.0)	anim	Trichard, et al (1995)
Verbal Fluency	Major Depression	23	12/11	47.00 (14.0)	n/a	29.0 d	28.0 (11.5)	35.0 (11.5)	MPD/ FAS	Trichard, et al (1995)

instrument	group	n	m/f	age	intervention	inter	t #1	t #2	note	citation
Verbal Fluency	MS	19	6/13	43.37	n/a	8 w	29.0 (3.1)	30.0 (2.5)	lett, *	Bever, et al (1995)
Verbal Fluency	MS w/ Depression	11	n/a	n/a	depressed/ euthymic	7 m	NR	0.27 c	presid	Schiffer, et al (1991)
Verbal Fluency	MS w/ Depression	11	n/a	n/a	depressed/ euthymic	7 m	NR	4.18 c	food	Schiffer, et al (1991)
Verbal Fluency	MS w/ Depression	11	n/a	n/a	depressed/ euthymic	7 m	NR	-3.18 c	F	Schiffer, et al (1991)
Verbal Fluency	Ocular Disease	50	27/23	42.00 (17.0)	steroid tx	~8 d	8.2 (3.0)	9.9 (3.7)	categ	Naber, et al (1996)
Verbal Fluency	Ocular Disease	50	27/23	42.00 (17.0)	steroid tx	~8 d	9.4 (3.6)	11.8 (4.3)	lett	Naber, et al (1996)
Verbal Fluency	Orthopedic Injury	25	14/11	10.03 (2.00)	n/a	4 m	16.6 (5.6)	15.0 (5.2)	anim	Chadwick, et al (1981)
Verbal Fluency	PD	4	3/1	53.50	fetal tissue implanted	12 m	17.2	14.3	2'	Sass, et al (1995)
Verbal Fluency	PD	20	9/11	57.90	posteroventral pallidotomy	3 m	40.9	37.0	FAS	Scott, et al (1998)
Verbal Fluency	PD	20	9/11	57.90	posteroventral pallidotomy	3 m	21.1	18.1	anim	Scott, et al (1998)
Verbal Fluency	PD	20	9/11	57.90	posteroventral pallidotomy	3 m	26.7	21.3	food	Scott, et al (1998)
Verbal Fluency	PD	19	13/6	54.30	pergolide	~6 w	18.2 (5.86)	17.8 (5.38)	categ	Stern, et al (1984)

instrument	group	n	m/f	age	intervention	inter	t #1	t #2	note	citation
Verbal Fluency	PD	19	13/6	54.30	pergolide	~6 w	14.4 (4.04)	13.3 (4.16)	FAS	Stern, et al (1984)
Verbal Fluency	PD/Tremor	13	8/5	56.00	right thalamotomy	~6 d	28.2	26.7	SA	Vilkki, et al (1974)
Verbal Fluency	PD/Tremor	12	7/5	56.00	left thalamotomy	~6 d	28.0	16.0	SA	Vilkki, et al (1974)
Verbal Fluency	PVD	20	18/2	56.80	major surgery	10 w	20.5 (4.9)	19.2 (5.2)	anim	Van Den Burg, et al (1985)
Verbal Fluency	PVD	20	18/2	56.80	major surgery	10 w	15.3 (4.8)	13.8 (3.8)	profes	Van Den Burg, et al (1985)
Verbal Fluency	Right AVM	16	5/11	34.00 (13.0)	surgery	4 m	23.7 (7.0)	25.6 (8.5)	*	Stabell, et al (1994)
Verbal Fluency	Schizophrenia	38	25/13	30.90 (8.73)	n/a	6 m	44.15 (11.45)	47.67 (10.12)	object, anim, bird/ color	Addington, et al (1991)
Verbal Fluency	Schizophrenia	10	8/2	71.00	risperidone	4 w	16.9 (12.0)	17.2 (10.4)	FAS	Berman, et al (1996)
Verbal Fluency	Schizophrenia	19	13/6	33.70 (6.30)	clozapine	10 w	42.9 (12.2)	46.9 (16.5)	categ	Buchanan, et al (1994)
Verbal Fluency	Schizophrenia	33	n/a	~33.7 (6.30)	clozapine	1 y	41.3 (14.0)	44.9 (15.2)	categ	Buchanan, et al (1994)
Verbal Fluency	Schizophrenia	19	15/4	34.00 (6.90)	haloperidol	10 w	44.3 (15.9)	35.4 (10.3)	categ	Buchanan, et al (1994)

instrument	group	n	m/f	age	intervention	inter	t #1	t #2	note	citation
Verbal Fluency	Schizophrenia	36	28/8	35.50 (9.80)	clozapine	6 w	39.7 (15.9)	41.9 (15.4)	street, anim, fruit & veg, *	Hagger, et al (1993)
Verbal Fluency	Schizophrenia	11	11/0	52.50 (11.5)	neuroleptic reduction	29.3 w	26.6 (6.3)	30.2 (9.0)	FAS	Seidman, et al (1993)
Verbal Fluency	Schizophrenia	18	12/6	37.90 (10.8)	n/a	84.3 d	8.27 (3.35)	10.25 (2.63)	lett	Verdoux, et al (1995)
Verbal Fluency	Schizophrenia (acute)	39	24/15	28.60 (8.60)	n/a	1 y	37.7 (12.4)	38.6 (12.5)	FAS	Sweeney, et al (1991)
Verbal Fluency	Spinal Cord Injury	67	54/13	32.00 (14.7)	n/a	38 w	40.44 (25.22)	46.9 (29.36)		Richards, et al (1988)
Verbal Fluency	Substance Abuse	15	8/7	21.10 (4.50)	outpt tx	4 w	34.3 (14.1)	37.2 (5.2)		Cosgrove, et al (1991)
Verbal Fluency	Substance Abuse (PCP)	15	8/7	21.10 (4.50)	outpt tx	4 w	36.5 (9.8)	35.1 (7.7)		Cosgrove, et al (1991)
Verbal Fluency	TBI	25	14/11	10.12 (2.60)	n/a	4 m	11.0 (4.9)	14.4 (5.9)	anim	Chadwick, et al (1981)
Verbal Fluency	TBI	15	15/0	18.0 - 56.0	n/a	1-1.5 d	24.07 (8.84)	24.40 (8.84)	PRW/C FL	desRosiers, et al (1987)
Verbal Fluency	TBI	15	15/0	18.0 - 56.0	n/a	1-1.5 d	23.80 (9.46)	24.67 (9.00)	CFL/ PRW	desRosiers, et al (1987)
Verbal Fluency	TBI	42	40/2	33.20 (11.2)	n/a	9 m	7.12 (4.6)	9.8 (3.7)	wood, round	Mukundan, et al (1987)

instrument	group	n	m/f	age	intervention	inter	t #1	t #2	note	citation
Verbal Fluency	TBI (mild - mod)	7	7/0	20.00	placebo	1 m	35.0	37.0	lett	Levin (1991)
Verbal Fluency	TBI (mild - mod)	7	7/0	25.00	CDP-choline	1 m	22.0	41.0	lett	Levin (1991)
Verbal Fluency	TIA	13	13/0	63.39	n/a	8 m	11.92 (2.90)	11.00 (3.76)	object	de Leo, et al (1987)
Verbal Fluency	TIA	25	25/0	63.32	CE	8 m	9.36 (3.81)	10.88 (3.33)	object	de Leo, et al (1987)
Verbal Fluency	TIA	25	25/0	63.32	CE	8 m	14.84 (4.53)	15.04 (3.82)	anim	de Leo, et al (1987)
Verbal Fluency	TIA	13	13/0	63.39	n/a	8 m	18.92 (5.54)	17.77 (5.60)	anim	de Leo, et al (1987)
Verbal Fluency	TIA	20	13/7	59.60	CE	10 w	13.5 (4.9)	13.9 (3.9)	profes	Van Den Burg, et al (1985)
Verbal Fluency	TIA	20	13/7	59.60	CE	10 w	19.3 (5.0)	17.8 (3.9)	anim	Van Den Burg, et al (1985)
Verbal Fluency (correct)	Neuropsych referrals	248	203/ 45	8.00 (1.70)	n/a	2.65 y	3.5 (3.0)	5.9 (3.2)		Brown, et al (1989)
Verbal Fluency- Written	Control	10	0/10	22.00	hypnosis induction	~15 min	31.9 (4.0)	32.6 (5.0)	categ	Gruzelier, et al (1993)
Verbal Fluency- Written	Control	10	0/10	22.00	hypnosis induction	~15 min	21.3 (3.7)	25.6 (4.7)	lett	Gruzelier, et al (1993)

instrument	group	n	m/f	age	intervention	inter	t #1	t #2	note	citation
Verbal Fluency-Written	Control (highly hypnotizable)	10	0/10	22.00	hypnosis induction	~15 min	32.0 (6.0)	31.3 (5.0)	categ	Gruzelier, et al (1993)
Verbal Fluency-Written	Control (highly hypnotizable)	10	0/10	22.00	hypnosis induction	~15 min	23.4 (5.6)	20.0 (4.7)	lett	Gruzelier, et al (1993)
Verbal Fluency-Written	Schizophrenia	38	25/13	30.90 (8.73)	n/a	6 m	37.95 (15.59)	41.08 (14.62)	S, 4-lett C	Addington, et al (1991)

Table 69. Visual Construction Tests

instrument	group	n	m/f	age	intervention	inter	t #1	t #2	note	citation
2-D/3-D drawings	CVD	33	23/10	64.00	CABG	8-10 d	NR	-0.30 c		Malheiros, et al (1995)
2-D/3-D drawings	CVD	48	34/14	62.00	CABG w/ complications	8-10 d	NR	-0.05 c		Malheiros, et al (1995)
clock drawing	CVD	33	23/10	64.00	CABG	8-10 d	NR	0.60 c		Malheiros, et al (1995)
clock drawing	CVD	48	34/14	62.00	CABG w/ complications	8-10 d	NR	0.25 c		Malheiros, et al (1995)
clock drawing [8]	CVA	19	n/a	~65.0	n/a	104.0 d	5.9	6.9		Bowler, et al (1994)
Copy a Cube	ALS	3	n/a	52.30 (8.10)	placebo	5 d	63.0 (34.5)	46.0 (23.3)	*	Poutiainen, et al (1994)

instrument	group	n	m/f	age	intervention	inter	t #1	t #2	note	citation
Copy a Cube	ALS	12	n/a	49.40 (11.8)	high dose interferon	5 d	37.5 (30.9)	58.1 (47.5)	*	Poutiainen, et al (1994)
Draw/Copy Clock/House [18]	Control	60	26/34	71.24 (5.96)	n/a	12 m	16.42 (1.75)	16.35 (1.58)		Olin, et al (1991)
House Drawing	Myotonic Dystrophy	15	n/a	35.40	n/a	12 y	15.1 (1.6)	13.7 (4.5)		Tuikka, et al (1993)
Rosen Drawing Test	CVA/Control	71	n/a	70.70	declined	9-12 m	NR	-0.6 (1.1) c		Desmond, et al (1995)
Rosen Drawing Test	CVA/Control	300	n/a	70.70	improved/ stable	9-12 m	NR	-0.1 (0.9) c		Desmond, et al (1995)

Table 70. Visual Search Tests (VST)

instrument	group	n	m/f	age	intervention	inter	t #1	t #2	note	citation
VST LVF (# of items)	TIA	12	6/6	63.40 (6.00)	RCE	60.7 d	9.7 (2.3)	9.3 (2.2)		Casey, et al (1989)
VST LVF (# of items)	TIA	12	6/6	66.00 (5.30)	LCE	59.8 d	9.8 (1.7)	9.9 (1.8)		Casey, et al (1989)
VST LVF (# of items)	TIA	12	6/6	59.20 (13.3)	n/a	59.1 d	9.9 (2.1)	10.3 (1.4)		Casey, et al (1989)
VST LVF (sec)	TIA	12	6/6	63.40 (6.00)	RCE	60.7 d	8.4 (6.1)	6.8 (4.0)		Casey, et al (1989)
VST LVF (sec)	TIA	12	6/6	59.20 (13.3)	n/a	59.1 d	7.3 (2.5)	5.9 (2.4)		Casey, et al (1989)

instrument	group	n	m/f	age	intervention	inter	t #1	t #2	note	citation
VST LVF (sec)	TIA	12	6/6	66.00 (5.30)	LCE	59.8 d	9.0 (4.4)	7.4 (3.9)		Casey, et al (1989)
VST RVF (# of items)	TIA	12	6/6	66.00 (5.30)	LCE	59.8 d	10.1 (1.5)	9.8 (1.6)		Casey, et al (1989)
VST RVF (# of items)	TIA	12	6/6	59.20 (13.3)	n/a	59.1 d	10.0 (2.1)	9.8 (1.4)		Casey, et al (1989)
VST RVF (# of items)	TIA	12	6/6	63.40 (6.00)	RCE	60.7 d	9.9 (2.0)	10.4 (2.2)		Casey, et al (1989)
VST RVF (sec)	TIA	12	6/6	59.20 (13.3)	n/a	59.1 d	5.7 (6.6)	7.2 (13.8)		Casey, et al (1989)
VST RVF (sec)	TIA	12	6/6	63.40 (6.00)	RCE	60.7 d	6.5 (2.3)	7.0 (4.6)		Casey, et al (1989)
VST RVF (sec)	TIA	12	6/6	66.00 (5.30)	LCE	59.8 d	8.0 (3.3)	7.3 (2.3)		Casey, et al (1989)
VST (errors)	HIV+ (asx)	20	15/5	36.70 (9.90)	n/a	7-10 d	1.4 (1.3)	1.0 (1.2)		McCaffrey, et al (1995)
VST (errors)	HIV+ (sx)	12	11/1	37.20 (6.40)	n/a	7-10 d	0.8 (1.4)	0.7 (1.2)		McCaffrey, et al (1995)
VST (errors)	HIV- ("At-Risk")	12	12/0	40.40 (13.0)	n/a	7-10 d	1.6 (1.1)	0.3 (0.5)		McCaffrey, et al (1995)
VST (time)	HIV+ (asx)	20	15/5	36.70 (9.90)	n/a	7-10 d	153.6 (57.3)	126.3 (45.4)		McCaffrey, et al (1995)
VST (time)	HIV+ (sx)	12	11/1	37.20 (6.40)	n/a	7-10 d	116.1 (39.2)	107.8 (31.2)		McCaffrey, et al (1995)

instrument	group	n	m/f	age	intervention	inter	t #1	t #2	note	citation
VST (time)	HIV- ("At-Risk")	12	12/0	40.40 (13.0)	n/a	7-10 d	135.3 (62.2)	101.0 (25.4)		McCaffrey, et al (1995)

Table 71. Wechsler Memory Scales (WMS)

instrument	group	n	m/f	age	intervention	inter	t #1	t #2	note	citation
WMS	Schizophrenia	10	n/a	36.00	DDAVP	3 w	93.8	101.8		Stein, et al (1984)
WMS	Schizophrenia	10	n/a	36.00	placebo	3 w	92.7	104.4		Stein, et al (1984)
WMS	Schizophrenia	11	n/a	36.00	DDAVP	3 w	70.2	77.2		Stein, et al (1984)
WMS	Schizophrenia	11	n/a	36.00	placebo	3 w	70.2	78.7		Stein, et al (1984)
WMS AMTC	Epilepsy	13	0/13	~30.0	RTL	12 m	25.3 (4.0)	25.0 (2.9)		McGlone (1994)
WMS AMTC	Epilepsy	12	12/0	~30.0	RTL	12 m	25.4 (3.3)	25.9 (2.2)		McGlone (1994)
WMS AMTC	Epilepsy	7	0/7	~32.0	LTL	12 m	23.5 (2.9)	24.0 (2.6)		McGlone (1994)
WMS AMTC	Epilepsy	9	9/0	~32.0	LTL	12 m	25.9 (3.1)	25.6 (2.2)		McGlone (1994)
WMS 20-1 Counting (sec)	ALS	12	n/a	49.40 (11.8)	high dose interferon	5 d	11.5 (2.9)	14.8 (7.7)	*	Poutiainen, et al (1994)
WMS 20-1 Counting (sec)	ALS	3	n/a	52.30 (8.10)	placebo	5 d	14.3 (5.9)	15.0 (4.0)	*	Poutiainen, et al (1994)
WMS Counting by 3's (sec)	ALS	3	n/a	52.30 (8.10)	placebo	5 d	33.3 (13.7)	28.3 (5.9)	*	Poutiainen, et al (1994)

instrument	group	n	m/f	age	intervention	inter	t #1	t #2	note	citation
WMS Counting by 3's (sec)	ALS	12	n/a	49.40 (11.8)	high dose interferon	5 d	29.5 (12.8)	37.1 (24.5)	*	Poutiainen, et al (1994)
WMS D Span	Age Related Cognitive Decline	24	13/11	64.10 (6.50)	n/a	2.0 y	9.2 (1.3)	9.5 (1.6)		Celsis, et al (1997)
WMS D Span	Alcoholic	10	10/0	33.05 (7.09)	lorazepam	1 h	11.1	10.9	I,II CB	Mallick, et al (1993)
WMS D Span	Alcoholic	10	10/0	33.05 (7.09)	placebo	1 h	10.6	11.1	I,II CB	Mallick, et al (1993)
WMS D Span	Alcoholic (brief abstin)	27	27/0	40.96	DGAVP	7 d	9.8 (2.1)	10.2 (1.9)	*	Korsic, et al (1991)
WMS D Span	Alcoholic (brief abstin)	27	27/0	43.07	placebo	7 d	9.9 (1.4)	9.9 (1.5)	*	Korsic, et al (1991)
WMS D Span	Alcoholic (long abstin)	26	26/0	41.40	placebo	7 d	10.0 (2.1)	10.1 (2.1)	*	Korsic, et al (1991)
WMS D Span	Alcoholic (long abstin)	23	23/0	46.26	DGAVP	7 d	9.9 (1.9)	10.2 (2.3)	*	Korsic, et al (1991)
WMS D Span	Bipolar Inpts	18	12/6	45.80 (13.7)	lithium	6 y	11.7 (2.3)	10.6 (1.8)		Engelsmann, et al (1988)
WMS D Span	Control	18	8/10	65.30 (6.00)	n/a	3.2 y	10.8 (1.8)	12.6 (1.5)		Celsis, et al (1997)
WMS D Span	Control	11	9/2	31.60 (5.00)	n/a	6 m	11.9 (1.1)	12.1 (1.4)		Di Stefano, et al (1996)
WMS D Span	Control	12	n/a	elderly	atropine	2 d	9.8 (1.6)	10.3 (2.1)		Inzelberg, et al (1990)

instrument	group	n	m/f	age	intervention	inter	t #1	t #2	note	citation
WMS D Span	Control	12	n/a	elderly	placebo	2 d	10.6 (0.9)	10.0 (1.3)		Inzelberg, et al (1990)
WMS D Span	Control	10	10/0	31.30 (6.14)	lorazepam	1 h	12.4	13.1	I, II CB	Mallick, et al (1993)
WMS D Span	Control	10	10/0	31.30 (6.14)	placebo	1 h	12.7	13.5	I, II CB	Mallick, et al (1993)
WMS D Span	Coronary Artery Disease	298	264/34	53.40 (7.40)	CABG	9.4 d	12.0 (1.84)	11.4 (2.14)		Shaw, et al (1986)
WMS D Span	DAT	18	11/7	65.30 (6.00)	n/a	3.0 y	9.6 (2.6)	8.7 (2.1)		Celsis, et al (1997)
WMS D Span	DAT	12	n/a	elderly	atropine	2 d	7.6 (1.7)	6.0 (0.4)		Inzelberg, et al (1990)
WMS D Span	DAT	12	n/a	elderly	placebo	2 d	8.0 (1.3)	8.0 (3.9)		Inzelberg, et al (1990)
WMS D Span	Depression	10	n/a	73.00 (6.00)	bilateral ECT	~3 w	9.7	10.3	*	Fraser, et al (1980)
WMS D Span	Depression	10	n/a	73.00 (6.00)	unilateral ECT	~3 w	8.9	10.1	*	Fraser, et al (1980)
WMS D Span	HD (at risk, + genetic marker)	8	1/7	26.20 (2.70)	n/a	2 y	12.6	12.4	*	Giordani, et al (1995)
WMS D Span	HD (at risk, - genetic marker)	8	1/7	28.40 (5.20)	n/a	2 y	12.0	12.1	*	Giordani, et al (1995)
WMS D Span	Hysterectomy/ Oophorectomy	9	0/9	48.20 (4.70)	placebo	9 w	6.6 (0.3)	6.9 (0.4)	I, II CB	Phillips, et al (1992)
WMS D Span	Hysterectomy/ Oophorectomy	10	0/10	48.20 (4.70)	estrogen tx	9 w	6.0 (0.4)	6.1 (0.4)	I, II CB	Phillips, et al (1992)

instrument	group	n	m/f	age	intervention	inter	t #1	t #2	note	citation
WMS D Span	MID	12	n/a	elderly	atropine	2 d	9.7 (1.5)	10.3 (1.1)		Inzelberg, et al (1990)
WMS D Span	MID	12	n/a	elderly	placebo	2 d	9.7 (2.1)	10.7 (1.5)		Inzelberg, et al (1990)
WMS D Span	Myotonic Dystrophy	15	n/a	35.40	n/a	12 y	9.8 (1.2)	9.1 (1.6)		Tuikka, et al (1993)
WMS D Span	PD	18	11/7	56.90 (8.90)	placebo	12 w	9.0 (1.7)	9.7 (1.2)		Hietanen (1991)
WMS D Span	PD	18	11/7	56.90 (8.90)	selegiline	12 w	9.2 (1.1)	9.1 (0.6)		Hietanen (1991)
WMS D Span	PD	12	n/a	elderly	atropine	2 d	11.0 (1.8)	11.5 (2.4)		Inzelberg, et al (1990)
WMS D Span	PD	12	n/a	elderly	placebo	2 d	10.2 (1.9)	9.5 (2.4)		Inzelberg, et al (1990)
WMS D Span	PD w/ Dementia	12	n/a	elderly	atropine	2 d	7.5 (1.3)	5.7 (4.9)		Inzelberg, et al (1990)
WMS D Span	PD w/ Dementia	12	n/a	elderly	placebo	2 d	6.8 (3.3)	7.8 (2.8)		Inzelberg, et al (1990)
WMS D Span	PVD	50	36/14	57.40 (6.40)	major surgery	7.5 d	11.79 (1.92)	12.08 (1.98)		Shaw, et al (1987)
WMS D Span	Schizophrenia (chronic)	14	n/a	30.75	benztropine/ placebo	4 w	8.9 (2.0)	10.6 (1.7)		Baker, et al (1983)
WMS D Span	Schizophrenia (chronic)	14	n/a	29.50	benztropine/ benztropine	4 w	10.3 (2.7)	9.6 (1.7)		Baker, et al (1983)
WMS D Span	Whiplash	21	8/13	35.50 (10.50)	n/a	6 m	10.6 (1.7)	10.5 (1.9)	*	Di Stefano, et al (1995)

instrument	group	n	m/f	age	intervention	inter	t #1	t #2	note	citation
WMS D Span	Whiplash	58	26/32	29.60 (8.90)	n/a	6 m	10.7 (1.9)	10.7 (11.8)		Di Stefano, et al (1996)
WMS D Span	Whiplash (asx at 6 mos)	67	28/36	29.00 (8.50)	n/a	6 m	10.7 (1.8)	10.8 (1.7)		Radanov, et al (1993)
WMS D Span	Whiplash (sx at 6 mos)	31	9/19	36.50 (10.20)	n/a	6 m	9.6 (1.6)	10.3 (2.1)		Radanov, et al (1993)
WMS D Span	Whiplash w/ continuing sx	21	8/13	35.40 (11.00)	n/a	6 m	9.9 (2.2)	10.2 (2.2)	*	Di Stefano, et al (1995)
WMS D Span	Whiplash w/ continuing sx	28	9/19	34.10 (10.20)	n/a	6 m	9.9 (1.7)	10.9 (2.5)		Di Stefano, et al (1996)
WMS D Span Backward	Alcoholic	10	10/0	33.05 (7.09)	placebo	1 h	4.2	4.6	I, II CB	Mallick, et al (1993)
WMS D Span Backward	Alcoholic	10	10/0	33.05 (7.09)	lorazepam	1 h	4.8	4.6	I, II CB	Mallick, et al (1993)
WMS D Span Backward	ALS	3	n/a	52.30 (8.10)	placebo	5 d	3.7 (1.5)	4.3 (2.1)	*	Poutiainen, et al (1994)
WMS D Span Backward	ALS	12	n/a	49.40 (11.80)	high dose interferon	5 d	4.7 (1.4)	3.8 (1.5)	*	Poutiainen, et al (1994)
WMS D Span Backward	Control	5	1/4	68.40 (6.10)	lorazepam	60 min	7.00 (0.00)	6.60 (2.79)	I, II	Kirkby, et al (1995)
WMS D Span Backward	Control	8	4/4	21.80 (4.20)	placebo	60 min	6.88 (1.55)	7.25 (2.05)	I, II	Kirkby, et al (1995)
WMS D Span Backward	Control	9	4/5	26.40 (7.70)	lorazepam	60 min	7.44 (1.59)	7.22 (1.09)	I, II	Kirkby, et al (1995)
WMS D Span Backward	Control	4	0/4	67.30 (0.50)	placebo	60 min	6.50 (1.29)	6.75 (1.71)	I, II	Kirkby, et al (1995)

instrument	group	n	m/f	age	intervention	inter	t #1	t #2	note	citation
WMS D Span Backward	Control	10	10/0	31.30 (6.14)	lorazepam	1 h	5.4	6.0	I, II CB	Mallick, et al (1993)
WMS D Span Backward	Control	10	10/0	31.30 (6.14)	placebo	1 h	5.7	6.0	I, II CB	Mallick, et al (1993)
WMS D Span Backward	Control (CDR-0)	30	15/15	70.9 (4.6)	n/a	1 y	5.3 (1.4)	4.8 (1.3)	*	Botwinick, et al (1986)
WMS D Span Backward	DAT	14	n/a	60.00 - 80.00	placebo	6 m	3.8 (1.4)	3.6 (1.5)		Sano, et al (1992)
WMS D Span Backward	DAT	13	n/a	60.00 - 80.00	acetyl levocarnitine	6 m	3.5 (0.7)	3.2 (0.8)		Sano, et al (1992)
WMS D Span Backward	DAT (CDR-1)	18	7/11	71.40 (4.40)	n/a	1 y	3.5 (1.4)	3.2 (1.5)	*	Botwinick, et al (1986)
WMS D Span Backward	Schizophrenia	11	11/0	52.50 (11.50)	neuroleptic reduction	29.3 w	4.2 (1.2)	4.3 (0.9)		Seidman, et al (1993)
WMS D Span Forward	Alcoholic	10	10/0	33.05 (7.09)	lorazepam	1 h	6.3	6.3	I, II CB	Mallick, et al (1993)
WMS D Span Forward	Alcoholic	10	10/0	33.05 (7.09)	placebo	1 h	6.4	6.5	I, II CB	Mallick, et al (1993)
WMS D Span Forward	Control	70	26/44	29.30 (1.15)	n/a	4 y	5.74 (1.0)	5.71 (1.0)		Amato, et al (1995)
WMS D Span Forward	Control	8	4/4	21.80 (4.20)	placebo	60 min	8.38 (2.07)	8.00 (1.60)	I, II	Kirkby, et al (1995)
WMS D Span Forward	Control	4	0/4	67.30 (0.50)	placebo	60 min	8.50 (1.29)	7.25 (1.89)	I, II	Kirkby, et al (1995)
WMS D Span Forward	Control	5	1/4	68.40 (6.10)	lorazepam	60 min	9.00 (1.41)	8.00 (1.58)	I, II	Kirkby, et al (1995)

instrument	group	n	m/f	age	intervention	inter	t #1	t #2	note	citation
WMS D Span Forward	Control	9	4/5	26.40 (7.70)	lorazepam	60 min	9.56 (1.81)	9.89 (1.54)	I, II	Kirkby, et al (1995)
WMS D Span Forward	Control	10	10/0	31.30 (6.14)	placebo	1 h	7.0	7.5	I, II CB	Mallick, et al (1993)
WMS D Span Forward	Control	10	10/0	31.30 (6.14)	lorazepam	1 h	7.0	7.1	I, II CB	Mallick, et al (1993)
WMS D Span Forward	Control (CDR-0)	30	15/15	70.9 (4.6)	n/a	1 y	6.8 (1.1)	6.6 (1.4)	*	Botwinick, et al (1986)
WMS D Span Forward	DAT	14	n/a	60.00 - 80.00	placebo	6 m	5.6 (1.1)	5.5 (1.2)		Sano, et al (1992)
WMS D Span Forward	DAT	13	n/a	60.00 - 80.00	acetyl levocarnitine	6 m	4.9 (1.0)	5.5 (1.3)		Sano, et al (1992)
WMS D Span Forward	DAT (CDR-1)	18	7/11	71.40 (4.40)	n/a	1 y	6.3 (1.2)	5.6 (1.8)	*	Botwinick, et al (1986)
WMS D Span Forward	MS	50	18/32	29.90 (8.48)	n/a	4 y	5.55 (1.7)	5.61 (1.7)		Amato, et al (1995)
WMS D Span Forward	PD	12	12/0	65.60	trihexyphen	1 m	7.03 (0.26)	6.92 (0.22)		Koller (1984)
WMS D Span Forward	Schizophrenia	11	11/0	52.50 (11.50)	neuroleptic reduction	29.3 w	5.7 (0.07)	5.7 (1.0)		Seidman, et al (1993)
WMS Delayed Memory (LM, VR, PAL)	Schizophrenia	10	10/0	34.80 (8.69)	clonidine	6 w	16.8 (9.55)	20.3 (6.86)		Fields, et al (1988)
WMS Info	Alcoholic	10	10/0	33.05 (7.09)	lorazepam	1 h	4.9	4.9	I, II CB	Mallick, et al (1993)

instrument	group	n	m/f	age	intervention	inter	t #1	t #2	note	citation
WMS Info	Alcoholic	10	10/0	33.05 (7.09)	placebo	1 h	5.0	5.1	I, II CB	Mallick, et al (1993)
WMS Info	Bipolar Inpts	18	12/6	45.80 (13.70)	lithium	6 y	5.8 (0.5)	5.0 (0.0)		Engelsmann, et al (1988)
WMS Info	Control	12	n/a	elderly	placebo	2 d	5.0 (1.0)	5.4 (1.1)		Inzelberg, et al (1990)
WMS Info	Control	12	n/a	elderly	atropine	2 d	4.8 (1.2)	5.1 (0.9)		Inzelberg, et al (1990)
WMS Info	Control	10	10/0	31.30 (6.14)	lorazepam	1 h	5.2	5.3	I, II CB	Mallick, et al (1993)
WMS Info	Control	10	10/0	31.30 (6.14)	placebo	1 h	5.3	5.2	I, II CB	Mallick, et al (1993)
WMS Info	Coronary Artery Disease	298	264/ 34	53.40 (7.40)	CABG	9.4 d	5.16 (0.74)	5.24 (0.77)		Shaw, et al (1986)
WMS Info	DAT	12	n/a	elderly	atropine	2 d	3.5 (1.7)	3.4 (2.4)		Inzelberg, et al (1990)
WMS Info	DAT	12	n/a	elderly	placebo	2 d	4.6 (1.1)	4.6 (1.5)		Inzelberg, et al (1990)
WMS Info	Depression	10	n/a	73.00 (6.00)	unilateral ECT	~3 w	4.3	5.0	*	Fraser, et al (1980)
WMS Info	Depression	10	n/a	73.00 (6.00)	bilateral ECT	~3 w	4.8	5.1	*	Fraser, et al (1980)
WMS Info	MID	12	n/a	elderly	placebo	2 d	4.9 (1.5)	4.2 (1.6)		Inzelberg, et al (1990)

instrument	group	n	m/f	age	intervention	inter	t #1	t #2	note	citation
WMS Info	MID	12	n/a	elderly	atropine	2 d	4.4 (1.5)	4.7 (1.6)		Inzelberg, et al (1990)
WMS Info	Myotonic Dystrophy	15	n/a	35.40	n/a	12 y	5.2 (0.9)	5.4 (0.8)		Tuikka, et al (1993)
WMS Info	PD	12	n/a	elderly	atropine	2 d	5.6 (0.5)	6.0 (0.0)		Inzelberg, et al (1990)
WMS Info	PD	12	n/a	elderly	placebo	2 d	3.9 (2.1)	5.5 (0.6)		Inzelberg, et al (1990)
WMS Info	PD w/ Dementia	12	n/a	elderly	atropine	2 d	5.2 (0.8)	5.7 (0.6)		Inzelberg, et al (1990)
WMS Info	PD w/ Dementia	12	n/a	elderly	placebo	2 d	4.3 (1.6)	5.1 (1.2)		Inzelberg, et al (1990)
WMS Info	PVD	50	36/14	57.40 (6.40)	major surgery	7.5 d	5.21 (0.58)	5.4 (0.54)		Shaw, et al (1987)
WMS Info	Schizophrenia (chronic)	14	n/a	30.75	benztropine/ placebo	4 w	3.6 (1.8)	3.7 (1.6)		Baker, et al (1983)
WMS Info	Schizophrenia (chronic)	14	n/a	29.50	benztropine/ benztropine	4 w	4.1 (1.5)	4.2 (1.2)		Baker, et al (1983)
WMS Info, Orient, MC	DAT	14	n/a	53.00 - 81.00	lithium carbonate	7 d	10.0 (2.0)	10.4 (2.1)	*	Brinkman, et al (1984)
WMS LM	AAMI	75	27/48	61.93 (6.05)	n/a	4.6 y	8.84 (2.79)	8.22 (2.22)		Youngjohn, et al (1993)
WMS LM	ALS	12	n/a	49.40 (11.80)	high dose interferon	5 d	13.0 (3.9)	10.4 (3.4)	*	Poutiainen, et al (1994)

instrument	group	n	m/f	age	intervention	inter	t #1	t #2	note	citation
WMS LM	ALS	3	n/a	52.30 (8.10)	placebo	5 d	14.3 (3.8)	9.5 (4.3)	*	Poutiainen, et al (1994)
WMS LM	Bipolar Inpts	18	12/6	45.80 (13.70)	lithium	6 y	9.3 (2.9)	9.6 (3.9)		Engelsmann, et al (1988)
WMS LM	Cardiac	60	35/25	44.30 (9.40)	open heart surgery	10 m	9.76 (3.33)	10.49 (4.03)		Joulasmaa, et al (1981)
WMS LM	Cardiac	245	198/ 47	54.70	CABG/ cardiac operation	6 m	7.99 (3.65)	8.42 (3.05)		Savageau, et al (1982)
WMS LM	Control	102	65/37	24.52	n/a	12 m	12.0	13.0	*	Dikmen, et al (1990)
WMS LM	Control	12	n/a	elderly	placebo	2 d	7.5 (3.2)	11.7 (2.6)		Inzelberg, et al (1990)
WMS LM	Control	12	n/a	elderly	atropine	2 d	7.2 (4.6)	11.3 (5.3)		Inzelberg, et al (1990)
WMS LM	Control	115	56/59	48.90 (19.30)	n/a	20.9 d	8.74 (2.33)	10.17 (2.56)		Youngjohn, et al (1992)
WMS LM	Control (CDR-0)	30	15/15	70.9 (4.6)	n/a	1 y	9.0 (2.2)	10.2 (2.7)	*	Botwinick, et al (1986)
WMS LM	Coronary Artery Disease	298	264/ 34	53.40 (7.40)	CABG	9.4 d	9.98 (3.28)	9.43 (3.1)		Shaw, et al (1986)
WMS LM	DAT	12	n/a	elderly	placebo	2 d	7.7 (1.5)	9.3 (2.2)		Inzelberg, et al (1990)
WMS LM	DAT	12	n/a	elderly	atropine	2 d	4.5 (0.7)	5.1 (0.7)		Inzelberg, et al (1990)
WMS LM	DAT	13	n/a	60.00 - 80.00	acetyl levocarnitine	6 m	2.8 (1.8)	3.0 (1.6)		Sano, et al (1992)

instrument	group	n	m/f	age	intervention	inter	t #1	t #2	note	citation
WMS LM	DAT	14	n/a	60.00 - 80.00	placebo	6 m	2.9 (1.6)	2.2 (2.1)		Sano, et al (1992)
WMS LM	DAT (CDR-1)	18	7/11	71.40 (4.40)	n/a	1 y	2.1 (1.7)	1.9 (2.5)	*	Botwinick, et al (1986)
WMS LM	Dementia	<35	n/a	66.00 (9.60)	n/a	19.0 m	9.7 (3.5)	9.1 (2.3)		Jones, et al (1992)
WMS LM	Dementia (2° to steroids)	6	6/0	49.67	steriods d/c or reduced	10.9 m	9.2	12.3		Varney, et al (1984)
WMS LM	Depression	10	n/a	73.00 (6.00)	bilateral ECT	~3 w	5.25	6.0	*	Fraser, et al (1980)
WMS LM	Depression	10	n/a	73.00 (6.00)	unilateral ECT	~3 w	2.85	4.15	*	Fraser, et al (1980)
WMS LM	Depression	33	14/19	37.40	antidepress	7 w	10.1 (4.1)	13.6 (12.7)		Fromm, et al (1984)
WMS LM	Depression	52	n/a	41.10	ECT 2 x wk	~3 w	NR	0.84 c	I/II, *	Stromgren, et al (1976)
WMS LM	Depression	51	n/a	40.80	ECT 4 x wk	~2 w	NR	1.00 c	II/II, *	Stromgren, et al (1976)
WMS LM	HD (at risk, + genetic marker)	8	1/7	26.20 (2.70)	n/a	2 y	10.1	9.6	*	Giordani, et al (1995)
WMS LM	HD (at risk, - genetic marker)	8	1/7	28.40 (5.20)	n/a	2 y	11.1	11.1	*	Giordani, et al (1995)
WMS LM	HIV+ (IVDU)	18	10/8	29.80 (5.40)	drug tx	17.7 m	9.2 (5.1)	8.3 (3.6)		Hestad, et al (1996)
WMS LM	HIV- (IVDU)	30	16/14	27.90 (4.90)	drug tx	14.9 m	9.0 (3.3)	10.3 (3.0)		Hestad, et al (1996)

instrument	group	n	m/f	age	intervention	inter	t #1	t #2	note	citation
WMS LM	Korsakoff's Syndrome	10	9/1	63.00 (10.00)	fluvoxamine	3 w	5.0 (2.0)	7.0 (2.0)	*	Martin, et al (1995)
WMS LM	MID	12	n/a	elderly	placebo	2 d	7.8 (1.9)	9.9 (1.1)		Inzelberg, et al (1990)
WMS LM	MID	12	n/a	elderly	atropine	2 d	5.6 (2.4)	7.4 (1.4)		Inzelberg, et al (1990)
WMS LM	Myotonic Dystrophy	15	n/a	35.40	n/a	12 y	12.5 (3.8)	9.0 (3.7)		Tuikka, et al (1993)
WMS LM	PD	18	11/7	56.90 (8.90)	selegiline	12 w	9.7 (3.4)	10.2 (4.1)		Hietanen (1991)
WMS LM	PD	18	11/7	56.90 (8.90)	placebo	12 w	9.0 (3.1)	12.3 (1.7)		Hietanen (1991)
WMS LM	PD	12	n/a	elderly	atropine	2 d	7.8 (3.9)	12.3 (3.5)		Inzelberg, et al (1990)
WMS LM	PD	12	n/a	elderly	placebo	2 d	5.2 (1.8)	10.3 (1.5)		Inzelberg, et al (1990)
WMS LM	PD	19	13/6	54.30	pergolide	~6 w	7.8 (3.02)	8.3 (2.99)		Stern, et al (1984)
WMS LM	PD w/ Dementia	12	n/a	elderly	placebo	2 d	6.5 (3.1)	8.3 (0.9)		Inzelberg, et al (1990)
WMS LM	PD w/ Dementia	12	n/a	elderly	atropine	2 d	5.8 (1.9)	8.5 (5.7)		Inzelberg, et al (1990)
WMS LM	PVD	50	36/14	57.40 (6.40)	major surgery	7.5 d	9.32 (2.74)	10.67 (2.6)		Shaw, et al (1987)
WMS LM	Pseudo-dementia	<35	n/a	66.00 (9.60)	n/a	19.0 m	11.1 (1.2)	12.1 (3.1)		Jones, et al (1992)

instrument	group	n	m/f	age	intervention	inter	t #1	t #2	note	citation
WMS LM	Schizophrenia	15	10/5	35.00	std neuroleptics	~15 m	7.3 (3.9)	7.0 (2.7)	II	Goldberg, et al (1993)
WMS LM	Schizophrenia (chronic)	14	n/a	30.75	benztropine/ placebo	4 w	4.3 (3.6)	6.8 (3.1)		Baker, et al (1983)
WMS LM	Schizophrenia (chronic)	14	n/a	29.50	benztropine/ benztropine	4 w	4.0 (2.7)	6.4 (3.6)		Baker, et al (1983)
WMS LM	TBI	31	20/11	24.16	n/a	12 m	6.0	9.5	*	Dikmen, et al (1990)
WMS LM	TBI	18	15/3	26.10 (8.30)	rehab	7.5 m	6.9	8.0		Prigatano, et al (1984)
WMS LM	TBI	17	15/2	23.50 (5.10)	n/a	12.6 m	7.0	6.8		Prigatano, et al (1984)
WMS LM	Temporal Lobe Epilepsy	17	11/6	29.00 (8.12)	LTL	1.8 y	6.53 (2.86)	5.71 (2.77)		Selwa, et al (1994)
WMS LM	Temporal Lobe Epilepsy	28	17/11	31.29 (9.52)	n/a	2.36 y	6.47 (2.28)	6.39 (2.77)		Selwa, et al (1994)
WMS LM	Temporal Lobe Epilepsy	14	6/8	31.36 (9.93)	RTL	1.93 y	8.36 (2.96)	8.39 (3.01)		Selwa, et al (1994)
WMS LM (ASS)	Epilepsy	35	17/18	28.40 (9.60)	RTL	9.4 m	10.6	10.3		Ivnik, et al (1987)
WMS LM (ASS)	Epilepsy	28	17/11	27.00 (5.90)	LTL	9.4 m	9.5	8.0		Ivnik, et al (1987)
WMS LM Delay	Alcoholic (brief abstin)	27	27/0	43.07	placebo	7 d	6.1 (4.2)	6.6 (4.1)	*	Korsic, et al (1991)
WMS LM Delay	Alcoholic (brief abstin)	27	27/0	40.96	DGAVP	7 d	4.4 (3.9)	6.1 (4.6)	*	Korsic, et al (1991)

instrument	group	n	m/f	age	intervention	inter	t #1	t #2	note	citation
WMS LM Delay	Alcoholic (long abstin)	26	26/0	41.40	placebo	7 d	6.9 (3.9)	6.8 (3.8)	*	Korsic, et al (1991)
WMS LM Delay	Alcoholic (long abstin)	23	23/0	46.26	DGAVP	7 d	7.1 (4.2)	8.0 (4.3)	*	Korsic, et al (1991)
WMS LM Delay	Cardiac	90	77/13	59.00 (10.59)	CABG/CPB	8 d	12.5 (3.9)	10.0 (5.1)	*	Townes, et al (1989)
WMS LM Delay	CAD	20	n/a	57.20 (7.20)	CE	6 m	11.6	13.6		Parker, et al (1983)
WMS LM Delay	CAD	17	n/a	57.20 (7.20)	n/a	6 m	11.9	12.6		Parker, et al (1983)
WMS LM Delay	CAD	17	n/a	57.90 (8.40)	n/a	6 m	12.2	13.1	*	Parker, et al (1986)
WMS LM Delay	CAD	36	n./a	61.10 (8.30)	CE	6 m	11.0	13.3	*	Parker, et al (1986)
WMS LM Delay	Control	16	10/6	64.00 (1.70)	n/a	1 w	7.3 (1.0)	7.8 (0.7)	*	Claus, et al (1991)
WMS LM Delay	Control	33	15/18	59.10 (9.30)	n/a	10 d	8.0 (3.0)	10.4 (3.0)		McCaffrey, et al (1993)
WMS LM Delay	Control	19	2/17	62.20 (2.50)	n/a	1 y	6.5 (3.0)	6.9 (2.7)	*	Mitrushina, et al (1991b)
WMS LM Delay	Control	40	6/34	68.20 (1.20)	n/a	1 y	6.8 (2.7)	7.2 (3.1)	*	Mitrushina, et al (1991b)
WMS LM Delay	Control	47	14/33	72.90 (1.40)	n/a	1 y	6.0 (3.2)	6.0 (3.6)	*	Mitrushina, et al (1991b)

instrument	group	n	m/f	age	intervention	inter	t #1	t #2	note	citation
WMS LM Delay	Control	16	4/12	78.30 (2.50)	n/a	1 y	6.6 (2.5)	4.8 (2.4)	*	Mitrushina, et al (1991b)
WMS LM Delay	Control	21	21/0	31.45 (5.53)	n/a	18 m	24.15 (5.02)	25.67 (5.69)		Saykin, et al (1991)
WMS LM Delay	Control	47	35/12	59.00 (9.81)	n/a	8 d	14.3 (3.0)	13.4 (2.7)	*	Townes, et al (1989)
WMS LM Delay	Control (Pain Pt/Volunteer)	15	5/10	33.90 (8.40)	n/a	20.7 d	15.1 (6.2)	22.4 (7.6)		Goulet Fisher, et al (1986)
WMS LM Delay	DAT	17	7/1	64.00 (1.70)	n/a	1 w	0.5 (0.2)	0.4 (0.2)	*	Claus, et al (1991)
WMS LM Delay	DAT (mild)	11	10/1	63.00 (8.00)	n/a	26 m	2.0 (4.0)	0.0 (1.0)		Haxby, et al (1990)
WMS LM Delay	DAT/MID	29	14/15	71.50 (1.30)	oxiracetam	6 m	1.4 (0.2)	1.2 (0.2)	*	Villardita, et al (1992)
WMS LM Delay	DAT/MID	30	15/15	71.70 (1.30)	oxiracetam	3 m	1.4 (0.2)	1.7 (0.2)	*	Villardita, et al (1992)
WMS LM Delay	DAT/MID	30	21/9	67.80 (1.50)	placebo	3 m	1.8 (0.3)	1.5 (0.2)	*	Villardita, et al (1992)
WMS LM Delay	Depression	15	6/9	28.50 (10.60)	inpt tx	19.5 d	12.4 (5.7)	19.8 (5.9)		Goulet Fisher, et al (1986)
WMS LM Delay	Epilepsy	40	23/17	32.20 (8.20)	n/a	~9 m	12.15 (5.59)	13.43 (5.78)		Hermann, et al (1996)
WMS LM Delay	Epilepsy	29	13/16	24.70 (8.30)	LTL	4 w	11.78 (7.58)	11.12 (6.00)		Powell, et al (1985)

instrument	group	n	m/f	age	intervention	inter	t #1	t #2	note	citation
WMS LM Delay	Epilepsy	30	21/9	26.30 (10.80)	RTL	4 w	13.84 (8.61)	15.50 (10.89)		Powell, et al (1985)
WMS LM Delay	Epilepsy	12	n/a	29.20 (7.70)	LTL	1.2 y	2.8 (2.1)	3.8 (2.8)		Rausch, et al (1993)
WMS LM Delay	Epilepsy	13	n/a	29.20 (7.70)	RTL	1.2 y	6.4 (2.1)	6.2 (2.3)		Rausch, et al (1993)
WMS LM Delay	HIV+ (IVDU)	42	31/11	27.00 (5.30)	n/a	12 m	7.9 (2.3)	8.2 (2.7)		Bono, et al (1996)
WMS LM Delay	HIV+/ARC	8	8/0	33.57 (6.35)	n/a	18 m	17.21 (6.62)	14.86 (6.30)		Saykin, et al (1991)
WMS LM Delay	HIV+/PGL	13	13/0	31.15 (4.91)	n/a	18 m	21.92 (5.56)	21.50 (5.21)		Saykin, et al (1991)
WMS LM Delay	HIV- (IVDU)	39	30/9	28.60 (4.90)	n/a	12 m	8.1 (2.9)	9.1 (2.5)		Bono, et al (1996)
WMS LM Delay	Hypertension	25	17/8	50.10 (14.00)	n/a	7-10 d	8.55 (2.65)	11.34 (3.39)		McCaffrey, et al (1992)
WMS LM Delay	Hypertension	35	n/a	76.10	bendrofluaz	24 w	4.7 (3.2)	5.2 (3.5)		Starr, et al (1996)
WMS LM Delay	Hypertension	34	n/a	76.10	captopril	24 w	4.2 (3.0)	5.5 (3.1)		Starr, et al (1996)
WMS LM Delay	Hysterectomy/ Oophorectomy	10	0/10	48.20 (4.70)	estrogen tx	9 w	15.9 (2.1)	21.1 (2.4)	I, II CB	Phillips, et al (1992)
WMS LM Delay	Hysterectomy/ Oophorectomy	9	0/9	48.20 (4.70)	placebo	9 w	16.7 (3.4)	21.2 (3.3)	I, II CB	Phillips, et al (1992)

instrument	group	n	m/f	age	intervention	inter	t #1	t #2	note	citation
WMS LM Delay	MS	13	n/a	36.20	placebo	2 y	15.7 (5.8)	15.1 (5.1)	I/ II	Pliskin, et al (1996)
WMS LM Delay	MS	9	n/a	38.90	high dose interferon	2 y	12.8 (9.8)	12.1 (7.1)	I/ II	Pliskin, et al (1996)
WMS LM Delay	MS	8	n/a	38.00	low dose interferon	2 y	12.6 (5.7)	12.4 (5.6)	I/ II	Pliskin, et al (1996)
WMS LM Delay	PD	4	3/1	53.50	fetal tissue implanted	12 m	9.8	13.3		Sass, et al (1995)
WMS LM Delay	Spinal Cord Injury	67	54/13	32.00 (14.70)	n/a	38 w	13.6 (7.5)	15.74 (7.93)		Richards, et al (1988)
WMS LM Delay	Surgical	17	n/a	57.20 (7.20)	surgery	6 m	14.0	15.8		Parker, et al (1983)
WMS LM Delay	Surgical	26	n/a	55.30 (6.80)	surgery (non-CE)	6 m	14.8	15.9	*	Parker, et al (1986)
WMS LM Delay (% forg)	HIV+ (IVDU)	42	31/11	27.00 (5.30)	n/a	12 m	13.2	13.7		Bono, et al (1996)
WMS LM Delay (% forg)	HIV- (IVDU)	39	30/9	28.60 (4.90)	n/a	12 m	13.8	9.1		Bono, et al (1996)
WMS LM Delay (% ret)	Alcoholic	10	10/0	33.05 (7.09)	lorazepam	1 h	80.1	51.7	I, II CB	Mallick, et al (1993)
WMS LM Delay (% ret)	Alcoholic	10	10/0	33.05 (7.09)	placebo	1 h	79.4	75.0	I, II CB	Mallick, et al (1993)
WMS LM Delay (% ret)	CAD	20	n/a	57.20 (7.20)	CE	6 m	71.1	79.4		Parker, et al (1983)

instrument	group	n	m/f	age	intervention	inter	t #1	t #2	note	citation
WMS LM Delay (% ret)	CAD	17	n/a	57.20 (7.20)	n/a	6 m	75.4	71.3		Parker, et al (1983)
WMS LM Delay (% ret)	CAD	36	n./a	61.10 (8.30)	CE	6 m	72.6	83.1	*	Parker, et al (1986)
WMS LM Delay (% ret)	CAD	17	n/a	57.90 (8.40)	n/a	6 m	78.5	75.1	*	Parker, et al (1986)
WMS LM Delay (% ret)	Control	10	10/0	31.30 (6.14)	lorazepam	1 h	87.8	53.8	I, II CB	Mallick, et al (1993)
WMS LM Delay (% ret)	Control	10	10/0	31.30 (6.14)	placebo	1 h	79.6	90.5	I, II CB	Mallick, et al (1993)
WMS LM Delay (% ret)	Depression	19	9/10	37.95 (12.70)	amitriptyline	4 d	43.18 (14.80)	45.76 (17.44)		Lamping, et al (1984)
WMS LM Delay (% ret)	Depression	21	12/9	31.19 (6.34)	clovoxamine	4 d	41.79 (15.37)	47.53 (18.46)		Lamping, et al (1984)
WMS LM Delay (% ret)	Epilepsy	40	23/17	32.20 (8.20)	n/a	~9 m	75.85 (20.81)	77.83 (18.03)		Hermann, et al (1996)
WMS LM Delay (% ret)	Epilepsy	30	21/9	26.30 (10.80)	RTL	4 w	72.65 (24.63)	73.96 (25.67)		Powell, et al (1985)
WMS LM Delay (% ret)	Epilepsy	29	13/16	24.70 (8.30)	LTL	4 w	66.37 (31.80)	73.46 (23.76)		Powell, et al (1985)
WMS LM Delay (% ret)	HD (at risk, + genetic marker)	8	1/7	26.20 (2.70)	n/a	2 y	79.4	82.5	*	Giordani, et al (1995)
WMS LM Delay (% ret)	HD (at risk, - genetic marker)	8	1/7	28.40 (5.20)	n/a	2 y	78.8	85.0	*	Giordani, et al (1995)

instrument	group	n	m/f	age	intervention	inter	t #1	t #2	note	citation
WMS LM Delay (% ret)	Myasthenia Gravis	11	7/4	49.00	prednisolone	3-11 m	81.0 (14.0)	84.0 (20.0)		Glennerster, et al (1996)
WMS LM Delay (% ret)	Schizophrenia	11	11/0	52.50 (11.50)	neuroleptic reduction	29.3 w	78.5 (29.3)	86.2 (19.7)		Seidman, et al (1993)
WMS LM Delay (% ret)	Spinal Cord Injury	67	54/13	32.00 (14.70)	n/a	38 w	76.49 (31.15)	87.11 (45.72)		Richards, et al (1988)
WMS LM Delay (% ret)	Surgical	17	n/a	57.20 (7.20)	surgery	6 m	77.9	85.1		Parker, et al (1983)
WMS LM Delay (% ret)	Surgical	26	n/a	55.30 (6.80)	surgery (non-CE)	6 m	81.8	86.1	*	Parker, et al (1986)
WMS LM Delay (% ret)	Temporal Lobe Epilepsy	17	11/6	29.00 (8.12)	LTL	1.8 y	64.53 (21.44)	63.18 (32.33)		Selwa, et al (1994)
WMS LM Delay (% ret)	Temporal Lobe Epilepsy	14	6/8	31.36 (9.93)	RTL	1.93 y	66.21 (19.22)	77.79 (14.84)		Selwa, et al (1994)
WMS LM Delay (% ret)	Temporal Lobe Epilepsy	28	17/11	31.29 (9.52)	n/a	2.36 y	58.07 (20.98)	51.96 (30.69)		Selwa, et al (1994)
WMS LM Delay (story A)	BZ Dependence	21	11/10	44.40 (9.40)	BZ tx & abstin	1 m	5.52 (3.44)	6.43 (4.25)	*	Tata, et al (1994)
WMS LM Delay (story A)	Control	21	11/10	43.10 (14.40)	n/a	1 m	12.52 (4.42)	12.81 (4.49)	*	Tata, et al (1994)
WMS LM Delay (story B)	BZ Dependence	21	11/10	44.40 (9.40)	BZ tx & abstin	1 m	5.67 (2.89)	6.57 (4.15)	*	Tata, et al (1994)
WMS LM Delay (story B)	Control	21	11/10	43.10 (14.40)	n/a	1 m	9.86 (5.04)	11.10 (3.65)	*	Tata, et al (1994)

instrument	group	n	m/f	age	intervention	inter	t #1	t #2	note	citation
WMS LM Imm	Alcoholic	10	10/0	33.05 (7.09)	placebo	1 h	7.1	8.25	I, II CB	Mallick, et al (1993)
WMS LM Imm	Alcoholic	10	10/0	33.05 (7.09)	lorazepam	1 h	7.45	7.0	I, II CB	Mallick, et al (1993)
WMS LM Imm	Alcoholic (brief abstin)	27	27/0	43.07	placebo	7 d	7.8 (4.2)	8.7 (4.4)	*	Korsic, et al (1991)
WMS LM Imm	Alcoholic (brief abstin)	27	27/0	40.96	DGAVP	7 d	5.7 (3.1)	7.3 (4.3)	*	Korsic, et al (1991)
WMS LM Imm	Alcoholic (long abstin)	26	26/0	41.40	placebo	7 d	8.8 (3.8)	8.0 (3.1)	*	Korsic, et al (1991)
WMS LM Imm	Alcoholic (long abstin)	23	23/0	46.26	DGAVP	7 d	8.3 (3.4)	9.4 (4.8)	*	Korsic, et al (1991)
WMS LM Imm	Cardiac	90	77/13	59.00 (10.59)	CABG/CPB	8 d	15.4 (2.9)	13.8 (4.5)	*	Townes, et al (1989)
WMS LM Imm	CAD	17	n/a	57.20 (7.20)	n/a	6 m	14.9	16.3		Parker, et al (1983)
WMS LM Imm	CAD	20	n/a	57.20 (7.20)	CE	6 m	14.7	16.7		Parker, et al (1983)
WMS LM Imm	CAD	17	n/a	57.90 (8.40)	n/a	6 m	15.0	16.5	*	Parker, et al (1986)
WMS LM Imm	CAD	36	n./a	61.10 (8.30)	CE	6 m	13.9	15.9	*	Parker, et al (1986)
WMS LM Imm	Control	16	10/6	64.00 (1.70)	n/a	1 w	9.4 (0.8)	9.5 (0.8)	*	Claus, et al (1991)

instrument	group	n	m/f	age	intervention	inter	t #1	t #2	note	citation
WMS LM Imm	Control	87	43/44	64.00 (3.10)	exercise program	1 y	11.51 (3.12)	11.57 (3.04)		Hill, et al (1993)
WMS LM Imm	Control	34	17/17	64.00 (3.10)	n/a	1 y	11.08 (2.98)	9.41 (2.56)		Hill, et al (1993)
WMS LM Imm	Control	10	10/0	31.30 (6.14)	lorazepam	1 h	10.3	8.35	I, II CB	Mallick, et al (1993)
WMS LM Imm	Control	10	10/0	31.30 (6.14)	placebo	1 h	9.7	9.25	I, II CB	Mallick, et al (1993)
WMS LM Imm	Control	33	15/18	59.10 (9.30)	n/a	10 d	9.6 (3.4)	11.0 (3.3)		McCaffrey, et al (1993)
WMS LM Imm	Control	19	2/17	62.20 (2.50)	n/a	1 y	9.7 (2.5)	9.3 (3.1)	*	Mitrushina, et al (1991b)
WMS LM Imm	Control	16	4/12	78.30 (2.50)	n/a	1 y	9.4 (2.2)	8.4 (1.8)	*	Mitrushina, et al (1991b)
WMS LM Imm	Control	47	14/33	72.90 (1.40)	n/a	1 y	9.2 (3.2)	8.9 (3.1)	*	Mitrushina, et al (1991b)
WMS LM Imm	Control	40	6/34	68.20 (1.20)	n/a	1 y	10.1 (2.6)	9.9 (3.0)	*	Mitrushina, et al (1991b)
WMS LM Imm	Control	21	21/0	31.45 (5.53)	n/a	18 m	27.35 (3.75)	27.42 (5.13)		Saykin, et al (1991)
WMS LM Imm	Control	47	35/12	59.00 (9.81)	n/a	8 d	16.2 (2.1)	16.1 (1.5)	*	Townes, et al (1989)
WMS LM Imm	Control (Pain Pt/Volunteer)	15	5/10	33.90 (8.40)	n/a	20.7 d	18.0 (6.1)	23.6 (7.0)		Goulet Fisher, et al (1986)

instrument	group	n	m/f	age	intervention	inter	t #1	t #2	note	citation
WMS LM Imm	DAT	17	7/1	64.00 (1.70)	n/a	1 w	1.4 (0.3)	1.6 (0.4)	*	Claus, et al (1991)
WMS LM Imm	DAT (mild)	11	10/1	63.00 (8.00)	n/a	26 m	11.0 (5.0)	5.0 (4.0)		Haxby, et al (1990)
WMS LM Imm	DAT/MID	30	21/9	67.80 (1.50)	placebo	3 m	1.6 (0.3)	1.6 (0.2)	*	Villardita, et al (1992)
WMS LM Imm	DAT/MID	30	15/15	71.70 (1.30)	oxiracetam	3 m	1.6 (0.2)	2.1 (0.2)	*	Villardita, et al (1992)
WMS LM Imm	DAT/MID	29	14/15	71.50 (1.30)	oxiracetam	6 m	1.7 (0.2)	1.8 (0.2)	*	Villardita, et al (1992)
WMS LM Imm	Depression	15	6/9	28.50 (10.60)	inpt tx	19.5 d	16.3 (6.6)	23.4 (5.8)		Goulet Fisher, et al (1986)
WMS LM Imm	Epilepsy	40	23/17	32.20 (8.20)	n/a	~9 m	15.37 (5.40)	16.87 (5.76)		Hermann, et al (1996)
WMS LM Imm	Epilepsy	30	21/9	26.30 (10.80)	RTL	4 w	17.28 (7.48)	19.35 (9.36)		Powell, et al (1985)
WMS LM Imm	Epilepsy	29	13/16	24.70 (8.30)	LTL	4 w	16.43 (6.71)	14.80 (6.52)		Powell, et al (1985)
WMS LM Imm	Epilepsy	12	n/a	29.20 (7.70)	LTL	1.2 y	7.8 (3.6)	5.4 (2.4)		Rausch, et al (1993)
WMS LM Imm	Epilepsy	13	n/a	29.20 (7.70)	RTL	1.2 y	9.3 (2.3)	9.4 (1.7)		Rausch, et al (1993)
WMS LM Imm	HIV+ (IVDU)	42	31/11	27.00 (5.30)	n/a	12 m	9.1 (2.1)	9.5 (2.4)		Bono, et al (1996)

instrument	group	n	m/f	age	intervention	inter	t #1	t #2	note	citation
WMS LM Imm	HIV+/ARC	8	8/0	33.57 (6.35)	n/a	18 m	19.43 (7.38)	18.79 (6.22)		Saykin, et al (1991)
WMS LM Imm	HIV+/PGL	13	13/0	31.15 (4.91)	n/a	18 m	23.69 (6.18)	23.65 (5.18)		Saykin, et al (1991)
WMS LM Imm	HIV- (IVDU)	39	30/9	28.60 (4.90)	n/a	12 m	9.4 (2.5)	9.9 (2.2)		Bono, et al (1996)
WMS LM Imm	Hypertension	25	17/8	50.10 (14.00)	n/a	7-10 d	10.23 (3.14)	12.36 (2.75)		McCaffrey, et al (1992)
WMS LM Imm	Hypertension	35	n/a	76.10	bendrofluaz	24 w	7.3 (3.5)	7.8 (3.3)		Starr, et al (1996)
WMS LM Imm	Hypertension	34	n/a	76.10	captopril	24 w	7.2 (3.0)	7.9 (3.0)		Starr, et al (1996)
WMS LM Imm	Hysterectomy/ Oophorectomy	9	0/9	48.20 (4.70)	placebo	9 w	23.1 (2.9)	24.6 (2.9)	I, II CB	Phillips, et al (1992)
WMS LM Imm	Hysterectomy/ Oophorectomy	10	0/10	48.20 (4.70)	estrogen tx	9 w	19.0 (2.3)	25.8 (2.2)	I, II CB	Phillips, et al (1992)
WMS LM Imm	MS	8	n/a	38.00	low dose interferon	2 y	16.1 (4.7)	16.8 (5.1)	I /II	Pliskin, et al (1996)
WMS LM Imm	MS	9	n/a	38.90	high dose interferon	2 y	16.8 (8.0)	18.7 (4.5)	I /II	Pliskin, et al (1996)
WMS LM Imm	MS	13	n/a	36.20	placebo	2 y	19.7 (5.5)	19.5 (4.5)	I /II	Pliskin, et al (1996)
WMS LM Imm	Myasthenia Gravis	11	7/4	49.00	prednisolone	3-11 m	10.0 (4.4)	12.2 (5.0)		Glennerster, et al (1996)

instrument	group	n	m/f	age	intervention	inter	t #1	t #2	note	citation
WMS LM Imm	PD	4	3/1	53.50	fetal tissue implanted	12 m	12.7	17.1		Sass, et al (1995)
WMS LM Imm	Spinal Cord Injury	67	54/13	32.00 (14.70)	n/a	38 w	17.43 (6.94)	18.66 (7.22)		Richards, et al (1988)
WMS LM Imm	Surgical	17	n/a	57.20 (7.20)	surgery	6 m	17.4	18.4		Parker, et al (1983)
WMS LM Imm	Surgical	26	n/a	55.30 (6.80)	surgery (non-CE)	6 m	17.4	18.2	*	Parker, et al (1986)
WMS LM Imm (story A)	BZ Dependence	21	11/10	44.40 (9.40)	BZ tx & abstin	1 m	7.19 (4.07)	8.76 (4.76)	*	Tata, et al (1994)
WMS LM Imm (story A)	Control	21	11/10	43.10 (14.40)	n/a	1 m	12.81 (3.37)	12.86 (3.72)	*	Tata, et al (1994)
WMS LM Imm (story B)	BZ Dependence	21	11/10	44.40 (9.40)	BZ tx & abstin	1 m	6.48 (3.09)	9.05 (3.62)	*	Tata, et al (1994)
WMS LM Imm (story B)	Control	21	11/10	43.10 (14.40)	n/a	1 m	9.81 (3.44)	11.19 (2.77)	*	Tata, et al (1994)
WMS MC	Alcoholic	10	10/0	33.05 (7.09)	placebo	1 h	7.9	7.9	I, II CB	Mallick, et al (1993)
WMS MC	Alcoholic	10	10/0	33.05 (7.09)	lorazepam	1 h	7.8	7.7	I, II CB	Mallick, et al (1993)
WMS MC	Bipolar Inpts	18	12/6	45.80 (13.70)	lithium	6 y	7.4 (1.9)	7.3 (1.9)		Engelsmann, et al (1988)
WMS MC	Control	12	n/a	elderly	atropine	2 d	5.7 (1.8)	5.8 (2.9)		Inzelberg, et al (1990)

instrument	group	n	m/f	age	intervention	inter	t #1	t #2	note	citation
WMS MC	Control	12	n/a	elderly	placebo	2 d	4.8 (2.6)	4.9 (2.2)		Inzelberg, et al (1990)
WMS MC	Control	10	10/0	31.30 (6.14)	lorazepam	1 h	8.4	8.1	I, II CB	Mallick, et al (1993)
WMS MC	Control	10	10/0	31.30 (6.14)	placebo	1 h	8.0	8.3	I, II CB	Mallick, et al (1993)
WMS MC	Control (CDR-0)	30	15/15	70.9 (4.6)	n/a	1 y	7.3 (1.8)	7.3 (1.6)	*	Botwinick, et al (1986)
WMS MC	Coronary Artery Disease	298	264/34	53.40 (7.40)	CABG	9.4 d	7.15 (1.83)	6.38 (2.11)		Shaw, et al (1986)
WMS MC	DAT	12	n/a	elderly	atropine	2 d	2.2 (2.2)	2.8 (3.0)		Inzelberg, et al (1990)
WMS MC	DAT	12	n/a	elderly	placebo	2 d	6.6 (1.8)	5.2 (2.3)		Inzelberg, et al (1990)
WMS MC	DAT (CDR-1)	18	7/11	71.40 (4.40)	n/a	1 y	4.9 (2.3)	3.9 (3.0)	*	Botwinick, et al (1986)
WMS MC	DAT/MID	30	15/15	71.70 (1.30)	oxiracetam	3 m	2.5 (0.3)	2.8 (0.3)	*	Villardita, et al (1992)
WMS MC	DAT/MID	30	21/9	67.80 (1.50)	placebo	3 m	2.5 (0.3)	2.3 (0.3)	*	Villardita, et al (1992)
WMS MC	DAT/MID	29	14/15	71.50 (1.30)	oxiracetam	6 m	2.6 (0.3)	3.0 (0.3)	*	Villardita, et al (1992)
WMS MC	Depression	10	n/a	73.00 (6.00)	bilateral ECT	~3 w	5.5	6.2	*	Fraser, et al (1980)

instrument	group	n	m/f	age	intervention	inter	t #1	t #2	note	citation
WMS MC	Depression	10	n/a	73.00 (6.00)	unilateral ECT	~3 w	4.2	5.9	*	Fraser, et al (1980)
WMS MC	Depression	33	14/19	37.40	antidepress	7 w	6.6 (2.3)	6.7 (1.5)		Fromm, et al (1984)
WMS MC	Depression	51	n/a	40.80	ECT 4 x wk	~2 w	NR	0.04 c	II/II, *	Stromgren, et al (1976)
WMS MC	Depression	52	n/a	41.10	ECT 2 x wk	~3 w	NR	0.13 c	I/II, *	Stromgren, et al (1976)
WMS MC	MID	12	n/a	elderly	atropine	2 d	3.7 (1.5)	4.0 (1.7)		Inzelberg, et al (1990)
WMS MC	MID	12	n/a	elderly	placebo	2 d	4.7 (1.5)	6.3 (2.5)		Inzelberg, et al (1990)
WMS MC	Myotonic Dystrophy	15	n/a	35.40	n/a	12 y	5.6 (1.2)	3.4 (2.0)		Tuikka, et al (1993)
WMS MC	PD	12	n/a	elderly	atropine	2 d	6.8 (1.7)	7.0 (1.7)		Inzelberg, et al (1990)
WMS MC	PD	12	n/a	elderly	placebo	2 d	5.0 (2.6)	5.5 (1.8)		Inzelberg, et al (1990)
WMS MC	PD w/ Dementia	12	n/a	elderly	atropine	2 d	5.3 (0.6)	5.3 (1.2)		Inzelberg, et al (1990)
WMS MC	PD w/ Dementia	12	n/a	elderly	placebo	2 d	4.2 (2.8)	4.8 (2.6)		Inzelberg, et al (1990)
WMS MC	PVD	50	36/14	57.40 (6.40)	major surgery	7.5 d	7.13 (1.91)	7.33 (1.69)		Shaw, et al (1987)

instrument	group	n	m/f	age	intervention	inter	t #1	t #2	note	citation
WMS MC	Schizophrenia (chronic)	14	n/a	29.50	benztropine/ benztropine	4 w	5.9 (2.1)	5.1 (2.1)		Baker, et al (1983)
WMS MC	Schizophrenia (chronic)	14	n/a	30.75	benztropine/ placebo	4 w	5.8 (2.3)	6.6 (1.7)		Baker, et al (1983)
WMS MC & D Span (avg std)	Cardiac	158	131/ 27	61.05	CABG w/ alpha-stat	7 d	-0.07 (0.89)	-0.21 (0.95)	*	Murkin, et al (1995)
WMS MC & D Span (avg std)	Cardiac	79	65/14	61.20 (7.80)	CABG w/ alpha-stat, nonpulsatile	7 d	-0.04 (0.91)	-0.14 (0.93)	*	Murkin, et al (1995)
WMS MC & D Span (avg std)	Cardiac	316	264/ 52	60.90 (8.30)	CABG	7 d	0.0 (0.86)	-0.17 (0.91)	*	Murkin, et al (1995)
WMS MC & D Span (avg std)	Cardiac	158	136/ 22	60.55	CABG w/ pulsatile	7 d	0.01 (0.88)	-0.21 (0.94)	*	Murkin, et al (1995)
WMS MC & D Span (avg std)	Cardiac	158	133/ 25	60.80	CABG w/ ph-stat	7 d	0.07 (0.82)	-0.13 (0.87)	*	Murkin, et al (1995)
WMS MC & D Span (avg std)	Cardiac	79	66/13	60.90 (8.70)	CABG w/ alpha-stat, pulsatile	7 d	-0.01 (0.88)	-0.28 (0.97)	*	Murkin, et al (1995)
WMS MC & D Span (avg std)	Cardiac	79	63/16	61.40 (8.40)	CABG w/ ph-stat, non-pulsatile	7 d	0.03 (0.76)	-1.3 (0.84)	*	Murkin, et al (1995)
WMS MC & D Span (avg std)	Cardiac	158	128/ 30	61.30	CABG w/ nonpulsatile	7 d	-0.01 (0.84)	-0.13 (0.88)	*	Murkin, et al (1995)
WMS MC & D Span (avg std)	Cardiac	79	70/9	60.20 (8.50)	CABG w/ ph-stat,pulsatile	7 d	0.11 (0.87)	-0.13 (0.91)	*	Murkin, et al (1995)
WMS MC & D Span (avg std)	Surgical	40	28/12	63.10 (8.40)	non-CABG surgery	7 d	0.0 (0.88)	0.06 (0.82)	*	Murkin, et al (1995)

instrument	group	n	m/f	age	intervention	inter	t #1	t #2	note	citation
WMS MC (ASS)	Epilepsy	28	17/11	27.00 (5.90)	LTL	9.4 m	11.4	11.1		Ivnik, et al (1987)
WMS MC (ASS)	Epilepsy	35	17/18	28.40 (9.60)	RTL	9.4 m	10.5	10.6		Ivnik, et al (1987)
WMS Memory Span	Depression	52	n/a	41.10	ECT 2 x wk	~3 w	NR	0.69 c	I/II, *	Stromgren, et al (1976)
WMS Memory Span	Depression	51	n/a	40.80	ECT 4 x wk	~2 w	NR	0.28 c	II/II, *	Stromgren, et al (1976)
WMS MQ	Alcoholic	10	10/0	37.70	n/a	1 m	89.6 (12.9)	95.7 (14.9)		Fish, et al (1980)
WMS MQ	Alcoholic	10	10/0	33.05 (7.09)	placebo	1 h	101.0	102.2	I, II CB	Mallick, et al (1993)
WMS MQ	Alcoholic	10	10/0	33.05 (7.09)	lorazepam	1 h	98.4	93.3	I, II CB	Mallick, et al (1993)
WMS MQ	Bipolar Inpts	18	12/6	45.80 (13.70)	lithium	6 y	112.4 (17.1)	112.8 (17.8)		Engelsmann, et al (1988)
WMS MQ	Cardiac	102	86/16	33.00 - 74.00	cardiac surgery	7 d	104.05 (15.55)	4.56 (11.6)c		Shealy, et al (1978)
WMS MQ	CAD	35	23/12	62.30 (8.30)	CE	50.9 d	111.54 (15.31)	121.26 (18.84)		Kelly, et al (1980)
WMS MQ	Control	102	65/37	24.52	n/a	12 m	118.0	118.0	*	Dikmen, et al (1990)
WMS MQ	Control	10	10/0	29.80	n/a	1 m	103.5 (12.9)	109.7 (14.9)		Fish, et al (1980)
WMS MQ	Control	102	~69/ 33	~26.00	n/a	12 m	118.0	119.0		Fraser, et al (1988)

instrument	group	n	m/f	age	intervention	inter	t #1	t #2	note	citation
WMS MQ	Control	10	10/0	31.30 (6.14)	lorazepam	1 h	114.5	105.1	I, II CB	Mallick, et al (1993)
WMS MQ	Control	10	10/0	31.30 (6.14)	placebo	1 h	111.8	108.9	I, II CB	Mallick, et al (1993)
WMS MQ	Control	34	20/14	34.60 (10.70)	n/a	14 d	110.1 (12.7)	117.3 (16.2)		Ryan, et al (1981)
WMS MQ	DAT	31	16/15	68.60 (4.80)	meclofenox	3 m	82.0 (6.5)	100.1 (11.3)		Predescu, et al (1994)
WMS MQ	DAT	32	17/15	70.80 (5.90)	antagonic-stress	3 m	81.3 (9.8)	108.6 (11.4)		Predescu, et al (1994)
WMS MQ	DAT	30	16/14	68.70 (4.80)	nicergoline	3 m	83.2 (6.0)	100.4 (7.9)		Predescu, et al (1994)
WMS MQ	Dementia	88	34/54	74.30	placebo	90 d	74.9 (16.67)	80.7 (19.07)		Ban, et al (1990)
WMS MQ	Dementia	87	39/48	76.10	nimodipine	90 d	71.6 (13.19)	85.4 (18.72)		Ban, et al (1990)
WMS MQ	Depression	33	14/19	37.40	antidepress	7 w	107.0 (19.1)	115.4 (19.3)		Fromm, et al (1984)
WMS MQ	Depression	52	n/a	41.10	ECT 2 x wk	~3 w	NR	0.98 c	I/II, *	Stromgren, et al (1976)
WMS MQ	Depression	51	n/a	40.80	ECT 4 x wk	~2 w	NR	2.36 c	II/II, *	Stromgren, et al (1976)
WMS MQ	Epilepsy	35	17/18	28.40 (9.60)	RTL	9.4 m	103.9	104.9		Ivnik, et al (1987)

instrument	group	n	m/f	age	intervention	inter	t #1	t #2	note	citation
WMS MQ	Epilepsy	28	17/11	27.00 (5.90)	LTL	9.4 m	96.1	92.4		Ivnik, et al (1987)
WMS MQ	Epilepsy	9	9/0	~32.00	LTL	12 m	100.3 (13.3)	92.6 (15)		McGlone (1994)
WMS MQ	Epilepsy	7	0/7	~32.00	LTL	12 m	95.4 (11.5)	91.3 (11.8)		McGlone (1994)
WMS MQ	Epilepsy	12	12/0	~30.00	RTL	12 m	104.3 (13.8)	106.6 (17.5)		McGlone (1994)
WMS MQ	Epilepsy	13	0/13	~30.00	RTL	12 m	94.2 (18.4)	96.6 (17.9)		McGlone (1994)
WMS MQ	HD (at risk, + genetic marker)	8	1/7	26.20 (2.70)	n/a	2 y	115.0	113.0	*	Giordani, et al (1995)
WMS MQ	HD (at risk, - genetic marker)	8	1/7	28.40 (5.20)	n/a	2 y	114.6	115.2	*	Giordani, et al (1995)
WMS MQ	HIV+ (IVDU)	18	10/8	29.80 (5.40)	drug tx	17.7 m	93.6 (17.6)	96.1 (18.6)		Hestad, et al (1996)
WMS MQ	HIV- (IVDU)	30	16/14	27.90 (4.90)	drug tx	14.9 m	96.2 (13.6)	100.9 (13.4)		Hestad, et al (1996)
WMS MQ	Korsakoff's Syndrome	10	9/1	63.00 (10.00)	fluvoxamine	3 w	96.0 (19.0)	104.0 (22.0)	*	Martin, et al (1995)
WMS MQ	Major Depression	7	n/a	46.80	unimproved post-ECT	11 d	89.7	77.0	*	Kurland, et al (1976)
WMS MQ	Major Depression	12	n/a	46.80	improved post-ECT	11 d	88.3	80.7	*	Kurland, et al (1976)

instrument	group	n	m/f	age	intervention	inter	t #1	t #2	note	citation
WMS MQ	Movement D/Os (non-PD)	9	n/a	49.00	l-dopa	47.0 d	104.0 (5.0)	107.0 (5.6)		Donnelly, et al (1973)
WMS MQ	Myotonic Dystrophy	15	n/a	35.40	n/a	12 y	105.6 (16.6)	99.0 (20.7)		Tuikka, et al (1993)
WMS MQ	Organic Amnestic D/O	31	22/9	67.10 (3.90)	placebo	3 m	78.1 (6.9)	83.9 (5.5)		Predescu, et al (1994)
WMS MQ	Organic Amnestic D/O	33	24/9	68.50 (4.30)	antagonic-stress	3 m	76.3 (6.6)	106.2 (11.1)		Predescu, et al (1994)
WMS MQ	PD	9	n/a	49.00	l-dopa	16.5 m	95.0 (5.7)	104.0 (6.0)		Donnelly, et al (1973)
WMS MQ	PD	13	n/a	49.00	l-dopa	51.0 d	90.0 (4.3)	98.0 (4.3)		Donnelly, et al (1973)
WMS MQ	PVD	17	14/3	61.40 (7.90)	PVD surgery	51.5 d	117.35 (19.52)	117.71 (19.46)		Kelly, et al (1980)
WMS MQ	Psychiatric/ Neurological	30	28/2	46.80 (13.30)	n/a	14.2 m	74.5 (20.5)	78.5 (17.6)		Ryan, et al (1981)
WMS MQ	Schizophrenia	10	10/0	34.80 (8.69)	clonidine	6 w	92.2 (19.22)	100.5 (14.94)		Fields, et al (1988)
WMS MQ	Schizophrenia	15	10/5	35.00	std neuroleptics	~15 m	96.4 (21.4)	90.4 (16.9)	II	Goldberg, et al (1993)
WMS MQ	Spinal Cord Injury	67	54/13	32.00 (14.70)	n/a	38 w	96.0 (17.66)	100.8 (17.37)		Richards, et al (1988)
WMS MQ	TBI	31	20/11	24.16	n/a	12 m	78.0	106.0	*	Dikmen, et al (1990)
WMS MQ	TBI	18	15/3	26.10 (8.30)	rehab	7.5 m	85.4	94.9		Prigatano, et al (1984)

instrument	group	n	m/f	age	intervention	inter	t #1	t #2	note	citation
WMS MQ	TBI	17	15/2	23.50 (5.10)	n/a	12.6 m	90.8	92.8		Prigatano, et al (1984)
WMS MQ	TBI (did not return to work)	13	3/10	24.00	n/a	12 m	92.0	105.0		Fraser, et al (1988)
WMS MQ	TBI (returned to work)	35	26/9	29.00	n/a	12 m	110.0	108.0		Fraser, et al (1988)
WMS MQ	Temporal Lobe Epilepsy	14	6/8	31.36 (9.93)	RTL	1.93 y	106.71 (14.52)	108.00 (15.44)		Selwa, et al (1994)
WMS MQ	Temporal Lobe Epilepsy	17	11/6	29.00 (8.12)	LTL	1.8 y	94.65 (15.26)	90.94 (11.45)		Selwa, et al (1994)
WMS MQ	Temporal Lobe Epilepsy	28	17/11	31.29 (9.52)	n/a	2.36 y	93.61 (14.38)	96.07 (14.78)		Selwa, et al (1994)
WMS MQ	TIA	12	6/6	66.00 (5.30)	LCE	59.8 d	108.5 (14.4)	112 (9.6)		Casey, et al (1989)
WMS MQ	TIA	12	6/6	59.20 (13.30)	n/a	59.1 d	107.8 (11.6)	108.3 (14.3)		Casey, et al (1989)
WMS MQ	TIA	12	6/6	63.40 (6.00)	RCE	60.7 d	103.8 (13.3)	110.2 (17.1)		Casey, et al (1989)
WMS Orientation	Alcoholic	10	10/0	33.05 (7.09)	placebo	1 h	5.0	5.0	I, II CB	Mallick, et al (1993)
WMS Orientation	Alcoholic	10	10/0	33.05 (7.09)	lorazepam	1 h	4.8	4.9	I, II CB	Mallick, et al (1993)
WMS Orientation	Bipolar Inpts	18	12/6	45.80 (13.70)	lithium	6 y	4.9 (0.2)	4.9 (0.2)		Engelsmann, et al (1988)
WMS Orientation	Control	12	n/a	elderly	atropine	2 d	4.3 (1.0)	4.9 (0.4)		Inzelberg, et al (1990)

instrument	group	n	m/f	age	intervention	inter	t #1	t #2	note	citation
WMS Orientation	Control	12	n/a	elderly	placebo	2 d	4.5 (0.8)	4.7 (0.8)		Inzelberg, et al (1990)
WMS Orientation	Control	10	10/0	31.30 (6.14)	lorazepam	1 h	5.0	5.0	I, II CB	Mallick, et al (1993)
WMS Orientation	Control	10	10/0	31.30 (6.14)	placebo	1 h	5.0	5.1	I, II CB	Mallick, et al (1993)
WMS Orientation	Coronary Artery Disease	298	264/ 34	53.40 (7.40)	CABG	9.4 d	4.93 (0.3)	4.85 (0.43)		Shaw, et al (1986)
WMS Orientation	DAT	12	n/a	elderly	atropine	2 d	3.2 (1.6)	3.4 (1.5)		Inzelberg, et al (1990)
WMS Orientation	DAT	12	n/a	elderly	placebo	2 d	5.0 (0.0)	4.5 (1.1)		Inzelberg, et al (1990)
WMS Orientation	Depression	10	n/a	73.00 (6.00)	bilateral ECT	~3 w	5.0	4.7	*	Fraser, et al (1980)
WMS Orientation	Depression	10	n/a	73.00 (6.00)	unilateral ECT	~3 w	4.6	4.7	*	Fraser, et al (1980)
WMS Orientation	Depression	52	n/a	41.10	ECT 2 x wk	~3 w	NR	0.38 c	I/II, *	Stromgren, et al (1976)
WMS Orientation	Depression	51	n/a	40.80	ECT 4 x wk	~2 w	NR	0.55 c	II/II, *	Stromgren, et al (1976)
WMS Orientation	MID	12	n/a	elderly	atropine	2 d	5.7 (2.9)	4.1 (2.9)		Inzelberg, et al (1990)
WMS Orientation	MID	12	n/a	elderly	placebo	2 d	3.0 (1.7)	3.0 (0.2)		Inzelberg, et al (1990)
WMS Orientation	Myotonic Dystrophy	15	n/a	35.40	n/a	12 y	4.9 (0.3)	4.7 (0.4)		Tuikka, et al (1993)

instrument	group	n	m/f	age	intervention	inter	t #1	t #2	note	citation
WMS Orientation	PD	12	n/a	elderly	atropine	2 d	4.8 (0.5)	4.8 (0.5)		Inzelberg, et al (1990)
WMS Orientation	PD	12	n/a	elderly	placebo	2 d	4.5 (0.6)	4.8 (0.4)		Inzelberg, et al (1990)
WMS Orientation	PD w/ Dementia	12	n/a	elderly	placebo	2 d	4.6 (0.9)	5.0 (0.0)		Inzelberg, et al (1990)
WMS Orientation	PD w/ Dementia	12	n/a	elderly	atropine	2 d	4.7 (0.6)	5.0 (0.0)		Inzelberg, et al (1990)
WMS Orientation	PVD	50	36/14	57.40 (6.40)	major surgery	7.5 d	4.9 (0.3)	5.0 (0.0)		Shaw, et al (1987)
WMS Orientation	Schizophrenia (chronic)	14	n/a	29.50	benztropine/ benztropine	4 w	4.6 (0.6)	4.4 (0.06)		Baker, et al (1983)
WMS Orientation	Schizophrenia (chronic)	14	n/a	30.75	benztropine/ placebo	4 w	4.2 (1.0)	4.6 (0.6)		Baker, et al (1983)
WMS PAL	AAMI	75	27/48	61.93 (6.05)	n/a	4.6 y	14.52 (3.18)	14.23 (3.61)		Youngjohn, et al (1993)
WMS PAL	Alcoholic	10	10/0	33.05 (7.09)	placebo	1 h	16.2	14.1	I, II CB	Mallick, et al (1993)
WMS PAL	Alcoholic	10	10/0	33.05 (7.09)	lorazepam	1 h	14.0	11.8	I, II CB	Mallick, et al (1993)
WMS PAL	Bipolar Inpts	18	12/6	45.80 (13.70)	lithium	6 y	15.4 (3.6)	16.1 (3.1)		Engelsmann, et al (1988)
WMS PAL	Cardiac	60	35/25	44.30 (9.40)	open heart surgery	10 m	16.97 (3.10)	15.83 (4.04)		Joulasmaa, et al (1981)
WMS PAL	Cardiac	158	128/30	61.30	CABG w/ nonpulsatile	7 d	22.5 (6.4)	20.6 (6.8)	*	Murkin, et al (1995)

instrument	group	n	m/f	age	intervention	inter	t #1	t #2	note	citation
WMS PAL	Cardiac	79	66/13	60.90 (8.70)	CABG w/ alpha-stat, pulsatile	7 d	23.6 (6.9)	20.5 (7.0)	*	Murkin, et al (1995)
WMS PAL	Cardiac	158	131/27	61.05	CABG w/ alpha-stat	7 d	23 (6.6)	20.7 (7.5)	*	Murkin, et al (1995)
WMS PAL	Cardiac	79	70/9	60.20 (8.50)	CABG w/ ph-stat,pulsatile	7 d	22.3 (6.0)	20.0 (6.0)	*	Murkin, et al (1995)
WMS PAL	Cardiac	79	63/16	61.40 (8.40)	CABG w/ ph-stat,non-pulsatile	7 d	22.5 (6.7)	20.3 (5.5)	*	Murkin, et al (1995)
WMS PAL	Cardiac	79	65/14	61.20 (7.80)	CABG w/ alpha-stat, nonpulsatile	7 d	22.4 (6.2)	21.0 (7.9)	*	Murkin, et al (1995)
WMS PAL	Cardiac	158	136/22	60.55	CABG w/ pulsatile	7 d	22.9 (6.5)	20.3 (6.5)	*	Murkin, et al (1995)
WMS PAL	Cardiac	158	133/25	60.80	CABG w/ ph-stat	7 d	22.4 (6.3)	20.2 (5.7)	*	Murkin, et al (1995)
WMS PAL	Cardiac	316	264/52	60.90 (8.30)	CABG	7 d	22.7 (6.5)	20.5 (6.6)	*	Murkin, et al (1995)
WMS PAL	Control	12	n/a	elderly	placebo	2 d	15.3 (4.3)	15.8 (3.9)		Inzelberg, et al (1990)
WMS PAL	Control	12	n/a	elderly	atropine	2 d	12.3 (5.2)	14.8 (4.9)		Inzelberg, et al (1990)
WMS PAL	Control	10	10/0	31.30 (6.14)	placebo	1 h	16.25	15.6	I, II CB	Mallick, et al (1993)
WMS PAL	Control	10	10/0	31.30 (6.14)	lorazepam	1 h	16.5	13.7	I, II CB	Mallick, et al (1993)

instrument	group	n	m/f	age	intervention	inter	t #1	t #2	note	citation
WMS PAL	Control	115	56/59	48.90 (19.30)	n/a	20.9 d	16.59 (3.7)	17.9 (3.48)		Youngjohn, et al (1992)
WMS PAL	Control (CDR-0)	30	15/15	70.9 (4.6)	n/a	1 y	13.5 (3.4)	13.9 (3.2)	*	Botwinick, et al (1986)
WMS PAL	Coronary Artery Disease	298	264/34	53.40 (7.40)	CABG	9.4 d	12.6 (3.56)	10.15 (3.82)		Shaw, et al (1986)
WMS PAL	DAT	12	n/a	elderly	atropine	2 d	8.2 (2.2)	7.5 (6.4)		Inzelberg, et al (1990)
WMS PAL	DAT	12	n/a	elderly	placebo	2 d	11.1 (4.5)	10.8 (4.4)		Inzelberg, et al (1990)
WMS PAL	DAT	14	n/a	60.00 - 80.00	placebo	6 m	6.3 (1.4)	6.4 (3.9)		Sano, et al (1992)
WMS PAL	DAT	13	n/a	60.00 - 80.00	acetyl levocarnitine	6 m	7.0 (2.0)	6.5 (1.9)		Sano, et al (1992)
WMS PAL	DAT (CDR-1)	18	7/11	71.40 (4.40)	n/a	1 y	6.0 (2.5)	5.4 (2.6)	*	Botwinick, et al (1986)
WMS PAL	Dementia	<35	n/a	66.00 (9.60)	n/a	19.0 m	8.5 (3.0)	8.0 (3.9)		Jones, et al (1992)
WMS PAL	Dementia (2° to steroids)	6	6/0	49.67	steriods d/c or reduced	10.9 m	7.0	12.3		Varney, et al (1984)
WMS PAL	Depression	10	n/a	73.00 (6.00)	bilateral ECT	~3 w	7.75	8.3	*	Fraser, et al (1980)
WMS PAL	Depression	10	n/a	73.00 (6.00)	unilateral ECT	~3 w	7.0	7.75	*	Fraser, et al (1980)

instrument	group	n	m/f	age	intervention	inter	t #1	t #2	note	citation
WMS PAL	Depression	33	14/19	37.40	antidepress	7 w	15.7 (4.0)	16.8 (4.0)		Fromm, et al (1984)
WMS PAL	Depression	51	n/a	40.80	ECT 4 x wk	~2 w	NR	-1.32 c	II/II, *	Stromgren, et al (1976)
WMS PAL	Depression	52	n/a	41.10	ECT 2 x wk	~3 w	NR	-2.40 c	I/II, *	Stromgren, et al (1976)
WMS PAL	Epilepsy	13	n/a	29.20 (7.70)	RTL	1.2 y	8.2 (3.2)	8.0 (2.9)		Rausch, et al (1993)
WMS PAL	Epilepsy	12	n/a	29.20 (7.70)	LTL	1.2 y	6.3 (0.3)	2.7 (2.1)		Rausch, et al (1993)
WMS PAL	HD (at risk, + genetic marker)	8	1/7	26.20 (2.70)	n/a	2 y	18.4	17.8	*	Giordani, et al (1995)
WMS PAL	HD (at risk, - genetic marker)	8	1/7	28.40 (5.20)	n/a	2 y	17.7	17.9	*	Giordani, et al (1995)
WMS PAL	HIV+	46	n/a	~33.00	n/a	7.4 m	10.0 (4.0)	10.0 (4.0)		McKegney, et al (1990)
WMS PAL	HIV+ (IVDU)	18	10/8	29.80 (5.40)	drug tx	17.7 m	15.1 (3.9)	15.6 (3.0)		Hestad, et al (1996)
WMS PAL	HIV+ (stage 2/3)	14	14/0	31.40 (8.54)	n/a	12.8 m	19.0 (2.5)	17.3 (4.0)		Burgess, et al (1994)
WMS PAL	HIV+ (stage 4)	6	6/0	36.20 (7.60)	n/a	12.8 m	14.0 (3.1)	13.8 (4.5)		Burgess, et al (1994)
WMS PAL	HIV-	41	41/0	31.50 (9.32)	n/a	12.8 m	16.5 (2.9)	16.5 (3.5)		Burgess, et al (1994)

instrument	group	n	m/f	age	intervention	inter	t #1	t #2	note	citation
WMS PAL	HIV-	45	n/a	~33.00	n/a	7.4 m	11.0 (4.0)	12.0 (4.0)		McKegney, et al (1990)
WMS PAL	HIV- (IVDU)	30	16/14	27.90 (4.90)	drug tx	14.9 m	17.6 (3.0)	17.6 (3.0)		Hestad, et al (1996)
WMS PAL	Hypertension	25	17/8	50.10 (14.00)	n/a	7-10 d	10.88 (2.73)	12.21 (2.39)		McCaffrey, et al (1992)
WMS PAL	Hypertension	34	n/a	76.10	captopril	24 w	12.1 (2.9)	12.1 (3.4)		Starr, et al (1996)
WMS PAL	Hypertension	35	n/a	76.10	bendrofluaz	24 w	12.4 (3.9)	12.0 (3.9)		Starr, et al (1996)
WMS PAL	Korsakoff's Syndrome	10	9/1	63.00 (10.00)	fluvoxamine	3 w	8.0 (3.0)	10.0 (4.0)	*	Martin, et al (1995)
WMS PAL	Medical	83	13/70	19.90 (5.60)	n/a	6.1 m	17.59 (2.47)	18.71 (1.89)		des Rosiers, et al (1988)
WMS PAL	Medical	64	20/44	21.90 (7.80)	n/a	5.4 m	16.87 (2.76)	18.6 (1.87)	II	des Rosiers, et al (1988)
WMS PAL	MID	12	n/a	elderly	atropine	2 d	9.5 (4.8)	10.7 (5.8)		Inzelberg, et al (1990)
WMS PAL	MID	12	n/a	elderly	placebo	2 d	9.0 (3.0)	8.2 (2.3)		Inzelberg, et al (1990)
WMS PAL	Myotonic Dystrophy	15	n/a	35.40	n/a	12 y	16.3 (4.8)	14.4 (4.4)		Tuikka, et al (1993)
WMS PAL	PD	18	11/7	56.90 (8.90)	selegiline	12 w	15.6 (3.2)	17.3 (3.0)		Hietanen (1991)

instrument	group	n	m/f	age	intervention	inter	t #1	t #2	note	citation
WMS PAL	PD	18	11/7	56.90 (8.90)	placebo	12 w	15.6 (3.6)	16.1 (3.8)		Hietanen (1991)
WMS PAL	PD	12	n/a	elderly	placebo	2 d	9.3 (2.6)	13.25 (3.4)		Inzelberg, et al (1990)
WMS PAL	PD	12	n/a	elderly	atropine	2 d	13.9 (1.9)	16.9 (4.6)		Inzelberg, et al (1990)
WMS PAL	PD	12	12/0	65.60	trihexyphen	1 m	12.7 (0.74)	10.7 (0.53)		Koller (1984)
WMS PAL	PD	19	13/6	54.30	pergolide	~6 w	14.6 (4.76)	13.8 (4.28)		Stern, et al (1984)
WMS PAL	PD w/ Dementia	12	n/a	elderly	placebo	2 d	10.8 (4.5)	10.6 (5.4)		Inzelberg, et al (1990)
WMS PAL	PD w/ Dementia	12	n/a	elderly	atropine	2 d	12.2 (2.9)	10.8 (10.5)		Inzelberg, et al (1990)
WMS PAL	PVD	50	36/14	57.40 (6.40)	major surgery	7.5 d	12.67 (3.76)	12.56 (3.7)		Shaw, et al (1987)
WMS PAL	Pseudo-dementia	<35	n/a	66.00 (9.60)	n/a	19.0 m	9.2 (3.7)	10.5 (6.2)		Jones, et al (1992)
WMS PAL	Schizophrenia	15	10/5	35.00	std neuroleptics	~15 m	13.1 (6.0)	12.9 (3.9)	II	Goldberg, et al (1993)
WMS PAL	Schizophrenia (chronic)	14	n/a	29.50	benztropine/ benztropine	4 w	11.0 (4.1)	9.8 (4.8)		Baker, et al (1983)
WMS PAL	Schizophrenia (chronic)	14	n/a	30.75	benztropine/ placebo	4 w	10.7 (4.5)	10.3 (4.8)		Baker, et al (1983)

instrument	group	n	m/f	age	intervention	inter	t #1	t #2	note	citation
WMS PAL	subjective memory impairment	12	6/6	72.00	methylphen	45 min	7.50	9.00		Crook, et al (1977)
WMS PAL	Surgical	40	28/12	63.10 (8.40)	non-CABG surgery	7 d	23.3 (5.7)	22.6 (7.7)	*	Murkin, et al (1995)
WMS PAL	Temporal Lobe Epilepsy	14	6/8	31.36 (9.93)	RTL	1.93 y	15.86 (3.28)	16.43 (3.98)		Selwa, et al (1994)
WMS PAL	Temporal Lobe Epilepsy	17	11/6	29.00 (8.12)	LTL	1.8 y	11.66 (3.49)	11.25 (3.25)		Selwa, et al (1994)
WMS PAL	Temporal Lobe Epilepsy	28	17/11	31.29 (9.52)	n/a	2.36 y	11.66 (4.34)	12.38 (3.81)		Selwa, et al (1994)
WMS PAL (ASS)	Epilepsy	35	17/18	28.40 (9.60)	RTL	9.4 m	11.4	11.6		Ivnik, et al (1987)
WMS PAL (ASS)	Epilepsy	28	17/11	27.00 (5.90)	LTL	9.4 m	9.9	8.5		Ivnik, et al (1987)
WMS PAL (transformed total score)	BZ Dependence	21	11/10	44.40 (9.40)	BZ tx & abstin	1 m	13.21 (3.62)	12.05 (3.97)	*	Tata, et al (1994)
WMS PAL (transformed score)	Control	21	11/10	43.10 (14.40)	n/a	1 m	16.60 (3.65)	16.14 (3.79)	*	Tata, et al (1994)
WMS PAL Delay	Alcoholic (brief abstin)	27	27/0	40.96	DGAVP	7 d	4.6 (1.5)	4.3 (1.5)	*	Korsic, et al (1991)
WMS PAL Delay	Alcoholic (brief abstin)	27	27/0	43.07	placebo	7 d	5.2 (1.3)	5.0 (1.7)	*	Korsic, et al (1991)

instrument	group	n	m/f	age	intervention	inter	t #1	t #2	note	citation
WMS PAL Delay	Alcoholic (long abstin)	26	26/0	41.40	placebo	7 d	4.9 (1.3)	4.8 (1.3)	*	Korsic, et al (1991)
WMS PAL Delay	Alcoholic (long abstin)	23	23/0	46.26	DGAVP	7 d	5.2 (1.7)	4.6 (1.3)	*	Korsic, et al (1991)
WMS PAL Delay	Control	16	10/6	64.00 (1.70)	n/a	1 w	5.5 (0.5)	5.8 (0.4)	*	Claus, et al (1991)
WMS PAL Delay	DAT	17	7/1	64.00 (1.70)	n/a	1 w	1.4 (0.3)	1.1 (0.2)	*	Claus, et al (1991)
WMS PAL Delay	Epilepsy	12	12/0	~30.00	RTL	12 m	6.9 (2.1)	8.4 (2.0)		McGlone (1994)
WMS PAL Delay	Epilepsy	13	0/13	~30.00	RTL	12 m	8.2 (1.5)	7.9 (2.0)		McGlone (1994)
WMS PAL Delay	Epilepsy	7	0/7	~32.00	LTL	12 m	7.4 (1.8)	6.6 (2.9)		McGlone (1994)
WMS PAL Delay	Epilepsy	9	9/0	~32.00	LTL	12 m	6.4 (1.9)	4.6 (1.7)		McGlone (1994)
WMS PAL Delay	Epilepsy	13	n/a	29.20 (7.70)	RTL	1.2 y	2.8 (1.3)	3.1 (1.4)		Rausch, et al (1993)
WMS PAL Delay	Epilepsy	12	n/a	29.20 (7.70)	LTL	1.2 y	1.8 (1.5)	0.7 (1.0)		Rausch, et al (1993)
WMS PAL Delay	Hysterectomy/ Oophorectomy	10	0/10	48.20 (4.70)	estrogen tx	9 w	11.8 (0.5)	12.3 (0.7)	I, II CB	Phillips, et al (1992)
WMS PAL Delay	Hysterectomy/ Oophorectomy	9	0/9	48.20 (4.70)	placebo	9 w	12.3 (0.7)	10.0 (0.9)	I, II CB	Phillips, et al (1992)
WMS PAL Delay (% ret)	Temporal Lobe Epilepsy	14	6/8	31.36 (9.93)	RTL	1.93 y	92.03 (10.18)	92.26 (15.61)		Selwa, et al (1994)

instrument	group	n	m/f	age	intervention	inter	t #1	t #2	note	citation
WMS PAL Delay (% ret)	Temporal Lobe Epilepsy	28	17/11	31.29 (9.52)	n/a	2.36 y	91.57 (18.84)	89.12 (16.10)		Selwa, et al (1994)
WMS PAL Delay (% ret)	Temporal Lobe Epilepsy	17	11/6	29.00 (8.12)	LTL	1.8 y	96.14 (20.25)	87.42 (14.21)		Selwa, et al (1994)
WMS PAL Delay Easy	Alcoholic	10	10/0	33.05 (7.09)	placebo	1 h	5.8	5.9	I, II CB	Mallick, et al (1993)
WMS PAL Delay Easy	Alcoholic	10	10/0	33.05 (7.09)	lorazepam	1 h	5.8	5.5	I, II CB	Mallick, et al (1993)
WMS PAL Delay Easy	Control	10	10/0	31.30 (6.14)	lorazepam	1 h	5.8	5.4	I, II CB	Mallick, et al (1993)
WMS PAL Delay Easy	Control	10	10/0	31.30 (6.14)	placebo	1 h	5.9	5.6	I, II CB	Mallick, et al (1993)
WMS PAL Delay Hard	Alcoholic	10	10/0	33.05 (7.09)	lorazepam	1 h	2.7	1.0	I, II CB	Mallick, et al (1993)
WMS PAL Delay Hard	Alcoholic	10	10/0	33.05 (7.09)	placebo	1 h	2.9	2.4	I, II CB	Mallick, et al (1993)
WMS PAL Delay Hard	Control	10	10/0	31.30 (6.14)	placebo	1 h	3.4	3.2	I, II CB	Mallick, et al (1993)
WMS PAL Delay Hard	Control	10	10/0	31.30 (6.14)	lorazepam	1 h	3.7	1.6	I, II CB	Mallick, et al (1993)
WMS PAL Easy	BZ Dependence	21	11/10	44.40 (9.40)	BZ tx & abstin	1 m	15.48 (2.91)	13.52 (2.54)	*	Tata, et al (1994)
WMS PAL Easy	Control	21	11/10	43.10 (14.40)	n/a	1 m	17.00 (1.41)	16.10 (2.36)	*	Tata, et al (1994)
WMS PAL Easy	Epilepsy	40	23/17	32.20 (8.20)	n/a	~9 m	16.25 (1.81)	16.60 (1.45)		Hermann, et al (1996)

instrument	group	n	m/f	age	intervention	inter	t #1	t #2	note	citation
WMS PAL Easy	Medical	64	20/44	21.90 (7.80)	n/a	5.4 m	16.31 (1.53)	16.55 (1.26)	II	des Rosiers, et al (1988)
WMS PAL Easy	Medical	83	13/70	19.90 (5.60)	n/a	6.1 m	17.28 (0.92)	17.45 (0.81)		des Rosiers, et al (1988)
WMS PAL Easy	PD	18	11/7	56.90 (8.90)	selegiline	12 w	16.6 (1.6)	17.9 (0.3)		Hietanen (1991)
WMS PAL Easy	PD	18	11/7	56.90 (8.90)	placebo	12 w	17.1 (0.8)	17.5 (0.8)		Hietanen (1991)
WMS PAL Hard	BZ Dependence	21	11/10	44.40 (9.40)	BZ tx & abstin	1 m	5.48 (2.82)	4.87 (3.31)	*	Tata, et al (1994)
WMS PAL Hard	Control	21	11/10	43.10 (14.40)	n/a	1 m	8.14 (3.28)	8.24 (2.77)	*	Tata, et al (1994)
WMS PAL Hard	Epilepsy	40	23/17	32.20 (8.20)	n/a	~9 m	5.73 (2.82)	6.48 (2.97)		Hermann, et al (1996)
WMS PAL Hard	Medical	83	13/70	19.90 (5.60)	n/a	6.1 m	8.95 (2.29)	9.99 (1.71)		des Rosiers, et al (1988)
WMS PAL Hard	Medical	64	20/44	21.90 (7.80)	n/a	5.4 m	8.71 (2.36)	10.32 (1.45)	II	des Rosiers, et al (1988)
WMS PAL Hard	PD	18	11/7	56.90 (8.90)	placebo	12 w	7.1 (2.4)	8.1 (2.5)		Hietanen (1991)
WMS PAL Hard	PD	18	11/7	56.90 (8.90)	selegiline	12 w	7.3 (3.1)	8.3 (3.0)		Hietanen (1991)
WMS PAL Hard	TBI	18	15/3	26.10 (8.30)	rehab	7.5 m	7.6	10.1		Prigatano, et al (1984)
WMS PAL Hard	TBI	17	15/2	23.50 (5.10)	n/a	12.6 m	7.9	9.3		Prigatano, et al (1984)

instrument	group	n	m/f	age	intervention	inter	t #1	t #2	note	citation
WMS PAL Imm	Alcoholic (brief abstin)	27	27/0	40.96	DGAVP	7 d	12.6 (3.8)	12.3 (3.7)	*	Korsic, et al (1991)
WMS PAL Imm	Alcoholic (brief abstin)	27	27/0	43.07	placebo	7 d	14.9 (3.9)	13.9 (4.1)	*	Korsic, et al (1991)
WMS PAL Imm	Alcoholic (long abstin)	26	26/0	41.40	placebo	7 d	13.7 (3.9)	12.8 (2.9)	*	Korsic, et al (1991)
WMS PAL Imm	Alcoholic (long abstin)	23	23/0	46.26	DGAVP	7 d	14.7 (4.2)	12.8 (3.9)	*	Korsic, et al (1991)
WMS PAL Imm	Control	16	10/6	64.00 (1.70)	n/a	1 w	16.5 (0.9)	15.9 (0.8)	*	Claus, et al (1991)
WMS PAL Imm	DAT	17	7/1	64.00 (1.70)	n/a	1 w	3.5 (0.8)	3.4 (0.5)	*	Claus, et al (1991)
WMS PAL Imm	Hysterectomy/ Oophorectomy	10	0/10	48.20 (4.70)	estrogen tx	9 w	31.7 (1.4)	31.3 (1.4)	I, II CB	Phillips, et al (1992)
WMS PAL Imm	Hysterectomy/ Oophorectomy	9	0/9	48.20 (4.70)	placebo	9 w	30.8 (1.6)	25.3 (1.7)	I, II CB	Phillips, et al (1992)
WMS Verbal Delay (LM + PAL)	Schizophrenia	38	25/13	30.90 (8.73)	n/a	6 m	10.85 (6.42)	9.51 (3.60)		Addington, et al (1991)
WMS Verbal Imm (LM + PAL)	Age Related Cognitive Decline	24	13/11	62.20 (8.80)	n/a	2.0 y	26.5 (7.1)	29.8 (4.8)		Celsis, et al (1997)
WMS Verbal Imm (LM + PAL)	Control	18	8/10	65.30 (6.00)	n/a	3.2 y	32.5 (4.5)	35.5 (1.8)		Celsis, et al (1997)

instrument	group	n	m/f	age	intervention	inter	t #1	t #2	note	citation
WMS Verbal Imm (LM + PAL)	DAT	18	11/7	65.30 (6.00)	n/a	3.0 y	19.8 (3.7)	12.2 (4.1)		Celsis, et al (1997)
WMS Verbal Imm (LM + PAL)	Schizophrenia	38	25/13	30.90 (8.73)	n/a	6 m	16.56 (5.88)	19.82 (6.85)		Addington, et al (1991)
WMS Verbal Recall (LM + PAL; % ret)	TIA	12	6/6	66.00 (5.30)	LCE	59.8 d	72.9 (12.0)	74.7 (18.3)	I, II CB	Casey, et al (1989)
WMS Verbal Recall (LM + PAL; % ret)	TIA	12	6/6	59.20 (13.30)	n/a	59.1 d	80.8 (20.1)	82.7 (17.8)	I, II CB	Casey, et al (1989)
WMS Verbal Recall (LM + PAL; % ret)	TIA	12	6/6	63.40 (6.00)	RCE	60.7 d	75.4 (17.3)	68.3 (22.1)	I, II CB	Casey, et al (1989)
WMS VR	Alcoholic Inpts	55	50/5	46.00	n/a	1 m	5.9	7.6	*	Clarke, et al (1975)
WMS VR	Bipolar Inpts	18	12/6	45.80 (13.70)	lithium	6 y	10.2 (3.6)	9.5 (3.9)		Engelsmann, et al (1988)
WMS VR	Cardiac	227	184/43	54.50	cardiac operation	10-12 d	11.22 (2.58)	11.16 (3.38)		Savageau, et al (1982b)
WMS VR	Cardiac	245	198/47	54.70	CABG/ cardiac operation	6 m	11.33 (2.483)	10.877 (2.627)		Savageau, et al (1982a)
WMS VR	Control	55	50/5	45.00	n/a	1 m	10.9	11.7	*	Clarke, et al (1975)
WMS VR	Control	102	65/37	24.52	n/a	12 m	13.0	12.0	*	Dikmen, et al (1990)

instrument	group	n	m/f	age	intervention	inter	t #1	t #2	note	citation
WMS VR	Control	12	n/a	elderly	placebo	2 d	4.6 (3.1)	6.1 (3.1)		Inzelberg, et al (1990)
WMS VR	Control	12	n/a	elderly	atropine	2 d	3.8 (3.7)	6.0 (4.6)		Inzelberg, et al (1990)
WMS VR	Coronary Artery Disease	298	264/ 34	53.40 (7.40)	CABG	9.4 d	11.1 (2.46)	11.5 (2.41)		Shaw, et al (1986)
WMS VR	DAT	12	n/a	elderly	atropine	2 d	1.0 (1.4)	0.8 (0.4)		Inzelberg, et al (1990)
WMS VR	DAT	12	n/a	elderly	placebo	2 d	4.0 (0.7)	5.2 (2.9)		Inzelberg, et al (1990)
WMS VR	DAT	14	n/a	60.00 - 80.00	placebo	6 m	1.8 (1.8)	2.1 (2.1)		Sano, et al (1992)
WMS VR	DAT	13	n/a	60.00 - 80.00	acetyl levocarnitine	6 m	1.4 (1.8)	1.2 (1.3)		Sano, et al (1992)
WMS VR	Depression	10	n/a	73.00 (6.00)	unilateral ECT	~3 w	1.9	4.8	*	Fraser, et al (1980)
WMS VR	Depression	10	n/a	73.00 (6.00)	bilateral ECT	~3 w	3.6	5.6	*	Fraser, et al (1980)
WMS VR	Depression	33	14/19	37.40	antidepress	7 w	8.9 (3.0)	10.3 (3.1)		Fromm, et al (1984)
WMS VR	Depression	52	n/a	41.10	ECT 2 x wk	~3 w	NR	1.46 c	I/II, *	Stromgren, et al (1976)
WMS VR	Depression	51	n/a	40.80	ECT 4 x wk	~2 w	NR	1.24 c	II/II, *	Stromgren, et al (1976)
WMS VR	HD (at risk, + genetic marker)	8	1/7	26.20 (2.70)	n/a	2 y	12.2	11.8	*	Giordani, et al (1995)

instrument	group	n	m/f	age	intervention	inter	t #1	t #2	note	citation
WMS VR	HD (at risk, - genetic marker)	8	1/7	28.40 (5.20)	n/a	2 y	11.7	10.8	*	Giordani, et al (1995)
WMS VR	HIV+ (IVDU)	18	10/8	29.80 (5.40)	drug tx	17.7 m	9.2 (2.0)	10.7 (1.6)		Hestad, et al (1996)
WMS VR	HIV+ (stage 2/3)	14	14/0	31.40 (8.54)	n/a	12.8 m	11.6 (1.9)	7.5 (8.3)		Burgess, et al (1994)
WMS VR	HIV+ (stage 4)	6	6/0	36.20 (7.60)	n/a	12.8 m	10.5 (2.8)	8.3 (1.0)		Burgess, et al (1994)
WMS VR	HIV-	41	41/0	31.50 (9.32)	n/a	12.8 m	10.7 (2.9)	8.2 (2.1)		Burgess, et al (1994)
WMS VR	HIV- (IVDU)	30	16/14	27.90 (4.90)	drug tx	14.9 m	9.1 (2.6)	9.8 (2.1)		Hestad, et al (1996)
WMS VR	MID	12	n/a	elderly	atropine	2 d	4.0 (3.6)	3.3 (4.9)		Inzelberg, et al (1990)
WMS VR	MID	12	n/a	elderly	placebo	2 d	4.3 (2.9)	4.0 (2.6)		Inzelberg, et al (1990)
WMS VR	Myotonic Dystrophy	15	n/a	35.40	n/a	12 y	7.7 (3.7)	7.3 (3.9)		Tuikka, et al (1993)
WMS VR	PD	18	11/7	56.90 (8.90)	placebo	12 w	9.0 (3.9)	8.8 (3.0)		Hietanen (1991)
WMS VR	PD	18	11/7	56.90 (8.90)	selegiline	12 w	7.9 (3.6)	8.0 (3.4)		Hietanen (1991)
WMS VR	PD	12	n/a	elderly	atropine	2 d	6.4 (4.9)	7.8 (5.5)		Inzelberg, et al (1990)
WMS VR	PD	12	n/a	elderly	placebo	2 d	2.8 (1.7)	4.8 (1.7)		Inzelberg, et al (1990)

instrument	group	n	m/f	age	intervention	inter	t #1	t #2	note	citation
WMS VR	PD w/ Dementia	12	n/a	elderly	placebo	2 d	2.6 (2.1)	3.8 (2.6)		Inzelberg, et al (1990)
WMS VR	PD w/ Dementia	12	n/a	elderly	atropine	2 d	6.7 (4.0)	7.0 (4.4)		Inzelberg, et al (1990)
WMS VR	PVD	50	36/14	57.40 (6.40)	major surgery	7.5 d	10.58 (1.93)	12.35 (1.67)		Shaw, et al (1987)
WMS VR	Schizophrenia	15	10/5	35.00	std neuroleptics	~15 m	9.0 (2.9)	7.6 (2.5)	II	Goldberg, et al (1993)
WMS VR	Schizophrenia (chronic)	14	n/a	29.50	benztropine/ benztropine	4 w	6.2 (3.6)	8.8 (3.9)		Baker, et al (1983)
WMS VR	Schizophrenia (chronic)	14	n/a	30.75	benztropine/ placebo	4 w	5.1 (4.0)	10.3 (2.8)		Baker, et al (1983)
WMS VR	TBI	31	20/11	24.16	n/a	12 m	8.0	12.0	*	Dikmen, et al (1990)
WMS VR	TBI	17	15/2	23.50 (5.10)	n/a	12.6 m	6.4	6.2		Prigatano, et al (1984)
WMS VR	TBI	18	15/3	26.10 (8.30)	rehab	7.5 m	4.3	5.6		Prigatano, et al (1984)
WMS VR	Temporal Lobe Epilepsy	28	17/11	31.29 (9.52)	n/a	2.36 y	10.25 (2.94)	10.43 (2.28)		Selwa, et al (1994)
WMS VR	Temporal Lobe Epilepsy	14	6/8	31.36 (9.93)	RTL	1.93 y	10.54 (2.90)	10.46 (2.11)		Selwa, et al (1994)
WMS VR	Temporal Lobe Epilepsy	17	11/6	29.00 (8.12)	LTL	1.8 y	10.79 (2.36)	9.91 (2.48)		Selwa, et al (1994)
WMS VR (% ret)	DAT (at risk)	32	32/0	83.30 (6.70)	n/a	2.0 y	51.2	54.3		Frank, et al (1996)

instrument	group	n	m/f	age	intervention	inter	t #1	t #2	note	citation
WMS VR (ASS)	Epilepsy	28	17/11	27.00 (5.90)	LTL	9.4 m	9.6	10.6		Ivnik, et al (1987)
WMS VR (ASS)	Epilepsy	35	17/18	28.40 (9.60)	RTL	9.4 m	10.9	10.9		Ivnik, et al (1987)
WMS VR Copy	Control	141	0/141	78.50 (6.60)	n/a	2.7 y	15.3	17.2		Frank, et al (1996)
WMS VR Copy	Control	101	101/0	78.50 (7.20)	n/a	2.6 y	14.8	17.1		Frank, et al (1996)
WMS VR Copy	CVA	19	n/a	~65.00	n/a	14.6 w	10.0	11.4		Bowler, et al (1994)
WMS VR Copy	DAT	34	34/0	83.90 (4.30)	n/a	2.1 y	13.4	14.7		Frank, et al (1996)
WMS VR Copy	DAT	34	34/0	83.90 (4.30)	n/a	2.1 y	13.0	14.2		Frank, et al (1996)
WMS VR Copy	DAT (at risk)	50	0/50	84.10 (5.10)	n/a	2.3 y	13.6	16.3		Frank, et al (1996)
WMS VR Copy	DAT (at risk)	32	32/0	83.30 (6.70)	n/a	2.0 y	14.3	17.2		Frank, et al (1996)
WMS VR Delay	Cardiac	90	77/13	59.00 (10.59)	CABG/CPB	8 d	6.3 (3.5)	4.3 (3.7)	*	Townes, et al (1989)
WMS VR Delay	CAD	17	n/a	57.20 (7.20)	n/a	6 m	4.6	5.1		Parker, et al (1983)
WMS VR Delay	CAD	20	n/a	57.20 (7.20)	CE	6 m	4.4	5.8		Parker, et al (1983)

instrument	group	n	m/f	age	intervention	inter	t #1	t #2	note	citation
WMS VR Delay	CAD	17	n/a	57.90 (8.40)	n/a	6 m	5.4	5.4	*	Parker, et al (1986)
WMS VR Delay	CAD	36	n./a	61.10 (8.30)	CE	6 m	4.0	5.4	*	Parker, et al (1986)
WMS VR Delay	Control	101	101/0	78.50 (7.20)	n/a	2.6 y	7.8	9.2		Frank, et al (1996)
WMS VR Delay	Control	141	0/141	78.50 (6.60)	n/a	2.7 y	6.5	7.7		Frank, et al (1996)
WMS VR Delay	Control	33	15/18	59.10 (9.30)	n/a	10 d	9.0 (3.5)	11.0 (2.9)		McCaffrey, et al (1993)
WMS VR Delay	Control	16	4/12	78.30 (2.50)	n/a	1 y	4.1 (4.0)	4.8 (3.8)	*	Mitrushina, et al (1991b)
WMS VR Delay	Control	47	14/33	72.90 (1.40)	n/a	1 y	4.9 (3.8)	5.8 (3.8)	*	Mitrushina, et al (1991b)
WMS VR Delay	Control	40	6/34	68.20 (1.20)	n/a	1 y	6.3 (3.5)	8.1 (3.6)	*	Mitrushina, et al (1991b)
WMS VR Delay	Control	19	2/17	62.20 (2.50)	n/a	1 y	5.8 (3.4)	7.4 (4.4)	*	Mitrushina, et al (1991b)
WMS VR Delay	Control	21	21/0	31.45 (5.53)	n/a	18 m	11.30 (2.15)	12.35 (1.35)		Saykin, et al (1991)
WMS VR Delay	Control	47	35/12	59.00 (9.81)	n/a	8 d	8.0 (2.9)	2.7 (2.7)	*	Townes, et al (1989)
WMS VR Delay	Control (Pain Pt/Volunteer)	15	5/10	33.90 (8.40)	n/a	20.7 d	8.6 (2.6)	10.4 (2.7)		Goulet Fisher, et al (1986)

instrument	group	n	m/f	age	intervention	inter	t #1	t #2	note	citation
WMS VR Delay	CVA	19	n/a	~65.00	n/a	14.6 w	7.7	8.4		Bowler, et al (1994)
WMS VR Delay	DAT	34	34/0	83.90 (4.30)	n/a	2.1 y	1.8	1.8		Frank, et al (1996)
WMS VR Delay	DAT	34	34/0	83.90 (4.30)	n/a	2.1 y	2.0	1.2		Frank, et al (1996)
WMS VR Delay	DAT (at risk)	32	32/0	83.30 (6.70)	n/a	2.0 y	3.3	5.3		Frank, et al (1996)
WMS VR Delay	DAT (at risk)	50	0/50	84.10 (5.10)	n/a	2.3 y	3.1	4.8		Frank, et al (1996)
WMS VR Delay	DAT (mild)	11	10/1	63.00 (8.00)	n/a	26 m	1.0 (1.0)	0.0 (1.0)		Haxby, et al (1990)
WMS VR Delay	Depression	15	6/9	28.50 (10.60)	inpt tx	19.5 d	5.7 (2.9)	8.4 (3.3)		Goulet Fisher, et al (1986)
WMS VR Delay	Epilepsy	40	23/17	32.20 (8.20)	n/a	~9 m	7.53 (2.76)	8.03 (3.01)		Hermann, et al (1996)
WMS VR Delay	Epilepsy	13	n/a	29.20 (7.70)	RTL	1.2 y	7.5 (3.2)	7.8 (3.4)		Rausch, et al (1993)
WMS VR Delay	Epilepsy	12	n/a	29.20 (7.70)	LTL	1.2 y	7.0 (3.3)	7.5 (3.9)		Rausch, et al (1993)
WMS VR Delay	HIV+ (IVDU)	42	31/11	27.00 (5.30)	n/a	12 m	9.8 (2.9)	10.1 (3.9)		Bono, et al (1996)
WMS VR Delay	HIV+/ARC	8	8/0	33.57 (6.35)	n/a	18 m	9.29 (3.09)	10.57 (2.88)		Saykin, et al (1991)

instrument	group	n	m/f	age	intervention	inter	t #1	t #2	note	citation
WMS VR Delay	HIV+/PGL	13	13/0	31.15 (4.91)	n/a	18 m	11.15 (2.27)	12.38 (2.14)		Saykin, et al (1991)
WMS VR Delay	HIV- (IVDU)	39	30/9	28.60 (4.90)	n/a	12 m	10.5 (2.0)	10.7 (2.0)		Bono, et al (1996)
WMS VR Delay	Hypertension	25	17/8	50.10 (14.00)	n/a	7-10 d	10.08 (3.51)	11.70 (2.37)		McCaffrey, et al (1992)
WMS VR Delay	Hysterectomy/ Oophorectomy	10	0/10	48.20 (4.70)	estrogen tx	9 w	8.7 (1.0)	8.5 (1.0)	I, II CB	Phillips, et al (1992)
WMS VR Delay	Hysterectomy/ Oophorectomy	9	0/9	48.20 (4.70)	placebo	9 w	9.3 (1.0)	7.1 (1.2)	I, II CB	Phillips, et al (1992)
WMS VR Delay	Mountain climbers	6	6/0	21.00 - 31.00	progressive decompress-ion	~43 d	10.14 (1.68)	7.00 (3.35)		Hornbein, et al (1989)
WMS VR Delay	Mountain climbers	35	34/1	24.00 - 45.00	Climb of 5,000-8,000 meters	~1 m	12.33 (1.96)	11.36 (1.88)		Hornbein, et al (1989)
WMS VR Delay	MS	9	n/a	38.90	high dose interferon	2 y	5.3 (4.1)	9.1 (3.5)	I/II	Pliskin, et al (1996)
WMS VR Delay	MS	13	n/a	36.20	placebo	2 y	7.6 (3.2)	8.0 (3.4)	I/II	Pliskin, et al (1996)
WMS VR Delay	MS	8	n/a	38.00	low dose interferon	2 y	5.8 (1.8)	7.6 (3.3)	I/II	Pliskin, et al (1996)
WMS VR Delay	Naphtha Exposure	185	n/a	36.00	n/a	1 y	7.80 (2.75)	10.12 (2.55)		White, et al (1994)
WMS VR Delay	PD	4	3/1	53.50	fetal tissue implanted	12 m	5.0	7.0		Sass, et al (1995)

instrument	group	n	m/f	age	intervention	inter	t #1	t #2	note	citation
WMS VR Delay	Schizophrenia	38	25/13	30.90 (8.73)	n/a	6 m	6.59 (4.63)	9.33 (4.13)		Addington, et al (1991)
WMS VR Delay	Surgical	17	n/a	57.20 (7.20)	surgery	6 m	5.6	6.4		Parker, et al (1983)
WMS VR Delay	Surgical	26	n/a	55.30 (6.80)	surgery (non-CE)	6 m	6.5	7.0	*	Parker, et al (1986)
WMS VR Delay (% forg)	HIV+ (IVDU)	42	31/11	27.00 (5.30)	n/a	12 m	9.1	9.8		Bono, et al (1996)
WMS VR Delay (% forg)	HIV- (IVDU)	39	30/9	28.60 (4.90)	n/a	12 m	10.2	9.3		Bono, et al (1996)
WMS VR Delay (% ret)	Alcoholic	10	10/0	33.05 (7.09)	placebo	1 h	64.9	68.0	I, II CB	Mallick, et al (1993)
WMS VR Delay (% ret)	Alcoholic	10	10/0	33.05 (7.09)	lorazepam	1 h	68.4	22.0	I, II CB	Mallick, et al (1993)
WMS VR Delay (% ret)	CAD	20	n/a	57.20 (7.20)	CE	6 m	77.2	89.7		Parker, et al (1983)
WMS VR Delay (% ret)	CAD	17	n/a	57.20 (7.20)	n/a	6 m	70.7	78.4		Parker, et al (1983)
WMS VR Delay (% ret)	CAD	17	n/a	57.90 (8.40)	n/a	6 m	80.2	78.4	*	Parker, et al (1986)
WMS VR Delay (% ret)	CAD	36	n./a	61.10 (8.30)	CE	6 m	82.9	86.2	*	Parker, et al (1986)
WMS VR Delay (% ret)	Control	141	0/141	78.50 (6.60)	n/a	2.7 y	67.8	62.2		Frank, et al (1996)

instrument	group	n	m/f	age	intervention	inter	t #1	t #2	note	citation
WMS VR Delay (% ret)	Control	101	101/0	78.50 (7.20)	n/a	2.6 y	74.7	69.1		Frank, et al (1996)
WMS VR Delay (% ret)	Control	10	10/0	31.30 (6.14)	lorazepam	1 h	83.3	22.1	I, II CB	Mallick, et al (1993)
WMS VR Delay (% ret)	Control	10	10/0	31.30 (6.14)	placebo	1 h	77.3	94.7	I, II CB	Mallick, et al (1993)
WMS VR Delay (% ret)	CVA	19	n/a	~65.00	n/a	14.6 w	116.0	119.0		Bowler, et al (1994)
WMS VR Delay (% ret)	DAT	34	34/0	83.90 (4.30)	n/a	2.1 y	41.0	28.7		Frank, et al (1996)
WMS VR Delay (% ret)	DAT	34	34/0	83.90 (4.30)	n/a	2.1 y	37.2	16.3		Frank, et al (1996)
WMS VR Delay (% ret)	DAT (at risk)	50	0/50	84.10 (5.10)	n/a	2.3 y	46.7	51.9		Frank, et al (1996)
WMS VR Delay (% ret)	Epilepsy	40	23/17	32.20 (8.20)	n/a	~9 m	83.57 (18.00)	82.25 (22.33)		Hermann, et al (1996)
WMS VR Delay (% ret)	Epilepsy	42	0/42	33.80 (8.90)	LTL	23.8 w	69.43 (28.76)	75.28 (25.01)		Trenerry, et al (1996)
WMS VR Delay (% ret)	Epilepsy	28	28/0	33.90 (10.30)	RTL	20.5 w	73.92 (24.0)	71.43 (23.59)		Trenerry, et al (1996)
WMS VR Delay (% ret)	Epilepsy	26	0/26	33.50 (10.40)	RTL	30.5 w	75.69 (24.14)	79.52 (25.06)		Trenerry, et al (1996)
WMS VR Delay (% ret)	Epilepsy	33	33/0	34.90 (8.90)	LTL	32.8 w	72.79 (29.39)	68.15 (26.33)		Trenerry, et al (1996)

instrument	group	n	m/f	age	intervention	inter	t #1	t #2	note	citation
WMS VR Delay (% ret)	HD (at risk, + genetic marker)	8	1/7	26.20 (2.70)	n/a	2 y	92.4	91.2	*	Giordani, et al (1995)
WMS VR Delay (% ret)	HD (at risk, - genetic marker)	8	1/7	28.40 (5.20)	n/a	2 y	86.4	89.4	*	Giordani, et al (1995)
WMS VR Delay (% ret)	Myasthenia Gravis	11	7/4	49.00	prednisolone	3-11 m	93.0 (12.0)	92.0 (10.0)		Glennerster, et al (1996)
WMS VR Delay (% ret)	Schizophrenia	11	11/0	52.50 (11.50)	neuroleptic reduction	29.3 w	70.6 (36.8)	90.4 (36.8)		Seidman, et al (1993)
WMS VR Delay (% ret)	Surgical	17	n/a	57.20 (7.20)	surgery	6 m	85.2	84.4		Parker, et al (1983)
WMS VR Delay (% ret)	Surgical	26	n/a	55.30 (6.80)	surgery (non-CE)	6 m	92.0	88.5	*	Parker, et al (1986)
WMS VR Delay (% ret)	Temporal Lobe Epilepsy	28	17/11	31.29 (9.52)	n/a	2.36 y	72.32 (20.93)	82.07 (20.43)		Selwa, et al (1994)
WMS VR Delay (% ret)	Temporal Lobe Epilepsy	14	6/8	31.36 (9.93)	RTL	1.93 y	82.79 (16.54)	79.50 (16.10)		Selwa, et al (1994)
WMS VR Delay (% ret)	Temporal Lobe Epilepsy	17	11/6	29.00 (8.12)	LTL	1.8 y	89.24 (11.86)	86.47 (22.67)		Selwa, et al (1994)
WMS VR Delay (% ret)	TIA	12	6/6	59.20 (13.30)	n/a	59.1 d	74.0 (28.6)	78.3 (23.6)		Casey, et al (1989)
WMS VR Delay (% ret)	TIA	12	6/6	63.40 (6.00)	RCE	60.7 d	68.6 (25.3)	77.2 (19.5)		Casey, et al (1989)
WMS VR Delay (% ret)	TIA	12	6/6	66.00 (5.30)	LCE	59.8 d	67.5 (36.6)	94.6 (82.0)		Casey, et al (1989)

instrument	group	n	m/f	age	intervention	inter	t #1	t #2	note	citation
WMS VR Imm	Alcoholic	10	10/0	33.05 (7.09)	placebo	1 h	10.5	10.6	I,II CB	Mallick, et al (1993)
WMS VR Imm	Alcoholic	10	10/0	33.05 (7.09)	lorazepam	1 h	10.0	9.4	I,II CB	Mallick, et al (1993)
WMS VR Imm	Cardiac	90	77/13	59.00 (10.59)	CABG/CPB	8 d	8.2 (3.2)	6.5 (3.7)	*	Townes, et al (1989)
WMS VR Imm	CAD	17	n/a	57.20 (7.20)	n/a	6 m	5.4	5.9		Parker, et al (1983)
WMS VR Imm	CAD	20	n/a	57.20 (7.20)	CE	6 m	5.8	6.4		Parker, et al (1983)
WMS VR Imm	CAD	17	n/a	57.90 (8.40)	n/a	6 m	6.1	6.4	*	Parker, et al (1986)
WMS VR Imm	CAD	36	n./a	61.10 (8.30)	CE	6 m	4.8	6.3	*	Parker, et al (1986)
WMS VR Imm	Control	101	101/0	78.50 (7.20)	n/a	2.6 y	9.9	12.8		Frank, et al (1996)
WMS VR Imm	Control	141	0/141	78.50 (6.60)	n/a	2.7 y	9.2	11.5		Frank, et al (1996)
WMS VR Imm	Control	10	10/0	31.30 (6.14)	lorazepam	1 h	12.0	10.7	I,II CB	Mallick, et al (1993)
WMS VR Imm	Control	10	10/0	31.30 (6.14)	placebo	1 h	12.5	11.0	I,II CB	Mallick, et al (1993)
WMS VR Imm	Control	33	15/18	59.10 (9.30)	n/a	10 d	9.7 (3.0)	11.2 (2.9)		McCaffrey, et al (1993)

instrument	group	n	m/f	age	intervention	inter	t #1	t #2	note	citation
WMS VR Imm	Control	40	6/34	68.20 (1.20)	n/a	1 y	8.8 (3.4)	10.3 (2.6)	*	Mitrushina, et al (1991b)
WMS VR Imm	Control	47	14/33	72.90 (1.40)	n/a	1 y	8.1 (3.0)	9.3 (2.9)	*	Mitrushina, et al (1991b)
WMS VR Imm	Control	19	2/17	62.20 (2.50)	n/a	1 y	8.8 (2.6)	10.3 (2.6)	*	Mitrushina, et al (1991b)
WMS VR Imm	Control	16	4/12	78.30 (2.50)	n/a	1 y	6.1 (3.6)	7.3 (3.7)	*	Mitrushina, et al (1991b)
WMS VR Imm	Control	21	21/0	31.45 (5.53)	n/a	18 m	12.45 (1.05)	12.80 (1.28)		Saykin, et al (1991)
WMS VR Imm	Control	47	35/12	59.00 (9.81)	n/a	8 d	9.3 (2.9)	9.3 (2.9)	*	Townes, et al (1989)
WMS VR Imm	Control (Pain Pt/Volunteer)	15	5/10	33.90 (8.40)	n/a	20.7 d	9.8 (2.7)	10.4 (2.3)		Goulet Fisher, et al (1986)
WMS VR Imm	CVA	19	n/a	~65.00	n/a	14.6 w	6.0	7.6		Bowler, et al (1994)
WMS VR Imm	DAT	34	34/0	83.90 (4.30)	n/a	2.1 y	5.3	5.5		Frank, et al (1996)
WMS VR Imm	DAT	22	0/22	83.10 (4.00)	n/a	2.0 y	5.1	6.0		Frank, et al (1996)
WMS VR Imm	DAT (at risk)	32	32/0	83.30 (6.70)	n/a	2.0 y	6.1	8.9		Frank, et al (1996)
WMS VR Imm	DAT (at risk)	50	0/50	84.10 (5.10)	n/a	2.3 y	6.2	8.3		Frank, et al (1996)

instrument	group	n	m/f	age	intervention	inter	t #1	t #2	note	citation
WMS VR Imm	DAT (mild)	11	10/1	63.00 (8.00)	n/a	26 m	7.0 (4.0)	4.0 (3.0)		Haxby, et al (1990)
WMS VR Imm	Depression	15	6/9	28.50 (10.60)	inpt tx	19.5 d	7.1 (2.9)	8.9 (2.6)		Goulet Fisher, et al (1986)
WMS VR Imm	Epilepsy	40	23/17	32.20 (8.20)	n/a	~9 m	8.83 (2.34)	9.67 (2.44)		Hermann, et al (1996)
WMS VR Imm	Epilepsy	13	n/a	29.20 (7.70)	RTL	1.2 y	9.5 (3.4)	9.9 (3.7)		Rausch, et al (1993)
WMS VR Imm	Epilepsy	12	n/a	29.20 (7.70)	LTL	1.2 y	9.7 (3.1)	10.4 (2.8)		Rausch, et al (1993)
WMS VR Imm	HIV+ (IVDU)	42	31/11	27.00 (5.30)	n/a	12 m	10.9 (2.1)	11.2 (3.4)		Bono, et al (1996)
WMS VR Imm	HIV+/ARC	8	8/0	33.57 (6.35)	n/a	18 m	10.29 (2.29)	10.71 (3.04)		Saykin, et al (1991)
WMS VR Imm	HIV+/PGL	13	13/0	31.15 (4.91)	n/a	18 m	12.23 (2.05)	12.77 (2.13)		Saykin, et al (1991)
WMS VR Imm	HIV- (IVDU)	39	30/9	28.60 (4.90)	n/a	12 m	11.7 (2.6)	11.8 (2.5)		Bono, et al (1996)
WMS VR Imm	Hypertension	25	17/8	50.10 (14.00)	n/a	7-10 d	11.17 (3.14)	12.17 (2.18)		McCaffrey, et al (1992)
WMS VR Imm	Hysterectomy/ Oophorectomy	9	0/9	48.20 (4.70)	placebo	9 w	11.3 (0.8)	10.1 (1.2)	I, II CB	Phillips, et al (1992)
WMS VR Imm	Hysterectomy/ Oophorectomy	10	0/10	48.20 (4.70)	estrogen tx	9 w	10.1 (0.7)	10.0 (0.8)	I, II CB	Phillips, et al (1992)

instrument	group	n	m/f	age	intervention	inter	t #1	t #2	note	citation
WMS VR Imm	MS	9	n/a	38.90	high dose interferon	2 y	6.4 (3.3)	9.9 (2.4)	I/ II	Pliskin, et al (1996)
WMS VR Imm	MS	8	n/a	38.00	low dose interferon	2 y	6.8 (2.2)	9.6 (2.7)	I/ II	Pliskin, et al (1996)
WMS VR Imm	MS	13	n/a	36.20	placebo	2 y	7.7 (3.5)	9.3 (2.6)	I/ II	Pliskin, et al (1996)
WMS VR Imm	Myasthenia Gravis	11	7/4	49.00	prednisolone	3-11 m	10.4 (3.1)	10.0 (2.5)		Glennerster, et al (1996)
WMS VR Imm	Naphtha Exposure	185	n/a	36.00	n/a	1 y	8.79 (2.45)	10.75 (2.42)		White, et al (1994)
WMS VR Imm	PD	4	3/1	53.50	fetal tissue implanted	12 m	7.4	7.5		Sass, et al (1995)
WMS VR Imm	Schizophrenia	38	25/13	30.90 (8.73)	n/a	6 m	6.77 (3.25)	11.97 (2.73)		Addington, et al (1991)
WMS VR Imm	Surgical	17	n/a	57.20 (7.20)	surgery	6 m	6.4	7.2		Parker, et al (1983)
WMS VR Imm	Surgical	26	n/a	55.30 (6.80)	surgery (non-CE)	6 m	7.0	7.6	*	Parker, et al (1986)
WMS x	Control	75	n/a	61.30 (8.03)	antigravity tx	12 m	62.00 (8.15)	65.65 (5.61)		Dubey, et al (1978)
WMS x LM (% ret)	Epilepsy	14	7/7	32.90 (8.30)	LTL	16.1 m	46.5 (18.7)	57.6 (39.5)		Phillips, et al (1995)
WMS x LM (% ret)	Epilepsy	24	12/13	28.40 (9.70)	RTL	16.1 m	50.5 (27.8)	54.7 (24.7)		Phillips, et al (1995)

instrument	group	n	m/f	age	intervention	inter	t #1	t #2	note	citation
WMS x LM (% ret)	Hydroceph (control pressure)	14	9/5	66.00 (14.16)	extracranial shunting	27.4 w	41.86 (36.4)	64.86 (17.86)		Stambrook, et al (1988)
WMS x LM (story A)	Asthma	8	n/a	6.00 - 12.00	placebo	2 w	9.0	9.62		Rappaport, et al (1989)
WMS x LM (story A)	Asthma	9	n/a	6.00 - 12.00	theophylline	2 w	8.55	9.92		Rappaport, et al (1989)
WMS x LM (story B)	Asthma	8	n/a	6.00 - 12.00	placebo	2 w	9.68	10.81		Rappaport, et al (1989)
WMS x LM (story B)	Asthma	9	n/a	6.00 - 12.00	theophylline	2 w	11.16	9.72		Rappaport, et al (1989)
WMS x LM Delay	Epilepsy	14	7/7	32.90 (8.30)	LTL	16.1 m	2.7 (1.7)	2.5 (1.9)		Phillips, et al (1995)
WMS x LM Delay	Epilepsy	24	12/13	28.40 (9.70)	RTL	16.1 m	3.2 (2.5)	3.5 (2.3)		Phillips, et al (1995)
WMS x LM Delay	Hydroceph (control pressure)	14	9/5	66.00 (14.16)	extracranial shunting	27.4 w	2.14 (1.68)	12.71 (9.55)		Stambrook, et al (1988)
WMS x LM Delay	Schizophrenia Inpts	35	29/6	23.71 (4.50)	neuroleptics	1-2 y	6.1 (5.0)	6.5 (3.6)		Nopoulos, et al (1994)
WMS x LM Delay (%ile)	Dyspepsia	6	3/3	53.00	ranitidine	8 w	43.0	42.0	*	Nwokolo, et al (1994)
WMS x LM Delay (%ile)	Dyspepsia	8	4/4	50.00	TDB	8 w	65.0	67.0	*	Nwokolo, et al (1994)

instrument	group	n	m/f	age	intervention	inter	t #1	t #2	note	citation
WMS x LM Imm	Epilepsy	24	12/13	28.40 (9.70)	RTL	16.1 m	5.6 (3.0)	5.9 (2.6)		Phillips, et al (1995)
WMS x LM Imm	Epilepsy	14	7/7	32.90 (8.30)	LTL	16.1 m	5.6 (2.3)	4.3 (1.6)		Phillips, et al (1995)
WMS x LM Imm	Hydroceph (control pressure)	14	9/5	66.00 (14.16)	extracranial shunting	27.37 w	6.57 (5.6)	17.57 (9.31)		Stambrook, et al (1988)
WMS x LM Imm	Schizophrenia Inpts	35	29/6	23.71 (4.50)	neuroleptics	1-2 y	7.6 (4.4)	8.4 (4.6)		Nopoulos, et al (1994)
WMS x LM Imm (%ile)	Dyspepsia	6	3/3	53.00	ranitidine	8 w	49.0	51.0	*	Nwokolo, et al (1994)
WMS x LM Imm (%ile)	Dyspepsia	8	4/4	50.00	TDB	8 w	78.0	78.0	*	Nwokolo, et al (1994)
WMS x PAL (% ret)	Epilepsy	24	12/13	28.40 (9.70)	RTL	16.1 m	55.7 (13.6)	56.2 (9.4)		Phillips, et al (1995)
WMS x PAL (% ret)	Epilepsy	14	7/7	32.90 (8.30)	LTL	16.1 m	54.8 (12.7)	55.6 (16.7)		Phillips, et al (1995)
WMS x PAL Delay	Epilepsy	24	12/13	28.40 (9.70)	RTL	16.1 m	7.6 (1.9)	8.1 (1.9)		Phillips, et al (1995)
WMS x PAL Delay	Epilepsy	14	7/7	32.90 (8.30)	LTL	16.1 m	6.8 (1.9)	5.5 (2.7)		Phillips, et al (1995)
WMS x PAL Easy	Schizophrenia Inpts	35	29/6	23.71 (4.50)	neuroleptics	1-2 y	15.2 (2.7)	15.3 (3.3)		Nopoulos, et al (1994)
WMS x PAL Hard	Schizophrenia Inpts	35	29/6	23.71 (4.50)	neuroleptics	1-2 y	5.7 (3.0)	7.0 (3.2)		Nopoulos, et al (1994)

instrument	group	n	m/f	age	intervention	inter	t #1	t #2	note	citation
WMS x PAL Imm	Epilepsy	24	12/13	28.40 (9.70)	RTL	16.1 m	14.2 (3.9)	14.5 (3.3)		Phillips, et al (1995)
WMS x PAL Imm	Epilepsy	14	7/7	32.90 (8.30)	LTL	16.1 m	12.5 (2.9)	10.0 (4.2)		Phillips, et al (1995)
WMS x VR (% ret)	Hydroceph (control pressure)	14	9/5	66.00 (14.16)	extracranial shunting	27.4 w	26.14 (38.31)	71.86 (30.45)		Stambrook, et al (1988)
WMS x VR Delay	Dyspepsia	6	3/3	53.00	ranitidine	8 w	19.0	16.0	*	Nwokolo, et al (1994)
WMS x VR Delay	Dyspepsia	8	4/4	50.00	TDB	8 w	24.0	19.0	*	Nwokolo, et al (1994)
WMS x VR Delay	HD	40	18/22	40.00 (10.30)	n/a	12 m	5.2 (0.4)	5.7 (0.4)		Bamford, et al (1995)
WMS x VR Delay	HD	26	12/14	39.00 (10.40)	n/a	12 m	5.4 (0.5)	5.4 (0.5)		Bamford, et al (1995)
WMS x VR Delay	Hydroceph (control pressure)	14	9/5	66.00 (14.16)	extracranial shunting	27.4 w	0.71 (0.95)	3.43 (3.66)		Stambrook, et al (1988)
WMS x VR Delay	mild Toxic Enceph	14	n/a	40.10 (6.00)	unimproved at retest	15.9 m	9.6 (4.5)	8.7 (3.5)		Morrow, et al (1991)
WMS x VR Delay	mild Toxic Enceph	13	n/a	36.40 (10.30)	improved at retest	18.1 m	7.2 (3.6)	10.5 (3.3)		Morrow, et al (1991)
WMS x VR Imm	Dyspepsia	8	4/4	50.00	TDB	8 w	29.0	39.0	*	Nwokolo, et al (1994)
WMS x VR Imm	Dyspepsia	6	3/3	53.00	ranitidine	8 w	26.0	19.0	*	Nwokolo, et al (1994)

instrument	group	n	m/f	age	intervention	inter	t #1	t #2	note	citation
WMS x VR Imm	HD	26	12/14	39.00 (10.40)	n/a	12 m	4.8 (0.4)	4.7 (0.5)		Bamford, et al (1995)
WMS x VR Imm	HD	40	18/22	40.00 (10.30)	n/a	12 m	4.5 (13.0)	5.4 (0.4)		Bamford, et al (1995)
WMS x VR Imm	Hydroceph (control pressure)	14	9/5	66.00 (14.16)	extracranial shunting	27.4 w	2.14 (2.27)	4.43 (3.55)		Stambrook, et al (1988)
WMS x VR Imm	mild Toxic Enceph	13	n/a	36.40 (10.30)	improved at retest	18.1 m	9.3 (4.2)	10.6 (3.7)		Morrow, et al (1991)
WMS x VR Imm	mild Toxic Enceph	14	n/a	40.10 (6.00)	unimproved at retest	15.9 m	11.1 (4.1)	9.6 (2.1)		Morrow, et al (1991)
WMS-III Auditory Delay	Control	156	78/78	55.00 - 89.00	n/a	35.6 d	98.5 (14.6)	108.7 (17.1)		Wechsler (1997)
WMS-III Auditory Delay	Control	141	71/70	16.00 - 54.00	n/a	35.6 d	101.9 (14.1)	110.6 (13.9)		Wechsler (1997)
WMS-III Auditory Imm	Control	141	71/70	16.00 - 54.00	n/a	35.6 d	101.7 (14.4)	111.5 (16.3)		Wechsler (1997)
WMS-III Auditory Imm	Control	156	78/78	55.00 - 89.00	n/a	35.6 d	97.3 (14.8)	107.2 (17.9)		Wechsler (1997)
WMS-III Auditory Recog Delay	Control	156	78/78	55.00 - 89.00	n/a	35.6 d	9.6 (2.7)	10.8 (3.2)		Wechsler (1997)
WMS-III Auditory Recog Delay	Control	141	71/70	16.00 - 54.00	n/a	35.6 d	10.1 (2.9)	11.4 (3.0)		Wechsler (1997)

instrument	group	n	m/f	age	intervention	inter	t #1	t #2	note	citation
WMS-III Auditory Recog Delay Index	Control	156	78/78	55.00 - 89.00	n/a	35.6 d	98.2 (13.7)	104.0 (16.2)		Wechsler (1997)
WMS-III Auditory Recog Delay Index	Control	141	71/70	16.00 - 54.00	n/a	35.6 d	100.6 (14.4)	106.9 (15.0)		Wechsler (1997)
WMS-III Faces I	Control	156	78/78	55.00 - 89.00	n/a	35.6 d	10.1 (3.1)	12.1 (3.8)		Wechsler (1997)
WMS-III Faces I	Control	141	71/70	16.00 - 54.00	n/a	35.6 d	10.5 (2.8)	13.2 (3.3)		Wechsler (1997)
WMS-III Faces II	Control	156	78/78	55.00 - 89.00	n/a	35.6 d	10.4 (3.0)	12.2 (3.8)		Wechsler (1997)
WMS-III Faces II	Control	141	71/70	16.00 - 54.00	n/a	35.6 d	10.6 (2.8)	12.8 (2.7)		Wechsler (1997)
WMS-III Family Pictures I	Control	156	78/78	55.00 - 89.00	n/a	35.6 d	9.7 (3.1)	11.1 (3.1)		Wechsler (1997)
WMS-III Family Pictures I	Control	141	71/70	16.00 - 54.00	n/a	35.6 d	10.5 (2.9)	12.4 (2.9)		Wechsler (1997)
WMS-III Family Pictures II	Control	156	78/78	55.00 - 89.00	n/a	35.6 d	10.0 (3.1)	11.3 (3.1)		Wechsler (1997)

instrument	group	n	m/f	age	intervention	inter	t #1	t #2	note	citation
WMS-III Family Pictures II	Control	141	71/70	16.00 - 54.00	n/a	35.6 d	10.4 (3.0)	12.6 (2.9)		Wechsler (1997)
WMS-III GMI	Control	156	78/78	55.00 - 89.00	n/a	35.6 d	99.1 (15.7)	110.6 (18.7)		Wechsler (1997)
WMS-III GMI	Control	141	71/70	16.00 - 54.00	n/a	35.6 d	102.5 (14.6)	115.4 (15.9)		Wechsler (1997)
WMS-III Imm Memory	Control	156	78/78	55.00 - 89.00	n/a	35.6 d	98.0 (16.9)	110.2 (19.8)		Wechsler (1997)
WMS-III Imm Memory	Control	141	71/70	16.00 - 54.00	n/a	35.6 d	102.8 (14.5)	117.6 (17.9)		Wechsler (1997)
WMS-III LM I	Control	141	71/70	16.00 - 54.00	n/a	35.6 d	10.2 (3.2)	12.1 (3.1)		Wechsler (1997)
WMS-III LM I	Control	156	78/78	55.00 - 89.00	n/a	35.6 d	9.6 (2.8)	11.3 (3.1)		Wechsler (1997)
WMS-III LM II	Control	141	71/70	16.00 - 54.00	n/a	35.6 d	10.2 (3.1)	12.5 (3.0)		Wechsler (1997)
WMS-III LM II	Control	156	78/78	55.00 - 89.00	n/a	35.6 d	9.9 (2.9)	12.1 (3.0)		Wechsler (1997)
WMS-III LNS	Control	141	71/70	16.00 - 54.00	n/a	35.6 d	10.3 (2.6)	10.7 (2.9)		Wechsler (1997)
WMS-III LNS	Control	156	78/78	55.00 - 89.00	n/a	35.6 d	10.0 (3.0)	10.3 (3.2)		Wechsler (1997)
WMS-III PA I	Control	156	78/78	55.00 - 89.00	n/a	35.6 d	9.6 (3.1)	11.1 (3.6)		Wechsler (1997)

instrument	group	n	m/f	age	intervention	inter	t #1	t #2	note	citation
WMS-III PA I	Control	141	71/70	16.00 - 54.00	n/a	35.6 d	10.4 (2.7)	11.8 (3.0)		Wechsler (1997)
WMS-III PA II	Control	156	78/78	55.00 - 89.00	n/a	35.6 d	9.6 (3.0)	10.8 (3.3)		Wechsler (1997)
WMS-III PA II	Control	141	71/70	16.00 - 54.00	n/a	35.6 d	10.5 (2.8)	11.1 (2.3)		Wechsler (1997)
WMS-III Spatial Span	Control	141	71/70	16.00 - 54.00	n/a	35.6 d	10.2 (2.7)	10.4 (2.6)		Wechsler (1997)
WMS-III Spatial Span	Control	156	78/78	55.00 - 89.00	n/a	35.6 d	10.0 (3.0)	10.0 (3.1)		Wechsler (1997)
WMS-III Visual Delay	Control	156	78/78	55.00 - 89.00	n/a	35.6 d	101.1 (15.4)	111.3 (18.9)		Wechsler (1997)
WMS-III Visual Delay	Control	141	71/70	16.00 - 54.00	n/a	35.6 d	103.0 (14.7)	117.4 (15.7)		Wechsler (1997)
WMS-III Visual Imm	Control	141	71/70	16.00 - 54.00	n/a	35.6 d	102.8 (13.7)	117.1 (16.2)		Wechsler (1997)
WMS-III Visual Imm	Control	156	78/78	55.00 - 89.00	n/a	35.6 d	99.3 (16.3)	109.6 (18.8)		Wechsler (1997)
WMS-III WMI	Control	156	78/78	55.00 - 89.00	n/a	35.6 d	100.0 (14.8)	101.0 (15.7)		Wechsler (1997)
WMS-III WMI	Control	141	71/70	16.00 - 54.00	n/a	35.6 d	100.8 (12.4)	103.1 (14.3)		Wechsler (1997)
WMS-R ACI	Alcohol Dependent	50	45/5	39.30 (10.00)	n/a	19.6 w	85.5 (16.7)	88.0 (18.2)		Bowden, et al (1995)

instrument	group	n	m/f	age	intervention	inter	t #1	t #2	note	citation
WMS-R ACI	Control	48	n/a	20.00 - 24.00	n/a	4-6 w	73.7 (11.8)	77.7 (12.3)		Wechsler (1987)
WMS-R ACI	Control	53	n/a	55.00 - 64.00	n/a	4-6 w	64.7 (10.2)	65.4 (10.2)		Wechsler (1987)
WMS-R ACI	Control	50	n/a	70.00 - 74.00	n/a	4-6 w	59.9 (12.5)	62.1 (12.5)		Wechsler (1987)
WMS-R ACI	Epilepsy	40	24/16	32.45 (8.04)	n/a	7.10 m	94.6 (16.7)	94.9 (18.9)		Chelune, et al (1993)
WMS-R ACI	Epilepsy	47	31/16	29.40 (7.56)	LTL	11.0 m	93.5 (14.2)	95.2 (13.0)		Chelune, et al (1993)
WMS-R ACI	Epilepsy	49	29/20	29.45 (7.28)	RTL	10.7 m	94.6 (17.5)	98.3 (15.8)		Chelune, et al (1993)
WMS-R ACI	Epilepsy	20	12/8	29.90 (10.10)	RTL	3.8 m	95.3	100.1		Ivnik, et al (1993)
WMS-R ACI	Epilepsy	20	8/12	34.60 (9.80)	LTL	4.1 m	92.0	91.5		Ivnik, et al (1993)
WMS-R ACI	Epilepsy	50	31/19	31.60 (8.20)	medical tx	7.8 m	65.6 (11.8)	66.1 (13.6)		McSweeney, et al (1993)
WMS-R ACI	Epilepsy	50	29/21	29.20 (7.60)	RTL	11.1 m	66.9 (12.9)	69.5 (12.1)		McSweeney, et al (1993)
WMS-R ACI	Epilepsy	47	31/16	29.40 (7.60)	LTL	11.0 m	66.2 (10.4)	67.2 (10.1)		McSweeney, et al (1993)
WMS-R D Span	Brain Tumor (post-surgery)	12	5/7	31.80 (8.60)	radiation tx	3 m	8.2 (2.0)	8.8 (1.4)	*	Armstrong, et al (1995)

instrument	group	n	m/f	age	intervention	inter	t #1	t #2	note	citation
WMS-R D Span	Control	63	8/55	56.22 (11.00)	n/a	~6 m	NR	0.06 (2.0) c		Bruggemans, et al (1997)
WMS-R D Span	Control	50	n/a	70.00 - 74.00	n/a	4-6 w	13.8 (4.0)	14.1 (3.7)		Wechsler (1987)
WMS-R D Span	Control	53	n/a	55.00 - 64.00	n/a	4-6 w	14.9 (3.3)	14.6 (3.5)		Wechsler (1987)
WMS-R D Span	Control	48	n/a	20.00 - 24.00	n/a	4-6 w	16.2 (3.4)	17.4 (3.5)		Wechsler (1987)
WMS-R D Span Backward	Control	17	n/a	~39.00	n/a	12 m	6.18	6.94		Hanly, et al (1994)
WMS-R D Span Backward	Control	50	n/a	70.00 - 74.00	n/a	4-6 w	6.0 (2.3)	6.3 (2.2)		Wechsler (1987)
WMS-R D Span Backward	Control	53	n/a	55.00 - 64.00	n/a	4-6 w	6.5 (2.1)	6.3 (2.2)		Wechsler (1987)
WMS-R D Span Backward	Control	48	n/a	20.00 - 24.00	n/a	4-6 w	7.1 (2.4)	8.0 (2.3)		Wechsler (1987)
WMS-R D Span Backward	Rheumatoid Arthritis	11	n/a	~39.00	n/a	12 m	7.18	7.18		Hanly, et al (1994)
WMS-R D Span Backward	SLE	59	n/a	39.60 (1.30)	n/a	12 m	6.44	6.81		Hanly, et al (1994)
WMS-R D Span Forward	Control	17	n/a	~39.00	n/a	12 m	8.18	8.24		Hanly, et al (1994)
WMS-R D Span Forward	Control	50	n/a	70.00 - 74.00	n/a	4-6 w	7.8 (2.0)	7.8 (2.0)		Wechsler (1987)

instrument	group	n	m/f	age	intervention	inter	t #1	t #2	note	citation
WMS-R D Span Forward	Control	53	n/a	55.00 - 64.00	n/a	4-6 w	8.4 (2.0)	8.3 (1.9)		Wechsler (1987)
WMS-R D Span Forward	Control	48	n/a	20.00 - 24.00	n/a	4-6 w	9.0 (1.7)	9.3 (1.8)		Wechsler (1987)
WMS-R D Span Forward	Rheumatoid Arthritis	11	n/a	~39.00	n/a	12 m	9.36	9.18		Hanly, et al (1994)
WMS-R D Span Forward	SLE	59	n/a	39.60 (1.30)	n/a	12 m	7.86	8.29		Hanly, et al (1994)
WMS-R DRI	Alcohol Dependent	50	45/5	39.30 (10.00)	n/a	19.6 w	92.8 (15.0)	98.9 (17.2)		Bowden, et al (1995)
WMS-R DRI	Control	64	21/43	28.80 (9.10)	n/a	2 w	109.4 (13.99)	124.49 (14.25)	*	Theisen, et al (1998)
WMS-R DRI	Control	48	n/a	20.00 - 24.00	n/a	4-6 w	79.6 (12.5)	91.5 (10)		Wechsler (1987)
WMS-R DRI	Control	53	n/a	55.00 - 64.00	n/a	4-6 w	66.1 (13.1)	75.7 (13.2)		Wechsler (1987)
WMS-R DRI	Control	50	n/a	70.00 - 74.00	n/a	4-6 w	52.6 (17.4)	59.3 (17.8)		Wechsler (1987)
WMS-R DRI	Control (avg IQ)	23	n/a	~28.80	n/a	2 w	111.65 (12.85)	128.43 (10.70)		Rapport, et al (1997a)
WMS-R DRI	Control (high avg IQ)	21	n/a	~28.80	n/a	2 w	116.62 (12.83)	130.57 (9.99)		Rapport, et al (1997a)
WMS-R DRI	Control (low avg IQ)	20	n/a	~28.80	n/a	2 w	99.50 (11.23)	113.90 (16.32)		Rapport, et al (1997a)

instrument	group	n	m/f	age	intervention	inter	t #1	t #2	note	citation
WMS-R DRI	Epilepsy	49	29/20	29.45 (7.28)	RTL	10.7 m	87.5 (18.4)	88.7 (19.3)		Chelune, et al (1993)
WMS-R DRI	Epilepsy	40	24/16	32.45 (8.04)	n/a	7.10 m	85.9 (18.6)	90.9 (21.3)		Chelune, et al (1993)
WMS-R DRI	Epilepsy	47	31/16	29.40 (7.56)	LTL	11.0 m	81.9 (15.5)	80.7 (14.6)		Chelune, et al (1993)
WMS-R DRI	Epilepsy	50	31/19	31.60 (8.20)	medical tx	7.8 m	67.3 (20.1)	70.0 (19)		McSweeney, et al (1993)
WMS-R DRI	Epilepsy	50	29/21	29.20 (7.60)	RTL	11.1 m	64.4 (20.6)	67.2 (19.1)		McSweeney, et al (1993)
WMS-R DRI	Epilepsy	47	31/16	29.40 (7.60)	LTL	11.0 m	61.9 (15.7)	59.8 (17.2)		McSweeney, et al (1993)
WMS-R DRI	Homeless	15	9/6	32.80 (6.10)	cognitive remediation	2-3 m	88.40 (13.90)	94.53 (12.68)		Cotman, et al (1997)
WMS-R DRI	Homeless	9	4/5	27.00 (5.80)	n/a	2-3 m	102.78 (19.90)	104.67 (18.08)		Cotman, et al (1997)
WMS-R FM	Control	50	n/a	70.00 - 74.00	n/a	4-6 w	5.8 (1.8)	6.5 (1.8)		Wechsler (1987)
WMS-R FM	Control	53	n/a	55.00 - 64.00	n/a	4-6 w	6.2 (1.4)	6.8 (1.3)		Wechsler (1987)
WMS-R FM	Control	48	n/a	20.00 - 24.00	n/a	4-6 w	7.2 (1.8)	7.9 (1.6)		Wechsler (1987)
WMS-R FM	Schizophrenia	19	13/6	33.70 (6.30)	clozapine	10 w	5.7 (2.01)	5.57 (1.88)		Buchanan, et al (1994)

instrument	group	n	m/f	age	intervention	inter	t #1	t #2	note	citation
WMS-R FM	Schizophrenia	19	15/4	34.00 (6.90)	haloperidol	10 w	6.1 (1.45)	5.74 (1.82)		Buchanan, et al (1994)
WMS-R FM	Schizophrenia	33	n/a	~33.70 (6.30)	clozapine	1 y	5.9 (1.8)	5.8 (1.9)		Buchanan, et al (1994)
WMS-R GMI	Alcohol Dependent	50	45/5	39.30 (10.00)	n/a	19.6 w	90.8 (15.7)	96.7 (17.2)		Bowden, et al (1995)
WMS-R GMI	Control	64	21/43	28.80 (9.10)	n/a	2 w	105.12 (14.0)	120.26 (15.07)	*	Theisen, et al (1998)
WMS-R GMI	Control	53	n/a	55.00 - 64.00	n/a	4-6 w	108.3 (17.2)	127.6 (16.9)		Wechsler (1987)
WMS-R GMI	Control	50	n/a	70.00 - 74.00	n/a	4-6 w	97.2 (23.3)	111.0 (24.6)		Wechsler (1987)
WMS-R GMI	Control	48	n/a	20.00 - 24.00	n/a	4-6 w	129.2 (18.4)	148.1 (17.2)		Wechsler (1987)
WMS-R GMI	Control (avg IQ)	23	n/a	~28.80	n/a	2 w	106.91 (11.42)	123.17 (12.30)		Rapport, et al (1997a)
WMS-R GMI	Control (high avg IQ)	21	n/a	~28.80	n/a	2 w	112.76 (13.19)	128.29 (9.29)		Rapport, et al (1997a)
WMS-R GMI	Control (low avg IQ)	20	n/a	~28.80	n/a	2 w	95.10 (12.31)	108.45 (16.46)		Rapport, et al (1997a)
WMS-R GMI	Epilepsy	40	24/16	32.45 (8.04)	n/a	7.1 m	92.9 (18.5)	99.7 (19.9)		Chelune, et al (1993)
WMS-R GMI	Epilepsy	47	31/16	29.40 (7.56)	LTL	11.0 m	88.7 (14.3)	82.2 (14.2)		Chelune, et al (1993)

instrument	group	n	m/f	age	intervention	inter	t #1	t #2	note	citation
WMS-R GMI	Epilepsy	49	29/20	29.45 (7.28)	RTL	10.7 m	90.9 (16.5)	93.2 (17.2)		Chelune, et al (1993)
WMS-R GMI	Epilepsy	20	8/12	34.60 (9.80)	LTL	4.1 m	83.7	80.5		Ivnik, et al (1993)
WMS-R GMI	Epilepsy	20	12/8	29.90 (10.10)	RTL	3.8 m	89.0	95.1		Ivnik, et al (1993)
WMS-R GMI	Epilepsy	47	31/16	29.40 (7.60)	LTL	11.0 m	113.5 (19.7)	104.1 (20.5)		McSweeney, et al (1993)
WMS-R GMI	Epilepsy	50	29/21	29.20 (7.60)	RTL	11.1 m	115.9 (22.1)	118.6 (22.4)		McSweeney, et al (1993)
WMS-R GMI	Epilepsy	50	31/19	31.60 (8.20)	medical tx	7.8 m	119.3 (26.2)	127.2 (25.1)		McSweeney, et al (1993)
WMS-R GMI	Homeless	9	4/5	27.00 (5.80)	n/a	2-3 m	99.33 (17.26)	100.22 (16.78)		Cotman, et al (1997)
WMS-R GMI	Homeless	15	9/6	32.80 (6.10)	cognitive program	2-3 m	89.47 (13.41)	94.27 (8.28)		Cotman, et al (1997)
WMS-R GMI	Schizophrenia	33	n/a	~33.70 (6.30)	clozapine	1 y	73.9 (18.9)	76.2 (21.7)		Buchanan, et al (1994)
WMS-R Info and Orient	Control	48	n/a	20.00 - 24.00	n/a	4-6 w	13.7 (0.4)	11.9 (0.3)		Wechsler (1987)
WMS-R Info and Orient	Control	50	n/a	70.00 - 74.00	n/a	4-6 w	13.3 (1.3)	11.4 (0.9)		Wechsler (1987)
WMS-R Info and Orient	Control	53	n/a	55.00 - 64.00	n/a	4-6 w	13.4 (0.6)	11.7 (0.5)		Wechsler (1987)

instrument	group	n	m/f	age	intervention	inter	t #1	t #2	note	citation
WMS-R LM Delay	Control	20	0/20	29.10 (4.70)	n/a	1 m	10.0 (3.5)	10.5 (3.9)	*	Harris, et al (1996)
WMS-R LM Delay	Control	64	21/43	28.80 (9.10)	n/a	2 w	24.23 (6.61)	32.59 (8.42)	*	Theisen, et al (1998)
WMS-R LM Delay	Control	53	n/a	55.00 - 64.00	n/a	4-6 w	17.8 (5.7)	24.6 (6.9)		Wechsler (1987)
WMS-R LM Delay	Control	48	n/a	20.00 - 24.00	n/a	4-6 w	22.1 (7.7)	31.5 (6.8)		Wechsler (1987)
WMS-R LM Delay	Control	50	n/a	70.00 - 74.00	n/a	4-6 w	14.7 (9.2)	19.3 (8.4)		Wechsler (1987)
WMS-R LM Delay	Pregnant	20	0/20	29.00 (4.60)	normal delivery	1 m	8.6 (4.3)	8.9 (3.3)	*	Harris, et al (1996)
WMS-R LM Delay (% ret)	Epilepsy	20	8/12	34.60 (9.80)	LTL	4.1 m	60.5	50.3		Ivnik, et al (1993)
WMS-R LM Delay (% ret)	Epilepsy	20	12/8	29.90 (10.10)	RTL	3.8 m	70.8	77.3		Ivnik, et al (1993)
WMS-R LM Imm	Control	64	21/43	28.80 (9.10)	n/a	2 w	27.8 (6.28)	34.6 (7.48)	*	Theisen, et al (1998)
WMS-R LM Imm	Control	53	n/a	55.00 - 64.00	n/a	4-6 w	22.1 (5.8)	27.9 (5.8)		Wechsler (1987)
WMS-R LM Imm	Control	48	n/a	20.00 - 24.00	n/a	4-6 w	25.7 (7.4)	33.1 (6.7)		Wechsler (1987)
WMS-R LM Imm	Control	50	n/a	70.00 - 74.00	n/a	4-6 w	20.9 (7.3)	24.1 (7.7)		Wechsler (1987)

instrument	group	n	m/f	age	intervention	inter	t #1	t #2	note	citation
WMS-R LM x	Control	45	n/a	68.80 (6.00)	n/a	9 m	24.42 (6.3)	26.04 (5.9)		Rasmusson, et al (1995)
WMS-R LM x	Schizophrenia	19	13/6	33.70 (6.30)	clozapine	10 w	29.2 (16.6)	28.7 (18.1)		Buchanan, et al (1994)
WMS-R LM x	Schizophrenia	19	15/4	34.00 (6.90)	haloperidol	10 w	35.4 (17.8)	34.5 (19.3)		Buchanan, et al (1994)
WMS-R LM x	Schizophrenia	33	n/a	~33.70 (6.30)	clozapine	1 y	30.7 (17.5)	34.7 (18.9)		Buchanan, et al (1994)
WMS-R MC	Control	50	n/a	70.00 - 74.00	n/a	4-6 w	4.9 (1.3)	4.8 (1.4)		Wechsler (1987)
WMS-R MC	Control	48	n/a	20.00 - 24.00	n/a	4-6 w	5.3 (0.9)	5.1 (0.9)		Wechsler (1987)
WMS-R MC	Control	53	n/a	55.00 - 64.00	n/a	4-6 w	4.9 (1.2)	5.2 (1.0)		Wechsler (1987)
WMS-R PA Delay	Control	64	21/43	28.80 (9.10)	n/a	2 w	7.8 (0.44)	7.88 (0.58)	*	Theisen, et al (1998)
WMS-R PA Delay	Control	48	n/a	20.00 - 24.00	n/a	4-6 w	7.7 (0.6)	7.8 (0.6)		Wechsler (1987)
WMS-R PA Delay	Control	53	n/a	55.00 - 64.00	n/a	4-6 w	6.9 (1.2)	7.4 (0.8)		Wechsler (1987)
WMS-R PA Delay	Control	50	n/a	70.00 - 74.00	n/a	4-6 w	6.7 (1.4)	6.7 (1.0)		Wechsler (1987)
WMS-R PA Imm	Control	64	21/43	28.80 (9.10)	n/a	2 w	19.86 (2.67)	22.25 (2.68)	*	Theisen, et al (1998)

instrument	group	n	m/f	age	intervention	inter	t #1	t #2	note	citation
WMS-R PA Imm	Control	50	n/a	70.00 - 74.00	n/a	4-6 w	16.8 (4.0)	19.0 (3.8)		Wechsler (1987)
WMS-R PA Imm	Control	53	n/a	55.00 - 64.00	n/a	4-6 w	17.9 (3.2)	20.1 (3.0)		Wechsler (1987)
WMS-R PA Imm	Control	48	n/a	20.00 - 24.00	n/a	4-6 w	21.8 (1.8)	23.0 (1.5)		Wechsler (1987)
WMS-R PA Trial 1	CVD	48	34/14	62.00	complicated CABG	8-10 d	NR	2.20 c		Malheiros, et al (1995)
WMS-R PA Trial 1	CVD	33	23/10	64.00	CABG	8-10 d	NR	1.73 c		Malheiros, et al (1995)
WMS-R PA Trial 2	CVD	48	34/14	62.00	complicated CABG	8-10 d	NR	0.90 c		Malheiros, et al (1995)
WMS-R PA Trial 2	CVD	33	23/10	64.00	CABG	8-10 d	NR	0.80 c		Malheiros, et al (1995)
WMS-R PA Trial 3	CVD	48	34/14	62.00	complicated CABG	8-10 d	NR	0.74 c		Malheiros, et al (1995)
WMS-R PA Trial 3	CVD	33	23/10	64.00	CABG	8-10 d	NR	0.80 c		Malheiros, et al (1995)
WMS-R PA x	Schizophrenia	33	n/a	~33.70 (6.30)	clozapine	1 y	15.5 (4.9)	15.6 (4.8)		Buchanan, et al (1994)
WMS-R PA x	Schizophrenia	19	13/6	33.70 (6.30)	clozapine	10 w	15.8 (5.3)	16.2 (4.7)		Buchanan, et al (1994)
WMS-R PA x	Schizophrenia	19	15/4	34.00 (6.90)	haloperidol	10 w	15.7 (4.7)	15.6 (5.6)		Buchanan, et al (1994)

instrument	group	n	m/f	age	intervention	inter	t #1	t #2	note	citation
WMS-R V Span	Brain Tumor (post-surgery)	12	5/7	31.80 (8.60)	radiation tx	3 m	9.2 (1.6)	9.1 (1.3)	*	Armstrong, et al (1995)
WMS-R V Span	Control	63	8/55	56.22 (11.00)	n/a	~6 m	NR	0.21 (2.3) c		Bruggemans, et al (1997)
WMS-R V Span Backward	Control	17	n/a	~39.00	n/a	12 m	6.82	7.12		Hanly, et al (1994)
WMS-R V Span Backward	Rheumatoid Arthritis	11	n/a	~39.00	n/a	12 m	7.91	6.82		Hanly, et al (1994)
WMS-R V Span Backward	SLE	59	n/a	39.60 (1.30)	n/a	12 m	7.12	6.42		Hanly, et al (1994)
WMS-R V Span Forward	Control	17	n/a	~39.00	n/a	12 m	8.12	8.18		Hanly, et al (1994)
WMS-R V Span Forward	Rheumatoid Arthritis	11	n/a	~39.00	n/a	12 m	8.73	7.55		Hanly, et al (1994)
WMS-R V Span Forward	SLE	59	n/a	39.60 (1.30)	n/a	12 m	7.93	7.97		Hanly, et al (1994)
WMS-R VeMI	Alcohol Dependent	50	45/5	39.30 (10.00)	n/a	19.6 w	93.9 (14.3)	98.3 (15.0)		Bowden, et al (1995)
WMS-R VeMI	Control	48	n/a	20.00 - 24.00	n/a	4-6 w	73.3 (15.7)	89.2 (14.0)		Wechsler (1987)
WMS-R VeMI	Control	53	n/a	55.00 - 64.00	n/a	4-6 w	62.2 (12.4)	75.9 (12.8)		Wechsler (1987)
WMS-R VeMI	Control	50	n/a	70.00 - 74.00	n/a	4-6 w	58.7 (17.1)	67.2 (17.8)		Wechsler (1987)

instrument	group	n	m/f	age	intervention	inter	t #1	t #2	note	citation
WMS-R VeMI	Epilepsy	47	31/16	29.40 (7.56)	LTL	11.0 m	89.2 (12.6)	81.1 (13.7)		Chelune, et al (1993)
WMS-R VeMI	Epilepsy	49	29/20	29.45 (7.28)	RTL	10.7 m	91.1 (14.9)	93.4 (14.9)		Chelune, et al (1993)
WMS-R VeMI	Epilepsy	40	24/16	32.45 (8.04)	n/a	7.1 m	94.5 (17.4)	102.5 (18.3)		Chelune, et al (1993)
WMS-R VeMI	Epilepsy	20	12/8	29.90 (10.10)	RTL	3.8 m	89.0	95.5		Ivnik, et al (1993)
WMS-R VeMI	Epilepsy	20	8/12	34.60 (9.80)	LTL	4.1 m	83.4	79.0		Ivnik, et al (1993)
WMS-R VeMI	Epilepsy	50	31/19	31.60 (8.20)	medical tx	7.8 m	67.8 (20.0)	75.1 (18.9)		McSweeney, et al (1993)
WMS-R VeMI	Epilepsy	50	29/21	29.20 (7.60)	RTL	11.1 m	63.4 (16.7)	65.9 (15.8)		McSweeney, et al (1993)
WMS-R VeMI	Epilepsy	47	31/16	29.40 (7.60)	LTL	11.0 m	61.8 (14.3)	51.3 (16.4)		McSweeney, et al (1993)
WMS-R VeMI	Epilepsy	30	18/12	28.70 (7.34)	LTL	11.1 m	90.83 (12.75)	81.87 (12.16)		Naugle, et al (1993)
WMS-R VeMI	Epilepsy	30	16/14	30.60 (8.08)	RTL	10.1 m	94.1 (14.47)	94.5 (16.01)		Naugle, et al (1993)
WMS-R VeMI	Epilepsy	50	31/19	31.60 (8.16)	n/a	7.82 m	95.66 (18.)	102.7 (18.11)		Naugle, et al (1993)
WMS-R VeMI	Homeless	15	9/6	32.80 (6.10)	cognitive remediation	2-3 m	87.07 (12.13)	90.40 (7.80)		Cotman, et al (1997)

instrument	group	n	m/f	age	intervention	inter	t #1	t #2	note	citation
WMS-R VeMI	Homeless	9	4/5	27.00 (5.80)	n/a	2-3 m	96.33 (13.60)	93.78 (19.04)		Cotman, et al (1997)
WMS-R ViMI	Alcohol Dependent	50	45/5	39.30 (10.00)	n/a	19.6 w	88.7 (14.3)	94.3 (15.6)		Bowden, et al (1995)
WMS-R ViMI	Control	50	n/a	70.00 - 74.00	n/a	4-6 w	38.5 (10.3)	43.8 (10.1)		Wechsler (1987)
WMS-R ViMI	Control	53	n/a	55.00 - 64.00	n/a	4-6 w	46.2 (7.7)	51.7 (7.2)		Wechsler (1987)
WMS-R ViMI	Control	48	n/a	20.00 - 24.00	n/a	4-6 w	55.9 (7.0)	58.9 (6.0)		Wechsler (1987)
WMS-R ViMI	Epilepsy	49	29/20	29.45 (7.28)	RTL	10.7 m	94.6 (18.6)	95.3 (18.11)		Chelune, et al (1993)
WMS-R ViMI	Epilepsy	47	31/16	29.40 (7.56)	LTL	11.0 m	93.4 (15.2)	95.2 (13.8)		Chelune, et al (1993)
WMS-R ViMI	Epilepsy	40	24/16	32.45 (8.04)	n/a	7.1 m	92.4 (16.3)	94.6 (19.0)		Chelune, et al (1993)
WMS-R ViMI	Epilepsy	20	12/8	29.90 (10.10)	RTL	3.8 m	93.0	96.1		Ivnik, et al (1993)
WMS-R ViMI	Epilepsy	20	8/12	34.60 (9.80)	LTL	4.1 m	91.1	93.6		Ivnik, et al (1993)
WMS-R ViMI	Epilepsy	47	31/16	29.40 (7.60)	LTL	11.0 m	51.7 (8.1)	52.7 (7.4)		McSweeney, et al (1993)
WMS-R ViMI	Epilepsy	50	29/21	29.20 (7.60)	RTL	11.1 m	52.3 (9.2)	52.8 (11.2)		McSweeney, et al (1993)

instrument	group	n	m/f	age	intervention	inter	t #1	t #2	note	citation
WMS-R ViMI	Epilepsy	50	31/19	31.60 (8.20)	medical tx	7.8 m	51.6 (8.5)	52.4 (9.1)		McSweeney, et al (1993)
WMS-R ViMI	Epilepsy	30	18/12	28.70 (7.34)	LTL	11.1 m	94.53 (14.41)	95.37 (14.66)		Naugle, et al (1993)
WMS-R ViMI	Epilepsy	50	31/19	31.60 (8.16)	n/a	7.82 m	94.04 (16.5)	96.44 (18.53)		Naugle, et al (1993)
WMS-R ViMI	Epilepsy	30	16/14	30.60 (8.08)	RTL	10.1 m	96.90 (18.48)	97.33 (18.97)		Naugle, et al (1993)
WMS-R ViMI	Homeless	15	9/6	32.80 (6.10)	cognitive remediation	2-3 m	100.60 (16.78)	103.53 (11.40)		Cotman, et al (1997)
WMS-R ViMI	Homeless	9	4/5	27.00 (5.80)	n/a	2-3 m	109.22 (19.95)	111.22 (13.59)		Cotman, et al (1997)
WMS-R Visual PA Delay	Control	48	n/a	20.00 - 24.00	n/a	4-6 w	5.7 (0.7)	5.9 (0.5)		Wechsler (1987)
WMS-R Visual PA Delay	Control	50	n/a	70.00 - 74.00	n/a	4-6 w	4.0 (1.9)	4.2 (1.8)		Wechsler (1987)
WMS-R Visual PA Delay	Control	53	n/a	55.00 - 64.00	n/a	4-6 w	4.6 (1.8)	5.2 (1.4)		Wechsler (1987)
WMS-R Visual PA Imm	Control	50	n/a	70.00 - 74.00	n/a	4-6 w	8.4 (4.3)	11.7 (4.3)		Wechsler (1987)
WMS-R Visual PA Imm	Control	53	n/a	55.00 - 64.00	n/a	4-6 w	11.2 (4.3)	14.7 (3.9)		Wechsler (1987)
WMS-R Visual PA Imm	Control	48	n/a	20.00 - 24.00	n/a	4-6 w	15.3 (2.9)	17.4 (1.1)		Wechsler (1987)

instrument	group	n	m/f	age	intervention	inter	t #1	t #2	note	citation
WMS-R Visual PA x	Schizophrenia	33	n/a	~33.70 (6.30)	clozapine	1 y	9.3 (4.2)	9.4 (5.3)		Buchanan, et al (1994)
WMS-R Visual PA x	Schizophrenia	19	15/4	34.00 (6.90)	haloperidol	10 w	9.9 (4.4)	10.1 (4.2)		Buchanan, et al (1994)
WMS-R Visual PA x	Schizophrenia	19	13/6	33.70 (6.30)	clozapine	10 w	9.7 (4.2)	11.0 (5.4)		Buchanan, et al (1994)
WMS-R VR Delay	Control	64	21/43	28.80 (9.10)	n/a	2 w	34.53 (5.22)	36.62 (3.88)	*	Theisen, et al (1998)
WMS-R VR Delay	Control	50	n/a	70.00 - 74.00	n/a	4-6 w	16.5 (8.3)	18.2 (10.2)		Wechsler (1987)
WMS-R VR Delay	Control	53	n/a	55.00 - 64.00	n/a	4-6 w	25.2 (7.2)	26.1 (7.0)		Wechsler (1987)
WMS-R VR Delay	Control	48	n/a	20.00 - 24.00	n/a	4-6 w	30.7 (6.2)	32.8 (4.9)		Wechsler (1987)
WMS-R VR Delay	Schizophrenia (acute)	39	24/15	28.60 (8.60)	n/a	1 y	32.2 (8.6)	31.8 (10.9)		Sweeney, et al (1991)
WMS-R VR Delay (% ret)	Epilepsy	20	12/8	29.90 (10.10)	RTL	3.8 m	81.3	77.0		Ivnik, et al (1993)
WMS-R VR Delay (% ret)	Epilepsy	20	8/12	34.60 (9.80)	LTL	4.1 m	74.4	70.4		Ivnik, et al (1993)
WMS-R VR Imm	Control	64	21/43	28.80 (9.10)	n/a	2 w	36.71 (3.85)	37.38 (3.24)	*	Theisen, et al (1998)
WMS-R VR Imm	Control	48	n/a	20.00 - 24.00	n/a	4-6 w	33.4 (5.3)	34.1 (4.8)		Wechsler (1987)

instrument	group	n	m/f	age	intervention	inter	t #1	t #2	note	citation
WMS-R VR Imm	Control	50	n/a	70.00 - 74.00	n/a	4-6 w	24.2 (7.3)	25.6 (7.1)		Wechsler (1987)
WMS-R VR Imm	Control	53	n/a	55.00 - 64.00	n/a	4-6 w	28.8 (5.2)	30.8 (4.8)		Wechsler (1987)
WMS-R VR Imm	Schizophrenia (acute)	39	24/15	28.60 (8.60)	n/a	1 y	34.8 (6.8)	35.8 (5.9)		Sweeney, et al (1991)
WMS-R VR x	Schizophrenia	33	n/a	~33.70 (6.30)	clozapine	1 y	25.7 (8.2)	25.0 (8.17)		Buchanan, et al (1994)
WMS-R VR x	Schizophrenia	19	15/4	34.00 (6.90)	haloperidol	10 w	26.3 (7.6)	25.0 (8.8)		Buchanan, et al (1994)
WMS-R VR x	Schizophrenia	19	13/6	33.70 (6.30)	clozapine	10 w	26.5 (8.9)	25.8 (8.4)		Buchanan, et al (1994)

Table 72. Western Aphasia Battery (WAB)

instrument	group	n	m/f	age	intervention	inter	t #1	t #2	note	citation
WAB Comp	Aphasia (chronic)	38	n/a	61.00	n/a	12-23 m	NR	9.39 ac		Shewan, et al (1980)
WAB Construction	Aphasia (chronic)	38	n/a	61.00	n/a	12-23 m	NR	4.07 ac		Shewan, et al (1980)
WAB Fluency	Aphasia (chronic)	38	n/a	61.00	n/a	12-23 m	NR	6.32 ac		Shewan, et al (1980)
WAB Info Content	Aphasia (chronic)	38	n/a	61.00	n/a	12-23 m	NR	8.68 ac		Shewan, et al (1980)

instrument	group	n	m/f	age	intervention	inter	t #1	t #2	note	citation
WAB Naming	Aphasia (chronic)	38	n/a	61.00	n/a	12-23 m	NR	8.58 ac		Shewan, et al (1980)
WAB Praxis	Aphasia (chronic)	38	n/a	61.00	n/a	12-23 m	NR	7.72 ac		Shewan, et al (1980)
WAB Reading	Aphasia (chronic)	38	n/a	61.00	n/a	12-23 m	NR	9.66 ac		Shewan, et al (1980)
WAB Reading Comp	Control	20	6/14	69.40 (4.20)	n/a	1 y	39.6 (1.9)	39.6 (1.9)	*	Fromm, et al (1991)
WAB Reading Comp	DAT	18	5/13	71.00 (9.40)	n/a	1 y	34.3 (9.7)	32.7 (5.9)	*	Fromm, et al (1991)
WAB Repetition	Aphasia (chronic)	38	n/a	61.00	n/a	12-23 m	NR	4.71 ac		Shewan, et al (1980)
WAB Writing	Aphasia (chronic)	38	n/a	61.00	n/a	12-23 m	NR	7.24 ac		Shewan, et al (1980)

Table 73. Wide Range Achievement Tests (WRAT)

instrument	group	n	m/f	age	intervention	inter	t #1	t #2	note	citation
WRAT Arithmetic	ALL	31	16/15	8.38 (3.19)	n/a	2.0 y	91.6 (10.8)	91.8 (11.8)		Berg, et al (1983)
WRAT Arithmetic	ALL	13	9/4	3.63	n/a	1 y	97.3 (11.3)	96.0 (10.8)	*	Stehbens, et al (1984)
WRAT Arithmetic	ALL	7	3/4	2.69	n/a	1 y	102.7 (7.7)	99.0 (4.9)	*	Stehbens, et al (1984)

instrument	group	n	m/f	age	intervention	inter	t #1	t #2	note	citation
WRAT Arithmetic	ALL	6	6/0	4.73	n/a	1 y	91.0 (12.0)	92.5 (14.9)	*	Stehbens, et al (1984)
WRAT Arithmetic	ALL	16	n/a	5.00 - 16.00	n.a	1 y	97.0 (10.9)	96.1 (11.4)		Stehbens, et al (1983)
WRAT Arithmetic	ALL (dx <8)	43	21/22	6.13 (1.07)	n/a	1 y	95.28 (15.18)	95.27 (20.23)		Moehle, et al (1985)
WRAT Arithmetic	ALL (dx >8)	34	20/14	12.05 (2.94)	n/a	1 y	89.50 (16.35)	90.78 (17.69)		Moehle, et al (1985)
WRAT Arithmetic	ADHD	128	128/0	10.60 (3.00)	n/a	4 y	96.8 (17.4)	93.4 (18.3)		Biederman, et al (1996)
WRAT Arithmetic	ALL w/ Somnolence	48	27/21	8.63 (3.15)	n/a	2.25 y	97.0 (13.0)	91.8 (11.8)		Berg, et al (1983)
WRAT Arithmetic	Brain Tumor	7	4/3	9.83	radiotherapy	11 m	90.2 (12.8)	88.2 (13.2)		Bordeaux, et al (1988)
WRAT Arithmetic	Brain Tumor	7	3/4	10.33	surgery	1 m	100.6 (8.9)	99.6 (8.9)		Bordeaux, et al (1988)
WRAT Arithmetic	Brain Tumor (post-surgery)	16	n/a	6.00 - 15.00	radiation tx	6 m	98.4	94.2		Mulhern, et al (1985)
WRAT Arithmetic	Control	109	109/0	11.60 (3.70)	n/a	4 y	111.3 (16.1)	109.5 (15.7)		Biederman, et al (1996)
WRAT Arithmetic	Control (Native American)	115	60/55	6.83 (0.80)	n/a	1 y	103.2 (10.7)	100.6 (10.2)	1978 ver	Naglieri, et al (1980)
WRAT Arithmetic	Control (Native American)	115	60/55	6.83 (0.80)	n/a	1 y	101.9 (11.8)	98.6 (9.3)	1965 ver	Naglieri, et al (1980)

instrument	group	n	m/f	age	intervention	inter	t #1	t #2	note	citation
WRAT Arithmetic	Depression w/ Melancholia	7	5/2	9.50	tricyclic antidepress	3 - 6 m	87.6 (8.1)	95.1 (21.4)		Stanton, et al (1981)
WRAT Arithmetic	Depression w/o Melancholia	4	4/2	11.00	tricyclic antidepress	3 - 6 m	86.0 (24.2)	85.3 (19.3)		Stanton, et al (1981)
WRAT Arithmetic	EMR	89	n/a	n/a	n/a	n/a	73.17 (11.31)	71.69 (8.95)		Givens, et al (1984)
WRAT Arithmetic	EMR	28	n/a	n/a	normal at retest	n/a	80.19 (6.95)	82.22 (8.29)		Givens, et al (1984)
WRAT Arithmetic	EMR	60	n/a	n/a	LD at retest	n/a	77.89 (7.91)	74.16 (10.19)		Givens, et al (1984)
WRAT Arithmetic	Hyperactivity	20	19/1	7.90	placebo	~8 w	1.93	2.22		Conners, et al (1980)
WRAT Arithmetic	Hyperactivity	20	18/2	7.90	methylphen	~8 w	2.24	2.58		Conners, et al (1980)
WRAT Arithmetic	Hyperactivity	18	18/0	7.90	pemoline	~8 w	2.59	2.72		Conners, et al (1980)
WRAT Arithmetic	Hyperactivity	72	72/0	10.20 (1.70)	n/a	2 y	91.01 (19.70)	89.40 (17.13)		Riddle, et al (1976)
WRAT Arithmetic	LD	128	n/a	n/a	n/a	n/a	83.47 (11.10)	75.93 (8.34)		Givens, et al (1984)
WRAT Arithmetic	LD	26	n/a	n/a	normal at retest	n/a	94.76 (11.95)	88.10 (10.70)		Givens, et al (1984)
WRAT Arithmetic	LD	31	15/16	8.10 (1.60)	F/T LD program	3 y	87.6 (8.4)	85.5 (12.4)		Kaye, et al (1987)

instrument	group	n	m/f	age	intervention	inter	t #1	t #2	note	citation
WRAT Arithmetic	LD	68	67/1	8.80 (1.50)	P/T LD program	3 y	90.0 (9.9)	86.1 (8.0)		Kaye, et al (1987)
WRAT Arithmetic	Neuropsych referrals	248	203/ 45	8.00 (1.70)	n/a	2.65 y	84.0 (14.5)	80.6 (10.3)		Brown, et al (1989)
WRAT Arithmetic	Psychiatric Inpts	50	21/29	15.02	n/a	82.0 d	86.4 (13.5)	90.8 (14.2)		Dura, et al (1989)
WRAT Arithmetic	Solid Tumor	11	6/5	4.56	n/a	1 y	97.5 (11.3)	92.8 (5.7)	*	Stehbens, et al (1984)
WRAT Arithmetic	Solid Tumor	3	2/1	2.95	n/a	1 y	108.7 (10.1)	92.3 (1.5)	*	Stehbens, et al (1984)
WRAT Arithmetic	Solid Tumor	8	4/4	5.16	n/a	1 y	93.4 (9.0)	93.0 (6.8)	*	Stehbens, et al (1984)
WRAT Arithmetic	Solid Tumor	17	n/a	5.00 - 16.00	n/a	1 y	97.7 (13.2)	96.3 (13.0)		Stehbens, et al (1983)
WRAT Arithmetic (gr)	LD	32	23/9	10.67 (1.30)	placebo	8 w	3.51 (0.11)	3.75 (0.15)		Gittleman-Klein, et al (1976)
WRAT Arithmetic (gr)	LD	29	24/5	10.83 (1.40)	methylphen	8 w	4.11 (0.12)	3.89 (0.15)		Gittleman-Klein, et al (1976)
WRAT Arithmetic (gr)	LD	35	n/a	10.00	n/a	15 y	3.9 (1.4)	5.5 (1.6)		Sarazin, et al (1986)
WRAT Arithmetic (gr)	LD (brain damage)	67	n/a	10.00	n/a	15 y	3.0 (1.6)	5.1 (2.1)		Sarazin, et al (1986)
WRAT Arithmetic (gr)	LD (min brain dysfunction)	73	n/a	10.00	n/a	15 y	3.4 (1.2)	5.0 (1.4)		Sarazin, et al (1986)

instrument	group	n	m/f	age	intervention	inter	t #1	t #2	note	citation
WRAT Arithmetic (raw)	Special Education	63	50/13	10.60 (1.60)	n/a	2 w	26.36	26.71		Woodward, et al (1975)
WRAT Arithmetic (raw)	Special Education	43	35/8	10.60 (1.30)	n/a	22 w	26.07	25.79		Woodward, et al (1975)
WRAT Reading	ALL	31	16/15	8.38 (3.19)	n/a	2.0 y	96.9 (13.7)	96.7 (18.6)		Berg, et al (1983)
WRAT Reading	ALL	6	6/0	4.73	n/a	1 y	93.3 (16.0)	93.7 (15.7)	*	Stehbens, et al (1984)
WRAT Reading	ALL	7	3/4	2.69	n/a	1 y	103.1 (9.0)	97.0 (6.7)	*	Stehbens, et al (1984)
WRAT Reading	ALL	13	9/4	3.63	n/a	1 y	98.6 (13.3)	95.5 (11.3)	*	Stehbens, et al (1984)
WRAT Reading	ALL	16	n/a	5.00 - 16.00	n.a	1 y	101.1 (13.3)	96.6 (11.3)		Stehbens, et al (1983)
WRAT Reading	ALL (dx <8)	43	21/22	6.13 (1.07)	n/a	1 y	95.51 (19.07)	94.40 (20.16)		Moehle, et al (1985)
WRAT Reading	ALL (dx >8)	34	20/14	12.05 (2.94)	n/a	1 y	99.29 (24.28)	101.15 (16.50)		Moehle, et al (1985)
WRAT Reading	ADHD	128	128/0	10.60 (3.00)	n/a	4 y	93.1 (16.8)	102.0 (16.3)	GORT /std	Biederman, et al (1996)
WRAT Reading	ALL w/ Somnolence	48	27/21	8.63 (3.15)	n/a	2.25 y	102.6 (12.9)	101.4 (14.5)		Berg, et al (1983)

instrument	group	n	m/f	age	intervention	inter	t #1	t #2	note	citation
WRAT Reading	Brain Tumor (post-surgery)	16	n/a	6.00 - 15.00	radiation tx	6 m	105.8	106.7		Mulhern, et al (1985)
WRAT Reading	Control	109	109/0	11.60 (3.70)	n/a	4 y	100.6 (10.1)	111.8 (10.0)	GORT /std	Biederman, et al (1996)
WRAT Reading	Control (Native American)	115	60/55	6.83 (0.80)	n/a	1 y	109.1 (14.3)	109.3 (16.7)	1965 ver	Naglieri, et al (1980)
WRAT Reading	Control (Native American)	115	60/55	6.83 (0.80)	n/a	1 y	110.9 (13.5)	109.8 (15.2)	1978 ver	Naglieri, et al (1980)
WRAT Reading	Depression w/ Melancholia	7	5/2	9.50	tricyclic antidepress	3 - 6 m	104.7 (7.2)	109.6 (11.6)		Stanton, et al (1981)
WRAT Reading	Depression w/o Melancholia	4	4/2	11.00	tricyclic antidepress	3 - 6 m	88.8 (12.5)	95.0 (23.1)		Stanton, et al (1981)
WRAT Reading	EMR	60	n/a	n/a	LD at retest	n/a	75.63 (10.07)	70.86 (9.31)		Givens, et al (1984)
WRAT Reading	EMR	89	n/a	n/a	n/a	n/a	71.24 (10.71)	68.68 (7.89)		Givens, et al (1984)
WRAT Reading	EMR	28	n/a	n/a	normal at retest	n/a	81.93 (8.58)	82.56 (10.38)		Givens, et al (1984)
WRAT Reading	Hyperactivity	72	72/0	10.20 (1.70)	n/a	2 y	97.54 (15.11)	97.65 (9.22)		Riddle, et al (1976)
WRAT Reading	LD	128	n/a	n/a	n/a	n/a	77.40 (14.13)	77.79 (12.84)		Givens, et al (1984)
WRAT Reading	LD	26	n/a	n/a	normal at retest	n/a	88.62 (11.65)	90.00 (14.11)		Givens, et al (1984)

instrument	group	n	m/f	age	intervention	inter	t #1	t #2	note	citation
WRAT Reading	LD	68	67/1	8.80 (1.50)	P/T LD program	3 y	85.0 (11.1)	87.1 (10.9)		Kaye, et al (1987)
WRAT Reading	LD	31	15/16	8.10 (1.60)	F/T LD program	3 y	78.4 (8.9)	76.8 (9.1)		Kaye, et al (1987)
WRAT Reading	Neuropsych referrals	248	203/ 45	8.00 (1.70)	n/a	2.65 y	82.5 (17.2)	82.4 (14.2)		Brown, et al (1989)
WRAT Reading	Psychiatric Inpts	50	21/29	15.02	n/a	82.0 d	100.4 (15.1)	103.6 (14.3)		Dura, et al (1989)
WRAT Reading	Schizophrenia	15	10/5	35.00	std neuroleptics	~15 m	100.5 (8.9)	99.3 (9.3)		Goldberg, et al (1993)
WRAT Reading	Solid Tumor	11	6/5	4.56	n/a	1 y	105.4 (13.7)	100.3 (12.8)	*	Stehbens, et al (1984)
WRAT Reading	Solid Tumor	3	2/1	2.95	n/a	1 y	110.0 (13.5)	102.9 (13.9)	*	Stehbens, et al (1984)
WRAT Reading	Solid Tumor	8	4/4	5.16	n/a	1 y	103.6 (14.2)	99.6 (13.2)	*	Stehbens, et al (1984)
WRAT Reading	Solid Tumor	17	n/a	5.00 - 16.00	n/a	1 y	104.2 (13.1)	100.1 (12.2)		Stehbens, et al (1983)
WRAT Reading	Special Education	63	50/13	10.60 (1.60)	n/a	2 w	48.32	48.84		Woodward, et al (1975)
WRAT Reading	Special Education	43	35/8	10.60 (1.30)	n/a	22 w	43.67	46.12		Woodward, et al (1975)
WRAT Reading (gr)	Hyperactivity	20	18/2	7.90	methylphen	~8 w	2.33	2.66		Conners, et al (1980)

instrument	group	n	m/f	age	intervention	inter	t #1	t #2	note	citation
WRAT Reading (gr)	Hyperactivity	18	18/0	7.90	pemoline	~8 w	2.60	2.88		Conners, et al (1980)
WRAT Reading (gr)	Hyperactivity	20	19/1	7.90	placebo	~8 w	2.35	2.56		Conners, et al (1980)
WRAT Reading (gr)	LD	29	24/5	10.83 (1.40)	methylphen	8 w	2.87 (0.09)	2.94 (0.08)		Gittleman-Klein, et al (1976)
WRAT Reading (gr)	LD	32	23/9	10.67 (1.30)	placebo	8 w	2.72 (0.09)	2.76 (0.08)		Gittleman-Klein, et al (1976)
WRAT Reading (gr)	LD	35	n/a	10.00	n/a	15 y	4.2 (2.3)	8.0 (1.6)		Sarazin, et al (1986)
WRAT Reading (gr)	LD (brain damage)	67	n/a	10.00	n/a	15 y	3.6 (2.3)	7.3 (2.6)		Sarazin, et al (1986)
WRAT Reading (gr)	LD (min brain dysfunction)	73	n/a	10.00	n/a	15 y	4.1 (2.2)	7.4 (2.0)		Sarazin, et al (1986)
WRAT Spelling	ALL	31	16/15	8.38 (3.19)	n/a	2.0 y	92.8 (10.1)	88.4 (17.8)		Berg, et al (1983)
WRAT Spelling	ALL (dx <8)	43	21/22	6.13 (1.07)	n/a	1 y	94.09 (18.16)	92.53 (22.42)		Moehle, et al (1985)
WRAT Spelling	ALL (dx >8)	34	20/14	12.05 (2.94)	n/a	1 y	95.52 (20.76)	95.56 (16.00)		Moehle, et al (1985)
WRAT Spelling	ALL w/ Somnolence	48	27/21	8.63 (3.15)	n/a	2.25 y	97.5 (16.5)	96.4 (14.8)		Berg, et al (1983)
WRAT Spelling	Brain Tumor	7	4/3	9.83	radiotherapy	11 m	99.4 (22.5)	100.2 (15.4)		Bordeaux, et al (1988)

instrument	group	n	m/f	age	intervention	inter	t #1	t #2	note	citation
WRAT Spelling	Brain Tumor	7	3/4	10.33	surgery	1 m	96.4 (7.0)	104.6 (9.6)		Bordeaux, et al (1988)
WRAT Spelling	Brain Tumor (post-surgery)	16	n/a	6.00 - 15.00	radiation tx	6 m	103.6	105.4		Mulhern, et al (1985)
WRAT Spelling	Control (Native American)	115	60/55	6.83 (0.80)	n/a	1 y	104.8 (12.5)	104.8 (13.4)	1965 ver	Naglieri, et al (1980)
WRAT Spelling	Control (Native American)	115	60/55	6.83 (0.80)	n/a	1 y	108.4 (12.1)	107.5 (12.3)	1978 ver	Naglieri, et al (1980)
WRAT Spelling	Depression w/ Melancholia	7	5/2	9.50	tricyclic antidepress	3 - 6 m	100.3 (8.3)	106.1 (11.5)		Stanton, et al (1981)
WRAT Spelling	Depression w/o Melancholia	4	4/2	11.00	tricyclic antidepress	3 - 6 m	87.3 (16.7)	85.0 (29.3)		Stanton, et al (1981)
WRAT Spelling	LD	68	67/1	8.80 (1.50)	P/T LD program	3 y	82.9 (9.6)	81.3 (9.4)		Kaye, et al (1987)
WRAT Spelling	LD	31	15/16	8.10 (1.60)	F/T LD program	3 y	80.8 (10.7)	75.6 (7.9)		Kaye, et al (1987)
WRAT Spelling	Neuropsych referrals	248	203/ 45	8.00 (1.70)	n/a	2.65 y	82.6 (15.2)	78.8 (12.6)		Brown, et al (1989)
WRAT Spelling	Psychiatric Inpts	50	21/29	15.02	n/a	82.0 d	98.6 (13.5)	98.7 (14.8)		Dura, et al (1989)
WRAT Spelling	Special Education	63	50/13	10.60 (1.60)	n/a	2 w	31.30	32.16		Woodward, et al (1975)
WRAT Spelling	Special Education	43	35/8	10.60 (1.30)	n/a	22 w	29.37	29.65		Woodward, et al (1975)

instrument	group	n	m/f	age	intervention	inter	t #1	t #2	note	citation
WRAT Spelling (gr)	Hyperactivity	18	18/0	7.90	pemoline	~8 w	2.38	2.57		Conners, et al (1980)
WRAT Spelling (gr)	Hyperactivity	20	18/2	7.90	methylphen	~8 w	2.09	2.37		Conners, et al (1980)
WRAT Spelling (gr)	Hyperactivity	20	19/1	7.90	placebo	~8 w	2.07	2.14		Conners, et al (1980)
WRAT Spelling (gr)	LD	32	23/9	10.67 (1.30)	placebo	8 w	2.74 (0.10)	3.75 (0.15)		Gittleman-Klein, et al (1976)
WRAT Spelling (gr)	LD	29	24/5	10.83 (1.40)	methylphen	8 w	2.83 (0.10)	2.84 (0.09)		Gittleman-Klein, et al (1976)
WRAT Spelling (gr)	LD	35	n/a	10.00	n/a	15 y	4.0 (2.7)	6.2 (2.2)		Sarazin, et al (1986)
WRAT Spelling (gr)	LD (brain damage)	67	n/a	10.00	n/a	15 y	3.3 (2.2)	6.1 (2.9)		Sarazin, et al (1986)
WRAT Spelling (gr)	LD (min brain dysfunction)	73	n/a	10.00	n/a	15 y	3.4 (1.5)	5.6 (2.2)		Sarazin, et al (1986)
WRAT-3 Arithmetic	Control	142	n/a	10.50 (4.00)	n/a	37.4 d	101.4 (14.7)	102.2 (14.0)		Wilkinson (1993)
WRAT-3 Arithmetic (Blue)	Control	142	n/a	10.50 (4.00)	n/a	37.4 d	99.9 (15.3)	101.7 (14.7)		Wilkinson (1993)
WRAT-3 Arithmetic (Tan)	Control	142	n/a	10.50 (4.00)	n/a	37.4 d	101.1 (14.8)	100.8 (13.8)		Wilkinson (1993)

instrument	group	n	m/f	age	intervention	inter	t #1	t #2	note	citation
WRAT-3 Reading	Control	142	n/a	10.50 (4.00)	n/a	37.4 d	101.9 (14.1)	102.9 (14.2)		Wilkinson (1993)
WRAT-3 Reading (Blue)	Control	142	n/a	10.50 (4.00)	n/a	37.4 d	101.6 (14.2)	102.8 (14.0)		Wilkinson (1993)
WRAT-3 Reading (Tan)	Control	142	n/a	10.50 (4.00)	n/a	37.4 d	101.0 (14.3)	101.9 (14.6)		Wilkinson (1993)
WRAT-3 Spelling	Control	142	n/a	10.50 (4.00)	n/a	37.4 d	101.6 (12.5)	102.7 (12.3)		Wilkinson (1993)
WRAT-3 Spelling (Blue)	Control	142	n/a	10.50 (4.00)	n/a	37.4 d	101.1 (13.0)	102.2 (12.3)		Wilkinson (1993)
WRAT-3 Spelling (Tan)	Control	142	n/a	10.50 (4.00)	n/a	37.4 d	101.3 (12.5)	102.7 (12.9)		Wilkinson (1993)
WRAT-R Arithmetic	BMT	25	14/11	~12.0	BMT	8.2 m	95.1 (17.2)	96.5 (17.7)		Phipps, et al (1995)
WRAT-R Arithmetic	Emotionally Disturbed	120	120/0	14.50	residential tx	1 y	85.46	88.72		Lorandos (1990)
WRAT-R Arithmetic	Epilepsy	40	23/17	32.20 (8.20)	n/a	~9 m	89.70 (16.70)	91.10 (17.60)		Hermann, et al (1996)
WRAT-R Reading	BMT	25	14/11	~12.0	BMT	8.2 m	95.4 (18.7)	96.0 (20.7)		Phipps, et al (1995)
WRAT-R Reading	BMT	25	14/11	~12.0	BMT	8.2 m	96.5 (20.4)	95.5 (18.9)		Phipps, et al (1995)
WRAT-R Reading	Emotionally Disturbed	120	120/0	14.50	residential tx	1 y	89.43	87.76		Lorandos (1990)

instrument	group	n	m/f	age	intervention	inter	t #1	t #2	note	citation
WRAT-R Reading	Epilepsy	40	23/17	32.20 (8.20)	n/a	~9 m	89.60 (19.00)	91.10 (19.60)		Hermann, et al (1996)
WRAT-R Reading	Epilepsy	40	23/17	32.20 (8.20)	n/a	~9 m	83.20 (17.50)	84.90 (17.50)		Hermann, et al (1996)
WRAT-R Reading	Epilepsy	28	13/15	30.40 (11.8)	RTL	12.8 m	88.6 (12.9)	90.5 (14.0)		McGlone (1994)
WRAT-R Reading	Epilepsy	19	10/9	32.60 (9.80)	LTL	12.9 m	86.2 (15.0)	82.7 (13.3)		McGlone (1994)
WRAT-R Reading	Neurological (declining)	13	5/8	43.92	n/a	~28.3 m	87.38 (13.79)	88.53 (15.65)		Johnstone, et al (1996)
WRAT-R Reading	Neurological (improving)	11	7/4	37.18	n/a	~28.3 m	90.36 (12.80)	99.82 (12.94)		Johnstone, et al (1996)
WRAT-R Reading	Neurological (stable)	15	11/4	45.67	n/a	~28.3 m	89.60 (17.30)	91.67 (17.63)		Johnstone, et al (1996)
WRAT-R Reading	Schizophrenia	11	11/0	52.50 (11.5)	neuroleptic reduction	29.3 w	101.8 (17.4)	103.3 (17.5)		Seidman, et al (1993)

Table 74. Wisconsin Card Sorting Test (WCST)

instrument	group	n	m/f	age	intervention	inter	t #1	t #2	note	citation
WCST (t)	Lung Cancer	11	n/a	~61.0	cranial irradiation	11 m	37.2	36.8		Komaki, et al (1995)
WCST Categories	AIDS Dementia Complex	30	29/1	33.80	zdv	6 m	5.83 (1.6)	8.33 (1.36)		Tozzi, et al (1993)

instrument	group	n	m/f	age	intervention	inter	t #1	t #2	note	citation
WCST Categories	Alcoholic Inpts	91	91/0	42.20 (10.0)	n/a	12-22 d	4.3 (2.2)	4.5 (2.2)		Eckardt, et al (1979)
WCST Categories	Autism	10	n/a	11.90 (2.70)	n/a	1.2 y	4.7 (1.6)	5.4 (1.3)	comp/ std	Ozonoff (1995)
WCST Categories	Control	20	9/11	28.15	n/a	8.41 m	5.05 (1.36)	5.25 (1.62)		Tate, et al (1998)
WCST Categories	Control	37	n/a	20.60 (5.00)	n/a	5 min	5.6 (1.2)	5.7 (0.8)	alt/std	Bowden, et al (1998)
WCST Categories	Control	38	n/a	20.60 (5.00)	n/a	5 min	5.1 (1.5)	5.5 (0.9)	std/alt	Bowden, et al (1998)
WCST Categories	Control	4	0/4	67.30 (0.50)	placebo	60 min	3.00 (0.82)	3.50 (1.73)	AF	Kirkby, et al (1995)
WCST Categories	Control	5	1/4	68.40 (6.10)	lorazepam	60 min	4.00 (1.23)	2.20 (0.45)	AF	Kirkby, et al (1995)
WCST Categories	Control	8	4/4	21.80 (4.20)	placebo	60 min	3.13 (1.13)	3.75 (1.58)	AF	Kirkby, et al (1995)
WCST Categories	Control	9	4/5	26.40 (7.70)	lorazepam	60 min	3.56 (1.67)	4.33 (1.12)	AF	Kirkby, et al (1995)
WCST Categories	Control	20	10/10	34.00 (12.4)	n/a	4 w	5.1 (1.6)	5.2 (1.8)		McGrath, et al (1997)
WCST Categories	Control	11	n/a	11.90 (1.30)	n/a	1.1 y	4.4 (2.1)	5.5 (1.2)	comp/ std	Ozonoff (1995)
WCST Categories	Control	216	106/ 110	7.91 (0.47)	n/a	2-3 y	2.92 (1.81)	4.17 (2.28)		Rebok, et al (1997)
WCST Categories	Control	18	12/6	37.20 (9.70)	n/a	76.5 d	5.0 (1.49)	5.76 (0.59)		Verdoux, et al (1995)

instrument	group	n	m/f	age	intervention	inter	t #1	t #2	note	citation
WCST Categories	Depression	33	14/19	37.40	antidepress	7 w	5.9 (1.8)	5.3 (1.5)		Fromm, et al (1984)
WCST Categories	Epilepsy	40	23/17	32.20 (8.20)	n/a	~9 m	4.63 (1.76)	4.65 (1.82)		Hermann, et al (1996)
WCST Categories	Mania	16	1/15	40.60 (12.8)	std tx	4 w	2.8 (2.5)	5.1 (1.5)		McGrath, et al (1997)
WCST Categories	Medical Inpts	20	20/0	45.60 (11.1)	n/a	12-22 d	3.2 (2.7)	4.2 (2.7)		Eckardt, et al (1979)
WCST Categories	MS	11	n/a	~38.0	total lymphoid irradiation	12 m	4.3 (2.1)	3.8 (2.5)	*	Wiles, et al (1994)
WCST Categories	MS	5	n/a	~39.0	placebo	12 m	4.6 (1.9)	6.0 (0.0)	*	Wiles, et al (1994)
WCST Categories	PD	20	11/9	63.30 (7.40)	levodopa	1 h	4.95 (1.5)	4.7 (1.7)	*	Kulisevsky, et al (1996)
WCST Categories	PD	19	13/6	54.30	pergolide	~6 w	4.5 (1.58)	5.4 (0.99)		Stern, et al (1984)
WCST Categories	Schizophrenia	38	25/13	30.90 (8.73)	n/a	6 m	2.95 (2.22)	3.74 (2.33)		Addington, et al (1991)
WCST Categories	Schizophrenia	15	10/5	35.00	std neuroleptics	~15 m	2.4 (1.2)	2.1 (1.8)		Goldberg, et al (1993)
WCST Categories	Schizophrenia	36	28/8	35.50 (9.80)	clozapine	6 w	3.0 (2.4)	2.9 (2.5)	*	Hagger, et al (1993)
WCST Categories	Schizophrenia	31	21/10	31.50 (8.90)	std tx	4 w	3.6 (2.3)	3.6 (2.4)		McGrath, et al (1997)
WCST Categories	Schizophrenia	12	10/2	28.70 (6.50)	n/a	3 y	3.3 (2.2)	2.6 (2.6)		Seidman, et al (1991)

instrument	group	n	m/f	age	intervention	inter	t #1	t #2	note	citation
WCST Categories	Schizophrenia	10	10/0	52.00 (11.9)	neuroleptic reduction	6 m	2.4 (2.8)	2.0 (2.4)		Seidman, et al (1991)
WCST Categories	Schizophrenia	11	11/0	52.50 (11.5)	neuroleptic reduction	29.3 w	2.4 (2.8)	2.0 (2.4)		Seidman, et al (1993)
WCST Categories	Schizophrenia	18	12/6	37.90 (10.8)	n/a	84.3 d	3.93 (2.13)	4.61 (1.6)		Verdoux, et al (1995)
WCST Categories	Schizophrenia (acute)	39	24/15	28.60 (8.60)	n/a	1 y	4.6 (1.7)	5.5 (1.2)		Sweeney, et al (1991)
WCST Categories	TBI (sev)	23	18/5	26.0 (8.94)	n/a	10.09 m	4.00 (1.54)	5.13 (1.79)		Tate, et al (1998)
WCST Categories	TBI	57	33/24	10.01	n/a	33.01 m	3.47	5.03		Levin, et al (1997)
WCST Concept Responses (%)	Control	20	9/11	28.15	n/a	8.41 m	69.6 (17.69)	73.01 (22.18)		Tate, et al (1998)
WCST Concept Responses (%)	TBI (sev)	23	18/5	26.0 (8.94)	n/a	10.09 m	51.74 (20.18)	66.89 (22.29)		Tate, et al (1998)
WCST Concept Responses (%)	TBI	57	33/24	10.01	n/a	33.01 m	50.32	65.48		Levin, et al (1997)
WCST Correct	Control	38	n/a	20.60 (5.00)	n/a	5 min	72.9 (9.9)	69.7 (7.7)	std/alt	Bowden, et al (1998)
WCST Correct	Control	37	n/a	20.60 (5.00)	n/a	5 min	71.1 (10.8)	67.0 (5.1)	alt/std	Bowden, et al (1998)

instrument	group	n	m/f	age	intervention	inter	t #1	t #2	note	citation
WCST Correct	Control	4	0/4	67.30 (0.50)	placebo	60 min	46.3 (8.30)	48.0 (11.4)	AF	Kirkby, et al (1995)
WCST Correct	Control	5	1/4	68.40 (6.10)	lorazepam	60 min	49.0 (7.52)	42.4 (5.77)	AF	Kirkby, et al (1995)
WCST Correct	Control	9	4/5	26.40 (7.70)	lorazepam	60 min	48.0 (4.33)	51.0 (9.27)	AF	Kirkby, et al (1995)
WCST Correct	Control	8	4/4	21.80 (4.20)	placebo	60 min	45.9 (6.45)	50.9 (4.82)	AF	Kirkby, et al (1995)
WCST Correct	Control	216	106/ 110	7.91 (0.47)	n/a	2-3 y	59.71 (17.66)	74.71 (19.63)		Rebok, et al (1997)
WCST Errors	Autism	10	n/a	11.90 (2.70)	n/a	1.2 y	37.4 (24.6)	23.0 (15.2)	comp/ std	Ozonoff (1995)
WCST Errors	Control	20	9/11	28.15	n/a	8.41 m	28.2 (20.2)	24.25 (22.91)		Tate, et al (1998)
WCST Errors	Control	38	n/a	20.60 (5.00)	n/a	5 min	30.9 (19.9)	27.0 (13.0)	std/alt	Bowden, et al (1998)
WCST Errors	Control	37	n/a	20.60 (5.00)	n/a	5 min	27.2 (18.5)	22.0 (11.0)	alt/std	Bowden, et al (1998)
WCST Errors	Control	4	0/4	67.30 (0.50)	placebo	60 min	17.8 (8.30)	16.0 (11.4)	AF	Kirkby, et al (1995)
WCST Errors	Control	5	1/4	68.40 (6.10)	lorazepam	60 min	15.0 (7.52)	21.4 (5.81)	AF	Kirkby, et al (1995)
WCST Errors	Control	8	4/4	21.80 (4.20)	placebo	60 min	18.1 (6.45)	11.9 (5.25)	AF	Kirkby, et al (1995)

instrument	group	n	m/f	age	intervention	inter	t #1	t #2	note	citation
WCST Errors	Control	9	4/5	26.40 (7.70)	lorazepam	60 min	16.0 (4.33)	13.0 (9.27)	AF	Kirkby, et al (1995)
WCST Errors	Control	11	n/a	11.90 (1.30)	n/a	1.1 y	47.6 (25.4)	23.5 (16.7)	comp/ std	Ozonoff (1995)
WCST Errors	Control	18	12/6	37.20 (9.70)	n/a	76.5 d	26.36 (19.56)	15.77 (14.06)		Verdoux, et al (1995)
WCST Errors	Depression	33	14/19	37.40	antidepress	7 w	29.8 (24.7)	20.1 (23.2)		Fromm, et al (1984)
WCST Errors	HIV+ (stage 2/3)	14	14/0	31.40 (8.54)	n/a	12.8 m	6.9 (6.9)	4.7 (3.9)		Burgess, et al (1994)
WCST Errors	HIV+ (stage 4)	6	6/0	36.20 (7.60)	n/a	12.8 m	15.8 (12.9)	8.6 (10.2)		Burgess, et al (1994)
WCST Errors	HIV-	41	41/0	31.50 (9.32)	n/a	12.8 m	7.0 (6.4)	4.7 (3.7)		Burgess, et al (1994)
WCST Errors	MS	5	n/a	~39.00	placebo	12 m	9.4 (4.8)	6.8 (8.5)	*	Wiles, et al (1994)
WCST Errors	MS	11	n/a	~38.00	total lymphoid irradiation	12 m	9.6 (8.7)	11.2 (9.3)	*	Wiles, et al (1994)
WCST Errors	PD	19	13/6	54.30	pergolide	~6 w	34.9 (15.72)	21.2 (15.93)		Stern, et al (1984)
WCST Errors	Schizophrenia	38	25/13	30.90 (8.73)	n/a	6 m	59.51 (24.31)	46.27 (27.64)		Addington, et al (1991)
WCST Errors	Schizophrenia	18	12/6	37.90 (10.8)	n/a	84.3 d	45.86 (27.31)	36.61 (25.07)		Verdoux, et al (1995)

instrument	group	n	m/f	age	intervention	inter	t #1	t #2	note	citation
WCST Errors	TBI (sev)	23	18/5	26.0 (8.94)	n/a	10.09 m	45.91 (21.78)	29.3 (23.74)		Tate, et al (1998)
WCST Failure to Maintain Set	Control	20	9/11	28.15	n/a	8.41 m	1.35 (1.53)	1.05 (1.28)		Tate, et al (1998)
WCST Failure to Maintain Set	Control	216	106/ 110	7.91 (0.47)	n/a	2-3 y	0.99 (1.09)	1.81 (5.14)		Rebok, et al (1997)
WCST Failure to Maintain Set	TBI (sev)	23	18/5	26.0 (8.94)	n/a	10.09 m	0.96 (1.22)	0.61 (0.78)		Tate, et al (1998)
WCST NPE	Control	20	9/11	28.15	n/a	8.41 m	14.1 (13.25)	13.3 (16.61)		Tate, et al (1998)
WCST NPE	Control	37	n/a	20.60 (5.00)	n/a	5 min	12.7 (6.9)	8.3 (9.6)	alt/std	Bowden, et al (1998)
WCST NPE	Control	38	n/a	20.60 (5.00)	n/a	5 min	15.0 (11.0)	10.6 (8.3)	std/alt	Bowden, et al (1998)
WCST NPE	Control	5	1/4	68.40 (6.10)	lorazepam	60 min	3.00 (2.35)	12.00 (7.91)	AF	Kirkby, et al (1995)
WCST NPE	Control	9	4/5	26.40 (7.70)	lorazepam	60 min	5.00 (1.32)	4.11 (6.99)	AF	Kirkby, et al (1995)
WCST NPE	Control	4	0/4	67.30 (0.50)	placebo	60 min	5.75 (3.40)	5.25 (4.50)	AF	Kirkby, et al (1995)
WCST NPE	Control	8	4/4	21.80 (4.20)	placebo	60 min	5.75 (2.38)	3.88 (2.64)	AF	Kirkby, et al (1995)
WCST NPE	TBI (sev)	23	18/5	26.0 (8.94)	n/a	10.09 m	15.39 (8.16)	13.22 (11.38)		Tate, et al (1998)

instrument	group	n	m/f	age	intervention	inter	t #1	t #2	note	citation
WCST PE	AIDS Dementia Complex	30	29/1	33.80	zdv	6 m	31.2 (25.2)	20.0 (23.5)		Tozzi, et al (1993)
WCST PE	Control	20	9/11	28.15	n/a	8.41 m	14.1 (10.84)	10.95 (8.42)		Tate, et al (1998)
WCST PE	Control	37	n/a	20.60 (5.00)	n/a	5 min	14.5 (13.8)	7.7 (6.8)	alt/std	Bowden, et al (1998)
WCST PE	Control	38	n/a	20.60 (5.00)	n/a	5 min	15.9 (10.4)	7.4 (5.4)	std/alt	Bowden, et al (1998)
WCST PE	Control	9	4/5	26.40 (7.70)	lorazepam	60 min	11.0 (5.00)	5.33 (2.55)	AF	Kirkby, et al (1995)
WCST PE	Control	8	4/4	21.80 (4.20)	placebo	60 min	12.4 (6.39)	8.00 (3.21)	AF	Kirkby, et al (1995)
WCST PE	Control	5	1/4	68.40 (6.10)	lorazepam	60 min	12.0 (7.38)	9.60 (3.78)	AF	Kirkby, et al (1995)
WCST PE	Control	4	0/4	67.30 (0.50)	placebo	60 min	12.0 (6.88)	11.00 (7.44)	AF	Kirkby, et al (1995)
WCST PE	Control	20	10/10	34.00 (12.4)	n/a	4 w	17.7 (12.1)	11.4 (11.1)		McGrath, et al (1997)
WCST PE	Control	216	106/ 110	7.91 (0.47)	n/a	2-3 y	35.46 (19.99)	31.88 (21.23)		Rebok, et al (1997)
WCST PE	Mania	16	1/15	40.60 (12.8)	std tx	4 w	41.4 (32.4)	22.4 (16.4)		McGrath, et al (1997)
WCST PE	PD	20	11/9	63.30 (7.40)	levodopa	1 h	8.6 (5.7)	9.05 (6.7)	*	Kulisevsky, et al (1996)

instrument	group	n	m/f	age	intervention	inter	t #1	t #2	note	citation
WCST PE	Schizophrenia	31	21/10	31.50 (8.90)	std tx	4 w	30.3 (21.8)	26.2 (23.6)		McGrath, et al (1997)
WCST PE	Schizophrenia (acute)	39	24/15	28.60 (8.60)	n/a	1 y	21.1 (10.4)	15.5 (8.9)		Sweeney, et al (1991)
WCST PE	TBI (sev)	23	18/5	26.0 (8.94)	n/a	10.09 m	30.52 (20.02)	16.04 (13.4)		Tate, et al (1998)
WCST PE (%)	Schizophrenia	19	13/6	33.70 (6.30)	clozapine	10 w	31.6 (20.9)	27.1 (19.0)		Buchanan, et al (1994)
WCST PE (%)	Schizophrenia	33	n/a	~33.7 (6.30)	clozapine	1 y	29.7 (20.6)	31.5 (18.6)		Buchanan, et al (1994)
WCST PE (%)	Schizophrenia	19	15/4	34.00 (6.90)	haloperidol	10 w	25.1 (15.8)	27.5 (18.2)		Buchanan, et al (1994)
WCST PE (%)	Schizophrenia	15	10/5	35.00	std neuroleptics	~15 m	19.6 (10.5)	20.1 (16.0)		Goldberg, et al (1993)
WCST PE (%)	Schizophrenia	36	28/8	35.50 (9.80)	clozapine	6 w	17.1 (12.7)	18.6 (13.8)	*	Hagger, et al (1993)
WCST PE (%)	TBI	57	33/24	10.01	n/a	33.01 m	19.66	12.70		Levin, et al (1997)
WCST PR	Autism	10	n/a	11.90 (2.70)	n/a	1.2 y	21.4 (17.5)	11.9 (9.1)	comp/ std	Ozonoff (1995)
WCST PR	Control	20	9/11	28.15	n/a	8.41 m	15.55 (12.21)	11.9 (10.03)		Tate, et al (1998)
WCST PR	Control	38	n/a	20.60 (5.00)	n/a	5 min	17.8 (11.7)	12.7 (8.8)	std/alt	Bowden, et al (1998)
WCST PR	Control	37	n/a	20.60 (5.00)	n/a	5 min	17.2 (17.7)	10.9 (8.4)	alt/std	Bowden, et al (1998)

Practitioner's Guide to Evaluating Change with Neuropsychological Assessment Instruments

instrument	group	n	m/f	age	intervention	inter	t #1	t #2	note	citation
WCST PR	Control	9	4/5	26.40 (7.70)	lorazepam	60 min	23.9 (6.39)	18.6 (9.54)	AF	Kirkby, et al (1995)
WCST PR	Control	8	4/4	21.80 (4.20)	placebo	60 min	25.5 (5.40)	20.9 (4.36)	AF	Kirkby, et al (1995)
WCST PR	Control	5	1/4	68.40 (6.10)	lorazepam	60 min	23.4 (9.37)	20.8 (6.94)	AF	Kirkby, et al (1995)
WCST PR	Control	4	0/4	67.30 (0.50)	placebo	60 min	25.8 (4.27)	24.3 (7.50)	AF	Kirkby, et al (1995)
WCST PR	Control	11	n/a	11.90 (1.30)	n/a	1.1 y	22.6 (15.3)	13.2 (9.4)	comp/ std	Ozonoff (1995)
WCST PR	Control	18	12/6	37.20 (9.70)	n/a	76.5 d	17.14 (15.1)	8.46 (9.34)		Verdoux, et al (1995)
WCST PR	Epilepsy	40	23/17	32.20 (8.20)	n/a	~9 m	14.30 (13.60)	12.90 (13.80)		Hermann, et al (1996)
WCST PR	Schizophrenia	38	25/13	30.90 (8.73)	n/a	6 m	28.51 (19.54)	22.81 (18.75)		Addington, et al (1991)
WCST PR	Schizophrenia	10	10/0	52.00 (11.9)	neuroleptic reduction	6 m	59.4 (49.9)	48.7 (45.5)		Seidman, et al (1991)
WCST PR	Schizophrenia	12	10/2	28.70 (6.50)	n/a	3 y	27.8 (23.4)	31.1 (19.5)		Seidman, et al (1991)
WCST PR	Schizophrenia	11	11/0	52.50 (11.5)	neuroleptic reduction	29.3 w	59.2 (50.1)	48.7 (45.5)		Seidman, et al (1993)
WCST PR	Schizophrenia	18	12/6	37.90 (10.8)	n/a	84.3 d	33.64 (29.01)	26.77 (25.73)		Verdoux, et al (1995)
WCST PR	TBI (sev)	23	18/5	26.0 (8.94)	n/a	10.09 m	37.35 (26.39)	18.04 (16.19)		Tate, et al (1998)

instrument	group	n	m/f	age	intervention	inter	t #1	t #2	note	citation
WCST Trials	Control	20	9/11	28.15	n/a	8.41 m	101.45 (23.47)	96.4 (22.37)		Tate, et al (1998)
WCST Trials	TBI (sev)	23	18/5	26.0 (8.94)	n/a	10.09 m	117.0 (19.76)	97.7 (20.61)		Tate, et al (1998)
WCST Trials to 1st Category	Schizophrenia	10	10/0	52.00 (11.9)	neuroleptic reduction	6 m	78.9 (56.1)	59.2 (60.1)		Seidman, et al (1991)
WCST Trials to 1st Category	Schizophrenia	12	10/2	28.70 (6.50)	n/a	3 y	34.3 (42.4)	57.3 (54.3)		Seidman, et al (1991)

Table 75. Woodcock Johnson-Revised (WJ-R)

instrument	group	n	m/f	age	intervention	inter	t #1	t #2	note	citation
WJ-R Broad Written Cluster	Control	20	10/10	~10.0	n/a	12-14 d	106.3 (12.8)	110.4 (13.0)		Shull-Senn, et al (1995)
WJ-R Applied Problems	Control	20	10/10	~10.0	n/a	12-14 d	106.3 (9.1)	107.1 (7.6)		Shull-Senn, et al (1995)
WJ-R Applied Problems	Control	20	10/10	~8.0	n/a	12-14 d	106.1 (14.6)	106.7 (15.2)		Shull-Senn, et al (1995)
WJ-R Applied Problems	Control	20	10/10	~6.0	n/a	12-14 d	100.2 (14.2)	101.7 (15.0)		Shull-Senn, et al (1995)
WJ-R Broad Math Cluster	Control	20	10/10	~10.0	n/a	12-14 d	110.0 (13.5)	113.5 (13.9)		Shull-Senn, et al (1995)
WJ-R Broad Math Cluster	Control	20	10/10	~8.0	n/a	12-14 d	112.4 (16.4)	114.9 (16.0)		Shull-Senn, et al (1995)
WJ-R Broad Math Cluster	Control	20	10/10	~6.0	n/a	12-14 d	97.7 (15.1)	101.4 (18.2)		Shull-Senn, et al (1995)

instrument	group	n	m/f	age	intervention	inter	t #1	t #2	note	citation
WJ-R Broad Reading Cluster	Control	20	10/10	~10.0	n/a	12-14 d	103.9 (13.4)	108.4 (16.5)		Shull-Senn, et al (1995)
WJ-R Broad Reading Cluster	Control	20	10/10	~8.0	n/a	12-14 d	106.5 (14.2)	107.5 (16.2)		Shull-Senn, et al (1995)
WJ-R Broad Reading Cluster	Control	20	10/10	~6.0	n/a	12-14 d	93.9 (19.6)	98.9 (19.6)		Shull-Senn, et al (1995)
WJ-R Broad Written Cluster	Control	20	10/10	~6.0	n/a	12-14 d	101.0 (6.7)	101.8 (8.5)		Shull-Senn, et al (1995)
WJ-R Broad Written Cluster	Control	20	10/10	~8.0	n/a	12-14 d	109.5 (12.8)	112.1 (15.4)		Shull-Senn, et al (1995)
WJ-R Calculation	Control	20	10/10	~10.0	n/a	12-14 d	111.7 (16.2)	114.5 (17.3)		Shull-Senn, et al (1995)
WJ-R Calculation	Control	20	10/10	~6.0	n/a	12-14 d	94.0 (14.2)	100.3 (18.5)		Shull-Senn, et al (1995)
WJ-R Calculation	Control	20	10/10	~8.0	n/a	12-14 d	113.8 (16.9)	117.6 (14.3)		Shull-Senn, et al (1995)
WJ-R Dictation	Control	20	10/10	~10.0	n/a	12-14 d	105.5 (11.6)	107.9 (11.8)		Shull-Senn, et al (1995)
WJ-R Dictation	Control	20	10/10	~8.0	n/a	12-14 d	110.3 (14.6)	113.2 (18.6)		Shull-Senn, et al (1995)
WJ-R Dictation	Control	20	10/10	~6.0	n/a	12-14 d	101.2 (7.94)	104.0 (12.1)		Shull-Senn, et al (1995)

instrument	group	n	m/f	age	intervention	inter	t #1	t #2	note	citation
WJ-R Letter-Word Identification	Control	20	10/10	~6.0	n/a	12-14 d	97.9 (16.5)	99.8 (17.7)		Shull-Senn, et al (1995)
WJ-R Letter-Word Identification	Control	20	10/10	~10.0	n/a	12-14 d	101.4 (13.5)	106.8 (15.8)		Shull-Senn, et al (1995)
WJ-R Letter-Word Identification	Control	20	10/10	~8.0	n/a	12-14 d	105.9 (14.6)	106.4 (14.7)		Shull-Senn, et al (1995)
WJ-R Passage Comp	Control	20	10/10	~6.0	n/a	12-14 d	92.7 (19.8)	99.6 (18.7)		Shull-Senn, et al (1995)
WJ-R Passage Comp	Control	20	10/10	~10.0	n/a	12-14 d	106.0 (9.7)	107.6 (11.5)		Shull-Senn, et al (1995)
WJ-R Passage Comp	Control	20	10/10	~8.0	n/a	12-14 d	104.5 (11.7)	107.5 (15.1)		Shull-Senn, et al (1995)
WJ-R Writing Samples	Control	20	10/10	~8.0	n/a	12-14 d	106.2 (12.1)	106.2 (11.4)		Shull-Senn, et al (1995)
WJ-R Writing Samples	Control	20	10/10	~6.0	n/a	12-14 d	101.6 (9.0)	100.5 (7.4)		Shull-Senn, et al (1995)
WJ-R Writing Samples	Control	20	10/10	~10.0	n/a	12-14 d	103.4 (10.6)	108.8 (11.5)		Shull-Senn, et al (1995)

References

Adams, K. M., Grant, I., & Reed, R. (1980). Neuropsychology in alcoholic men in their late thirties: One-year follow-up. American Journal of Psychiatry, 137(8), 928-931.

Addington, J., Addington, D., & Maticka-Tyndale, E. (1991). Cognitive functioning and positive and negative symptoms in schizophrenia. Schizophrenia Research, 5, 123-134.

Agnoli, A., Fabbrini, G., Fioravanti, M., & Martucci, N. (1992). CBF and cognitive evaluation of Alzheimer type patients before and after IMAO-B treatment: A pilot study. European Neuropsychopharmacology, 2, 31-35.

Ahles, T. A., Tope, D. M., Furstenberg, C., Hann, D., & Mills, L. (1996). Psychologic and neuropsychologic impact of autologous bone marrow transplantation. Journal of Clinical Oncology, 14, 1457-1462.

Aldenkamp, A. P., Overweg, J., Smakman, J., Beun, A. M., Diepman, L., Edelbroek, P., Gutter, T., Mulder, O. G., Slot, B. v. t., & Vledder, B. (1995). Effect of Sabeluzole (R58735) on memory functions in patients with elderly. Neuropsychobiology, 32, 37-44.

Alder, A. G., Adam, J., & Arenberg, D. (1990). Individual-differences assessment of the relationship between change in and initial level of adult cognitive functioning. Psychology and Aging, 5(4), 560-568.

Amato, M. P., Ponziani, G., Pracucci, G., Bracco, L., Siracusa, G., & Amaducci, L. (1995). Cognitive impairment in early-onset multiple sclerosis. Archives of Neurology, 52, 168-172.

Anastasi, A. (1988). Psychological Testing. (6th ed.). New York: Macmillan Publishing Company.

Anastasi, A., & Urbina, S. (1997). Psychological Testing. (7th ed.). Upper Saddle River, NJ: Prentice Hall.

Anstey, K. J., Smith, G. A., & Lord, S. (1997). Test-retest reliability of a battery of sensory, motor, and physiological measures of aging. Perceptual and Motor Skills, 84, 831-834.

Applebaum, H. (1978). Stability of Portable Rod-and-Frame Test scores. Perceptual and Motor Skills, 47, 1153-1154.

Armstrong, C., Ruffer, J., Corn, B., DeVries, K., & Mollman, J. (1995). Biphasic patterns of memory deficits following moderate-dose partial-brain irradiation: Neuropsychologic outcome and proposed mechanisms. Journal of Clinical Oncology, 13, 2263-2271.

Atlas, J. A., Fortunato, M., & Lavin, V. (1990). Stability and concurrent validity of the PPVT-R in hospitalized psychotic adolescents. Psychological Reports, 67, 554.

Baker, L. A., Cheng, L. Y., & Amara, I. B. (1983). The withdrawal of benztropine mesylate in chronic schizophrenia patients. British Journal of Psychiatry, 143, 584-590.

Bamford, K. A., Caine, E. D., Kido, D. K., Cox, C., & Shoulson, I. (1995). A prospective evaluation of cognitive decline in early Huntington's disease: Functional and radiographic correlates. Neurology, 45, 1867-1873.

Ban, T. A., Morey, L., Aguglia, E., Azzarelli, O., Balsano, F., Marigliano, V., Caglieris, N., Sterlicchio, M., Capruso, A., Tomasi, N. A., Crepaldi, G., Volpe, D., Palmieri, G., Ambrosi, G., Polli, E., Cortellaro, M., Zanussi, C., & Froldi, M. (1990). Nimodipine in the treatment of old age dementias. Progress in

Neuro-Psychopharmacology and Biological Psychiatry, 14, 525-551.

Banks, G. K., & Beran, R. G. (1991). Neuropsychological assessment in lamotrigine treated epileptic patients. Clinical and Experimental Neurology, 28, 230-237.

Barth, J.T., Gideon, D.A., Scieara, A.D., Hulsey, P.H., & Anchor, K.N. (1986). Forensic aspects of mild head trauma. Journal of Head Trauma Rehabilitation, 1, 63-70.

Becker, J. T., Huff, F. J., Nebes, R. D., Holland, A., & Boller, F. (1988). Neuropsychological function in Alzheimer's disease: Pattern of impairment and rates of progression. Archives of Neurology, 45, 263-268.

Bell, F.O., Hoff, A.L., & Hoyt, K.B. (1964). Answer sheets do make a difference. Personnel Psychology, 17, 65-71.

Benton, A.L., deS. Hamsher, K., Varney, N.R., & Spreen, O. (1983). Contributions to Neuropsychological Assessment: A Clinical Manual. New York: Oxford University Press.

Berg, R. A., Ch'ien, L. T., Lancaster, W., Williams, S., & Cummins, J. (1983). Neuropsychological sequelae of postradiation somnolence syndrome. Developmental and Behavioral Pediatrics, 4(2), 103-107.

Bergamasco, B., Scarzella, L., & Commare, P. L. (1994). Idebenone, a new drug in the treatment of cognitive impairment in patients with dementia of the Alzheimer type. Functional Neurology, 9, 161-168.

Berman, I., Merson, A., Rachov-Pavlov, J., Allan, E., Davidson, M., & Losonczy, M. F. (1996). Risperidone in elderly schizophrenic patients. The American Journal of Geriatric Psychiatry, 4(2), 173-179.

Berry, D. T. R., Allen, R. S., & Schmitt, F. A. (1991). Rey-Osterriety Complex Figure: Psychometric characteristics in a geriatric sample. The Clinical Neuropsychologist, 5(2), 143-153.

Bever, C. T., Jr., Grattan, L., Panitch, H. S., & Johnson, K. P. (1995). The brief repeatable battery of neuropsychological tests for multiple sclerosis: A preliminary serial study. Multiple Sclerosis, 1, 165-169.

Biederman, J., Faraone, S., Milberger, S., Guite, J., Mick, E., Chen, L., Mennin, D., Marrs, A., Ouellette, C., Moore, P., Spencer, T., Norman, D., Wilens, T., Kraus, I., & Perrin, J. (1996). A prospective 4-year follow-up study of attention-deficit hyperactivity and related disorders. Archives of General Psychiatry, 53, 437-446.

Bono, G., Mauri, M., Sinforiani, E., Barbarini, G., Minoli, L., & Fea, M. (1996). Longitudinal neuropsychological evaluation of HIV-infected intravenous drug users. Addiction, 91(2), 263-268.

Bordeaux, J. D., Dowell, R. E., Jr., Copeland, D. R., Fletcher, J. M., Francis, D. J., & van Eys, J. (1988). A prospective study of neuropsychological sequelae in children with brain tumors. Journal of Child Neurology, 3, 63-68.

Bornstein, R. A., Baker, G. B., & Douglass, A. B. (1987). Short-term retest reliability of the Halstead-Reitan Battery in a normal sample. Journal of Nervous and Mental Disease, 175, 229-232.

Botwinick, J., Storandt, M., & Berg, L. (1986). A longitudinal, behavioral study of senile dementia of the Alzheimer's type. Archives of Neurology, 43, 1124-1127.

Bowden, S. C., Fowler, K. S., Bell, R. C., Whelan, G., Clifford, C. C., Ritter, A. J., & Long, C. M. (1998). The reliability and internal validity of the

Wisconsin Card Sorting Test. Neuropsychological Rehabilitation, 8(3), 243-254.

Bowden, S. C., Whelan, G., Long, C. M., & Clifford, C. C. (1995). Temporal stability of the WAIS-R and WMS-R in a heterogeneous sample of alcohol dependent clients. The Clinical Neuropsychologist, 9(2), 194-197.

Bowler, J. V., Hadar, Y., & Wade, J. P. H. (1994). Cognition in stroke. Acta Neruologica Scandinavia, 90, 424-429.

Brinkman, S. D., Pomara, N., Barnett, N., Block, R., Domino, E. F., & Gershon, S. (1984). Lithium-induced increases in red blood cell chloine and memory performance in Alzheimer's-type dementia. Biological Psychiatry, 19, 157-164.

Brooks, B., Kayser, L., Jorgensen, B., Danielson, U., Hansen, J. E. M., & Perrild, H. (1988). Three-week-beta-adrenergic blockade does not impair or improve general intellectual function in young healthy males. Clinical Cardiology, 11, 5-8.

Brookshire, B. L., Fletcher, J. M., Bohan, T. P., & Landry, S. H. (1995). Verbal and nonverbal skill discrepancies in children with hydroencephalus: A five-year longitudinal follow-up. Journal of Pediatric Psychology, 20(6), 785-800.

Brouwers, P. & Mohr, E. (1989). A metric for the evaluation of change in clinical trials. Clinical Neuropharmacology, 12, 129-133.

Brown, S. J., Rourke, B. P., & Cicchetti, D. V. (1989). Reliability of tests and measures used in the neuropsychological assessment of children. Clinical Neuropsychologists, 3, 353-368.

Bruggemans, E. F., Vijver, F. J. R. V. d., & Huysmans, H. A. (1997). Assessment of congitive deterioration in individual patients following cardiac surgery: Correcting for measurement error and practice effects. Journal of Clinical and Experimental Neuropsychology, 19(4), 543-559.

Bryant, C. K., & Roffe, M. W. (1978). A reliability study of the McCarthy Scales of Children's Abilities. Journal of Clinical Psychology, 34(2), 401-406.

Buchanan, R. W., Holstein, C., & Breier, A. (1994). The comparative efficacy and long-term effect of clozapine. Biological Psychiatry, 36, 717-725.

Burgess, A. P., Riccio, M., Jadresic, D., Pugh, K., Catalan, J., Hawkins, D. A., Baldeweg, T., Lovett, E., Gruzelier, J., & Thompson, C. (1994). A longitudinal study of the neuropsychiatric consequences of HIV-1 infection in gay men. I. Neuropsychological performance and neurological status at baseline and at 12-month follow-up. Psychological Medicine, 24, 885-895.

Burt, D. B., Loveland, K. A., Chen, Y.-W., Chuang, A., Lewis, K. R., & Cherry, L. (1995). Aging in adults with Down Syndrome: Report from a longitudinal study. American Journal on Mental Retardation, 100(3), 262-270.

Casey, J. E., Ferguson, G. G., Kimura, D., & Hachinski, V. C. (1989). Neuropsychological improvement versus practice effect following unilateral carotid endarterectomy in patients without stroke. Journal of Clinical and Experimental Neuropsychology, 11, 461-470.

Catron, D.W. (1978). Immediate test-retest changes in WAIS scores among college males. Psychological Reports, 43, 279-290.

Catron, D.W., & Thompson, C.C. (1979). Test-retest gains in WAIS scores after four retest intervals. Journal of Clinical Psychology, 35(2), 352-357.

Celsis, P., Agniel, A., Cardebat, D., Demonet, J. F., Ousset, P. J., & Puel, M. (1997). Age related cognitive decline: A clinical entity? A longitudinal study of cerebral blood flow and memory performance. Journal of Neurology, Neurosurgery, and Psychiatry, 62, 601-608.

Chadwick, O., Rutter, M., Shaffer, D., & Shrout, P. E. (1981). A prospective study of children with head injuries: IV. Specific cognitive deficits. Journal of Clinical Neuropsychology, 3(2), 101-120.

Chelune, G., Naugle, R. I., Lunders, H., Sedlak, J., & Awad, I.A. (1993). Individual differences after epilepsy surgery: Practice effects and base-rate information. Neuropsychology, 7, 41-52.

Choca, J., & Morris, J. (1992). Administering the Category Test by computer: Equivalence of results. The Clinical Neuropsychologist, 6(1), 9-15.

Claiborn, J. M., & Greene, R. L. (1981). Neuropsychological changes in recovering men alcoholics. Journal of Studies on Alcohol, 42(9), 757-?

Clark, C., & Klonoff, H. (1988). Reliability and construct validity of the six-block Tactual Performance Test in an adult sample. Journal of Clinical and Experimental Neuropsychology, 10(2), 175-184.

Clarke, J., & Haughton, H. (1975). A study of intellectual impairment and recovery rates in heavy drinkers in Ireland. British Journal of Psychiatry, 126, 178-184.

Claus, J. J., Mohr, E., & Chase, T. N. (1991). Clinical trials in dementia: Learning effects with repeated testing. Journal of Psychiatry and Neuroscience, 16, 1-4.

Clifford, C., & Rim, C.S. (1976, Feb.). Neuropsychological criteria for anticonvulsant drug treatment. Presented at the Annual Meeting of the International Neuropsychology Society, Toronto, Canada.

Coblentz, G.M., Mattis, S., Zingesser, L.H., Kasoff, S.S., Wisniewski, H.M., & Katzman, R. (1973). Presenile dementia: Clinical aspects and evaluation of cerebrospinal fluid dynamics. Archives of Neurology, 29, 299-308.

Conners, C. K., & Taylor, E. (1980). Pemoline, methylphenidate, and placebo in children with minimal brain dysfunction. Archives of General Psychiatry, 37, 922-930.

Connor, A., Franzen, M., & Sharp, B. (1988). Effects of practice and differential instructions on Stroop performance. The International Journal of Clinical Neuropsychology, 10, 1-4.

Cook, M. J., Holder-Brown, L., Johnson, L. J., & Kilgo, J. L. (1989). An examination of the stability of the Bayley Scales of Infant Development with high-risk infants. Journal of Early Intervention, 13(1), 45-49.

Cook, M. R., Bergman, F. J., Cohen, H. D., Gerkovich, M. M., Graham, C., Harris, R. K., & Siemann, L. G. (1991). Effects of methanol vapor on human neurobehavioral measures. Research Report of the Health Efficacy Institute, 42, 1-45.

Cooper, S. A., Anthony, J. E., Mopsik, E., Moore, M. S., Sullivan, D. C., & Kruger, G. O. (1978). A techniques for investigating the intensity and duration of human psychomotor impairment after intravenous diazepam. Oral Surgery, Oral Medicine, and Oral Pathology, 45(4), 493-502.

Cosgrove, J., & Newell, T. G. (1991). Recovery of neuropsychological functions during reduction in use of phencyclidine. Journal of Clinical Psychology, 47(159-169).

Cotman, A., & Sandman, C. (1997). Cognitive deficits and their remediation in the homeless. Journal of Cognitive Rehabilitation, 15(1), 16-23.

Coutts, R.L., Lichstein, L., Bermudez, J.M., Daigle, M., Mann, D.P., Charbonnel, T.S., Michaud, R., & Williams, C.R. (1987). Treatment assessment of learning disabled children. Is there a role for frequently repeated neuropsychological testing? Archives of Clinical Neuropsychology, 2, 237-244.

Crawford, J. R., Parker, D. M., Stewart, L. E., Besson, J. O. A., & De Lacey, G. (1989). Prediction of WAIS IQ with the National Adult Reading Test: Cross-validation and extension. British Journal of Clinical Psychology, 28, 267-273.

Crawford, J. R., Stewart, L. E., & Moore, J. W. (1989). Demonstration of savings on the AVLT and development of a parallel form. Journal of Clinical and Experimental Neuropsychology, 11, 975-981.

Crook, T., Ferris, S., Sathananthan, G., Raskin, A., & Gershon, S. (1977). The effect of methylphenidate on test performance in the cognitively impaired aged. Psychopharmacology, 52, 251-255.

Crossen, J. R., & Weins, A. N. (1994). Comparison of the Auditory-Verbal Learning Test (AVLT) and California Verbal Learning Test (CVLT) in a sample of normal subjects. Journal of Clinical and Experimental Neuropsychology, 16(2), 190-194.

Curran, H. V., Sakulsriprong, M., & Lader, M. (1988). Antidepressants and human memory: An investigation of four drugs with different sedative and anticholinergic profiles. Psychopharmacology, 95, 520-527.

Cushman, L., Brinkman, S.D., Gnaji, S., & Jacobs, L.A. (1984). Neuropsychological impairment after carotid endarterectomy correlates with intraoperative ischemia. Cortex, 20, 403-412.

Davis, E. E., & Slettedahl, R. W. (1976). Stability of the McCarthy Scales over a 1-year period. Journal of Clinical Psychology, 32, 798-800.

Davis, K. L., Thal, L. J., Gamzu, E. R., Davis, C. S., Woolson, R. F., Gracon, S. I., Drachman, D. A., Schneider, L. S., Whitehouse, P. J., Hoover, T. M., Morris, J. C., Kawas, C. H., Knopman, D. S., Earl, N. L., Klumar, V., Doody, R. S., & Group, T. C. S. (1992). A double-blind, placebo-controlled multicenter study of tacrine for Alzheimer's disease. The New England Journal of Medicine, 327, 1253-1259.

de Beaurepaire, C., de Beaurepaire, R., Cleau, M., & Borenstein, P. (1993). Bromocriptine improves digit symbol substitution test scores in neuroleptic-treated chronic schizophrenic patients. European Psychiatry, 8, 89-93.

De Leo, D., Serraiotto, L., Pellegrini, C., Magni, G., Franceschi, L., & Deriu, G. P. (1987). Outcome from carotid endarterectomy. Neuropsychological performances, depressive symptoms and quality of life: 8-month follow-up. International Journal of Psychiatry in Medicine, 17(4), 317-325.

Delaney, R. C., Prevey, M. L., Cramer, J., Mattson, R. H., & Group, V. E. C. S. R. (1992). Test-retest comparability and control subject data for the Rey-Auditory Verbal Learning Test and Rey-Osterrieth/Taylor Complex Figures. Archives of Clinical Neuropsychology, 7, 523-528.

Delis, D. C., Kramer, J. H., Kaplan, E., & Ober, B. A. (1987). California Verbal Learning Test. San Antonio, TX: The Psychological Corporation.

Delis, D. C., Massman, P. J., Kaplan, E., McKee, R., Kramer, J. H., & Gettman, D. (1991). Alternate form of the California Verbal Learning Test: Development and reliability. The Clinical Neuropsychologist, 5(154-162).

Della Sala, S., Laiacona, M., Spinnler, H., & Ubezio, C. (1992). A cancellation test: Its reliability in assessing attentional deficits in Alzheimer's disease. Psychological Medicine, 22(885-901).

Denney, N. W., & Heidrich, S. M. (1990). Training effects on Raven's Progressive Matrices in young, middle-aged, and elderly adults. Psychology and Aging, 5(1), 144-145.

Desmond, D. W., Tatemichi, T. K., Stern, Y., & Stano, M. (1995). The determination of clinically meaningful cognitive decline: Development and use of an alternative method. Archives of Clinical Neuropsychology, 10(6), 535-542.

desRosiers, G., & Ivison, D. (1988). Paired associate learning: Form 1 and Form 2 of the Wechsler Memory Scale. Archives of Clinical Neuropsychology, 3, 47-67.

desRosiers, G., & Kavanagh, D. (1987). Cognitive assessment in closed head injury: Stability, validity and parallel forms for two neuropsychological measures of recovery. The International Journal of Clinical Neuropsychology, 9, 162-171.

Desrosiers, J., Herbert, R., Bravo, R. H., & Dutil, E. (1995). The Purdue Pegboard Test: Normative data for people aged 60 and over. Disability and Rehabilitation, 17(5), 217-224.

Di Stefano, G., & Radanov, B. P. (1995). Course of attention and memory after common whiplash: A two-years prospective study with age, education and gender pair-matched patients. Acta Neurologica Scandinavia, 91, 346-352.

Di Stefano, G., & Radanov, B. P. (1996). Quantitative and qualitative aspects of learning and memory in common whiplash patients: A 6-month follow-up study. Archives of Clinical Neuropsychology, 11(8), 661-676.

Dikmen, S., Machamer, J., Temkin, N., & McClean, A. (1990). Neuropsychological recovery in patients with moderate to severe head injury: 2 year follow-up. Journal of Clinical and Experimental Neuropsychology, 12, 507-519.

Dikmen, S., Reitan, R. M., & Temkin, N. R. (1983). Neuropsychological recovery in head injury. Archives of Neurology, 40, 333-338.

Dodrill, C. B., & Thoreson, N. S. (1993). Reliability of the Lateral Dominance Examination. Journal of Clinical and Experimental Neuropsychology, 15(2), 183-190.

Dodrill, C. B., & Troupin, A. (1975). Effects of repeated administrations of a comprehensive neuropsychological battery among chronic epileptics. The Journal of Nervous and Mental Disease, 161, 185-190.

Dodrill, C. B., Arnett, J. L., Sommerville, K. W., & Sussman, N. M. (1995). Effects of differing dosages of Vigabatrin (Sabril) on congitive abilities and quality of life in epilepsy. Epilepsia, 36(2), 164-173.

Donnelly, E. F., & Chase, T. N. (1973). Intellectual and memory function in parkinsonian and non-parkinsonian patients treated with l-dopa. Diseases of the Nervous System, 34, 119-122.

Drudge, O. W., Williams, J. M., Kessler, M., & Gomes, F. B. (1984). Recovery from severe closed head injuries: Repeat testings with the Halstead-Reitan Neuropsychological Battery. Journal of Clinical Psychology, 40(1), 259-265.

Dubey, B. L., Singh, S., & Boparai, T. S. (1978). Can we control aging and memory deterioration. Indian Journal of Clinical Psychology, 5, 85-88.

Duff, K., Westervelt, H. J., Haase, R. F., & McCaffrey, R. J. (1999). The viability of dual baseline assessments with the CVLT in an HIV sample. Archives of Clinical Neuropsychology, 14, 105-106.

Dura, J. R., Myers, E. G., & Freathy, D. T. (1989). Stability of the Wide Range Achievement Test in an adolescent psychiatric inpatient setting. Educational and Psychological Measurement, 49, 253-256.

Dyche, G. M., & Johnson, D. A. (1991). Development and evaluation of CHIPASAT, an attention test for children: II. Test-retest reliability and practice effect for a normal sample. Perceptual and Motor Skills, 72, 563-572.

Eagger, S., Morant, N., Levy, R., & Sahakian, B. (1992). Tacrine in Alzheimer's Disease: Time course of changes in cognitive function and practice effects. British Journal of Psychiatry, 160, 36-40.

Eckardt, M. J., & Matarazzo, J. D. (1981). Test-retest reliability of the Halstead Impairment Index in hospitalized alcoholic and nonalcoholic males with mild to moderate neuropsychological impairment. Journal of Clinical Neuropsychology, 3(3), 257-269.

Eckardt, M. J., Parker, E. S., Noble, E. P., Pautler, C. P., & Gottschalk, L. A. (1979). Changes in neuropsychological performance during treatment for alcoholism. Biological Psychiatry, 14(6), 943-954.

Eisen, E. A., Letz, R. A., Wegman, D. H., Baker, E. L., Jr., & Pothier, L. (1988). Defining measurement precision for effort dependent tests: The case of three neurobehavioural tests. International Journal of Epidemiology, 17(4), 920-926.

Elias, M. F., Robbins, M. A., Schultz, N. R., Jr., & Streeten, D. H. P. (1986). A longitudinal study of neuropsychological test performance for hypertensive and normotensive adults: Initial findings. Journals of Gerontology, 41(4), 503-505.

Elias, M. F., Schultz, N. R., Jr., Robbins, M. A., & Elias, P. K. (1989). A longitudinal study of neuropsychological performance by hypertensives and normotensives: A third measurement point. Journal of Gerontology: Psychological Sciences, 44(1), P25-28.

Enderby, P., Broeckx, J., Hospers, W., Schildermans, F., & Deberdt, W. (1994). Effect of Piracetam and recovery and rehabilitation after stroke: A double-blind, placebo-controlled study. Clinical Neuropharmacology, 17, 320-331.

Engelsmann, F., Katz, J., Ghadirian, A. M., & Schachter, D. (1988). Lithium and memory: A long-term follow-up study. Journal of Clinical Psychopharmacology, 8(3), 207-212.

Ewert, J., Levin, H. S., Watson, M. G., & Kalisky, Z. (1989). Procedural memory during posttraumatic amnesia in survivors of severe closed head injury. Archives of Neurology, 46, 911-916.

Fakouhi, T. D., Jhee, S. S., Sramek, J. J., Benes, C., Schwartz, P., Hantsburger, G., Herting, R., Swabb, E. A., & Cutler, N. R. (1995). Evaluation of cycloserine in the treatment of Alzheimer's Disease. Journal of Geriatric Psychiatry and Neurology, 8, 226-230.

Farmer, R. H. (1973). Functional changes during early weeks of abstinence, measured by the Bender-Gestalt. Quarterly Journal of Studies on Alcohol, 34, 786-796.

Farnill, D., & Hayes, S. C. (1995). Retest reliabililty of the Woodcock Language Proficiency Battery. Perceptual and Motor Skills, 81, 1147-1152.

Fields, R. B., Van Kammen, D. P., Peters, J. L., Rosen, J., Van Kammen, W. B., Nugent, A., Stipetic, M., & Linnoila, M. (1988). Clonidine improves memory functioning in schizophrenia independently from change in psychosis. Schizophrenia Research, 1, 417-423.

Fish, J. M., & Sinkel, P. (1980). Correlation of scores on Wechsler Memory Scale and Wechsler Adult Intelligence Scale for chronic alcoholics and normals. Psychological Reports, 47, 940-942.

Flanagan, J. L., & Jackson, S. T. (1997). Test-retest reliability of three aphasia tests: Performance of non-brain-damaged older adults. Journal of Communication Disorders, 30, 33-43.

Flicker, C., Ferris, S. H., & Reisberg, B. (1993). A longitudinal study of cognitive function in elderly persons with subjective memory complaints. Journal of the American Geriatric Society, 41, 1029-1032.

Folstein, M. F., Folstein, S. E., & McHugh, P. R. (1975). "Mini-Mental State": A practical method for grading the cognitive state of patients for the clinician. Journal of Psychiatric Research, 12, 189-198.

Frank, R., Wiederholt, W. C., Kritz-Silerstein, D., Salmon, D. P., & Barrett-Connor, E. (1996). Effects of sequential neuropsychological testing of an elderly community-based sample. Neuroepidemiology, 15, 257-268.

Franzen, M. D., Paul, D., & Iverson, G. L. (1996). Reliability of alternate forms of the Trail Making Test. The Clinical Neuropsychologist, 10(2), 125-129.

Franzen, M. D., Tishelman, A. C., Sharp, B. H., & Friedman, A. G. (1987). An investigation of the test-retest reliability of the Stroop Color-Word Test across two intervals. Archives of Clinical Neuropsychology, 2, 265-272.

Franzen, M. D., Tishelman, A. C., Smith, S., Sharp, B. H., & Friedman, A. G. (1989). Preliminary data concerning the test-retest and parallel-forms reliability of the Randt Memory Test. The Clinical Neuropsychologist, 3(1), 25-28.

Fraser, R., Dikmen, S., McLean, A., Jr., Miller, B., & Temkin, N. (1988). Employability of head injury survivors: First year post-injury. Rehabilitation Counseling Bulletin, 31, 276-288.

Freides, D., Engen, L., Miller, D., & Londa, J. B. (1996). Narative and visual-spatial recall: Alternate forms, learning trial effects, and geriatric performance. The Clinical Neuropsychologist, 10(4), 407-418.

Fromm, D., & Schopflocher, D. (1984). Neuropsychological test performance in depressed patients before and after drug therapy. Biological Psychiatry, 19(1), 55-72.

Fromm, D., Holland, A. L., Nebes, R. D., & Oakley, M. A. (1991). A longitudinal study of word-reading ability in Alzheimer's Disease: Evidence from the National Adult Reading Test. Cortex, 27, 367-376.

Fudge, J. L., Perry, P. J., Garvey, M. J., & Kelly, M. W. (1990). A comparison of the effect of fluoxetine and trazadone on the cognitive functioning of depressed outpatients. Journal of Affective Disorders, 18, 275-280.

Gallassi, R., Morreale, A., Lorusso, S., Procaccianti, G., Lugaresi, E., & Baruzzi, A. (1988). Carbamazepine and phenytoin: Comparison of cognitive effects in epileptic patients during monotherapy and withdrawal. Archives of Neurology, 45, 892-894.

Ganguli, M., Seaberg, E. C., Ratcliff, G. C., Belle, S. H., & DeKosky, S. T. (1996). Cognitive stability over 2 years in a rural elderly population: The MoVIES project. Neuroepidemiology, 15, 42-50.

Geffen, G. M., Butterworth, P., & Geffen, L. B. (1994). Test-retest reliability of a new form of the Auditory Verbal Learning Test (AVLT). Archives of Clinical Neuropsychology, 9, 303-316.

Geisler, M. W., Sliwinski, M., Coyle, P. K., Masur, D. M., Doscher, C., & Krupp, L. B. (1996). The effects of amantadine and pemoline on cognitive functioning in multiple sclerosis. Archives of Neurology, 53, 185-188.

Giambra, L. M., Arenberg, D., Zonderman, A. B., Kawas, C., & Costa, P. T., Jr. (1995). Adult life span changes in immediate visual memory and verbal intelligence. Psychology and Aging, 10(1), 123-139.

Gigli, G. L., Maschio, M. C. E., Diomedi, M., Moroni, M., Dell'Orso, S., Placidi, F., & Marciani, M. G. (1993). Brotizolam and cognitive performance: A double-blind, crossover study versus placebo in a population of shift workers. Current Therapuetic Research, 53, 129-136.

Giordani, B., Berent, S., Boivin, M. J., Penney, J. B., Lehtinen, S., Markel, D. S., Hollingsworth, Z., Butterbaugh, G., Hichwa, R. D., Gusella, J. F., & Young, A. B. (1995). Longitudinal neuropsychological and genetic linkage analysis of persons at risk for Huntington's disease. Archives of Neurology, 52, 59-64.

Gittleman-Klein, R., & Klein, D. F. (1976). Methylphendate effects in learning disabilities. Archives of General Psychiatry, 33, 655-664.

Givens, T. S., & Davis, J. R. (1984). The stability of special education categorical assignments. Journal of Psychoeducational Assessment, 2, 131-139.

Glennerster, A., Palace, J., Warburton, D., Oxbury, S., & Newsom-Davis, J. (1996). Memory in myasthenia gravis: Neuropsychological tests of central cholinergic function before and after effective immunological treatment. Neurology, 46, 1138-1142.

Goldberg, T. E., Greenberg, R. D., Griffin, S. J., Gold, J. M., Kleiman, J. E., Pickar, D., Schulz, S. C., & Weinberger, D. R. (1993). The effect of clozapine on cognition and psychiatric symptoms in patients with schizophrenia. Brisith Journal of Psychiatry, 162, 43-48.

Golden, C. J., Berg, R. A., & Graber, B. (1982). Test-retest reliability of the Luria-Nebraska Neuropsychological Battery in stable, chronically impaired patients. Journal of Consulting and Clinical Psychology, 50(3), 452-454.

Golden, P. L., Warner, P. E., Fleishaker, J. C., Jewell, R. C., Millikin, S., Lyon, J., & Brouwer, K. L. R. (1994). Effects of probenecid on the pharmacokinetics and pharmacodynamics of adinazolam in humans. Clinical Pharmacology and Therapeutics, 56, 133-141.

Goldman, M. S., Williams, D. L., & Klisz, D. K. (1983). Recoverability of psychological functioning following alcohol abuse: Prolonged visual-spatial dysfunction in older alcoholics. Journal of Consulting and Clinical Psychology, 51(3), 370-378.

Gooday, R., Hayes, P. C., Bzeizi, K., & O'Carroll, R. E. (1995). Benzodiazepine receptor antagonism improves reaction time in latent hepatic encephalopathy. Psychopharmacology, 119, 295-298.

Goulet Fisher, D., Sweet, J.J., & Pfaelzer-Smith, E.A. (1986). Influence of depression on repeated neuropsychological testing. International Journal of Clinical Neuropsychology, 8(1), 14-18.

Green, J. B., Elder, W. W., & Freed, D. M. (1995). The P1 component of the middle latency auditory evoked potential predicts a practice effect during clinical trials in Alzheimer's disease. Neurology, 45, 962-966.

Green, R. C., Goldstein, F. C., Auchus, A. P., Presley, R., Clark, W. S., Tuyl, L. V., Green, J., Hersch, S. M., & Karp, H. R. (1992). Treatment trial of oxiracetam in Alzheimer's disease. Archives of Neurology, 49, 1135-1136.

Gregory, S. J., Davies, A. D. M., & Binks, M. G. (1983). The improvements of verbal fluency in the elderly: The effects of practice on the Set Test and an alternate form. Educational Gerontology, 9, 139-146.

Greiffenstein, M. F., Brinkman, S., Jacobs, L., & Braun, P. (1988). Neuropsychological improvement following endarterectomy as a function of outcome measure and reconstructed vessel. Cortex, 24, 223-230.

Gruzelier, J., & Warren, K. (1993). Neuropsychological evidence of reductions on left frontal tests with hypnosis. Psychological Medicine, 23, 93-101.

Guarnaccia, V. J., Daniels, L. K., & Sefick, W. J. (1975). Comparison of automated and standard administration of the Purdue Pegboard with mentally retarded adults. Perceptual and Motor Skills, 40, 371-374.

Haaland, K. Y., Temkin, N., Randahl, G., & Dikmen, S. (1994). Recovery of simple motor skills after head injury. Journal of Clinical and Experimental Neuropsychology, 16(3), 448-456.

Hagger, C., Buckley, P., Kenny, J. T., Friedman, L., Ubogy, D., & Meltzer, H. Y. (1993). Improvement in cognitive functions and psychiatric symptoms in treatment-refractory schizophrenic patients recieving clozapine. Biological Psychiatry, 34, 702-712.

Halperin, J.J., Pass, H.L., Anand, A.K., Luft, B.J., Volkman, D.J., & Dattwyler, R.J. (1988). Nervous sytem abnormalities in Lyme disease. Annals of the New York Academy of Sciences, 539, 24-34.

Hamazaki, T., Sawazaki, S., Itomura, M., Asaoka, E., Nagao, Y., Nishimura, N., Yazawa, K., Kuwamori, T., & Kobayashi, M. (1996). The effect of docosahexaenoic acid on aggression in young adults. A placebo-controlled double-blind study. Journal of Clinical Investigation, 97(4), 1129-1133.

Hamby, S.L., Bardi, C.A., & Wilkins, J.W. (1993). Practice effects differ as a function of vocabulary and age. Paper presented at 13th Annual Conference of the National Academy of Neuropsychologists, Phoenix, AZ.

Hanly, J. G., Fisk, J. D., Sherwood, G., & Eastwood, B. (1994). Clinical course of cognitive dysfunction in systemtic lupus erythematosus. Journal of Rheumatology, 21, 1825-1831.

Hannay, H. J., & Levin, H. S. (1985). Selective Reminding Test: An examination of the equivalence of four sheets. Journal of Clinical and Experimental

Neuropsychology, 7, 251-263.

Harrington, R. G., & Jennings, V. (1986). A comparison of three short forms of the McCarthy Scales of Children's Abilities. Contemporary Educational Psychology, 11, 109-116.

Harris, N. D., Deary, I. J., Harris, M. B., Lees, M. M., & Wilson, J. A. (1996). Peripartal cognitive impairment: Secondary to depression? British Journal of Health Psychology, 1, 127-136.

Hatsukami, D. K., Mitche, J. E., Morley, J. E., Morgan, S. F., & Levine, A. S. (1986). Effect of naltrexone on mood and cognitive functioning among overweight men. Biological Psychiatry, 21, 293-300.

Haxby, J. V., Grady, C. L., Koss, E., Horwitz, B., Heston, L., Schapiro, M., Friedland, R. P., & Rapoport, S. I. (1990). Longitudinal study of cerebral metabolic asymmetries and associated neuropsychological patterns in early dementia of the Alzheimer's type. Archives of Neurology, 47, 753-760.

Hayes, W.L. (1988). Statistics. (4th ed.) New York: Holt, Rinehart, & Wilson.

Hermann, B. P., Seidenberg, M., Schoenfeld, J., Peterson, J., Leveroni, C., & Wyler, A. R. (1996). Empirical techniques for determining the reliability, magnitude, and pattern of neuropsychological change after epilepsy surgery. Epilepsia, 37(10), 942-950.

Hermann, B. P., Wyler, A. R., Bush, A. J., & Tabatabai, F. R. (1992). Differential effects of left and right anterior temporal lobectomy on verbal learning and memory performance. Epilepsia, 33(2), 289-297.

Hestad, K., Aukrust, P., Ellersten, B., & Klove, H. (1996). Neuropsychological deficits in HIV-1 seropositive and seronegative intravenous drug users (IVDUs): A follow-up study. Journal of the International Neuropsychological Society, 2, 126-133.

Heyer, E. J., Delphin, E., Adams, D. C., Rose, E. A., Smith, C. R., Todd, G. J., Ginsburg, M., Haggerty, R., & McMahon, D. J. (1995). Cerebral dysfunction after cardiac operations in elderly patients. Annals of Thoracic Surgery, 60, 1716-1722.

Hietanen, M. H. (1991). Selegiline and cognitive function in Parkinson's disease. Acta Neurologica Scandinavica, 84, 407-410.

Hill, R. D., Storandt, M., & Malley, M. (1993). The impact of long-term exercise training on psychological function in older adults. Journal of Gerontology: Psychological Sciences, 48(1), P12-P17.

Hinkin, C. H., van Gorp, W. G., Mandelkern, M. A., Gee, M., Satz, P., Holston, S., Marcotte, T. D., Evans, G., Paz, D. H., Ropchan, J. R., Quinones, N., Khonsary, A., & Blahd, W. H. (1995). Cerebral metabolic change in patients with AIDS: Report of a six-month follow-up using positron-emission tomography. The Journal of Neuropsychiatry and Clinical Neurosciences, 7, 180-187.

Hird, J. S., Landers, D. M., Thomas, J. R., & Horan, J. J. (1981). Physical practice is superior to mental practice in enhancing cognitive and motor task performance. Journal of Sport & Exercise Psychology, 8, 281-293.

Hopp, G. A., Dixon, R. A., Grut, M., & Backman, L. (1997). Longitudinal and psychometric profiles of two cognitive status tests in very old adults. Journal of Clinical Psychology, 53(7), 673-686.

Hornbein, T. F., Townes, B. D., Schoene, R. B., Sutton, J. R., & Houston, C. S. (1989). The cost to the central nervous system of climbing to extremely high altitude. New England Journal of Medicine, 321(25), 1714-1719.

Inzelberg, R., Shapira, T., & Korczyn, A. D. (1990). Effects of atropine on learning and memory functions in dementia. Clinical Neuropharmacology, 13(3), 241-247.

Ivnik, R. J., Malec, J. F., Sharbrough, F. W., Cascino, G. D., Hirschorn, K. A., Crook, T. H., & Larrabee, G. J. (1993). Traditional and computerized assessment procedures applied to the evaluation of memory change after temporal lobectomy. Archives of Clinical Neuropsychology, 8, 69-81.

Ivnik, R. J., Sharbrough, F. W., & Jr., E. R. L. (1987). Effects of anterior temporal lobectomy on cognitive function. Journal of Clinical Psychology, 43(1), 128-137.

Jacobson, N.S., & Traux, P. (1991). Clinical significance: A statistical approach to defining meaningful change in psychotherapy research. Journal of Consulting and Clinical Psychology, 59, 12-19.

Jalan, R., Gooday, R., O'Carroll, R. E., Redhead, D. N., Elton, R. A., & Hayes, P. C. (1995). A prospective evaluation of changes in neuropsychological and liver function tests following transjugular intrahepatic portosystemic stent-shunt. Journal of Hepatology, 23, 697-705.

Johnson-Greene, D., Adams, K. M., Gilman, S., Koeppe, R. A., Junck, L., Kluin, K. J., Martorello, S., & Heumann, M. (1997). Effects of abstinence and relapse upon neuropsychological function and cerebral glucose metabolism in severe chronic alcoholism. Journal of Clinical and Experimental Neuropsychology, 19(3), 378-385.

Johnstone, B., & Wilhelm, K. L. (1996). The longitudinal stability of the WRAT-R Reading subtest: Is it an appropriate estimate of premorbid intelligence? Journal of the International Neuropsychological Society, 2, 282-285.

Jones, R. D., Tranel, D., Benton, A., & Paulsen, J. (1992). Differentiating dementia from "pseudodementia" early in the clinical course: Utility of neuropsychological tests. Neuropsychology, 6(1), 13-21.

Juolasmaa, A., Outakoski, J., Hirvenoja, R., Tienari, P., Sotaniemi, K., & Takkunen, J. (1981). Effect of open heart surgery on intellectual performance. Journal of Clinical Neuropsychology, 3(3), 181-197.

Kaye, D. B., & Baron, M. B. (1987). Long-term stability of intelligence and achievement scores in specific-learning-dsabilities samples. Journal of Psychoeducational Assessment, 3, 257-266.

Kazdin, A.E. (1992). Research Design in Clinical Psychology. (2nd ed.). Boston: Allyn and Bacon.

Kazdin, A.E. (1998). Research Design in Clinical Psychology. (3rd ed.). Boston: Allyn and Bacon.

Kelland, D. Z., & Lewis, R. F. (1996). The Digit Vigilance Test: Reliability, validity, and sensitivity to diazepam. Archives of Clinical Neuropsychology, 11(4), 339-344.

Kelly, M. P., Garron, D. C., & Javid, H. (1980). Carotid artery disease, carotid endarterectomy, and behavior. Archives of Neurology, 37, 743-748.

Kepner, M. D., & Neimark, E. D. (1984). Test-retest reliability and differential patterns of score change on the Group Embedded Figures Test. Journal of Personality and Social Psychology, 46(6), 1405-1413.

Kilburn, K.H., Warsaw, R.H., & Shields, M.G. (1989). Neurobehavioral dysfunction in firemen exposed to polychlorinated biphenyls (PCBs): Possible improvement after detoxification. Archives of Environmental Health, 44, 345-350.

Killian, G. A., Holzman, P. S., Davis, J. M., & Gibbons, R. (1984). Effects of psychotropic medication on selected cognitive and perceptual measures. Journal of Abnormal Psychology, 93(1), 58-70.

King, G. D., Gideon, D. A., Haynes, C. D., Dempsey, R. L., & Jenkins, C. W. (1977). Intellectual and personality changes associated with carotid endarterectomy. Journal of Clinical Psychology, 33(1), 215-?

Kirkby, K. C., Montgomery, I. M., Badcock, R., & Daniels, B. A. (1995). A comparison of age-related deficits in memory and frontal lobe function following oral lorazepam administration. Journal of Psychopharmacology, 9, 319-325.

Klonoff, H., Clark, C., Kavanagh-Gray, D., Mizgala, H., & Munro, I. (1989). Two-year follow-up study of coronary bypass surgery. Journal of Thorasic and Cardiovascular Surgery, 97, 78-85.

Knight, R.G. & Shelton, E.J. (1983). Tables for evaluating predicted retest changes in Wechsler Adult Intelligence Scale scores. British Journal of Clinical Psychology, 22, 77-81.

Knights, R. M., Richardson, D. H., & McNarry, L. R. (1973). Automated vs. clinical administration of the Peabody Picture Vocabulary Test and the Coloured Progressive Matrices. American Journal of Mental Deficiency, 78(2), 223-225.

Knotek, P. C., Bayles, K. A., & Kaszniak, A. W. (1990). Response consistency on a semantic memory task in persons with dementia of the Alzheimer type. Brain-Language, 3(8), 4665-475.

Koller, W. C. (1984). Disturbance of recent memory function in parkinsonian patients on anticholinergic therapy. Cortex, 20, 307-311.

Komaki, R., Meyers, C. A., Shin, D. M., Garden, A. S., Byrne, K., Nickens, J. A., & Cox, J. D. (1995). Evaluation of cognitive function in patients with limited small cell lung cancer prior to and shortly following prophylactic cranial irradiation. International Journal of Radiation, Oncology, Biology, and Physics, 33, 179-182.

Korsic, M., Jokic, N., Ilic-Supek, D., Skocilic, Z., Lovric, M., Bacic, J., Jakovljevic, M., Maslo, K., & Trbovic, M. (1991). Effects of (desgly9-arg8) vasopressin on cognitive processes in alcoholic patients. Acta med. iug., 45, 223-230.

Kronfol, Z., Hamsher, K. d., Digre, K., & Waziri, R. (1978). Depression and hemispheric functions: Changes associated with unilateral ECT. British Journal of Psychiatry, 132, 560-567.

Kulisevsky, J., Avila, A., Barbanoj, M., Antonijoan, R., Berthier, M. L., & Gironell, A. (1996). Acute effects of levodopa on neuropsychological performance in stable and fluctuating Parkinson's disease patients at different levodopa plasma levels. Brain, 119, 2121-2132.

Kurland, A. A., Turek, I. S., Brown, C. C., & Wagman, A. M. I. (1976). Electroconvulsive therapy and EEG correlates in depressive disorders. Comprehensive Psychiatry, 17(5), 581-589.

La Rue, A., O'Hara, R., Matsyama, S. S., & Jarvik, L. F. (1995). Cognitive changes in young-old adults: Effect of family history of dementia. Journal of Clinical and Experimental Neuropsychology, 17(1), 65-70.

Lamping, D. L., Spring, B., & Gelenberg, A. J. (1984). Effects of tow antidepressants on memory performance in depressed outpatients: A double-blind study. Psychopharmacology, 84, 254-261.

Lehmann, H.E., & Kral, V.A. (1968). Psychological tests: Practice effect in geriatric patients. Geriatrics, Feb., 160-163.

Levenson, R. L., & Lasher-Adelman, V. (1988). Stability of the Peabody Picture Vocabulary Test-Revised for emotionally handicapped middle-school-age children. Perceptual and Motor Skills, 67, 392-394.

Levin, H. S. (1991). Treatment of postconcussional symptoms with CDP-choline. Journal of the Neurological Sciences, 103, S39-S42.

Levin, H. S., High, W. M., Jr., Ewing-Cobbs, L., Fletcher, J. M., Eisenberg, H. M., Miner, M. E., & Goldstein, F. C. (1988). Memory functioning during the first year after closed head injury in children and adolescents. Neurosurgery, 22(6, Pt. 1), 1043-1052.

Levin, H. S., Song, J., Scheibel, R. S., Fletcher, J. M., Harward, H., Lilly, M., & Goldstein, F. (1997). Concept formation and problem-solving following closed head injury in children. Journal of the International Neuropsychological Society, 3, 598-607.

Lezak, M.D. (1995). Neuropsychological Assessment. (3rd ed.). New York: Oxford University Press.

Linde, L., & Bergstron, M. (1992). The effect of one night without sleep on problem-solving and immediate recall. Psychological Research, 54(2), 127-136.

Lloyd, C., Hafner, R. J., & Holme, G. (1995). Behavioral disturbance in dementia. Journal of Geriatric Psychiatry and Neurology, 8, 213-216.

Long, J. A., & McLachlan, J. F. C. (1974). Abstract reasoning and perceptual-motor efficiency in alcoholics: Impairment and reversibility. Quarterly Journal of Studies on Alcohol, 35, 1220-1229.

Lorandos, D. A. (1990). Change in adolescent boys at teen ranch: A five-year study. Adolescence, 25(99), 509-516.

Loring, D. W., Meador, K. J., & Lee, G. P. (1994). Effects of temporal lobectomy on generative fluency and other language functions. Archives of Clinical Neuropsychology, 9(3), 229-238.

Ludgate, J., Keating, J., O'Dwyer, R., & Callaghan, N. (1985). An improvement in cognitive function following polypharmacy reduction in a group of epileptic patients. Acta Neurologica Scandinavia, 71, 448-452.

Lynch, J.K., & McCaffrey, R.J. (1997). Premorbid intellectual functioning and the determination of cognitive loss. In R.J. McCaffrey, A.D. Williams, J.M. Fisher & L.C. Laing (Eds.), The Practice of Forensic Neuropsychology: Meeting Challenges in the Courtroom. (pp. 91-116). New York: Plenum.

Macciocchi, S. N. (1990). "Practice makes perfect:" Retest effects in college athletes. Journal of Clinical Psychology, 46(5), 628-631.

MacInnes, W.D., Paull, D., Uhl, H.S.M., & Schima, E. (1987). Longitudinal neuropsychological changes in a "normal" elderly group. Archives of Clinical Neuropsychology, 2, 273-282.

Maddocks, D., & Saling, M. (1996). Neuropsychological deficits following concussion. Brain Injury, 10(2), 99-103.

Malheiros, S. M. F., Brucki, S. M. D., Gabbai, A. A., Bertolucci, P. H. F., Juliano, Y., Carvalho, A. C., & Buffolo, E. (1995). Neurological outcome in coronary artery surgery with and without cardiopulmonary bypass. Acta Neurologica Scandinavica, 92, 256-260.

Mallick, J. L., Kirkby, K. C., Martin, F., Philp, M., & Hennessy, M. J. (1993). A comparison of the amnesic effects of lorazepam in alcoholics and non-alcoholics. Psychopharmacology, 110, 181-?

Malloy, F. W., Small, I. F., Miller, M. J., Milstein, V., & Stout, J. R. (1982). Changes in neuropsychological test performance after electroconvulsive therapy. Biological Psychiatry, 17(1), 61-?

Maltby, N., Broe, G. A., Creasey, H., Jorm, A. F., Christensen, H., & Brooks, W. S. (1994). Efficacy of tacrine and lecithin in mild to moderate Alzheimer's disease: Double blind trial. British Medical Journal, 308, 879-883.

Martin, P. R., Adinoff, B., Lane, E., Stapleton, J. M., Bone, G. A. H., Weingartner, H., Linnoila, M., & Eckardt, M. J. (1995). Fluvoxamine treatment of alcoholic amnestic disorder. European Neuropsychopharmacology, 5, 27-33.

Matarazzo, R. G., Matarazzo, J. D., Gallo, A. E., Jr., & Wiens, A. N. (1979). IQ and neuropsychological changes following carotid endarterectomy. Journal of Clinical Neuropsychology, 1(2), 97-116.

Mattis, S. (1988). Dementia Rating Scale: Professional Manual. Odessa, FL: Psychological Assessment Resources.

McCaffrey, R. J., Krahula, M. M., & Heimberg, R. G. (1989). An analysis of the significance of performance errors on the Trail Making Test in polysubstance users. Archives of Clinical Neuropsychology, 4, 393-398.

McCaffrey, R. J., Ortega, A., & Haase, R. F. (1993). Effects of repeated neuropsychological assessments. Archives of Clinical Neuropsychology, 8, 519-524.

McCaffrey, R. J., Ortega, A., Orsillo, S. M., Nelles, W. B., & Haase, R. F. (1992). Practice effects in repeated neuropsychological assessments. The Clinical Neuropsychologist, 6, 32-42.

McCaffrey, R. J., Steckler, R. A., Gansler, D. A., & Roman, L. O. (1987). An experimental evaluation of the efficacy of suloctidil in the treatment of Primary Degenerative Dementia. Archives of Clinical Neuropsychology, 2, 155-161.

McCaffrey, R.J., & Westervelt, H.J. (1995). Issues associated with repeated neuropsychological assessments. Neuropsychology Review, 5(3), 203-221.

McCaffrey, R.J., Cousins, J.P., Westervelt, H.J., Martynowicz, M., Remick, S.C., Szebenyi, S., Wagle, W.A., Bottomley, P.A., Hardy, C.J., & Haase, R.F. (1995). Practice effects with the NIMH AIDS abbreviated neuropsychological battery. Archives of Clinical Neuropsychology, 10(3), 241-250.

McCrimmon, R. J., Deary, I. J., Huntly, B. J. P., MacLeod, K. J., & Frier, B. M. (1996). Visual information processing during controlled hypoglycaemia in humans. Brain, 119, 1277-1287.

McGlone, J. (1994). Memory complaints before and after temporal lobectomy: Do they predict memory performance or lesion laterality? Epilepsia, 35(3), 529-539.

McGrath, J., Scheldt, S., Welham, J., & Clair, A. (1997). Performance on tests sensitive to impaired executive ability in schizophrenia, mania and well controls: Acute and subacute phases. Schizophrenia Research, 26, 127-137.

McKegney, F. P., O'Dowd, M. A., Feiner, C., Selwyn, P., Drucker, E., & Friedland, G. H. (1990). A prospective comparison of neuropsychologic function in HIV-seropositive and seronegative methadone-maintained patients. AIDS, 4(565-569).

McSweeny, A.J., Naugle, R.I., Chelune, G.J., & Luders, H. (1993). "T score for change": An illustration of a regression approach to depicting change in clinical neuropsychology. The Clinical Neuropsychologist, 7, 300-312.

Meador, K. J., Loring, D. W., Allen, M. E., Zamrini, E. Y., Moore, E. E., Abney, O. L., & King, D. W. (1991). Comparative cognitive effects of carbamazepine and phenytoin in healthy adults. Neurology, 41, 1537-1540.

Meredith, W. & Tisak, J. (1990). Latent curve analysis. Psychometrika, 55, 107-122.

Merrill, L. L., Lewandowski, L. J., & Kobus, D. A. (1994). Selective attention skills of experienced sonar operators. Perceptual and Motor Skills, 78, 803-812.

Meyers, C. A., Weitzner, M., Byrne, K., Valentine, A., Champlin, R. E., & Przepiorka, D. (1994). Evaluation of the neurobehavioral functioning of patients before, during, and after bone marrow transplantation. Journal of Clinical Oncology, 12, 820-826.

Miller, M. J., Small, I. F., Milstein, V., Malloy, F., & Stout, J. R. (1981). Electrode placement and cognitive change with ECT: Male and female response. American Journal of Psychiatry, 138(3), 384-385.

Mitrushina, M., & Satz, P. (1991a). Changes in cognitive functioning associated with normal aging. Archives of Clinical Neuropsychology, 6, 49-60.

Mitrushina, M., & Satz, P. (1991b). Effects of repeated administration of a neuropsychological battery in the elderly. Journal of Clinical Psychology, 47, 790-801.

Mitrushina, M., & Satz, P. (1995). Repeated testing of normal elderly with the Boston Naming Test. Aging Clinical and Experimental Research, 7, 123-127.

Moehle, K. A., & Berg, R. A. (1985). Academic achievement and intelligence test performance in children with cancer at diagnosis and one year later. Developmental and Behavioral Pediatrics, 6(2), 62-64.

Mohr, E. & Brouwers, P. (Eds.) (1991). Handbook of Clinical Trials: The Neurobehavioral Approach. Netherlands: Swets & Zeitlinger.

Morgan, S. F. (1982). Measuring long-term memory storage and retrieval in children. Journal of Clinical Neuropsychology, 4(1), 77-85.

Morris, J. C., Edland, S., Clark, C., Galasko, D., Koss, E., Mohs, R., van Belle, G., Fillenbaum, G., & Heyman, A. (1993). The Consortium to Establish a Registry for Alzheimer's Disease (CERAD): Part IV. Rates of cognitive change in the longitudinal assessment of probable Alzheimer's disease. Neurology, 43, 2457-2465.

Morris, J. C., Heyman, A., Mohs, R. C., Hughes, J. P., van Belle, G., Fillenbaum, G., Mellits, E. D., Clark, C., & investigators, C. (1989). The Consortium to Establish a Registry for Alzheimer's Disease (CERAD): Part I. Clinical and neuropsychological assessment of Alzheimer's disease. Neurology, 39, 1159-1165.

Morrow, L. A., Ryan, C. M., Hodgson, M. J., & Robin, N. (1991). Risk factors associated with persistence of neuropsychological deficits in persons with organic solvent exposure. The Journal of Nervous and Mental Disease, 179, 540-545.

Mukundan, C. R., Reddy, G. N. N., Hegde, A. S., Shankar, J., & Kaliaperumal, V. G. (1987). Neuropsychological and clinical recovery in patients with head trauma. National Institute of Mental Health and Neuro Sciences Journal, 5(1), 23-31.

Mulhern, R. K., & Kun, L. E. (1985). Neuropsychologic function in children with brain tumors: III. Interval changes in the six months following treatment. Medical and Pediatric Oncology, 13, 318-324.

Murkin, J. M., Martzke, J. S., Buchan, A. M., Bentley, C., & Wong, C. J. (1995). A randomized study of the influence of perfusion technique and pH management strategy in 316 patients undergoing coronary artery bypass surgery: II. Neurologic and cognitive outcomes. The Journal of Thoracic and Cardiovascular Surgery, 110, 349-362.

Naber, D., Sand, P., & Heigl, B. (1996). Psychopathological and neuropsychological effects of 8-days' corticosteriod treatment: A prospective study. Psychoneuroendocrinology, 21(1), 25-31.

Naglieri, J. A., & Parks, J. C. (1980). Wide Range Achievement Test: A one-year stability study. Psychological Reports, 47, 1028-1030.

Naugle, R. I., Chelune, G. J., Cheek, R., Luders, H., & Awad, I. A. (1993). Detection of changes in material-specific memory following temporal lobectomy using the Wechsler Memory Scale-Revised. Archives of Clinical Neuropsychology, 8, 381-395.

Netherton, S. D., Elias, J. W., Albrecht, N. N., Acosta, C., Hutton, J. T., & Albrecht, J. W. (1989). Changes in the performance of parkinsonian patients and normal aged on the Benton Visual Retention Test. Experimental Aging Research, 15(1), 13-18.

Neyens, L. G. J., & Aldenkamp, A. P. (1996). Stability of cognitive measures in children of average ability. Child Neuropsychology, 2(3), 161-170.

Noble, J., Jones, J. G., & Davis, E. J. (1993). Cognitive function during moderate hypoxaemia. Anaesthia and Intensive Care, 21, 180-184.

Nopoulos, P., Flashman, L., Flaum, M., Arndt, S., & Andreasen, N. (1994). Stability of cognitive functioning early in the course of schizophrenia. Schizophrenia Research, 14, 29-37.

Nwokolo, C. U., Fitzpatrick, J. D., Paul, R., Dyal, R., Smits, B. J., & Loft, D. E. (1994). Lack of evidence of neurotoxicity following 8 weeks of treatment

Practitioner's Guide to Evaluating Change with Neuropsychological Assessment Instruments

531

with tripotassium dicitrato bismuthate. Ailment Pharmacological Therapy, 8, 45-53.

O'Carroll, R. E., Baikie, E. M., & Whittick, J. E. (1987). Does the National Adult Reading Test hold in dementia? British Journal of Clinical Psychology, 26, 315-316.

Oken, B. S., Kishiyama, S. S., & Salinsky, M. C. (1995). Pharmacologically induced changes in arousal: Effects on behavioral and electrophysiologic measures of alertness and attention. Electroencephalography and Clinical Neurophysiology, 95, 359-371.

O'Leary, M., Radford, L. M., Chaney, E. F., & Schau, E. J. (1977). Assessment of cognitive recovery in alcoholics by use of the Trail-Making Test. Journal of Clinical Psychology, 33(2), 579-582.

Olin, J. T., & Zelinski, E. M. (1991). The 12-month reliability of the Mini-Mental State Examination. Psychological Assessment, 3, 427-432.

Overton, G. W., & Scott, K. G. (1972). Automated and manual intelligence testing: Data on parallel forms of the Peabody Picture Vocabulary Test. American Journal of Mental Deficiency, 76(6), 639-643.

Ozonoff, S. (1995). Reliability and validity of the Wisconsin Card Sorting Test in studies of autism. Neuropsychology, 9, 491-500.

Palazzini, E., Soliveri, P., Filippini, G., Fetoni, V., Zappacosta, B., Scigliano, G., Monza, D., Caraceni, T., & Girotti, F. (1995). Progression of motor and cognitive impairment in Parkinson's disease. Journal of Neurology, 242, 535-540.

Paolo, A. M., Troster, A. I., & Ryan, J. J. (1997). Test-retest stability of the California Verbal Learning Test in older persons. Neuropsychology, 11(4), 613-616.

Paolo, A. M., Troster, A. I., & Ryan, J. J. (1998). Test-retest stability of the Continuous Visual Memory Test in elderly persons. Archives of Clinical Neuropsychology, 13(7), 617-621.

Parker, J. C., Granberg, B. W., Nichols, W. K., Jones, J. G., & Hewett, J. E. (1983). Mental status outcomes following carotid endarterectomy: A six-month analysis. Journal of Clinical Neuropsychology, 5(4), 345-353.

Parker, J. C., Smarr, K. L., Granberg, B. W., Nichols, W. K., & Hewett, J. E. (1986). Neuropsychological parameters of carotid endarterectomy: A two-year prospective analysis. Journal of Consulting and Clinical Psychology, 54(5), 676-681.

Pass, H.L., Dattwyler, R., Ollo, C., & Mitchell, M. (1987). Neuropsychological measures of a reversible dementia in Lyme disease. Journal of Clinical and Experimental Neuropsychology, 9, 75.

Payne, J. S., Hallahan, D. P., Ball, D. W., & Obenauf, P. A. (1972). Sex differences in reliability and congruent validity of Stanford-Binet short forms and Peabody Picutre Vocabulary Test. Psychological Reports, 31, 934.

Peak, D. T. (1970). A replication study of changes in short-term memory in a group of aging community residents. Journal of Gerontology, 25(4), 316-319.

Pettegrew, J. W., Klunk, W. E., Panchalingam, K., Kanfer, J. N., & McClure, R. J. (1995). Clinical and neurochemical effects of acetyl-L-carnitine in Alzheimer's disease. Neurobiology of Aging, 16, 1-4.

Phillips, N. A., & McGlone, J. (1995). Grouped data do not tell the whole story: Individual analysis of cognitive change after temporal lobectomy. Journal of Clinical and Experimental Neuropsychology, 17(5), 713-724.

Phillips, S. M., & Sherwin, B. B. (1992). Effects of estrogen on memory function in surgically menopausal women. Psychoneuroendocrinology, 17(5), 485-495.

Phipps, S., Brenner, M., Heslop, H., Krance, R., Jayawardene, D., & Mulhern, R. (1995). Psychological effects of bone marrow transplantation on children and adolescents: Preliminary report of a longitudinal study. Bone Marrow Transplantation, 15, 829-835.

Piccini, C., Bracco, L., Falcini, M., Pracucci, G., & Amaducci, L. (1995). Natural history of Alzheimer's disease: Prognostic value of plateaux. Journal of the Neurological Sciences, 131, 177-182.

Pieters, M. S. M., Jennekens-Schinkel, A., Stijnen, T., Edelbroek, P. M., Brouwer, O. F., Liauw, L., Heyer, A., Lanser, J. B. K., & Peters, A. C. B. (1992). Carbamazepine (CBZ) controlled release compared with conventional CBZ: A controlled study of attention and vigilance in children with epilepsy. Epilepsia, 33(6), 1137-1144.

Plaisted, J. R., & Golden, C. J. (1982). Test-retest reliability of teh Clinical, Factor, and Localization Scales of the Luria-Nebraska Neuropsychological Battery. International Journal of Neurosciences, 17, 163-167.

Pliskin, N. H., Hamer, D. P., Goldstein, D. S., Towle, V. L., Reder, A. T., Noronha, A., & Arnason, B. G. W. (1996). Improved delayed visual reproduction test performance in multiple sclerosis patients receiving inteferon B-1b. Neurology, 47, 1463-1468.

Porter, M. D., & Fricker, P. A. (1996). Controlled prospective neuropsychological assessment of active experienced amateur boxers. Clinical Journal of Sport Medicine, 6, 90-96.

Poutiainen, E., Hokkanen, L., Niemi, M. L., & Farkkila, M. (1994). Reversible cognitive decline during high dose a-interferon treatment. Pharmacology Biochemistry and Behavior, 47(4), 901-905.

Powell, G. E., Polkey, C. E., & McMillan, T. (1985). The new Maudsley series of temporal lobectomy: I. Short-term cognitive effects. British Journal of Clinical Psychology, 24, 109-124.

Predescu, V., Riga, D., Riga, S., Turlea, J., Barbat, I. M., & Botezat-Antonescu, L. (1994). Antagonic-stress: A new treatment in gerontopsychiatry and for a healthy productive life. Annals of New York Academy of Sciences, 717, 315-331.

Prevey, M. L., Delaney, R. C., Cramer, J. A., Cattanach, L., Collins, J. F., & Mattson, R. H. (1996). Effect of valproate on cognitive functioning: Comparison with carbamazepine. Archives of Neurology, 53, 1008-1016.

Prigatano, G. P., Fordyche, D., Zeiner, H. K., Roueche, J. R., Pepping, M., & Wood, B. C. (1984). Neuropsychological rehabilitation after closed head injury in young adults. Journal of Neurology, Neruosurgery, and Psychiatry, 47, 505-513.

Pulliainen, V., & Jokelainen, M. (1994). Effects of phenytoin and carbamazepine on cognitive functions in newly diagnosed epileptic patients. Acta Neurologica Scandinavica, 89, 81-86.

Putnam, S.H., Adams, K.M., & Schneider, A.M. (1992). One-day test-retest reliability of neuropsychological tests in a personal injury case. Psychological Assessment, 4, 312-316.

Radanov, B. P., Stefano, G. D., Schnidrig, A., Sturzenegger, M., & Augustiny, K. F. (1993). Cognitive functioning after common whiplash: A controlled follow-up study. Archives of Neurology, 50, 87-91.

Rappaport, L., Coffman, H., Guare, R., Fenton, T., DeGraw, C., & Twarog, F. (1989). Effects of theophylline on behavior and learning in children with asthma. AJDC, 143, 368-372.

Rapport, L. J., Axlerod, B. N., Theisen, M. E., Brines, B., Kalechstein, A. D., & Ricker, J. H. (1997a). Relationship of IQ to verbal learning and memory:

Test and retest. Journal of Clinical and Experimental Neuropsychology, 19(5), 655-666.

Rapport, L. J., Brines, D. B., Axelrod, B. N., & Theisen, M. E. (1997b). Full scale IQ as mediator of practice effects: The rich get richer. The Clinical Neuropsychologist, 11(4), 375-380.

Raskin, L. M., & Fong, L. J. (1970). Temporal stability of the PPVT in normal children and educable-retarded children. Psychological Reports, 26, 547-549.

Rasmusson, D. X., Bylsma, F. W., & Brandt, J. (1995). Stability of performance on the Hopkins Verbal Learning Test. Archives of Clinical Neuropsychology, 10, 21-26.

Ratner, D. P., Adams, K. M., Levin, N. W., & Rourke, B. P. (1983). Effects of hemodialysis on the cognitive and sensory-motor functioning of the adult chronic hemodialysis patient. Journal of Behavioral Medicine, 6(3), 291-311.

Rausch, R., & Babb, T. L. (1993). Hippocampal neuron loss and memory scores before and after temporal lobe surgery for epilepsy. Archives of Neurology, 50, 812-817.

Raven, J. C., Court, J. H., & Raven, J. (1977). Manual for Raven's Progressive Matrices and Vocabulary Scales. London: H.K. Lewis & Co. LTD.

Rawlings, D. B., & Crewe, N. M. (1992). Test-retest practice effects and test score changes of the WAIS-R in recovering traumatically brain-injured survivors. The Clinical Neuropsychologist, 6, 415-430.

Rebok, G. W., Smith, C. B., Pascualvaca, D. M., Mirsky, A. F., Anthony, B. J., & Kellman, S. G. (1997). Developmental changes in attentional performance in urban children from eight to thirteen years. Child Neuropsychology, 3(1), 28-46.

Rebok, G., Brandt, J., & Folstein, M. (1990). Longitudinal cognitive decline in patients with Alzheimer's disease. Journal of Geriatric Psychiatry and Neurology, 3, 91-97.

Reddon, J. R., Gill, D. M., Gauk, S. E., & Maerz, M. D. (1988). Purdue Pegboard: Test-retest estimates. Perceptual and Motor Skills, 66, 503-506.

Reich, J. N., Kaspar, J. C., Puczynski, M. S., Puczynski, S., Cleland, J. W., Dell'Angela, K., & Emanuele, M. A. (1990). Effect of hypoglycemic episode on neuropsychological functioning in diabetic children. Journal of Clinical and Experimental Neuropsychology, 12(4), 613-626.

Reisberg, B., Ferris, S. H., Anand, R., Mir, P., Geibel, V., & DeLeon, M. J. (1983). Effects of naloxone in senile dementia: A double-blind trial. New England Journal of Medicine, 308, 721-722.

Reitan, R. M., & Wolfson, D. (1996). The question of validity of neuropsychological test scores among head-injured litigants: Development of a dissimulation index. Archives of Clinical Neuropsychology, 11(7), 573-580.

Rennick, P.M., Keiser, T., Rodin, E., Rim, C., & Lennox, K. (1974, Dec.). Carbamazepine (Tegretol): Behavioral side effects in temporal lobe epilepsy during short-term comparison with placebo. Presented at the Annual Meeting of the American Epilepsy Society, New York.

Rich, J. B., Rasmusson, D. X., Folstein, M. F., Carson, K. A., Kawas, C., & Brandt, J. (1995). Nonsteriodal anti-inflammatory drugs in Alzheimer's disease. Neurology, 45, 51-55.

Richards, J. S., Brown, L., Hagglund, K., Bua, G., & Reeder, K. (1988). Spinal cord injury and concomitant traumatic brain injury: Results of a longitudinal investigation. American Journal of Physical Medicine and Rehabilitation, 67, 211-216.

Richards, M., Sano, M., Goldstein, S., Mindry, D., Todak, G., & Stern, Y. (1992). The stability of neuropsychological test performance in a group of parenteral drug users. Journal of Substance Abuse Treatment, 9, 371-377.

Richardson, J. S., Miller, P. S., Lemay, J. S., Jyu, C. A., Neil, S. G., Kilduff, C. J., & Keegan, D. L. (1985). Mental dysfunction and the blockade of muscarinic receptors in the brains of the normal elderly. Progress in Neuro-Psychopharmacology and Biological Psychiatry, 9, 651-654.

Riddle, K. D., & Rapoport, J. L. (1976). A 2-year follow-up of 72 hyperactive boys: Classroom behavior and peer acceptance. The Journal of Nervous and Mental Disorders, 162(2), 126-?

Roberts, P., & Dorze, G. L. (1994). Semantic verbal fluency in aphasia: A quantitative and qualitative study in test-retest conditions. Aphasiology, 8(6), 569-582.

Roehrich, L., & Goldman, M. S. (1993). Experience-dependent neuropsychological recovery and the treatment of alcoholism. Journal of Consulting and Clinical Psychology, 61(5), 812-821.

Roman, D. D., Kubo, S. H., Ormaza, S., Francis, G. S., Bank, A. J., & Shumway, S. J. (1997). Memory improvement following cardiac transplantation. Journal of Clinical and Experimental Neuropsychology, 19(5), 692-697.

Ruff, R. M., Light, R. H., & Parker, S. B. (1996). Benton Controlled Word Association Test: Reliability and updated norms. Archives of Clinical Neuropsychology, 11(4), 329-338.

Ruzicka, E., Roth, J., Spackova, N., Mecir, P., & Jech, R. (1994). Apomorphine induced cognitive changes in Parkinson's disease. Journal of Neurology, Neurosurgery, and Psychiatry, 57, 998-1001.

Ryan, J. J., Geisser, M. E., Randall, D. M., & Georgemiller, R. J. (1986). Alternate form reliability and equivalency of the Rey Auditory Verbal Learning Test. Journal of Clincial and Experimental Neuropsychology, 8(5), 611-616.

Ryan, J. J., Morris, J., Yaffa, S., & Peterson, L. (1981). Test-retest reliability of the Wechsler memory Scale, Form I. Journal of Clinical Psychology, 37(4), 847-848.

Sacks, E.L. (1952). Intelligence scores as a function of experimentally established social relationships between the child and examiner. Journal of Abnormal and Social Psychology, 47, 354-358.

Sacks, T. L., Clark, C. R., Pols, R. G., & Geffen, L. B. (1991). Comparability and stability of performance of six alternate forms of the Dodrill-Stroop Colour-Word Test. The Clinical Neuropsychologist, 5, 220-225.

Sano, M., Bell, K., Cote, L., Dooneief, G., Lawton, A., Legler, L., Marder, K., Naini, A., Stern, Y., & Mayeux, R. (1992). Double-blind parallel design pilot study of acetyl levocarnitine in patients with Alzheimer's disease. Archives of Neurology, 49, 1137-1141.

Sarazin, F. F.-A., & Spreen, O. (1986). Fifteen-year stability of some neuropsychological tests in learning disabled subjects with and without neurological impairment. Journal of Clinical and Experimental Neuropsychology, 8(3), 190-200.

Sass, K. J., Buchanan, C. P., Westerveld, M., Marek, K. L., Farhi, A., Robbins, R. J., Naftolin, F., Vollmer, T. L., Leranth, C., Roth, R. L., Price, L. H., Bunney, B. S., Elsworth, J. D., Hoffer, P. B., Redmond, E., & Spencer, D. D. (1995). General cognitive ability following unilateral and bilateral fetal ventral mesencephalic tissue transplantation for treatment of Parkinson's disease. Archives of Neurology, 52, 680-686.

Sattler, J.M. (1990). Assessment of Children. (3rd ed.). San Diego: Sattler.

Savageau, J. A., Stanton, B. A., Jenkins, D., & Frater, R. W. M. (1982). Neuropsychological dysfunction following elective cardiac operation: II. A six-month reassessment. Journal of Thorasic and Cardiovascular Surgery, 84, 595-600.

Savageau, J. A., Stanton, B. A., Jenkins, D., & Klein, M. D. (1982). Neuropsychological dysfunction following elective cardiac operation: I. Early assessment. Journal of Thorasic and Cardiovascular Surgery, 84, 585-594.

Sawrie, S.M., Marson, D.C., Boothe, A.L., & Harrell, L.E. (1999). A method for assessing clinically relevant individual cognitive change in older adult populations. Journal of Gerontology: Psychological Sciences, 54, 116-124.

Saykin, A. J., Janssen, R. S., Sprehn, G. C., Kaplan, J. E., Spira, T. J., & O'Connor, B. (1991). Longitudinal evaluation of neuropsychological function in homosexual men with HIV infection: 18-month follow-up. The Journal of Neuropsychiatry and Clinical Neurosciences, 3, 286-298.

Schain, R. J., Ward, J. W., & Guthrie, D. (1977). Carbamazepine as an anticonvulsant in children. Neurology, 27, 476-480.

Schain, R.J., Ward, J.W., & Guthrie, D. (1977). Carbamazepine as an anticonvulsant in children. Neurology, 27, 476-480.

Schau, E. J., O'Leary, M. R., & Chaney, E. F. (1980). Reversiblity of cognitive deficit in alcoholics. Journal of Studies on Alcohol, 41(7), 733-?

Schiffer, R. B., & Caine, E. D. (1991). The interaction between depressive affective disorder and neuropsychological test performance in multiple sclerosis patients. The Journal of Neuropsychiatry and Clinical Neurosciences, 3, 28-32.

Schludermann, E. H., Schludermann, S. M., Merryman, P. W., & Brown, B. W. (1983). Halstead's studies in the neuropsychology of aging. Archives of Gerontology and Geriatrics, 2, 49-172.

Schmand, B., Lindeboom, J., Launer, L., Dinkgreve, M., Hooijer, C., & Jonker, C. (1995). What is a significant score change on the Mini-Mental State Examination? International Journal of Geriatric Psychiatry, 10, 411-414.

Scott, R., Gregory, R., Hines, N., Carroll, C., Hyman, N., Papanassiasiou, V., Leather, C., Rowe, J., Silburn, P., & Aziz, T. (1998). Neuropsychological, neurological and functional outcome following palidotomy for Parkinson's disease: A consecutive series of eight simultaneous bilateral and twelve unilateral procedures. Brain, 121, 659-675.

Scottish, S. R. G. (1988). The Scottish Fist Episode Schizophrenia Study: V. One-year follow-up. British Journal of Psychiatry, 152, 470-476.

Seidenberg, M., O'Leary, D. S., Giordani, B., Berent, S., & Boll, T. J. (1981). Test-retest IQ changes of epilepsy patients: Assessing the influence of practice effects. Journal of Clinical Neuropsychology, 3, 237-255.

Seidman, L. J., Pepple, J. R., Faraone, S. V., Kremen, W. S., Cassens, G., McCarley, R. W., & Tsuang, M. T. (1991). Wisconsin Card Sorting Test performance over time in schizophrenia: Preliminary evidence from clinical follow-up and neuroleptic reduction studies. Schizophrenia Research, 5, 233-242.

Seidman, L. J., Pepple, J. R., Faraone, S. V., Kremen, W. S., Green, A. I., Brown, W. A., & Tsuang, M. T. (1993). Neuropsychological performance in chronic schizophrenia in response to neuroleptic dose reduction. Biological Psychiatry, 33, 575-584.

Selnes, O. A., McArthur, J. C., Royal, W., III, Updike, M. L., Nance-Sproson, T., Concha, M., Gordon, B., Solomon, L., & Vlahov, D. (1992). HIV-1 infection and intravenous drug use: Longitudinal neuropsychological evaluation of asymptomatic subjects. Neurology, 42, 1924-1930.

Selnes, O. A., Miller, E., McArthur, J., Gordon, B., Munoz, A., Sheridan, K., Fox, R., Saah, A. J., & Study, M. A. C. (1990). HIV-1 infection: No evidence of cognitive decline during the asymptomatic stages. Neurology, 40, 204-208.

Selwa, L. M., Berent, S., Giodani, B., Henry, T. R., Buchtel, H. A., & Ross, D. A. (1994). Serial cognitive testing in temporal lobe epilepsy: Longitudinal changes with medical and surgical therapies. Epilepsia, 35, 743-749.

Serafetinides, E. A., & Clark, M. L. (1973). Psychological effects of single-dose antipsychotic medication. Biological Psychiatry, 7(3), 263-?

Shatz, M.W. (1981). WAIS practice effects in clinical neuropsychology. Journal of Clinical Neuropsychology, 3, 171-179.

Shaw, P. J., Bates, D., Cartlidge, N. E. F., French, J. M., Heaviside, D., Julian, D. G., & Shaw, D. A. (1987). Neurologic and neuropsychological morbidity following major surgery: Comparison of coronary artery bypass and peripheral vascular surgery. Stroke, 18, 700-707.

Shealy, A. E., & Walker, D. R. (1978). Minnesota Multiphasic Personality Inventory prediction of intellectual changes following cardiac surgery. The Journal of Nervous and Mental Disease, 166(4), 263-267.

Shewan, C. M., & Kertesz, A. (1980). Reliability and validity characteristics of the Western Aphasia Battery (WAB). Journal of Speech and Hearing Disorders, 45, 308-324.

Shull-Senn, S., Weatherly, M., Morgan, S. K., & Bradley-Johnson, S. (1995). Stability reliability for elementary-age students on the Woodcock-Johnson Psychoeducational Battery-Revised (Achievement Section) and the Kaufman Test of Educational Achievement. Psychology in the Schools, 32, 86-92.

Silberstein, C. H., O'Dowd, M. A., Chartock, P., Schoenbaum, E. E., Freidland, G., Hartel, D., & McKegney, F. P. (1993). A prospective four-year follow-up of neuropsychological function in HIV seropositive and seronegative methadone-maintained patients. General Hospital Psychiatry, 15, 351-359.

Small, B. J., Basun, H., & Backman, L. (1998). Three-year changes in cognitive performance as a function of apolipoprotein E genotype: Evidence from very old adults without dementia. Psychology and Aging, 13(1), 80-87.

Smith, A. (1982). Symbol Digit Modalities Test Manual (rev.). Los Angeles: Western Psychological Services.

Soewondo, S. (1995). The effect of iron deficiency and mental stimulation on Indonesian children's cognitive performance and development. Kobe Journal of Medical Science, 41(1), 1-17.

Sotaniemi, K. A., Mononen, H., & Hokkanen, T. E. (1981). Neurologic outcome after open-heart surgery. Archives of Neurology, 38, 2-8.

Stabell, K. E., & Nornes, H. (1994). Prospective neuropsychological investigation of patients with supratentorial artiovenous malformations. Acta Neurochirurgica, 131, 32-44.

Stambrook, M., Cardoso, E., Hawryluk, G. A., Eirikson, P., Piatek, D., & Sicz, G. (1988). Neuropsychological changes following the neurosurgical treatment of normal pressure hydrocephalus. Archives of Clinical Neuropsychology, 3, 323-330.

Stanton, R. D., Wilson, H., & Brumback, R. A. (1981). Cognitive improvement associated with tricyclic antidepressant treatment of childhood major depressive illness. Perceptual and Motor Skills, 53, 219-234.

Starr, J. M., Whalley, L. J., & Deary, I. J. (1996). The effects of antihypertensive treatment on cognitive function: Results from the HOPE study. Journal of the Amercian Geriatric Society, 44, 411-415.

Stehbens, J. A., & Kisker, C. T. (1984). Intelligence and achievement testing in childhood cancer: Three years postdiagnosis. Developmental and Behavioral Pediatrics, 5(4), 184-188.

Stehbens, J. A., Kisker, C. T., & Wilson, B. K. (1983). Achievement and intelligence test-retest performance in pediatric cancer patients at diagnosis and one year later. Journal of Pediatric Psychology, 8, 47-56.

Stein, D., Bannet, J., Averbuch, I., Landa, L., Chazan, S., & Belmaker, R. H. (1984). Ineffectiveness of vasopressin in the treatment of memory impairment in chronic schizophrenia. Psychopharmacology, 84, 566-568.

Stern, Y., Mayeux, R., Ilson, j., Fahn, S., & Cote, L. (1984). Pergolide therapy for Parkinson's disease: Neurobehavioral changes. Neurology, 34, 201-204.

Stromgren, L. S., Christensen, A. L., & Fromholt, P. (1976). The effects of unilateral brief-interval ECTon memory. Acta Psychiatrica Scandinavica, 54, 336-346.

Sturm, W., & Willmes, K. (1991). Efficacy of a reaction training on various attentional and cognitive functions in stroke patients. Neuropsychological Rehabilitation, 1(4), 259-280.

Stuss, D. T., Stethem, L. L., & Pelchat, G. (1988). Three tests of attention and rapid information processing: An extension. The Clinical Neuropsychologist, 2(3), 246-250.

Stuss, D. T., Stethem, L. L., Hugenholtz, H., & Richard, M. T. (1989). Traumatic brain injury: A comparison of three clinical tests, and analysis of recovery. The Clinical Neuropsychologist, 3(2), 146-156.

Stuss, S. T., Stethem, L. L., & Poirier, C. A. (1987). Comparison of three tests of attention and rapid information processing across six age groups. The Clinical Neuropsychologist, 1, 139-152.

Suvanto, S., Huuhtanen, P., Nygard, C.-H., & Ilmarinen, J. (1991). Performance efficiency and its changes among aging municipal employees. Scandinavian Journal of Work and Environmental Health, 17(Suppl. 1), 118-121.

Sweeney, J. A., Haas, G. L., Kelip, J. G., & Long, M. (1991). Evaluation of the stability of neuropsychological functioning after acute episodes of schizophrenia: One-year followup study. Psychiatry Research, 38, 63-76.

Szmuckler, G. I., Andrewes, D., Kingston, K., Chen, L., Stargatt, R., & Stanley, R. (1992). Neuropsychological impairment in anorexia nervosa: Before and after refeeding. Journal of Clinical and Experimental Neuropsychology, 14(2), 347-352.

Tarter, R. E., & Jones, B. M. (1971). Motor impairment in chronic alcoholics. Diseases of the Nervous System, 32, 632-636.

Tarter, R. E., Switala, J., Arria, A., Plail, J., & Van Theil, D. H. (1990). Subclinical hepatic encephalopathy: Comparisons before and after othotopic liver transplantation. Transplantation, 50(4), 632-637.

Tata, P. R., Rollings, J., Collins, M., Pickering, A., & Jacobson, R. R. (1994). Lack of cognitive recovery following withdrawal from long-term benzodiazepine use. Psychological Medicine, 24, 203-213.

Tate, R.L., Perdices, M., & Maggiotto, S. (1998). Stability of the Wisconsin Card Sorting Test and the determination of reliability of change in scores. The Clinical Neuropsychologist, 12(3), 348-357.

Taylor, K. I., Salmon, D. P., Rice, V. A., Bondi, M. W., Hill, L. R., Ernesto, C. R., & Butters, N. (1996). Longitudinal examination of American National Adult Reading Test (AMNART) performance in dementia of the Alzheimer's type (DAT): Validation and correction based on degree of cognitive decline. Journal of Clinical and Experimental Neuropsychology, 18(6), 883-891.

Temple, R. M., Deary, I. J., & Winney, R. J. (1995). Recombinant erthropoietin improves cognitive function in patients maintained on chronic ambulatory peritoneal dialysis. Nephrology Dialysis Transplantation, 101, 1733-1738.

Thal, L. J., Grundman, M., & Golden, R. (1986). Alzheimer's disease: A correlational analysis of the Blessed Information-Memory-Concentration Test and the Mini-Mental State Exam. Neurology, 36, 262-264.

Thapa, P. B., Meador, K. G., Gideon, P., Fought, R. L., & Ray, W. A. (1994). Effects of antipsychotic withdrawal in elderly nursing home residents. Journal of the American Geriatric Society, 42, 280-286.

Theisen, M. E., Rapport, L. J., Axelrod, B. N., & Brines, D. B. (1998). Effects of practice in repeated administrations of the Wechsler Memory Scale-Revised in normal adults. Assessment, 5(1), 85-92.

Thomas, L., & Trimble, M. (1996). The effects of vigabatrin on attention, concentration and mood: An investigation in healthy volunteers. Seizure, 5, 205-208.

Tisak, J. & Meredith, W. (1989). Exploratory longitudinal factor analysis in multiple populations. Psychometrika, 54, 261-281.

Tomer, R., & Flor-Henry, P. (1989). Neuroleptics reverse attention asymmetries in schizophrenia patients. Biological Psychiatry, 25, 852-860.

Townes, B. D., Bashein, G., Hornbein, T. F., Coppel, D. B., Goldstein, D. E., Davis, K. B., Nessly, M. L., Bledsoe, S. W., Veith, R. C., Ivey, T. D., & Cohen, M. A. (1989). Neurobehavioral outcomes in cardiac operations: A prospective controlled study. ?, ?, 774-782.

Tozzi, V., Narciso, P., Galgani, S., Sette, P., Balestra, P., Gerace, C., Pau, F. M., Pigorini, F., Volpini, V., Camporiondo, M. P., Giulianelli, M., & Visco, G. (1993). Effects of zidovudine in 30 patients with mild to end-stage AIDS dementia complex. AIDS, 7, 683-692.

Traxler, A.E. & Hilkert, R.N. (1942). Effect of type of desk on results of machine-scored test. School and Society, 56, 277-296.

Trenerry, M. R., Jack, C. R., Cascino, G. D., Sharbrough, F. W., & Ivnik, R. J. (1996). Sex differences in the relationship between visual memory and MRI hippocampal volumes. Neuropsychology, 10(3), 343-351.

Trichard, C., Martinot, J. L., Alagille, M., Masure, M. C., Hardy, P., Ginestet, D., & Feline, A. (1995). Time course of prefrontal lobe dysfunction in severely depressed in-patients: A longitudinal neuropsychological study. Psychological Medicine, 25, 79-85.

Tsudzuki, A., Hata, Y., & Kuze, T. (1957). (A study of rapport between examiner and subject.) Japanese Journal of Psychology, 27, 22-28.

Tuikka, R. A., Laaksonen, R. K., & Somer, H. V. K. (1993). Cognitive function in myotonic dystropy: A follow-up study. European Neurology, 33, 436-441.

Tuma, J.M., & Applebaum, A.S. (1980). Reliability and practice effects of WISC-R IQ estimates in a normal population. Educational and Psychological Measurement, 40, 671-678.

Uchiyama, C. L., D'Elia, L. F., Dellinger, A. M., Becker, J. T., Selnes, O. A., Wesch, J. E., B.B., C., Satz, P., van Gorp, W., & Miller, E. N. (1995). Alternate forms of the Auditory Verbal Learning Test: Issues of test comparability, longitudinal reliability, and moderating demographic variables. Archives of Clinical Neuropsychology, 10, 133-145.

Uchiyama, C. L., D'Elia, L. F., Dellinger, A. M., Selnes, O. A., Becker, J. T., Wesch, J. E., Chen, B. B., Satz, P., van Gorp, W., & Miller, E. N. (1994). Longitudinal comparison of alternate versions of the Symbol Digit Modalities Test: Issues of form comparability and moderating demographic variables. The Clinical Neuropsychologist, 8(2), 209-218.

Udwin, O., Davies, M., & Howlin, P. (1996). A longitudinal study of cognitive abilities and educational attainment in Williams syndrome. Developmental Medicine and Child Neurology, 38, 1020-1029.

Unkenstein, A. E., & Bowden, S. C. (1991). Predicting the course of neuropsychological status in recently abstinent alcoholics: A pilot study. The Clinical Neuropsychologist, 5(1), 24-32.

Valencia, R. R. (1983). Stability of the McCarthy Scales of Children's Abilities over a one-year period for Mexican-American children. Psychology in the Schools, 20, 29-34.

Vance, H.B., Blixt, S., Ellis, R., & Debell, S. (1981). Stability of the WISC-R for a sample of exceptional children. Journal of Clinical Psychology, 37(2), 397-399.

Van Den Burg, W., Saan, R. J., Van Zomeren, A. H., Boontje, A. H., Haaxma, R., & Wichmann, T. E. (1985). Carotid endarterectomy: Does it improve cognitive or motor functioning? Psychological Medicine, 15, 341-346.

van Dyck, C. H., McMahon, T. J., Rosen, M. I., O'Malley, S. S., O'Connor, P. G., Lin, C. H., Pearsall, H. R., Woods, S. W., & Kosten, T. R. (1997). Sustained-release methylphenidate for cognitive impairment in HIV-1-infected drug abusers: A pilot study. The Journal of Neuropsychiatry and Clinical Neurosciences, 9, 29-36.

van Oosterhout, A. G. M., Boon, P. J., Houx, P. J., ten Velde, G. P. M., & Twijnstra, A. (1995). Follow-up of cognitive functioning in patients with small cell lung cancer. International Journal of Oncology Biology Physics, 31(4), 911-914.

Varney, N. R., Alexander, B., & MacIndoe, J. H. (1984). Reversible steriod dementia in patients without steriod psychosis. American Journal of Psychiatry, 141, 369-372.

Verdoux, H., Magnin, E., & Bourgeois, M. (1995). Neuroleptic effects on neuropsychological test performance in schizophrenia. Schizophrenia Research, 14, 133-139.

Vilkki, J., & Laitinen, L. V. (1974). Differential effects of left and right ventrolateral thalamotomy on receptive and expressive verbal performances and face-matching. Neuropsychologia, 12, 11-19.

Villardita, C., Grioli, S., Lomeo, C., Cattaneo, C., & Parini, J. (1992). Clinical studies with oxiracetam in patients with dementia of the Alzheimer's type and multi-infarct dementia of mild to moderate degree. Neuropsychobiology, 25, 24-28.

Vingerhoets, G., Jannes, C., De Soete, G., & Van Nooten, G. (1996). Prospective evaluation of verbal memory performance after cardiopulmonary bypass surgery. Journal of Clinical and Experimental Neuropsychology, 18(2), 187-196.

Webster, L., Wood, R. W., Eicher, C., & Hoag, C. L. (1989). A preschool language tutoring project: Family support--the essential factor. Early Childhood Research Quarterly, 4, 217-224.

Wechsler, D. (1987). Wechsler Memory Scale-Revised Manual. New York: Psychological Corporation.

Wechsler, D. (1997). WAIS-III-WMS-III Technical Manual. San Antonio, TX: The Psychological Corporation.

Welford, A.T. (1985). Practice effects in relation to age: A review and a theory. Developmental Neuropsychology, 1, 173-190.

Welford, A.T. (1987). On rates of improvement with practice. Journal of Motor Behavior, 19, 401-415.

Westervelt, H. J., McCaffrey, R. J., Cousins, J. P., Wagle, W. A., & Haase, R. F. (1997). Longitudinal analysis of olfactory deficits in HIV infection. Archives of Clinical Neuropsychology, 12(6), 557-565.

White, R. F., Robins, T. G., Proctor, S., Echeverria, D., & Rocskay, A. S. (1994). Neuropsychological effects of exposure to naphtha among automotive workers. Occupational and Environmental Medicine, 51, 102-112.

Wickes, T.A., Jr. (1956). Examiner influence in a testing situation. Journal of Consulting Psychology, 20, 23-26.

Wiles, C. M., Omar, L., Swan, A. V., Sawle, G., Frankel, J., Grunewald, R., Joannides, T., Jones, P., Laing, H., Richardson, P. H., Hambin, A. S., Harris, J., Thomas, G., Miller, D. H., Moseley, I. F., McDonald, W. I., & MacManus, D. G. (1994). Total lymphoid irradiation in multiple sclerosis. Journal of Neurology, Neurosurgery, and Psychiatry, 57, 154-163.

Wilkinson, G. S. (1993). WRAT-3 Administration Manual. Wilmington, DE: Wide Range.

Williams, K. T., & Wang, J.-J. (1997). Technical References to the Peabody Picture Vocabulary Test-Third Edition (PPVT-III). Circle Pines, MN: American Guidance Services.

Williams-Russo, P., Sharrock, N. E., Mattis, S., Szatrowski, T. P., & Charlson, M. E. (1995). Cognitive effects after epidural vs general anesthesia in older adults: A randomized trial. Journal of the American Medical Association, 274, 44-50.

Willis, J., Nelson, A., Black, F. W., Borges, A., An, A., & Rice, J. (1997). Barbituate anticonvulsants: A neuropsychological and quantitative electroencephalographic study. Journal of Child Neurology, 12, 169-171.

Woo, E., Proulx, S. M., & Greenblatt, D. J. (1991). Differential side effect profile of triazolam versus flurazepam in elderly patients undergoing rehabilitation therapy. Journal of Clinical Pharmacology, 31, 168-173.

Woodward, C. A., Santa-Barbara, J., & Roberts, R. (1975). Test-retest reliability of the Wide Range Achievement Test. Journal of Clinical Psychology, 13(1), 81-84.

Youngjohn, J. R., & Crook, T. H., III. (1993). Stability of everyday memory in age-associated memory impairment: A longitudinal study. Neuropsychology, 7(3), 406-416.

Zegers, F.E., & Hafkenscheid, A. (1994). The Ultimate Reliable Change Index: An Alternative to the Hageman & Arrindell Approach. Groningen, The Netherlands: University of Groningen.

Zigler, E., Abelson, W. D., & Seitz, V. (1973). Motivational factors in the performance of economically disadvantaged children on the Peabody Picture Vocabulary Test. Child Development, 44, 294-303.

Index